Cancer Exposomics and Environmental Influences on Carcinogenesis

Ramya Raghavan
Sri Sathya Sai University for Human Excellence, India

IGI Global
Scientific Publishing
Publishing Tomorrow's Research Today

Vice President of Editorial — Melissa Wagner
Director of Acquisitions — Mikaela Felty
Director of Book Development — Jocelynn Hessler
Production Manager — Mike Brehm
Cover Design — Jose Rosado

Published in the United States of America by
IGI Global Scientific Publishing
701 East Chocolate Avenue
Hershey, PA, 17033, USA
Tel: 717-533-8845
Fax: 717-533-7115
Website: https://www.igi-global.com E-mail: cust@igi-global.com

Library of Congress Cataloging-in-Publication Data

Names: Raghaven, Ramya, 1975- editor
Title: Cancer exposomics and environmental influences on carcinogenesis / edited by Ramya Raghaven.
Description: Hershey, PA : IGI Global Scientific Publlishing, [2026] | Includes bibliographical references and index. | Summary: "This book aims to advance our understanding the link between the exposome and cancer"-- Provided by publisher.
Identifiers: LCCN 2025013641 (print) | LCCN 2025013642 (ebook) | ISBN 9798337321653 hardcover | ISBN 9798337321660 paperback | ISBN 9798337321677 ebook
Subjects: LCSH: Carcinogenesis | Cancer--Environmental aspects | Environmentally induced diseases | Carcinogens
Classification: LCC RC268.5 .C325 2026 (print) | LCC RC268.5 (ebook)
LC record available at https://lccn.loc.gov/2025013641
LC ebook record available at https://lccn.loc.gov/2025013642

British Cataloguing in Publication Data
A Cataloguing in Publication record for this book is available from the British Library.

Table of Contents

Detailed Table of Contents

There is an intricate relationship between the exposome and critical periods of gametogenesis, teratogenesis, and cancer development. Developmental Origins of Health and Disease (DOHaD) framework to cancer susceptibility examines the hypothesis that early-life environmental exposures can program long-term cancer risk. The authors review epidemiological studies demonstrating associations between developmental exposures and increased cancer risk. Case studies beginning from gametogenesis, debates on biological mechanisms, epigenetic modifications, and altered tissue development are discussed. The chapter also critically analyzes key controversies such as methodological limitations, the etiological complexity of cancer, issues of generalizability, and translational hurdles. This work demonstrates how environmental factors influence gamete formation, embryonic development, and carcinogenesis to highlight the need for addressing parental health and reducing health disparities.

The chapter explores the transformative role of omics technologies in elucidating the complex pathways and mechanisms involved in xenobiotic metabolism. The chapter incorporates the metabolomics role in profiling xenobiotic-induced metabolic alterations, facilitating the identification of biomarkers, transcriptomic analyses uncovering dynamic gene expression patterns, and the application of high-throughput sequencing techniques to identify genetic variations influencing drug

Gene-environment interactions play a crucial role in tumor initiation by influencing cellular and tissue plasticity. Environmental and internal factors influence carcinogenesis by acting on specific sensing genes and pathways, leading to epigenetic, genetic, and metabolic changes that shape the TME. Understanding the exposome can inform gene expression, epigenetic changes, and immune responses, particularly for the reproductive health and cancer prevention. The authors discuss the latest methodologies in exposome assessment, challenges in defining and measuring harmful environmental impacts. Exposome applications in public health policy face challenges and also opportunities in translating exposome research into actionable measures. Gene-environment interactions are shown by analyzing case studies, emerging debates in research, and clinical practice. This work highlights the transformative potential of exposome informed policies in addressing global health challenges and reducing health disparities.

The microbiome refers to the complex community of microorganisms dwelling in and on the human body. Especially, the gut microbiota is involved in modulating a host of crucial physiological processes such as immunity development, anabolism, and nutrient uptake. Diverse ecological exposures ranging from environmental pollutants to dietary components and infectious agents may influence the microbiome to either promote carcinogenesis by inducing chronic inflammation and producing toxic metabolites or exert anticancer effects by boosting the host immune response. This

Preface

Welcome to the Exposome, the groundbreaking science that reveals how every breath you take, every bite you eat, and every environment you inhabit profoundly shapes your well-being. Cancer exposomics move beyond single causes to expose cumulative effect of our environment. In an era where environmental factors increasingly influence human health and disease, understanding the complex interplay between xenobiotic exposures and biological systems has become paramount. Recent developments in environmental toxicology and multi-omics integration have revolutionized our ability to understand the molecular changes in biological systems due to environmental exposures. This book reveals how genomics, proteomics, metabolomics, show the etiology of congenital tumors, breast cancer, prostate cancer, and cervical cancer.

Cancer exposomics approaches promises a more comprehensive understanding of cancer biology. The pervasive burden of cancer necessitates comprehensive strategies for prevention and control. This aligns cancer exposomics with the United Nations Sustainable Development Goals (SDGs). Cancer Exposome, reflects the totality of exposures chemical, physical, and biological agents. It includes endogenous factors, lifestyle choices, and socio-economic determinants from conception to death. The totality of environmental exposures, chemical pollutants, dietary habits, occupational hazards, lifestyle factors, biological agents (viruses, bacteria, mycobiome influences). The toxicants endocrine disruptors, and xenobiotics also increase cancer risk. The technological innovations drive omics platforms, environmental exposure assessment, and data analysis methods. The book contents cater to pharmaceuticals, data mining scientists, researchers, clinicians, public health professionals, and policymakers. This book isn't just about understanding the problem; it's about empowering you with knowledge. It's an essential guide for public health professionals, researchers, healthcare providers, and students alike, offering a comprehensive overview of the latest exposome research.

This comprehensive volume also serves as a resource for a diverse readership, from high school to graduate students embarking on careers in environmental health sciences, toxicology, epidemiology, and precision medicine. Its pedagogical approach ensures accessibility for adolescents and young adults grappling with health decisions. The contents robust scientific depth caters aspiring parents seeking to optimize preconception health and fetal development. Grandparents, caregivers, and anyone seeking to understand the environmental influences on their health will find invaluable insights within these pages. We demystify complex concepts, paving the way for individuals across the lifespan interested in risk factors, disease susceptibility for promoting cancer awareness.

Section 1 lays the foundational concepts in exposomics and early life origins. The escalating incidence of cancers, underscores the influence of environmental factors on as cancer risk from gametogenesis to ageing. This book particularly emphasizes the role of early-life exposures linked to genomic instability and cancer risk. Epigenetic modifications in sperm and egg cells affect offspring cancer susceptibility and early development The altered germline mutation rates are demonstrated by projects such as the Human Early Life Exposome (HELIX). In the introductory section to the field of exposomics, contents focus on the parental and fetal exposures that influence genetic variation and carcinogenesis. Discover how simple awareness and informed decisions can lead to profound differences, helping you, your family, and your community thrive. The contents go beyond traditional toxicology and discuss teratogenesis, carcinogenesis, immunomodulation. The chapters explore cancer risk starting before conception influencing fetal programming, immune system maturation, and early tissue development. Several examples are provided for a compelling exploration of the paternal and maternal factors potentially setting the stage for later cancer risk, altered tumor microenvironment (TME).

From there, we navigate xenobiotic metabolism, unraveling how our bodies process foreign compounds and oncometabolites. Section 2 demonstrates that environmental influences include exogenous chemicals, lifestyle choices, endogenous factors, and biological systems. Section 2 delves on xenobiotic metabolism, gene-environment interactions, and microbiome and environmental toxins that can increased risk of cancers, leukemia, brain tumors. We learn how gene-environment interactions dictate biomarkers of exposure and regulates cellular antioxidant response. The gut microbiome can also play a role in heavy metal toxicity, affect cancer risk through metabolic pathways. The hormone-like substances, endocrine disruptor chemicals alter the microbiome. Accumulation of somatic mutations, epigenetic alterations, chronic inflammation leading to a pro-tumorigenic TME. The epidemiology studies link environmental factors to early marker of DNA damage and disease patterns in populations. The multi-omics advancements in high throughput technologies, on angiogenesis and metastasis, continue suppression of anti-tumor immunity is reported to play an essential role.

Section 3 begins by consolidating the key takeaways from the preceding sections, to identify cancer stem-like cells. The imperative of integrative omics and systems biology approaches show cumulative exposures and age-related changes can lead to genomic instability, chronic inflammation. Consequently, contribute to tumor initiation and progression by disrupting the mechanisms that maintain tissue architecture and cellular identity. We will explore biotechnology tools, in vitro models and sophisticated computational approaches, are transforming our understanding of gene-environment interactions. Experimental techniques pave the way to simulate risk assessment to decipher the complexities of gene-environment interactions. Several case studies demonstrate advanced methodologies and challenges in research. The biomarkers, gene expression profiles and molecular features indicate how exposure to environmental chemicals affects biological processes. These developments will likely lead to new insights into genetic predisposition, ultimately contributing to improved cancer outcomes and public health strategies.

Section 4 provides a review on disease-specific applications and health disparities. The contents delve into innovative research approaches and practical case studies. Health disparities research provides critical insights into why certain communities bear a disproportionate burden of environmentally-linked diseases. Why do certain places seem to foster wellness, while others carry hidden risks? Health disparities research emphasizes how socioeconomic status and environmental exposures contribute to differences in cancer incidence. It aligns with the core principles of public health by promoting prevention, addressing health disparities, and improving population health. Social determinants of health advocate for prevention of DNA damage, chronic inflammation and hormonal imbalances. The final section will serve as a vital resource for researchers, clinicians, and public health professionals, bridging the gap between scientific research and practical applications in global health.

Developmental Origins of Health and Disease: Maternal and Paternal Exposures in Carcinogenesis

Chapter 1 of exposomics, aim to illuminate Developmental Origins of Health and Disease (DOHaD) to discover how exposures in the womb and early childhood can program lifelong health. Why do some of us face health challenges that others don't, even when our genes seem similar? An adolescent navigating new independence, a young adult building a career, a parent raising a family, or an elder reflecting on a lifetime of experiences, the answers to these questions resonate deeply. The time between exposure and cancer development can be decades. The Developmental Origins of Health and Disease concept has historically emphasized maternal environmental influences on offspring phenotypes. Recent investigation expands this framework to include paternal contributions. DOHaD examines mechanisms by which paternal health status and environmental exposures, prior to and at conception, affect offspring development. Focus areas include the paternal exposome, gamete quality, and epigenetic inheritance, as they relate to long-term offspring health and disease risk. This chapter establishes the father's role in developmental programming, advocating a comprehensive, intergenerational perspective on health outcomes.

Omics Integration in Understanding Xenobiotic Metabolism: Systems Biology Insights

Chapter 2, Xenobiotic Metabolism is about how your body processes foreign chemicals and why it matters for detoxification and disease prevention. Organisms adapt to their environment through xenobiotic-metabolizing pathways (XMP), which are responsible for detecting, metabolizing, and eliminating xenobiotics, but can also produce reactive toxic intermediates. Understanding xenobiotic metabolism requires a systems-level approach to molecular interactions and regulatory networks. This chapters provides details of diverse omics datasets. Emphasis is placed on the functional roles of cytochrome P450 enzymes and the influence of microbiome-derived metabolites in xenobiotic processing pathways.

Systems Biology and Integrative Omics Decoding Xenobiotic Metabolism in Environmental Carcinogenesis

Chapter 3 focuses on the application of systems biology and integrative omics approaches Many XMP proteins exhibit low specificity, allowing them to interact with a wide range of chemicals, leading to potential negative outcomes such as cross-inhibition, inefficient metabolism, and the release of toxic intermediates. to decode tumor heterogeneity, and epigenetic toxicants. It specifically addresses enzymes and signaling pathways in tumorigenesis, and their inhibition is potentially beneficial for anticancer drug designs.

The Cancer Exposome: Gene-Environment Interactions (GxE) in Carcinogenesis

In Chapter 4, GxE research demonstrates vulnerable subgroups with genetic susceptibility to environmental exposures. The genome, remains relatively stable over time, the exposome is a highly dynamic and constantly evolving as individuals interact with their surroundings from the prenatal period onwards. The profound justification for the intensive study of gene-environment interactions (GxE) in carcinogenesis lies in the recognition that genetic predispositions rarely operate in isolation. While germline mutations in high-penetrance genes contribute to a minority of familial cancers, the vast majority of sporadic cancers are attributable to a complex interplay between an individual's genetic landscape and a lifetime of environmental exposures. Exposure to chemicals (Bisphenol A, nickel chloride, radiation) can disrupt the tumor microenvironment by affecting stromal cells, immune cells, and signaling molecules. Additionally, there are ethical, legal, and societal implications (ELSI) inherent in leveraging exposomic data for prevention.

Insights on the Role of the Microbiome in Influencing How Ecological Exposures Affect Cancer Risk: Microbiome's Role in Influencing Cancer Risk

The microbiome can also play a role in how environmental exposures affect cancer risk through metabolic pathways, highlighting the complex interactions between the exposome and biological systems. This section introduces the microbiome, encompassing the diverse community of microorganisms including bacteria, viruses, archaea, fungi, and parasites. Its role as a critical environmental factor influencing human health and disease is explored.. The diet, pollution, and lifestyle, can alter the microbiome and immune system, which in turn modulate the tumor microenvironment and gene expression profiles. The microbiome action on the chemicals produces numerous metabolites that can either help metabolize xenobiotics or result in toxic derivatives. Establishing causal relationships between specific environmental exposures and cancer outcomes remains a challenge, necessitating more robust epidemiological studies.

Cutting-Edge In Vitro Models and Multi-Omics Approaches for Carcinogen Exposome Studies

Chapter 6 explores advanced in vitro models and microfluidics in carcinogenesis research. This chapter focuses on cutting-edge toxicological techniques for investigating carcinogen effects. Studies show that prenatal exposure to phthalates, BPA, metals, and other toxicants leads to significant changes in DNA methylation and gene expression in the placenta and fetal tissues. It addresses concepts of bioaccumulation and persistence through the application of in vitro studies, including the use of cell lines and organoids. Furthermore, the integration of proteomics and transcriptomics is highlighted as a means to understand the spatial organization of molecules within tissues. These technologies offer critical insights into the tumor microenvironment and cell-cell interactions, thereby enhancing the understanding of cancer biology.

Environmental DNA And RNA Metabarcoding: Advancing Insights in Cancer Research

Chapter 7, is on environmental nucleic acids in carcinogenesis assessment. It explores the application of environmental DNA (eDNA) and environmental RNA (eRNA). In the assessment of carcinogenesis, metabarcoding, utilizes high-throughput sequencing, for characterization of microbial ecosystems. Enhanced detection technologies will enable the identification of previously unknown environmental carcinogens and facilitate the accurate assessment of exposure levels in diverse ecosystems. Metabarcoding technique facilitates the detection of potential carcinogenic exposures and elucidates their interactions with human health.

Digital Exposome. A Digital Age Approach To Environmental Exposure And Cancer Risk Assessment

Chapter 8, addresses key challenges in multi-omics data analysis, specifically focusing on data heterogeneity and format inconsistencies. Given the increasing scale of datasets, the need for high-performance computing resources for efficient data processing and analysis are discussed. This section addresses the increasing application of artificial intelligence (AI) and machine learning (ML) algorithms in multi-omics data analysis within cancer research.

Conclusion

The book emphasizes that the exposome is not a singular entity but a interdisciplinary collaboration from applied environment fields. The integration of cancer exposomics with the SDGs offers a synergistic approach to global health. Exposomics research directly informs several SDGs, notably SDG 3 (Good Health and Well-being) by identifying preventable risk factors, SDG 6 (Clean Water and Sanitation) and SDG 11 (Sustainable Cities and Communities) by addressing environmental pollutants, and SDG 10 (Reduced Inequalities) by highlighting disproportionate exposure burdens. This comprehensive resource is designed for researchers, clinicians, and advanced students in environmental health, toxicology, oncology, and related fields. By fostering collaboration across disciplines, we can pave the way for a future where we can prevent disease, promote well-being, and create a healthier world.

Several examples demonstrate the challenges and opportunities in exposomics research. The importance of collaboration, data sharing, and ethical considerations is the way forward to reach the Sustainable Developmental Goals, public health and medical services. Cancer exposome can guide interventions that mitigate cancer risk, promote environmental stewardship, and foster equitable health outcomes. Future advancements in cancer prevention and public health depend on this integrated perspective. This necessitates an immediate, collaborative effort to translate scientific advancements into tangible reductions in cancer incidence and improved public health outcomes globally. The call to action for cancer prevention extends beyond the exposome research community, resonating with a broader audience invested in health equity and disease prevention.

Ramya Raghavan
Sri Sathya Sai University for Human Excellence, India

Chapter 1 Developmental Origins of Health and Disease: Maternal and Paternal Exposures in Carcinogenesis

Ramya Raghavan
https://orcid.org/0000-0002-9953-543X
Sri Sathya Sai University for Human Excellence, Kalaburagi, India

Shadab Ahamad
https://orcid.org/0000-0003-0788-4817
Sri Sathya Sai Sanjeevani Research Foundation, Palwal, India

ABSTRACT

There is an intricate relationship between the exposome and critical periods of gametogenesis, teratogenesis, and cancer development. Developmental Origins of Health and Disease (DOHaD) framework to cancer susceptibility examines the hypothesis that early-life environmental exposures can program long-term cancer risk. The authors review epidemiological studies demonstrating associations between developmental exposures and increased cancer risk. Case studies beginning from gametogenesis, debates on biological mechanisms, epigenetic modifications, and altered tissue development are discussed. The chapter also critically analyzes key controversies such as methodological limitations, the etiological complexity of cancer, issues of generalizability, and translational hurdles. This work demonstrates how environmental factors influence gamete formation, embryonic development, and carcinogenesis to highlight the need for addressing parental health and reducing health disparities.

DOI: 10.4018/979-8-3373-2165-3.ch001

BACKGROUND ON DEVELOPMENTAL ORIGINS OF HEALTH AND DISEASE (DOHAD)

Lamarck's early theories on inheritance and environmental adaptation have influenced the concepts of the Developmental Origins of Health and Disease (DOHaD) (Zambrano & Ibáñez, 2025). DOHaD is the idea that environmental exposures during critical periods of development (in utero, infancy, early childhood) are essential. DOHaD believes that internal and external early life exposures can have epigenetic effects.

Exposome research purports that exposures of biological, environmental, and chemical origin influence human health. There are debates on Lamarckian ideas that also argue the link between DOHaD and cancer susceptibility. Arguments focus on how molecular markers for internal and external exposure vary in time and interact in complex ways. The tumorigenic effects can be cumulative, and the diagnosis of phenotypic plasticity based on morphological, physiological, and behavioral adaptations is obscure (Vineis & Dagnino, 2024). The eighth annual US DOHAD meeting calls for birth cohort studies, longitudinal cohorts, and innovative methodologies (Non, 2025). It aims to gain a modern understanding of how early-life environmental factors impact carcinogenesis across an individual's lifetime and future generations.

Exposome measurements examine colorectal cancer (CRC) risk using data from the UK Biobank. Findings revealed that risk factors such as ecosystem, healthy lifestyles, tobacco or alcohol use, socioeconomic status, and insufficient social support. Certain dietary factors, such as high intake of fat, red meat, processed meat, and dietary fiber, influence the risk of colorectal cancer. Conversely, nutritional variables like higher linolenic acid intake and lower coffee consumption are associated with squamous cell carcinoma. Cultural Practices, such as the use of betel quid, have been linked to increased oral and esophageal cancer risk. Poor living conditions that cause chronic inflammation, such as inflammatory bowel disease (IBD) and chronic hepatitis, can increase the risk of cancer development in affected tissues (Tortolero et al., 2024).

Figure 1. Etiology of Pediatric Cancer: Genetic, Exogenous, Environmental Risks

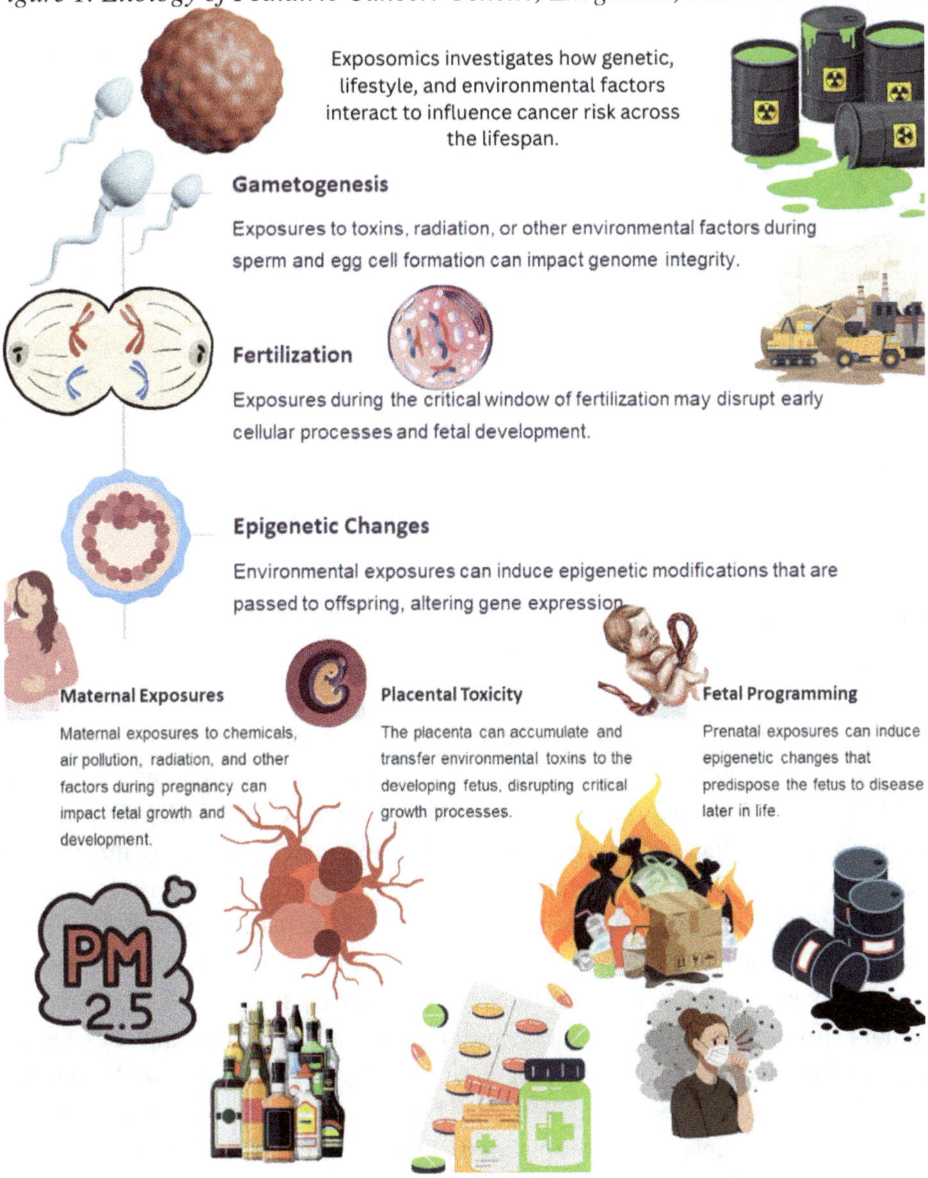

Table 1. Toxic Exposures at Every Life Stage have an Impact on Carcinogenesis and Tumor Microenvironment

Life Stage	Exposure	Tumor Microenvironment Impact (TME)	Reference
Gametogenesis	Parental Exposures (Chemical, Physical, Biological, Lifestyle)	Epigenetic modifications in sperm and egg cells alter germline mutation rates.	(Krausová et al., 2023) (Gu et al., 2025)
Prenatal Neonatal	In Utero Exposures (Maternal Diet, Environmental Toxins, Infections, Stress), Early Life Exposures (Air pollution, Infections)	Influencing Fetal Programming, Immune System Maturation, Tissue Development	(Coste et al., 2020) (Paul et al., 2023)
Childhood Adolescence	Environmental Exposures (Pollution, Pesticides), Diet, Infections, Radiation (pharmaceutical), Lifestyle	Increased risk of childhood cancers (leukemia, brain tumors) Suppression Of Anti-Tumor Immunity	(Kaltsas et al., 2025) (Msallem et al., 2025)
Adulthood	Occupational, Lifestyle Factors (Diet, Smoking, Alcohol), Chronic Infections, Reproductive Factors, Pollution, Stress	Accumulation of Somatic Mutations, Epigenetic Alterations, Chronic Inflammation Pro-Tumorigenic TME, Promotion of Angiogenesis and Metastasis,	(Coste et al., 2020) (Young et al., 2025)
Aging	Cumulative Lifetime Exposures, Hormones, Microbiome	Decline in immune surveillance, chronic low-grade inflammation, Impaired detoxification and DNA repair, altered metabolic landscape	(Vineis & Dagnino, 2024) (Feng et al., 2024) (Weinberg et al., 2025)

DOHaD as Cancer Risk

The etiology of cancer is linked to genetic, exogenous, and environmental risk factors. The field of exposomics presents a hypothesis that early-life exposures can influence tumor microenvironment (TME), Epithelial-Mesenchymal Transition (EMT) Extracellular matrix (ECM) remodeling. Based on the DOHaD, exposure to gametogenesis and critical developmental periods can significantly impact fetal health outcomes (Table 1). The prenatal exposure changes during critical embryological periods of development, when combined with postnatal exposure at developmental milestones, disrupt growth and health. The most common types of pediatric cancers include leukemias, brain tumors, lymphomas, sarcomas, and embryonal tumors (Boysen et al., 2025). The exposome as cancer risk encompasses factors influencing cancer initiation and progression. In the case of tumors, understanding of early-life health impacts is challenged. There is a bias towards short-term effects and contesting complex data from parental exposures and social determinants. There is a pressing need to improve prenatal care globally, as deprioritizing paternal and maternal health could have detrimental effects on the health of parents today and children in the future.

From preconception through infancy, the early-life period depends on nutrition, toxicant impacts, and metabolic microenvironment. Some consensus exists to explain potential epigenetic modifications and altered tissue development to link environmental exposure to cancer risk. It does acknowledge that the DOHaD framework's application to cancer is not without debate. There is a lacuna clearly to synthesizing the research data and controversies surrounding the DOHaD link to cancer. This paper will explore the evidence suggesting a role for developmental origins in cancer susceptibility. The main objective is to critically examine the methodological challenges and etiological complexities that fuel ongoing arguments about the environmental influences of cancer.

Prenatal and perinatal toxic exposures may lead to permanent metabolic derangements in offspring and the functional diversity of TME populations. They have been linked to altered histone and DNA methylation, which can impact EMT. Chlorinated solvents and chemical compounds used in various industrial processes have been associated with increased ECM changes in childhood brain tumors. This underscores the importance of minimizing pesticide, plastic, endocrine, and metabolic disruptor exposure to protect fetal development and long-term health outcomes (Paul et al., 2023).

Congenital Anomaly-Cancer Associations

Environmental exposures contribute to cancer through carcinogenic agents affecting critical developmental periods, including preconception, transplacental, and postnatal stages. Evidence suggests that certain environmental exposures, particularly during critical developmental periods, can lead to increased cancer risks in children. One of the critical windows of susceptibility to chemical exposures is during the embryo-fetal stages. Incorporation of novel exposure assessment methodologies is needed, as some chemicals and pollutants can cross the placenta, affecting fetal growth and development. Dietary factors and anti-nutritional exposure can result in complications such as low birth weight, preterm birth, and developmental delays. Ethanol in alcoholic beverages is metabolized to acetaldehyde, a known carcinogen. The viruses and bacteria, such as human papillomavirus (HPV), hepatitis B and C viruses, and Helicobacter pylori, are known to contribute to the development of cancers. The relationship between childhood leukemia and the role of environmental pollutants, such as secondhand smoke, particulate matter, chemicals, DDT, organophosphates, and heavy metals, reflects significant environmental risk factors for congenital tumors.

Congenital anomaly-cancer associations, such as choanal atresia linked to acute leukemia and congenital heart defects associated with neuroblastoma, show cancer predisposition syndromes. The phenylalanine/tyrosine ratio, tyrosine, and thyroxine were the analytes most consistently associated with various congenital disabilities. The relationships between newborn screening analytes and congenital disabilities may provide insights into the underlying mechanisms of congenital disability etiology (Lupo et al., 2024). The genetic and viral factors contribute to acute myeloid leukemia (AML), focusing on the role of germline mutations and viral infections in developing the disease. To study correlation for identifying new congenital anomaly-pediatric cancer patterns, analyzing germline whole-genome sequencing data to help find pleiotropic genes and somatic alterations in cancers linked to these variants. The identified variants included genes associated with both anomalies and cancer (WT1, USP9X, PTPN1, LZTR1), established cancer predisposition genes (TP53, PAX5), and genes linked to anomalies (MMUT, FBN1, COL3A1, KAT6B). With a gene-based analysis, significant evidence for KAT6B as a novel neuroblastoma susceptibility gene shows enrichment of rare, predicted deleterious variants in neuroblastoma cases compared to controls (Gu et al., 2025). Funding for pooled international prospective studies on environmental carcinogens can offer new insights into cancers of the liver, breast, and esophagus. Establishing causal relationships between known carcinogens can change global public health policies to prevent infections.

Epidemiological Studies

Parental exposures can induce epigenetic changes in germ cells. Epigenetics shows that altering the expression of key developmental regulators in the offspring leads to increased cancer susceptibility and developmental defects. Congenital abnormalities and cancer risk share common pathways affecting tissue organization and cell differentiation. The cohort studies and case-control studies have link early-life exposures (maternal nutrition, gestational diabetes, low birth weight, exposure to environmental toxins) to increased cancer risk in adulthood. Examples of the cumulative parental and fetal effects leading to cancer are reported for pre-pubertal DDT exposure, breast cancer, and gene-environment interactions with endocrine and metabolic disruptors (Gu et al., 2025). The risk of pediatric carcinomas, with non-syndromic anomalies and chromosomal or genetic link, is shown. Pesticides also have an increased hazard of developing hepatocellular and renal carcinomas. Research has shown that prenatal stressors, traumatic events during pregnancy, and pathogenetic mechanisms of umbilical cord (UC) anomalies are all connected to adverse outcomes. Specifically, the hazard ratios indicate a significant risk for cancer among affected children compared to unaffected peers (Schraw et al., 2025).

Animal Models

Mechanistic insights are gained from animal models on the environmental influences of cancer. Studies indicate that prenatal exposure to pesticides is associated with a higher risk of neuroblastoma in children, with an Odds Ratio (OR): 1.6 (1.1-2.3; $p = 0.013$). Perinatal exposure to the herbicide amitrole and the antithyroid drug MMI on thyroid hormone levels and testis development in Sprague-Dawley rats, revealing that both chemicals significantly reduced TH levels. The detrimental effects of several commonly encountered EDCs, including bisphenol A (BPA), phthalates, polychlorinated biphenyls (PCBs), parabens, pesticides, and heavy metals, impact the hypothalamic-pituitary-gonadal (HPG) axis. The reproductive dysfunction caused by the organophosphate pesticide malathion in adolescent male mice highlights its effects at environmentally relevant concentrations. Malathion exposure for eight weeks resulted in reduced testis weight, hormonal disorders, and damage to the testicular spermatogenic epithelium, along with increased oxidative stress. Malathion activates the HIF-1/MAPK/PI3K signaling pathways, leading to increased expression of HIF-1α and disruption of steroid hormone biosynthesis, contributing to spermatogenesis dysfunction (Xiao et al., 2024).

Table 2. Developmental Origins of Health and Disease and Genes in Carcinogenesis

DOHaD	Carcinogenesis Pathways	Common Genes	Reference
Fertilization Cleavage	Cell Proliferation Genomic Stability Epigenetic Programming	DNMTs (DNA methyltransferases), Histone Modifying Enzymes HMTs miRNAs	(Wu et al., 2024) (Paul et al., 2023)
Gastrulation Germ Cell Formation	Pattern Formation Cell Fate Specification Axial Development	IGF1/2 ERBB2 VEGFA Immune-related genes (cytokines, chemokines)	(Benavent et al., 2025) (Krausová et al., 2023).
Neurulation Tissue and Immune cell Brain Spinal cord Nervous System	Tissue Folding and Fusion Cell-Cell Interactions Immune System Development Influencing Tissue Homeostasis	MYC RB1 TP53 DNA Repair Genes Immune Checkpoint Regulators	(Coste et al., 2020) (Paul et al., 2023)
Histogenesis Tissue Differentiation, Apoptosis, and Organogenesis	Cell Proliferation Differentiation Branching Morphogenesis Angiogenesis Cell Proliferation	Oncogenes (KRAS, PIK3CA), Tumor Suppressor Genes (PTEN, APC), Inflammatory cytokines (IL-6, TNF-α) ECM remodeling genes (MMPs)	(Maria et al., 2023) (Borankova et al., 2023)
Aging Apoptosis Autophagy DNA Repair Mechanisms	Tissue Remodeling and Repair Cellular Senescence Maintenance Of Tissue Homeostasis	Senescence-associated secretory phenotype (SASP) genes (IL-6 IL-8 MMPs) Immune checkpoint ligands (PD-L1) Metabolic regulators Antioxidant defense genes	(Lupo et al., 2024) (Gu et al., 2025)

Epigenetic Inheritance and Transgenerational Effects

Epigenetic modifications in sperm and egg cells potentially influence offspring cancer susceptibility and early development; altered germline mutation rates. The heritability of environmentally induced epigenetic changes across generations remains controversial. In utero and early life exposures to environmental toxins can disrupt hormonal signaling and developmental pathways. Literature has strong evidence in animal models to show tissue organization, cell growth, and differentiation being altered. Interestingly increasing the risk of developmental abnormalities and also predisposing tissues to later oncogenic transformation by altering the foundational tissue structure. However, growing recognition of paternal contributions, particularly through epigenetic pathways, has limited human data to support and refute transgenerational effects.

Paternal Exposure as a Risk Factor

Environmental exposures during gamete formation (spermatogenesis) can introduce mutations and epigenetic alterations that influence the early stages of embryonic development. For instance, exposure to air pollutants during sperm formation has been linked to adverse birth outcomes, such as low birth weight and congenital disabilities. More infant biomonitoring studies are needed, including a broad range of xenobiotics and household natural toxins. Paternal lifestyle and environmental factors, such as diet, smoking, and exposure to endocrine-disrupting chemicals, influence the sperm epigenome. The significance of the loss of imprinting (LOI) of genomic imprinting genes in cancer and its role in tumorigenesis is affected by sperm fertilizing ability in embryo development. Epigenetic mechanisms, including DNA methylation, histone modifications, and non-coding RNA activity, are essential for spermatogenesis and sperm maturation, influencing male reproductive health. The epigenetic alterations caused by oxidative stress can be inherited, potentially affecting the health and fertility of offspring and future generations, raising concerns about hereditary infertility and disease predisposition (Kaltsas et al., 2025). There are several questions about the extent to which future generations can inherit epigenetic changes affecting cancer risk.

Hormonal Programming

The environmental risk factors associated with Wilms tumor (WT) in children include high birth weight, cesarean section, and parental occupational exposure to pesticides. Conversely, breastfeeding and maternal intake of vitamins and folic acid during pregnancy were found to have protective effects (Onyije et al., 2024). Parental occupational exposure to hazardous medical agents, particularly anticancer drugs, increases the risk of childhood cancer, specifically leukemia and brain tumors, in offspring. The use of specific goods with greater amounts of phthalates may play a role in early hormone exposures in shaping cancer risk in hormone-sensitive tissues. Consumer products, such as hair relaxers and skin-whitening products marketed to Black consumers, represent a social factor influencing chemical exposure.

Molecular docking studies demonstrated that malathion interacts with HIF-1α and steroid hormone synthases, indicating a mechanism by which malathion induces reproductive toxicity and spermatogenesis impairment. These factors explain the potential influence of paternal occupational and environmental exposures on offspring health outcomes, particularly cancer risk. Present findings from animal studies that demonstrate how in-utero or early postnatal exposures can lead to increased tumor development or altered susceptibility to carcinogens later in life. Spatial variable genes (SVGs) are crucial in mapping this intricate tumor heterogeneity, providing insights into the spatial organization. The timing of exposure is critical, with perinatal and in-utero exposures being particularly influential in determining cancer risk. Spatial omics research has demonstrated that early-life exposures can have long-lasting effects on health, potentially leading to congenital tumors (Coste et al., 2020).

Brain Tumors

Congenital brain tumors have an incidence of 1.1-3.6 per 100,000 live births and account for 0.5-2% of all pediatric cancers. The congenital gliomas neuroblastoma in newborns exhibit sepsis-like symptoms or unexplained metabolic acidosis and hypertension and have a poor prognosis. The mortality rates for congenital glioblastoma are high, with 29% of affected infants dying on the first day of life, 38% within the first week, and 56% within the first two months, while the average survival length is only two years. Previous studies indicate maternal stress can affect the fetal hypothalamic-pituitary-adrenal (HPA) axis (Benavent et al., 2025). Interference with neurulation can lead to neural tube defects and stress hormones leading to changes in fetal immune function. The signaling pathways that govern early tissue morphogenesis and cell identity are similar to carcinogenesis (Table 2). In the nervous system, disruption due to stress-related hormones released affects neurulation. Thus, providing a biological basis for the connection between maternal stress and CNS or PNS cancer risk in offspring. The exposomics of high-grade tumors, particularly in the pediatric population, highlights the significance of histone mutations and gene amplifications in understanding tumor biology. The most prevalent mutations in these aggressive tumors (WHO grades III and IV) include H3F3A mutations (specifically H3K27M and H3.3G34R/V) and amplifications of genes such as PDGFRA, EGFR, MYC, MYCN, and MDM4. Notably, the H3K27M mutation is found in only about 6% of brain tumors documented in the literature, indicating its rarity yet importance in tumor characterization (Maria et al., 2023).

Altered Tissue Development and Hematopoietic Tumors

Maternal pesticide exposure, birth weight, parental smoking, and pharmaceuticals cause genetic changes in hematopoietic progenitor/stem cells. Key prenatal factors that influence the preleukemic lesions include parental age, ethnicity, maternal diet, folate intake, and alcohol consumption. X-ray exposure, pesticides, and perinatal infections affect cell proliferation, differentiation, and the establishment of stem cell populations. and fetal growth. Investigating the relationship between maternal lifestyle factors and genetic lesions associated with childhood leukemia is essential (Benítez et al., 2024). Significant associations were found between maternal coffee consumption (more than 2 cups/day) and non-Hodgkin lymphoma (NHL), as well as maternal alcohol consumption and Burkitt NHL, along with paternal smoking during preconception/pregnancy and NHL (Msallem et al., 2025).

Figure 2. Paternal Epigenetics Play A Significant Role in Carcinogenesis

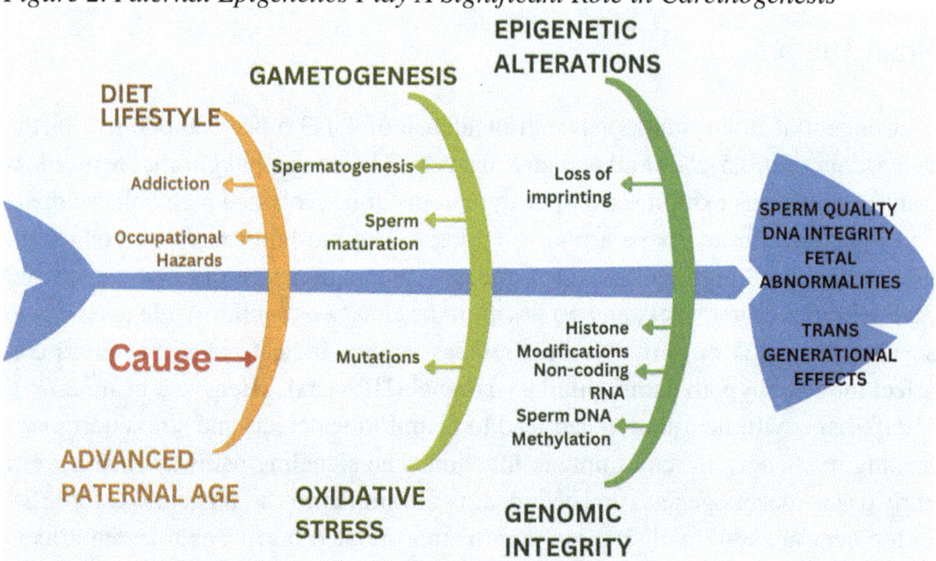

Endocrine Disruptors and DNA methylation, histone modifications, and non-coding RNAs.

According to data from the Japan Environment and Children's Study, there is an association between maternal exposure to per- and polyfluoroalkyl substances (PFAS) and the prevalence of chromosomal abnormalities in offspring. PFAS compounds, particularly perfluorononanoic acid (PFNA) and perfluorooctane sulfonic acid (PFOS), were found to have positive associations with chromosomal abnormalities (Hasegawa et al., 2024). Disruption of hormonal signaling and growth factor pathways during organogenesis can lead to malformations. Cancer studies show that altering the cellular composition of developing tissues is analogous to tumor microenvironment changes. Data gaps on prenatal and infant exposure to xenobiotic mixtures, including natural biotoxins, and synthetic toxicants. A more holistic assessment of the chemical exposome requires incorporating these less-studied contaminants.

Loss of Imprinting

Genomic imprinting is crucial for mammalian growth and development. Loss of imprinting (LOI) can impact various epigenetic processes, including tumor susceptibility. Oxidative stress disrupts epigenetic mechanisms essential for spermatogenesis, leading to male infertility and the risk of childhood leukemia (Kaltsas et al., 2025). Exposure to teratogens, toxins, and heavy metals during embryonic development led to epigenetic changes. Exposures during active tissue differentiation and growth periods can disrupt the balance between cell proliferation and apoptosis. Thereby promoting chronic inflammation that alters the tissue microenvironment, and pre-cancerous lesions affecting tissue maturation. LOI of imprinted genes is recognized as an early event in gametogenesis and is also involved in cancer progression, with over 120 imprinted genes identified in humans. Maternal nutritional status around the time of conception affects DNA methylation, and tobacco, alcohol, and drugs influence cancer risk. Exposure routes include prenatal placental transfer and postnatal oral, parenteral, inhalation, and dermal exposure. Placental transfer is influenced by molecular weight, pKa, lipid solubility, and protein binding, with small lipophilic compounds passing via passive diffusion or carrier proteins (Krausová et al., 2023). Additionally, accumulating harmful substances in placental tissue may disrupt the fetus's development and nutrient and oxygen delivery.

- Paternal occupational exposure to carcinogens such as pesticides has deleterious effects on fetal development, linked to congenital malformations and neuroblastoma in children (Onyije et al., 2022).

- Endocrine disruptors can interfere with neuroendocrine systems, causing developmental, reproductive, neurological, and immune effects (Krausová et al., 2023).

Maternal vs. Paternal Cancer Risk Contributions

Traditional emphasis has been on maternal effects due to the direct biological connection during gestation. Exposures during periods of rapid growth and tissue development can interfere with normal development. The signaling pathways can potentially lead to abnormal cell proliferation, altered vascularization of developing tissues, and chronic inflammation, creating a microenvironment susceptible to tumorigenesis.

There is a debate over whether maternal factors have a more direct impact due to gestational environment versus paternal influences through genetic/epigenetic pathways. The cancer risk is influenced by the xenobiotics exposed during the fetal stage by maternal, fetal, and environmental interactions. Data shows that maternal coffee and alcohol consumption during pregnancy, as well as paternal smoking, may increase the risk of childhood non-Hodgkin lymphoma. Tobacco smoke, when exposed during pregnancy, leads to permanent metabolic derangements in offspring, emphasizing an exposomic approach to understanding cancer risk (Msallem et al., 2025). Early life exposures include dietary factors, pollutants, occupational hazards, lifestyle choices, infectious agents, and social determinants of health (Krausová et al., 2023). Therefore, single-cell omics technology to study spatially variable genes (SVGs) is becoming increasingly relevant to linking the complexities of cause and effect in cancer biology (Biradar, Suresh, et al., 2025). SVGs allow the understanding of the tumor microenvironment (TME). TME includes mutation burden, variants disrupting transcriptional activity, chromatin state, and non-coding cis-regulatory regions between tumor cells and surrounding healthy cells. Several studies present the challenges in applying DOHaD concepts to contemporary scientific research in cancer. The hour needs longitudinal cohort studies on exposome to study SVGs in cancer development and metastasis.

Table 3. Parental Exposures Alter Genes in Development Leading to Cancers

Examples of Parental Exposures	Genes	Pathways in Development Leading to Cancers	Reference
Parental Smoking, Occupational Chemical Endocrine Disruptors, Radiation Parental Diet	Hox Genes Wnt Signaling (WNT3 FZD) Shh (SHH PTCH1) DNA Methyltransferases (DNMTs)	Pattern Formation, Cell Fate Determination Tissue Polarity Epigenetic Regulation Of Developmental Genes	(Akhatova et al., 2025) (Kaltsas et al., 2025) (Di Renzo et al., 2024)
Exposure To BPA Phthalates Dioxins Hormones Early Exposure To Particulate Matter	TGF-β (TGFB1 SMADs) RTKs (Receptor Tyrosine Kinases EGFR FGFR) Cell Adhesion (Cadherins Integrins) Hedgehog	Cell Proliferation Differentiation Migration Cell-Cell; Cell-Matrix Interactions Tissue Architecture	(Gu et al., 2025) (Maria et al., 2023) (Benavent et al., 2025)
Phthalates Viral Infections Maternal Nutritional Deficiencies Maternal Stress	IGF (IGF1R) NF-kappa B Angiogenic Factor(VEGF) Notch	Growth Development Inflammatory Responses Angiogenesis	(Chu et al., 2025) (Onyije et al., 2024)
Asbestos Benzene Inflammatory Conditions (IBD) High Estrogen Or Testosterone	EMT (Snail Twist) Matrix Metalloproteinases (MMPs) WNT/β-CATENIN PI3K/AKT/ mTOR	Epithelial-Mesenchymal Transition (EMT) ECM Remodeling (Tissue Morphogenesis) Cell Growth ; Metabolism	(Maria et al., 2023) (Tortolero et al., 2024) (Huoi et al., 2014)

Polycyclic Aromatic Hydrocarbons (PAH)

Interestingly, when a father experiences high levels of stress due to environmental factors, it may affect his partner's health and, consequently, the health of the developing fetus. Extensive longitudinal cohort studies on occupational exposure to Polycyclic Aromatic Hydrocarbons (PAH) diesel motor exhaust (DME), asbestos, crystalline silica, and metals are needed to show the high risk of childhood brain tumors (Huoi et al., 2014). Parental Occupational Exposure to polycyclic aromatic hydrocarbons (PAH) and an increased risk of childhood brain tumors, with specific odds ratios indicating a higher likelihood of developing these tumors. Increased risks of brain tumors may also correlate with broader environmental pollutants. Further highlighting the standardization of exposure assessments to improve understanding of industrial and occupational exposures. Prenatal pesticide exposure increases the risk of neuroblastoma in children, demonstrating the diverse impact of parental occupational hazards. The specific types of brain tumors associated with these exposures include astroglial tumors and other nervous system tumors.

Socioeconomic factors often exacerbate the teratogenicity of rubella virus infection during pregnancy. The potential of rubella virus infection to cause congenital malformations also reflects disparities that influence exposure levels and access to healthcare. Thus, a holistic approach is crucial for understanding the complex interactions, such as medical drug abuse in parents and unhealthy lifestyle behaviors that adversely influence prenatal development. Synthetic biology offers powerful tools to dissect the complex interplay between environmental exposures and tumor biology (Ananthakumar et al., 2024). AI can be leveraged to analyze vast datasets of environmental exposures, including microbial volatile organic compounds, pollutants, and dietary factors, correlating them with cancer incidence and spatial gene expression patterns (GVS et al., 2025). Computational biology tools allow for identifying critical exposure windows and specific environmental factors that contribute to tumorigenesis (Lakshmaiah et al., 2025).

Maternal Stress

Adult exposures can reactivate or dysregulate developmental pathways like EMT and ECM remodeling, which are usually tightly controlled in mature tissues (Table 3). This dysregulation can promote invasion, metastasis, and angiogenesis in tumors, mirroring processes involved in tissue remodeling during development. There is an association between maternal stressful life events during pregnancy and congenital pathologies with the risk of developing neuroblastoma (NB) in children. Data was collected from 56 mothers through interviews and Health System databases, indicating that stressful life events during pregnancy and specific congenital pathologies are independently linked (Benavent et al., 2025). The mitonuclear balance is crucial during early embryo development. The mismatches between mitochondrial and nuclear genomes can impede embryo progression, possibly leading to early miscarriage abnormalities, including congenital pathologies and tumors. Mitochondrial mosaicism is a key factor influencing health, biological efficiency, and fertility, as it determines the functionality of the respiratory chain. Even minor alterations, such as a single amino acid change, can have significant health implications. For example, the MYC gene is associated with mitochondrial control and mitonuclear imbalance. In high-risk NB patients, MYCN gene amplification correlates with a poor prognosis.

In contrast, non-MYCN-amplified high-risk NB patients show elevated levels of c-MYC expression and its target genes. MYC-driven NB cells rely on effective mitochondrial ribosome processes. They are prone to cell death when inhibiting mitochondrial translation—the mitochondrial translation machinery is a novel target for overcoming multidrug resistance in MYC-driven neuroblastoma. Inhibition of mitochondrial ribosomes leads to cell death in these cancer cells by activating the integrated stress response, which downregulates c-MYC/N-MYC proteins (Borankova et al., 2023). Cumulative exposures and stress-related changes can lead to genomic instability, chronic inflammation, and EMT contributing to tumor initiation.

Paternal Developmental Origins in Cancer Susceptibility

Several environmental and lifestyle factors in men have been found to alter sperm epigenetics, which can regulate gene expression during early embryonic development. The effects of paternal exposure to p,p'-DDE, and a high-fat diet on male offspring's fertility and epigenetic modifications, explicitly focusing on sperm Igf2 DMR2 methylation. Paternal exposure to p,p'-DDE did not directly impair male fertility in offspring but was associated with decreased sperm quality and increased testicular apoptosis when combined with a high-fat diet. The combination of paternal p,p'-DDE exposure, and a pre-pubertal high-fat diet led to hypo-methylation of sperm Igf2 DMR2. It reduced gene expression in male offspring (Lu et al., 2024).

The continuous production of sperm from spermatogonia stem cells throughout a man's adult life, and the presence of spermatogonia stem cells outside the blood-testis barrier, make them susceptible to environmental insults. Furthermore, altered sperm DNA methylation patterns can be maintained throughout development and ultimately result in impairments, which could predispose offspring to disease (Greeson et al., 2023). The accumulation of damage and chronic inflammation in tissues can disrupt the delicate balance of cell proliferation and death that maintains tissue homeostasis, potentially reactivating developmental programs inappropriately and contributing to uncontrolled growth and tumor formation. In aged males, SASP factors released by senescent cells can also influence the TME in ways that resemble developmental signaling cues.

Sperm Quality and DNA Integrity

Paternal exposures to environmental toxins, such as heavy metals, pesticides, and endocrine disruptors, can negatively affect sperm quality. This can lead to compromised DNA integrity in sperm, which may result in developmental issues in offspring, such as congenital malformations and neurodevelopmental disorders. DNA methylation in sperm is associated with changes in sperm quality and fertilization ability, potentially through the regulation of specific signaling pathways. Paternal exposure to endocrine-disrupting chemicals (EDCs) can lead to transgenerational health issues, including infertility and metabolic disorders. High paternal occupational exposure to crystalline silica was significantly associated with an increased risk of childhood acute lymphoblastic leukemia (ALL) and acute myeloid leukemia (AML), with odds ratios of 2.20 and 2.03, respectively (Onyije et al., 2022).

The environmental toxic heavy metals impact epigenetics during gametogenesis and embryonic development. Military pollution includes using materials like depleted uranium, emphasizing the risk due to heavy metal exposure. Testicular and breast cancer may arise from prenatal or early childhood exposures. The Developmental Origins of Health and Disease (DOHaD) theory suggests that exposure to environmental chemicals (methylmercury, cadmium, arsenic, and lead) during embryonic development can lead to epigenetic changes. To gain mechanistic insights into the metabolism, transfer, and biological effects of the chemical exposome in early life, in vitro toxicity assessments in advanced human models (organoids) should be strengthened.

Paternal Oxidative Stress

Excessive reactive oxygen species lead to oxidative stress, disrupting epigenetic processes, impairing sperm function, abnormal gene expression, and compromised genomic integrity. However, the challenges in the long latency period from initial mutation to diagnosis present new opportunities in studying how early life exposures influence cancer risk. Understanding the mechanisms of oxidative stress and epigenetic dysregulation is crucial for developing therapeutic strategies to mitigate toxicological damage. Restore epigenetic homeostasis to enhance male reproductive health, emphasizing personalized diagnostics and multi-omics approaches.

Paternal Obesity

The potential for parental preconception exposure to alter gametes and for these alterations to be passed on to offspring and negatively affect embryo growth and development is of concern. Influencing fetal programming, immune system maturation, and early tissue development. For offspring, setting the stage for later cancer risk begins as altered TME composition in early life. The study investigates the association between pre-conceptional paternal obesity and the risk of congenital urogenital anomalies in offspring, highlighting a gap in existing research focused primarily on maternal obesity (Achkar et al., 2024). A case-control study was conducted with 179 newborns, where 91 had congenital urogenital abnormalities (cases) and 88 were without abnormalities (controls), excluding various confounding factors. Significant differences in paternal BMI were observed between cases and controls, with overweight and obese fathers showing increased odds of having offspring with congenital malformations, particularly with odds ratios of 4.44 for overweight and 8.62 for obese Class I fathers compared to normal-weight fathers. The findings indicate that higher paternal BMI during the preconception period is linked to an increased risk of urogenital malformations in offspring. Increased risk of childhood cancers by influencing the immune system shaping the baseline TME. Thus suggesting the need for addressing paternal obesity in preventive health strategies (Achkar et al., 2024).

Dietary Risk Factors

The Western diet, characterized by a high intake of fat, red meat, ; processed meat, has emerged as an important contributor to colorectal cancer. High consumption of red meats, smoked foods, cold cuts, or canned foods is believed to contribute to carcinogenesis (Nagashri et al., 2024). Conversely, dietary factors involved in one-carbon metabolism influence DNA methylation, a process essential for maintaining cellular function, ; changes in methylation patterns may contribute to cancer development. Lower socioeconomic status is associated with higher cancer incidence ; mortality, often due to factors like limited access to healthcare, unhealthy lifestyle choices, ; environmental exposures (Di Renzo et al., 2024). Accumulation of somatic mutations, epigenetic alterations, chronic inflammation leading to a pro-tumorigenic TME, promotion of angiogenesis and metastasis, suppression of anti-tumor immunity.

Notably, dietary supplements may have harmful effects ; are associated with an increased risk of cancer. Food additives, artificial sweeteners, and preservatives have raised concerns regarding their potential carcinogenic effects. Nutritional deficiencies in essential nutrients, such as folate, vitamin D, may contribute to cancer risk by impairing DNA repair mechanisms. The gut microbiome can influence cancer risk through the inflammation metabolism of dietary components. Dysbiosis may be linked to colorectal cancer (Weinberg et al., 2025). In some cultures, particularly in parts of India and the Middle East, saffron is traditionally given to pregnant women. Saffron, bioactive compounds like crocin and crocetin, have shown promising anti-cancer properties. *Crocus sativus* can influence cell proliferation, inducing apoptosis as an antioxidant (Korrapati et al., 2024).

Figure 3. Environmental Exposures, During Critical Developmental Periods, Lead To Increased Cancer Risks

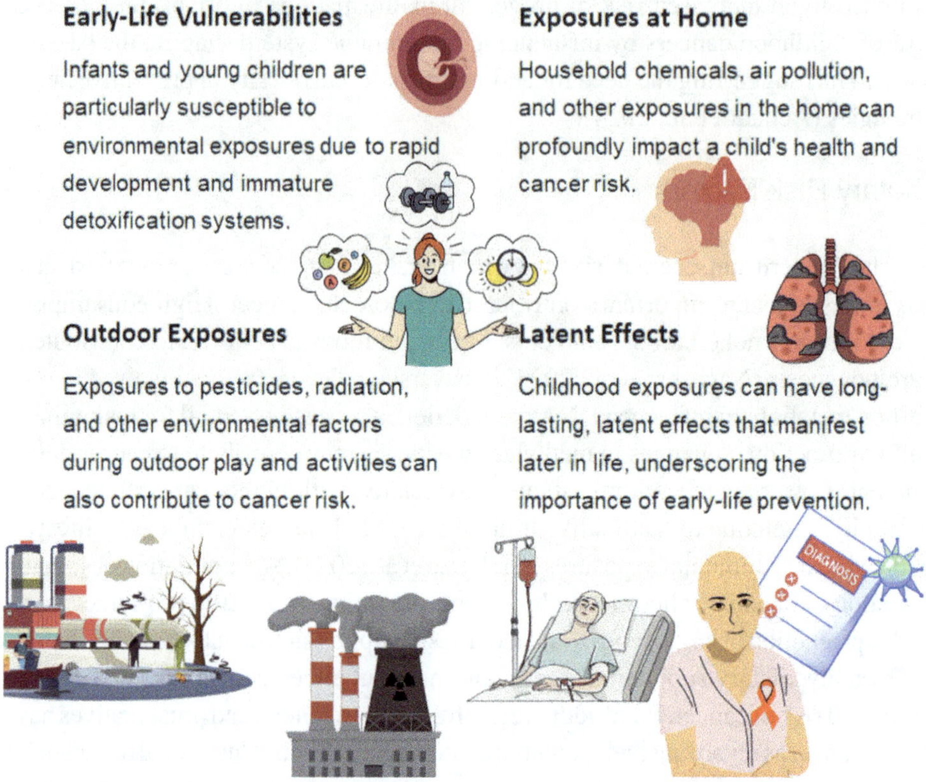

Dietary patterns, such as the Mediterranean diet, healthful plant-based index, Healthy Eating Index (HEI)/alternate HEI (AHEI), and Dietary Approaches to Stop Hypertension (DASH), showed limited evidence for lower CRC risk The dietary patterns like the Empirical Dietary Pattern for Hyperinsulinemia (EDIH) and Empirical Dietary Inflammatory Pattern (EDIP) indicated evidence for increased CRC risk. The dietary patterns influence CRC risk associations, particularly regarding exposure-mortality pairs and dietary pattern outcomes, demonstrating the need for further research in this area (Chu et al., 2025). Lack of large-scale studies covering a broad range of xenobiotics is gaining momentum. Current research often focuses on a narrow range of priority substances, hindering a holistic risk assessment.

Translational Challenges in the DOHaD-Cancer Associations

This upcoming research area will take time to translate DOHaD findings into effective cancer prevention strategies. Advanced paternal age, lifestyle choices, environmental toxins, and assisted reproductive techniques (ART). Chemotherapy is linked to an increased rate of germline DNMs, which can negatively affect pregnancy outcomes and offspring health (Dehghanbanadaki et al., 2024). Parental factors and the immediate post-fertilization environment can influence the zygote's initial cell divisions and epigenetic landscape. DOHaD-Cancer Associations increase susceptibility to developmental errors and later cancer by affecting cell cycle regulation and DNA integrity. Data on the relative importance of genetic versus epigenetic factors is available. Germline de novo mutations (DNMs) are spontaneous mutations that occur during gametogenesis and can be passed to the next generation, affecting offspring health. While maternal exposures have been widely studied, recent research emphasizes the significant impact of paternal factors on the germline DNM burden in spermatozoa.

Etiological Complexity of Cancer

Literature acknowledges that cancer is a multifactorial disease with diverse subtypes and underlying genetic and molecular mechanisms. Parental and postnatal biological pathways via early-life programming can influence cancer development. Exposure to teratogens and endocrine disruptors during gastrulation can disrupt the precise signaling required for germ layer formation and body axis specification. Congenital Anomaly-Cancer Associations show developmental defects increasing the risk of cancers arising from tissues with disrupted embryonic origins.

Long Latency Periods to Identify Biomarkers for Placental Toxicity

The decades-long gap between early exposure and cancer diagnosis makes establishing direct causal links challenging. Tobacco contains numerous carcinogens, including polycyclic aromatic hydrocarbons and nitrosamines. Smoking is a well-established risk factor for multiple cancers, including lung, throat, and bladder cancer. In living or working conditions, air exposure can lead to changes in gene expression and increased oxidative stress. Prenatal exposure can affect brain development, but limited knowledge about the placental exposome exists. The prenatal risk factors associated with childhood leukemia highlight the significance of parental age, ethnicity, maternal diet, folate intake, alcohol consumption, X-ray exposure, pesticides, perinatal infections, and fetal growth in the development of preleukemic lesions (Benítez et al., 2024). Results demonstrate indirect placenta-mediated fetotoxicity leading to neurodevelopmental disorders and cognitive deficits. The decline in immune surveillance, chronic low-grade inflammation contributing to increased susceptibility to environmental carcinogens due to impaired detoxification, DNA repair, favoring tumor growth. Discovering novel genes linked to these conditions can improve care and provide insights for at-risk populations.

Indirect Effects: Paternal Interaction with Pregnant Mothers

Paternal exposures can also indirectly affect child development by influencing maternal health and behavior. Secondhand tobacco smoke by the mother and child has been shown to increase the risk of respiratory diseases, potentially leading to compromised lung function and chronic conditions later in life. Father smoking during pregnancy is also associated with an increased risk of various congenital anomalies, including neural tube defects and associated congenital tumors. Exposure to air pollutants, particularly during critical developmental periods such as pregnancy, has been linked to various adverse health outcomes, including certain types of cancers. Air Pollution, such as particulate matter, nitrogen oxides, and volatile organic compounds, can lead to oxidative stress, inflammation, and lung cancer (Park et al., 2017). There is difficulty in establishing whether epigenetic changes are direct responses to environmental factors or consequences of other cellular processes.

Retrospective Exposure Assessment Challenges

Pre and Postnatal exposure is typically linked with environmental factors, such as residential pesticide use. Specifically, there is an increased risk for health-related radiation, biological fields, and fathers working in environments with hazardous dioxins and hazardous air pollutants (HAPs) exposures (Guth et al., 2023). Paternal exposure to solvents, cutting oils, paints, dust, and fumes increases the risk of testicular cancer.

There is a methodological difficulty in accurately reconstructing past exposures, especially in utero.

- Childhood Brain Tumors Paternal pre-conceptional occupational exposure to Polycyclic Aromatic Hydrocarbons (PAH) was associated with increased risks of childhood brain tumors (Odds Ratio (OR): 1.3, 95% Confidence Interval (CI): 1.1, 1.6) and astroglial tumors (OR: 1.4, 95% CI: 1.1, 1.7) (Huoi et al., 2014).

Enzyme levels involved in xenobiotic metabolism (CYPs, UGTs) tend to be lower during birth than in adulthood. More testing about exposing fetuses and young infants to higher doses of xenobiotics and toxins is warranted. Current in vitro models must capture the human placenta's complex physiologic structure, function, and dynamics as valuable prescreening tools.

Functional Exposomics and Confounding Factors

The complex interplay of genetic, environmental, and lifestyle factors in the sample population can influence cancer risk. Functional exposomics aims to study the role of environmental pollutants as potential risk factors. Geographical and socioeconomic influences indicate that cancer-related disparities often correlate with geographical areas, such as a higher population of non-Hispanic Black individuals in the USA. Further, higher poverty rates and rurality collectively impact access to care and treatment options. The chemical exposome is vast, and its definition and categorization are not straightforward. The impact of cosmetic chemical exposure on female fertility particularly focuses on racial/ethnic disparities. Long-term exposures to chemicals that affect ovarian function and reproductive health face the limitations of cross-sectional studies in establishing causality. Significant differences in breast cancer incidence and mortality rates among various racial and ethnic groups. Endocrine Disruptors (EDCs), such as bisphenol A (BPA) and phthalates, interfere with hormonal systems. EDCs influence cancer risk, particularly hormone-related cancers like breast and prostate cancer. Investigating the per- and poly-fluoroalkyl substances (PFAS) exposure and breast cancer risk in a diverse multiethnic cohort is challenging. A recent study utilized pre-diagnostic plasma samples and integrated genetics and metabolomic profiles (Hasegawa et al., 2024). Mixed findings exist on links between PFASs and various cancers.

Reverse Causality and Racial Disparities

Maternal health is an increased risk of tumors, reflecting that exposomics has become increasingly important in understanding health disparities. Key factors include maternal education level, maternal age, annual per capita income, number of pregnancies, and congenital abnormalities. Female adolescents and young adults (AYAs) with cancer from non-Hispanic Blacks have significantly lower 10-year cumulative incidence of live birth compared to other racial/ethnic groups. Specifically, Black AYAs are less likely to have a live birth after cancer, particularly in cases of gynecologic cancers, lymphomas, and thyroid cancers, highlighting the need for research and initiatives to address childbearing equity post-cancer (Betts et al., 2024).

African American women have a higher mortality rate from breast cancer (28 per 100,000) compared to White women (20.3 per 100,000) and Asian/Pacific Islander women (11.5 per 100,000). Inherited genetic mutations, such as BRCA1 and BRCA2, significantly increase the risk of breast and ovarian cancers, highlighting the role of genetic predisposition in carcinogenesis. Although Black women have a somewhat lower incidence rate (126.7 per 100,000) compared to White women (130.8 per 100,000), they experience the highest mortality and more aggressive forms of breast cancer (Neagu et al., 2024).

Germline and Somatic Mutations

Understanding genetic and non-genetic factors is crucial for developing effective prevention strategies and mitigating the global cancer burden. Research has shown that epigenomic interactions between multiple co-occurring determinants of cancer disparities can be unraveled through exposomic studies (Xie et al., 2024). Socioeconomic factors also link several cancers, including breast and colon cancer. Poor dietary habits lead to excess body weight. They are linked to endometrial, breast, and colorectal cancers, likely due to inflammation and hormonal changes. Radiation exposure to ionizing radiation from sources like X-rays and radon gas can damage DNA and increase the risk of leukemia and thyroid cancer. The longer extended gene sequences are more susceptible to mutations. Analysis of whole genome sequencing datasets reveals radiation- and polycyclic aromatic hydrocarbons (PAH) induced mutations in tumorigenic genes.

In contrast, increased gene expression correlates with a lower mutation rate in coding sequences. A higher GC content is linked to increased mutation rates in coding sequences. The findings suggest that environmental radiation pollution may contribute to the genetic etiology of neurodevelopmental disorders through both germline and somatic mutations (Baker et al., 2023).

Isolating Early-Life Exposure Effects

Further, there are challenges in isolating the specific contribution of early-life exposures. Emerging evidence suggests a potential link between maternal smoking and neurological issues, contributing to developmental disorders in children. Various environmental factors, including parental exposures, can influence brain tumors in children. Some studies show clear links to certain cancers, while others find negative or unclear associations. Research has shown that exposure to environmental pollutants during critical developmental windows can increase the risk of congenital tumors. For instance, studies have linked parental exposure to pesticides with an increased risk of childhood brain tumors. The data outline differences in how pesticide exposure affects children's health depending on whether the exposure occurs prenatally (during pregnancy) or postnatally (after birth).

Maternal Smoking vs. Secondhand Smoke

Maternal tobacco use is strongly associated with low birth weight, which can result in increased neonatal morbidity and long-term health complications. Smoking during pregnancy is also linked to an increased risk of preterm birth. Ongoing controversy needs more data on the connection between maternal smoking. Testicular cancer risks Sudden Infant Death Syndrome (SIDS), which highlights the critical need for smoking cessation interventions for pregnant women and their partners to protect maternal and fetal health.

Debates about the relationship between maternal smoking and specific cancer types need work on and biological responses in cancer initiation. The placental explant cultures cannot determine maternal-fetal transfer rates due to the lack of two separate circulations. More complex coculture systems are needed to fully understand the health hazards of xenobiotics and their mixtures to the developing fetus in vitro by assessing both direct and indirect embryo-fetotoxicity and the cross-talk between placental and embryonic tissues (Biradar, Korrapati, et al., 2025). This integrated approach would allow researchers to quantify biomarkers related to chemical exposure.

Generalizability and Heterogeneity

The variability in individual responses to early-life exposures due to genetic background and social factors cannot be generalized. Parental occupational exposure, chemical exposures, social determinants, lifestyle factors, and biomonitoring data are often limited to specific geographical regions. Due to differing exposure temporal and spatial patterns, bioaccumulation effects may not represent the global population. Biomarkers of environmental etiology show the application of the exposome in cancer epidemiology (Young et al., 2025). The family should be considered related to interventions during pregnancy or early childhood.

Primary healthcare workers need training to increase the feasibility of identifying individuals at higher risk based on early-life exposures. A multidisciplinary approach is essential for effective disease management, involving specialists from various fields such as hematology, obstetric medicine, and maternal-fetal medicine. The Australasian working group recommends diagnosis, imaging safety, therapy, supportive care, oncofertility, management of pregnancy and birth, and clinical practice guidelines (Mills et al., 2025). The impact of neighborhood social vulnerability on survival among women with epithelial ovarian cancer in Pennsylvania is linked to later-stage diagnoses, reduced access to standard treatments, and a 13% increased mortality hazard. The research found a strong association between social vulnerability and all-cause mortality, with an adjusted hazard ratio of 1.55 for the highest versus lowest quintile, indicating a need for interventions to address neighborhood disparities to improve survival equity among AYAs (Tortolero et al., 2024)

By integrating epidemiologic and genomic data, scientists seek to identify new patterns of congenital anomaly-pediatric cancer associations. Challenges in selecting appropriate controls in case-control studies often cause generalizability issues. The findings from specific populations or models cannot be broadly generalized to human cancer development. There is insufficient biomonitoring data from infants and pregnant women. In particular, longitudinal sampling and data from various biological matrices for natural contaminants and toxins are missing.

Timing of Exposures- Preconception vs. During Pregnancy

The etiology of congenital tumors and their association with paternal exposures is an emerging area of research that highlights significant health disparities. The childbirth and perinatal outcomes among male adolescents and young adults (AYAs) diagnosed with cancer between ages 15-39 had a higher prevalence of preterm birth (8.9% vs. 8.0%) and low birth weight (6.0% vs. 5.3%) compared to offspring of men without cancer (Murphy et al., 2025). The ongoing debate is about whether preconception or during-pregnancy exposures have a more significant impact on offspring cancer risk.

Understanding how the male environment contributes to the development of tumors in offspring also focuses on the potential risks of cancer treatment during childbearing years. Advanced paternal age is associated with an increased risk of psychiatric and developmental disorders in offspring, primarily due to genetic mutations, particularly de novo single nucleotide variants (dnSNVs) (Taylor et al., 2019). The epidemiologic associations with older fatherhood may be influenced by factors that do not necessarily increase with paternal age, but due to the cumulative effect of endocrine disruptors. Plastics can disrupt the endocrine balance, particularly during fetal development, requiring public health strategies to reduce micro-nano plastic-related cancer susceptibility in future generations. The questions about critical windows of vulnerability for both maternal and paternal exposures are met with complexity in studying the long-term effects of different exposure timing periods.

Environmental Exposures and Chemical Exposures

Conflicting evidence regarding associations between chemical exposures and cancer risk exists. Depleted uranium is a heavy metal associated with environmental pollution, demonstrating public health concerns. Naturally occurring contaminants in food generated during food processing and xenobiotics in ambient air are to be studied. The ecological chemicals from everyday products and data on exposure to natural contaminants are often outdated. It is even scarcer for perinatal and paternal exposures that are associated with an increased risk of cancer in children. Exposure to heavy metals is associated with various cancers and developmental issues in children. Certain paternal occupations, including roles as service workers, transport equipment operators, and specialized farmers, along with maternal jobs in secondary education, appear to be linked to an increased risk of testicular germ cell tumors (TGCT). The association varies based on the histological type of TGCT based on occupational exposures, such as pesticides, solvents, or heavy metals (Paul et al., 2023). Literature synthesizes findings related to paternal exposures and genetic alterations in sperm. The relationship between epigenetic aging of semen and inflammation reveals that age-related changes in the semen methylome are linked to inflammatory genes (Feng et al., 2024). Literature also has inconsistent results across different populations and study types regarding epigenetic molecular pathways involved in cancer susceptibility.

Methodological Challenges

Fetal-Placental Barrier

Acute leukemia is the most common pediatric cancer, with a peak incidence between 2-5 years of age, and it often has a prenatal origin following a two-hit carcinogenesis model. Research on phytotoxins or aquatic toxins and their potential to cross the placenta is currently lacking. While some mycotoxins have been shown to cross the placenta in human placental perfusion and animal models, more data on maternal and cord blood levels from biomonitoring studies are needed. Breast milk offers some protection against chemical exposure, and the transfer of chemicals depends on their properties. The infants' low body weight can lead to a higher body burden of persistent organic pollutants (POPs) than their healthy cohorts. Studies on the contamination of infant formula and food with natural toxins such as mycotoxins highlight a problem worldwide requiring ongoing investigation.

Study Design Issues

Paternal epigenetics plays a significant role in influencing the health and developmental trajectory of offspring. Controlling for multiple confounding variables impedes intergenerational paternal epigenetic inheritance in mammals, particularly through environmental exposures and lifestyle choices before conception. Environmental and lifestyle factors can lead to alterations in the epigenetic state of sperm, including changes in DNA methylation and histone modifications, which may have transgenerational effects (Wu et al., 2024). These epigenetic changes can affect gene expression regulation in offspring and may increase the risk of certain diseases. Significant associations with stillbirth were found for various pesticides, including cyfluthrin, zeta-cypermethrin, organophosphates, malathion, carbaryl, and propamocarb hydrochloride during preconception, and fenpropathrin, permethrin, acephate, and formetanate hydrochloride during the first trimester. The results were consistent across different measures of exposure. Difficulties in achieving sufficient statistical power for rare cancers indicate that both preconception and first-trimester pesticide exposures may be linked to an increased risk of stillbirth (Furlong et al., 2024).

Control and Confounding Factors

Paternal exposure to pesticides is associated with the risk of developing cancers, particularly testicular cancer and leukemia, lymphomas, CNS, and non-CNS solid tumors (Coste et al., 2020). Paternal occupational exposure to pesticides has Debates about the effectiveness of different methods to control confounding. Specifically noted for pesticides being linked to nervous system tumors and other cancers in children. There is a significant association between parental pesticide exposure, particularly paternal exposure, and an increased risk of acute leukemia (AL) in children. The odds ratios (OR) suggest that parental exposure has an OR: 1.75 (95% CI: 1.08-2.85), while paternal exposure has an OR: 1.20 (95% CI: 1.07-1.35) (Karalexi et al., 2021). Neonicotinoids are widely used insecticides that target various insects and are found in agricultural systems, home gardens, and veterinary pharmaceuticals, leading to routine exposure in humans and animals. At the same time, neonicotinoid exposure has been linked to various toxic effects (genotoxicity, neurotoxicity, hepatotoxicity, and immunotoxicity) in non-target species. However, their specific impact on mammalian reproductive systems remains largely understudied. Understanding paternal exposures before conception is essential for making informed reproductive decisions (Oladosu & Flaws, 2024). Literature has examined paternal preconception occupational exposures and their effect on the risk and anticipating health risks for future generations. Mechanistic debates surround the role of DNA methylation and histone modifications from low-level general population exposure to environmental toxicants. Paternal exposure to solvents, cutting oils, paints, dust, and fumes is linked to increased risks of leukemia and Testicular germ cell tumors (TGCT) in offspring. Transmission mechanisms show uncertainty about the exact mechanisms by which parental exposures affect offspring cancer risk. Exposure to petroleum-based solvents and groups of oxygenated or chlorinated solvents showed OR 0.89 (95% CI 0.68-1.15) has resolved issues with matching techniques in case-control studies on TGCT risk (Guth et al., 2023). In summary, our work synthesized findings on parental exposomics, environmental exposures, and germline transmission, and their implications for cancer susceptibility in future generations.

CONCLUSION

Carcinogenesis is characterized by its biological and clinical heterogeneity, with a variety of associated risk factors. Environmental exposures play a significant role in cancer development, with various key exposomic factors identified. Early developmental exposures are particularly significant, highlighting the importance of prevention. Innovative approaches using primary teeth and dried blood spots for exposomic studies can enhance the understanding of environmental exposures in pediatric populations (Lupo et al., 2024). This work examined epidemiological studies linking cancer to environmental agents. Recent advances in epigenomics have improved our understanding of cancer etiology, particularly concerning exposure to chemicals, radiation, paints, solvents, and infectious agents. Key exposomic factors involve timing, dose, parental occupational exposures, and socioeconomic status, which require further investigation. Incorporating epigenetics and metabolomics into studies can provide insights into gene-environment interactions that may lead to cancer. While the focus on parental environmental factors is crucial, other unknown factors may also play a significant role in tumor development. Evidence suggests strong associations with leukemia, central nervous system tumors, and testicular cancer, revealing significant associations with air pollution and pesticides. Parental behaviors such as alcohol consumption and smoking generally show associations with cancer risk. Additionally, factors like low socioeconomic status and the cumulative effects of maternal and paternal exposures may further contribute to cancer risk in children. This work advocates for longitudinal and case-control studies in the future to assess environmental exposures and their implications on public health.

REFERENCES

Achkar, M. E., Atieh, O., Ghadban, C., Awad, T., Ghadban, E., Grandjean, V., Yarkiner, Z., Raad, G., & Khalife, M.-C. F. (2024). Preconceptional paternal obesity may increase the risk of congenital urogenital anomalies in offspring: A case–control study. *Andrology*. DOI: 10.1111/andr.13673

Akhatova, A., Jones, C., Coward, K., & Yeste, M. (2025). How do lifestyle and environmental factors influence the sperm epigenome? Effects on sperm fertilising ability, embryo development, and offspring health. *Clinical Epigenetics*, *17*(1), 1. Advance online publication. DOI: 10.1186/s13148-025-01815-1 PMID: 39819375

Ananthakumar, B., Nanjundeshwara, N., Lakshmaiah, A., & Raghavan, R. (2024). Synthetic Gene Circuits as a Promising Approach in Cancer Immunotherapy. *Critical Developments in Cancer Immunotherapy*, 391–418. DOI: 10.4018/979-8-3693-3976-3.ch011

Baker, B. H., Zhang, S., Simon, J. M., McLarnan, S. M., Chung, W. K., & Pearson, B. L. (2023). Environmental carcinogens disproportionally mutate genes implicated in neurodevelopmental disorders. *Frontiers in Neuroscience*, *17*, 1106573. Advance online publication. DOI: 10.3389/fnins.2023.1106573 PMID: 37599994

Benavent, N., Cañete, A., Moreno, L., Gros, L., Verdú-Amorós, J., Salinas, J. A., Navarro, S., Álvaro, T., Carbonell-Asins, J. A., & Noguera, R. (2025). Risk of developing neuroblastoma influenced by maternal stressful life events during pregnancy and congenital pathologies. *Pediatric Blood & Cancer*, *72*(2), e31402. DOI: 10.1002/pbc.31402 PMID: 39618320

Benítez, L., Castro-Barquero, S., Crispi, F., Youssef, L., Crovetto, F., Fischer, U., Kameri, E., Bueno, C., Camos, M., Menéndez, P., Heinäniemi, M., Borkhardt, A., & Gratacós, E. (2024). Maternal Lifestyle and Prenatal Risk Factors for Childhood Leukemia: A Review of the Existing Evidence. *Fetal Diagnosis and Therapy*, *51*(4), 395–410. DOI: 10.1159/000539141 PMID: 38710162

Betts, A. C., Roth, M. E., Albritton, K., Pruitt, S. L., Lupo, P. J., Wang, J. S., Shay, L. A., Allicock, M. A., & Murphy, C. C. (2024). Racialized inequities in live birth after cancer: A population-based study of 63,000 female adolescents and young adults with cancer. *Cancer*, *130*(17), 2928–2937. DOI: 10.1002/cncr.35341 PMID: 38696087

Biradar, S., Korrapati, C., Krishna, R. J., & Nanjundeshwara, N. (2025). Spatial Omics and Gene Circuits: The Future in Cancer Biology. *Spatially Variable Genes in Cancer: Development, Progression, and Treatment Response*, 383–408. DOI: 10.4018/979-8-3693-7728-4.ch014

Biradar, S., Suresh, C., Nanjundeshwara, N., & Raghavan, R. (2025). Spatially Variable Genes. *Spatially Variable Genes in Cancer*, 1–28. DOI: 10.4018/979-8-3693-7728-4.ch001

Borankova, K., Krchniakova, M., Leck, L. Y. W., Kubistova, A., Neradil, J., Jansson, P. J., Hogarty, M. D., & Skoda, J. (2023). Mitoribosomal synthetic lethality overcomes multidrug resistance in MYC-driven neuroblastoma. *Cell Death & Disease*, *14*(11), 1–17. DOI: 10.1038/s41419-023-06278-x PMID: 37973789

Boysen, G., Alexandrov, L. B., Rahbari, R., Nookaew, I., Ussery, D., Chao, M.-R., Hu, C.-W., & Cooke, M. S. (2025). Investigating the origins of the mutational signatures in cancer. *Nucleic Acids Research*, *53*(1), gkae1303. Advance online publication. DOI: 10.1093/nar/gkae1303 PMID: 39778866

Chu, A. H., Lin, K., Croker, H., Kefyalew, S., Becerra-Tomás, N., Dossus, L., González-Gil, E. M., Ahmadi, N., Park, Y., Krebs, J., Weijenberg, M. P., Baskin, M. L., Copson, E., Lewis, S. J., Seidell, J. C., Chowdhury, R., Hill, L., Chan, D. S., Lee, D. H., & Giovannucci, E. L. (2025). Dietary patterns and colorectal cancer risk: Global Cancer Update Programme (CUP Global) systematic literature review. *The American Journal of Clinical Nutrition*, *121*(5), 999–1016. Advance online publication. DOI: 10.1016/j.ajcnut.2025.02.021 PMID: 40010692

Coste, A., Bailey, H. D., Kartal-Kaess, M., Renella, R., Berthet, A., & Spycher, B. D. (2020). Parental occupational exposure to pesticides and risk of childhood cancer in Switzerland: A census-based cohort study. *BMC Cancer*, *20*(1), 819. DOI: 10.1186/s12885-020-07319-w PMID: 32859175

Dehghanbanadaki, H., Jimbo, M., Fendereski, K., Kunisaki, J., Horns, J. J., Ramsay, J. M., Gross, K. X., Pastuszak, A. W., & Hotaling, J. M. (2024). Transgenerational effects of paternal exposures: The role of germline de novo mutations. *Andrology*, *n/a*(n/a). DOI: 10.1111/andr.13609

Di Renzo, L., Gualtieri, P., Frank, G., Cianci, R., Caldarelli, M., Leggeri, G., Raffaelli, G., Pizzocaro, E., Cirillo, M., & De Lorenzo, A. (2024). Exploring the Exposome Spectrum: Unveiling Endogenous and Exogenous Factors in Non-Communicable Chronic Diseases. *Diseases (Basel, Switzerland)*, *12*(8), 176. DOI: 10.3390/diseases12080176 PMID: 39195175

Feng, J., Rubbi, L., Kianian, R., Mills, J. N., Osadchiy, V., Sigalos, J. T., Eleswarapu, S. V., & Pellegrini, M. (2024). Epigenetic aging of semen is associated with inflammation. *Epigenetics*, *19*(1), 2436304. DOI: 10.1080/15592294.2024.2436304 PMID: 39637179

Furlong, M. A., Paul, K. C., Parra, K. L., Fournier, A. J., Ellsworth, P. C., Cockburn, M. G., Arellano, A. F., Bedrick, E. J., Beamer, P. I., & Ritz, B. (2024). Pre-Conception And First Trimester Exposure To Pesticides And Associations With Stillbirth. *American Journal of Epidemiology*, kwae198. Advance online publication. DOI: 10.1093/aje/kwae198 PMID: 39013781

Greeson, K. W., Crow, K. M. S., Edenfield, R. C., & Easley, C. A.IV. (2023). Inheritance of paternal lifestyles and exposures through sperm DNA methylation. *Nature Reviews. Urology*, *20*(6), 356–370. DOI: 10.1038/s41585-022-00708-9 PMID: 36653672

Gu, H., Yu, Y., Sisoudiya, S. D., Mishra, P., Li, H., Schraw, J. M., Scheurer, M. E., Muzny, D. M., Mitchell, D., Taylor, O., Jhangiani, S. N., Dugan-Perez, S., Wu, Y., Doddapaneni, H., Bhamidipati, S. V., Gingras, M.-C., Posey, J. E., Gibbs, R. A., Huff, C. D., & Sabo, A. (2025). An evaluation of genetic predisposition to congenital anomalies and pediatric cancer supports KAT6B as a novel neuroblastoma susceptibility gene. *Genetics in Medicine Open*, *3*, 101901. Advance online publication. DOI: 10.1016/j.gimo.2024.101901

Guth, M., Lefevre, M., Pilorget, C., Coste, A., Ahmadi, S., Danjou, A., Dananché, B., Praud, D., Koscinski, I., Papaxanthos, A., Blagosklonov, O., Fauque, P., Pérol, O., Schüz, J., Bujan, L., Olsson, A., Fervers, B., & Charbotel, B.TESTIS study group. (2023). Parental occupational exposure to solvents and risk of developing testicular germ cell tumors among sons: A French nationwide case-control study (TESTIS study). *Scandinavian Journal of Work, Environment & Health*, *49*(6), 405–418. DOI: 10.5271/sjweh.4102 PMID: 37649372

GVS, A. C., Ananthakumar, B., & Raghavan, R. (2025). Enhancing Assistive Technologies With Neuromorphic Computing. *Revolutionizing AI with Brain-Inspired Technology: Neuromorphic Computing*, 207–232. DOI: 10.4018/979-8-3693-6303-4.ch009

Hasegawa, K., Motoki, N., Inaba, Y., Toubou, H., Shibazaki, T., Nakayama, S. F., Kamijima, M., Tsukahara, T., & Nomiyama, T.Japan Environment and Children's Study Group. (2024). Maternal Exposure to Per- and Polyfluoroalkyl Substances and Offspring Chromosomal Abnormalities: The Japan Environment and Children's Study. *Environmental Health Perspectives*, *132*(9), 097004. DOI: 10.1289/EHP13617 PMID: 39258902

Huoi, C., Olsson, A., Lightfoot, T., Roman, E., Clavel, J., Lacour, B., Kaatsch, P., Kromhout, H., Vermeulen, R., Peters, S., Bailey, H. D., & Schüz, J. (2014). Parental occupational exposure and risk of childhood central nervous system tumors: A pooled analysis of case-control studies from Germany, France, and the UK. *Cancer Causes & Control, 25*(12), 1603–1613. DOI: 10.1007/s10552-014-0465-4 PMID: 25281325

Kaltsas, A., Markou, E., Kyrgiafini, M.-A., Zikopoulos, A., Symeonidis, E. N., Dimitriadis, F., Zachariou, A., Sofikitis, N., & Chrisofos, M. (2025). Oxidative-Stress-Mediated Epigenetic Dysregulation in Spermatogenesis: Implications for Male Infertility and Offspring Health. *Genes, 16*(1), 1. Advance online publication. DOI: 10.3390/genes16010093 PMID: 39858640

Karalexi, M. A., Tagkas, C. F., Markozannes, G., Tseretopoulou, X., Hernández, A. F., Schüz, J., Halldorsson, T. I., Psaltopoulou, T., Petridou, E. T., Tzoulaki, I., & Ntzani, E. E. (2021). Exposure to pesticides and childhood leukemia risk: A systematic review and meta-analysis. *Environmental Pollution (Barking, Essex: 1987), 285*, 117376. DOI: 10.1016/j.envpol.2021.117376

Korrapati, C., Yaraladdi, A. B., Vaddi, H., & Raghavan, R. (2024). Applications of the Saffron European Kitchen Spice Crocus sativus. *Therapeutic and Pharmacological Applications of Ethnobotany*, 98–127. DOI: 10.4018/979-8-3693-1986-4.ch005

Krausová, M., Braun, D., Buerki-Thurnherr, T., Gundacker, C., Schernhammer, E., Wisgrill, L., & Warth, B. (2023). Understanding the Chemical Exposome During Fetal Development and Early Childhood: A Review. *Annual Review of Pharmacology and Toxicology, 63*(1), 517–540. DOI: 10.1146/annurev-pharmtox-051922-113350 PMID: 36202091

Lakshmaiah, A., Korrapati, C., Suresh, C., & Raghavan, R. (2025). Synthetic Biology and AI. *Spatially Variable Genes in Cancer*, 265–290. DOI: 10.4018/979-8-3693-7728-4.ch010

Lu, L., Cheng, Y., Wu, W., Wang, L., Li, S., Li, Q., Chen, L., Zhang, J., Chen, R., Tan, X., Hong, Y., Yang, L., & Song, Y. (2024). Paternal p,p′-DDE exposure and pre-pubertal high-fat diet increases the susceptibility to fertility impairment and sperm *Igf2* DMR2 hypo-methylation in male offspring. *Ecotoxicology and Environmental Safety, 271*, 115999. DOI: 10.1016/j.ecoenv.2024.115999 PMID: 38262096

Lupo, P. J., Archer, N. P., Harris, R. D., Marengo, L. K., Schraw, J. M., Hoyt, A. T., Tanksley, S., Lee, R., Drummond-Borg, M., Freedenberg, D., Shetty, P. B., Agopian, A. J., Shumate, C., Rasmussen, S. A., Langlois, P. H., & Canfield, M. A. (2024). Newborn screening analytes and structural birth defects among 27,000 newborns. *PLoS One, 19*(7), e0304238. DOI: 10.1371/journal.pone.0304238 PMID: 38968308

Maria, O. M., Weronika, P. K., Beata, B.-D., Ewa, G.-I., & Bożena, K.-N. (2023). Congenital glioblastoma – prenatal diagnosis becoming a diagnostic challenge after birth: A case report. *Case Reports in Perinatal Medicine*, *12*(1), 20230008. Advance online publication. DOI: 10.1515/crpm-2023-0008 PMID: 40041279

Mills, G., Shand, A., Kennedy, D., Lowe, S., Bilsland, V., Cutts, B., McBride, B., Brown, W., Bolisetty, S., Wegner, E. A., & Kidson-Gerber, G. (2025). Position statement on the diagnosis and management of acute leukaemia and aggressive lymphomas in pregnancy. *The Lancet. Haematology*, *12*(2), e151–e162. DOI: 10.1016/S2352-3026(24)00309-0 PMID: 39761682

Msallem, E., Pacquement, H., Olivier, L., Brugières, L., Landman Parker, J., Garnier, N., Lambilliotte, A., Faure, L., Clavel, J., & Bonaventure, A. (2025). Association Between Perinatal Factors and Childhood Lymphoma—A Pooled Analysis of the ESCALE and ES LE Studies (SFCE). *Pediatric Blood & Cancer*, *72*(2), e31439. DOI: 10.1002/pbc.31439 PMID: 39579109

Murphy, C. C., Wang, J. S., Betts, A. C., Lupo, P. J., Shay, L. A., Allicock, M. A., Kirk, C. L., & Pruitt, S. L. (2025). Childbirth after cancer among 42 896 male adolescents and young adults: A population-based study. *Journal of the National Cancer Institute*, *117*(5), djae347. Advance online publication. DOI: 10.1093/jnci/djae347 PMID: 39752327

Nagashri, N., Archana, L., & Raghavan, R. (2024). Microbial Volatile Compounds (MVOCs) in Food Industries and Food Safety Applications. *Innovations, Securities, and Case Studies Across Healthcare, Business, and Technology*, 75–96. DOI: 10.4018/979-8-3693-1906-2.ch005

Neagu, A.-N., Bruno, P., Johnson, K. R., Ballestas, G., & Darie, C. C. (2024). Biological Basis of Breast Cancer-Related Disparities in Precision Oncology Era. *International Journal of Molecular Sciences*, *25*(7), 4113. DOI: 10.3390/ijms25074113 PMID: 38612922

Non, A. L. (2025). The eighth annual US DOHAD meeting: Promising approaches in epigenetics research of early life exposures. *Epigenomics*, *17*(4), 209–211. DOI: 10.1080/17501911.2025.2459550 PMID: 39874076

Oladosu, J. I., & Flaws, J. A. (2024). The Impact of Neonicotinoid Pesticides on Reproductive Health. *Toxicological Sciences*, kfae138. Advance online publication. DOI: 10.1093/toxsci/kfae138 PMID: 39460954

Onyije, F. M., Dolatkhah, R., Olsson, A., Bouaoun, L., & Schüz, J. (2024). Environmental risk factors of Wilms tumour: A systematic review and meta-analysis. *EJC Paediatric Oncology*, *4*, 100178. Advance online publication. DOI: 10.1016/j.ejcped.2024.100178 PMID: 39678930

Onyije, F. M., Olsson, A., Erdmann, F., Magnani, C., Petridou, E., Clavel, J., Miligi, L., Bonaventure, A., Ferrante, D., Piro, S., Peters, S., Vermeulen, R., Kromhout, H., & Schüz, J. (2022). Parental occupational exposure to combustion products, metals, silica and asbestos and risk of childhood leukaemia: Findings from the Childhood Cancer and Leukaemia International Consortium (CLIC). *Environment International*, *167*, 107409. DOI: 10.1016/j.envint.2022.107409 PMID: 35908390

Park, A. S., Ritz, B., Ling, C., Cockburn, M., & Heck, J. E. (2017). Exposure to ambient dichloromethane in pregnancy and infancy from industrial sources and childhood cancers in California. *International Journal of Hygiene and Environmental Health*, *220*(7), 1133–1140. DOI: 10.1016/j.ijheh.2017.06.006 PMID: 28720343

Paul, A., Danjou, A. M. N., Deygas, F., Guth, M., Coste, A., Lefevre, M., Dananché, B., Kromhout, H., Spinosi, J., Béranger, R., Pérol, O., Boyle, H., Hersant, C., Loup-Cabaniols, V., Veau, S., Bujan, L., Olsson, A., Schüz, J., Fervers, B., & Charbotel, B. (2023). Parental occupations at birth and risk of adult testicular germ cell tumors in offspring: A French nationwide case-control study. *Frontiers in Public Health*, *11*, 1303998. DOI: 10.3389/fpubh.2023.1303998 PMID: 38292387

Schraw, J. M., Tark, J. Y., Desrosiers, T. A., Chambers, T. M., Shumate, C. J., Nembhard, W. N., Yazdy, M. M., Nestoridi, E., Malone, M. F. W., Laetsch, T. W., Widemann, B. C., Janitz, A. E., Tanner, J. P., Kirby, R. S., Salemi, J. L., Spector, L. G., Huff, C. D., Plon, S. E., & Lupo, P. J. (2025). Risk of carcinomas among children and adolescents with birth defects. *Cancer Epidemiology*, *95*, 102748. DOI: 10.1016/j.canep.2025.102748 PMID: 39848200

Taylor, J. L., Debost, J.-C. P. G., Morton, S. U., Wigdor, E. M., Heyne, H. O., Lal, D., Howrigan, D. P., Bloemendal, A., Larsen, J. T., Kosmicki, J. A., Weiner, D. J., Homsy, J., Seidman, J. G., Seidman, C. E., Agerbo, E., McGrath, J. J., Mortensen, P. B., Petersen, L., Daly, M. J., & Robinson, E. B. (2019). Paternal-age-related de novo mutations and risk for five disorders. *Nature Communications*, *10*(1), 3043. DOI: 10.1038/s41467-019-11039-6 PMID: 31292440

Tortolero, G. A., Betts, A. C., Suragh, T. A., Pruitt, S. L., Roth, M. E., & Murphy, C. C. (2024). Social vulnerability and survival in 112000 adolescents and young adults with cancer: A population-based study. *Journal of the National Cancer Institute*, *116*(12), 2003–2008. DOI: 10.1093/jnci/djae170 PMID: 39084675

Vineis, P., & Dagnino, S. (2024). An evolutionary perspective for the exposome. *Exposome*, *4*(1), osae008. Advance online publication. DOI: 10.1093/exposome/osae008 PMID: 39867564

Weinberg, B. A., Murphy, C. C., Freyer, D. R., Greathouse, K. L., Blancato, J. K., Stoffel, E. M., Drewes, J. L., Blaes, A., Salsman, J. M., You, Y. N., Arem, H., Mukherji, R., Kanth, P., Hu, X., Fabrizio, A., Hartley, M. L., Giannakis, M., & Marshall, J. L. (2025). Rethinking the rise of early-onset gastrointestinal cancers: A call to action. *JNCI Cancer Spectrum*, *9*(1), pkaf002. Advance online publication. DOI: 10.1093/jncics/pkaf002 PMID: 39814070

Wu, D., Zhang, K., Guan, K., Khan, F. A., Pandupuspitasari, N. S., Negara, W., Sun, F., & Huang, C. (2024). Future in the past: Paternal reprogramming of offspring phenotype and the epigenetic mechanisms. *Archives of Toxicology*, *98*(6), 1685–1703. DOI: 10.1007/s00204-024-03713-6 PMID: 38460001

Xiao, S., Cui, J., Cao, Y., Zhang, Y., Yang, J., Zheng, L., Zhao, F., Liu, X., Zhou, Z., Liu, D., & Wang, P. (2024). Adolescent exposure to organophosphate insecticide malathion induces spermatogenesis dysfunction in mice by activating the HIF-1/MAPK/PI3K pathway. *Environmental Pollution*, *363*, 125209. DOI: 10.1016/j.envpol.2024.125209 PMID: 39476999

Xie, G., Si, Q., Zhang, G., Fan, Y., Li, Q., Leng, P., Qiao, F., Liang, S., Yu, R., & Wang, Y. (2024). The role of imprinting genes' loss of imprints in cancers and their clinical implications. *Frontiers in Oncology*, *14*, 1365474. Advance online publication. DOI: 10.3389/fonc.2024.1365474 PMID: 38812777

Young, A. S., Mullins, C. E., Sehgal, N., Vermeulen, R. C. H., Kolijn, P. M., Vlaanderen, J., Rahman, M. L., Birmann, B. M., Barupal, D., Lan, Q., Rothman, N., & Walker, D. I. (2025). The need for a cancer exposome atlas: A scoping review. *JNCI Cancer Spectrum*, *9*(1), pkae122. Advance online publication. DOI: 10.1093/jncics/pkae122 PMID: 39700422

Zambrano, E., & Ibáñez, C. A. (2025). Celebrating 280 birth years of Lamarck: Revisiting his legacy in the concept of Developmental Origins of Health and Disease. *Journal of Developmental Origins of Health and Disease*, *16*, e8. DOI: 10.1017/S2040174425000030 PMID: 39950302

Chapter 2
Omics Integration in Understanding Xenobiotic Metabolism: Systems Biology Insights

Ankur Bhardwaj
https://orcid.org/0000-0003-0687-8810
Shri Vaishnav Vidyapeeth Vishwavidyalaya, Indore, India

Surendra Prakash Gupta
https://orcid.org/0000-0002-4873-6346
Shri Vaishnav Vidyapeeth Vishwavidyalaya, Indore, India

ABSTRACT

The chapter explores the transformative role of omics technologies in elucidating the complex pathways and mechanisms involved in xenobiotic metabolism. The chapter incorporates the metabolomics role in profiling xenobiotic-induced metabolic alterations, facilitating the identification of biomarkers, transcriptomic analyses uncovering dynamic gene expression patterns, and the application of high-throughput sequencing techniques to identify genetic variations influencing drug metabolism enzymes and transporters, thereby shaping individual responses to xenobiotics. Integration of these omics datasets through systems biology approaches enhances our understanding of xenobiotic metabolism as a complex network of molecular interactions and regulatory circuits. Emphasis is placed on cytochrome P450 enzymes, role of microbiome-derived metabolites, and their contribution to xenobiotic processing. The future of xenobiotic metabolism research lies in harnessing artificial intelligence (AI) and multi-omics integration to provide holistic insights into system-wide responses.

DOI: 10.4018/979-8-3373-2165-3.ch002

1. INTRODUCTION

Xenobiotics are chemical substances that are foreign to a biological system. They are not naturally produced by an organism or expected to be part of its normal metabolic processes. These compounds can be beneficial, like drugs, or harmful, like pollutants and toxins (Bojić et al., 2024). Xenobiotics enter the body through various environmental and dietary sources, including medications like antibiotics, pain relievers, and chemotherapy drugs, food additives and contaminants: preservatives, pesticides, artificial colours, and flavour enhancers, heavy metals, plasticizers, hydrocarbons, and dioxins from industrial waste, vehicle emissions, and chemical spills (Priya et al., 2024; De Filippis et al., 2024). Lifestyle-related compounds like alcohol, nicotine, caffeine, and recreational drugs also adds the list.

Xenobiotics can have both beneficial and toxic effects, depending on their nature, dose, and duration of exposure (Vicidomini et al., 2024). Many drugs (Table 1) act as xenobiotics, interacting with biological targets to treat diseases. For instance, antibiotics target bacterial infections, while chemotherapy drugs kill cancer cells (Panebianco et al., 2018). Some xenobiotics (Table 1) can cause cellular damage, leading to toxicity, organ failure, or cancer (Shreenidhi et al., 2024). Persistent organic pollutants (POPs) like dioxins and polychlorinated biphenyls (PCBs) can accumulate in the environment and living organisms, disrupting hormonal balance and increasing disease risk (Beigh, 2024). Some xenobiotics (heavy metals – Pb, Hg, Cd, As, Cr and persistent chemicals – Polychlorinated Biphenyls, Dioxins & Furans, Organochlorines, Perfluorinated Compounds, Phthalates) accumulate in organisms and move up the food chain, posing ecological and health risks (Edo et al., 2024; Beigh, 2024). To counteract their potential toxicity, the body metabolizes xenobiotics primarily in the liver through Phase I (modification) and Phase II (conjugation) reactions, making them more water-soluble for excretion via urine or bile (Stanley, 2024). Understanding xenobiotics and their metabolism is crucial for drug development, toxicology, and environmental health, ensuring safety in medicine, food, and industrial practices.

Table 1. Categories of Xenobiotic Drugs and Their Metabolic Pathways

Drug Category	Instances	Diseases/Conditions Caused as Xenobiotics	Metabolic Pathway	References
Alcohols	Ethanol	Liver cirrhosis, Alcoholic hepatitis	Alcohol dehydrogenase → Acetaldehyde → Acetate	Gaither et al., 2025
Benzodiazepines	Diazepam, Lorazepam	Dependence, Cognitive impairment	Glucuronidation, Oxidation	Bernardo and Valentão, 2024
Opioids	Morphine, Codeine	Respiratory depression, Addiction	Glucuronidation, Oxidation, Conjugation with glucuronic acid	Makmor et al., 2024
Nonsteroidal Anti-inflammatory Drugs (NSAIDs)	Ibuprofen, Naproxen	Gastric ulcers, Kidney damage	Oxidation, Conjugation with glucuronic acid	Show and Halder, 2024
Antibiotics	Penicillin, Ciprofloxacin	Antibiotic resistance, Allergic reactions	Hydrolysis, Oxidation, Conjugation with glucuronic acid	Khmaissa et al., 2024
Antidepressants	Fluoxetine, Sertraline	Serotonin syndrome, Liver toxicity	Oxidation, Conjugation with glucuronic acid	Khalil et al., 2024
Antipsychotics	Haloperidol, Risperidone	Tardive dyskinesia, Metabolic syndrome	Oxidation, Conjugation with glucuronic acid	Hart et al., 2024
Antihypertensives	Atenolol, Lisinopril	Hypotension, Kidney damage	Oxidation, Conjugation with glucuronic acid	Dharmarathne et al., 2024
Statins	Simvastatin, Atorvastatin	Rhabdomyolysis, Liver toxicity	Oxidation, Glucuronidation	Shi and Han, 2025
Steroids	Prednisone, Testosterone	Cushing's syndrome, Hormonal imbalance	Hydroxylation, Conjugation with glucuronic acid	Pecori et al., 2024
Antivirals	Acyclovir, Oseltamivir	Kidney toxicity, Neurotoxicity	Oxidation, Glucuronidation	Rodríguez et al., 2024

1.1 Overview of Xenobiotic Metabolism and Its Biological Importance

Xenobiotic metabolism refers to the process by which the body metabolizes and detoxifies foreign compounds, known as xenobiotics, that enter the body. The metabolism of xenobiotics primarily occurs in the liver, although other organs like the intestines and kidneys also play roles.

- **Phase I Metabolism**: Involves reactions like oxidation, reduction, and hydrolysis, often catalysed by enzymes like cytochrome P450 enzymes. These reactions generally make the xenobiotics more reactive and prepare them for further metabolism (Mahanayak, 2024).
- **Phase II Metabolism**: In this phase, conjugation reactions occur where the reactive products from Phase I are combined with endogenous molecules like glucuronic acid, sulphate, or glutathione. This conjugation makes the xenobiotics more water-soluble and facilitates their excretion from the body (Li, 2025).
- **Biological Importance**: Metabolism of xenobiotic substances is crucial for detoxifying harmful substances that could damage cells and tissues and further influences the efficacy and toxicity of pharmaceutical drugs (Vicidomini et al., 2024). Different individuals may metabolize drugs differently, affecting their therapeutic outcomes. It also helps in processing environmental pollutants, thus reducing their harmful effects on ecosystems and human health (Gupta et al., 2024). Some xenobiotics (furanocoumarins in grapefruit juice, heavy metals, polycyclic aromatic hydrocarbons, polybrominated biphenyls) can interfere with nutrient absorption or utilization, and metabolism helps mitigate these effects (Li et al., 2024). Advancements in understanding xenobiotic metabolism are important for drug development, environmental health, and understanding how our bodies interact with the chemicals in our environment and diet.

1.2 Limitations of Traditional Approaches in Understanding Xenobiotic Pathways

Traditional approaches in understanding xenobiotic pathways, while foundational, have several limitations Many traditional methods focus on studying one xenobiotic compound at a time, which may not reflect real-world exposure scenarios where multiple xenobiotics interact simultaneously (Motsinger-Reif et al., 2024). Limited scope of these approaches often prioritizes known pathways and mechanisms, potentially overlooking novel pathways or interactions that could be significant

(Ouma et al., 2024). Traditional approaches may provide a static snapshot rather than dynamic insights into how xenobiotics and their metabolites change over time and in different biological contexts (Cassotta et al., 2024).

Species-specific studies often rely on model organisms or human-derived cell lines, which may not fully represent the diversity of biological responses across different species or populations (Himmel et al., 2022). Some methods (Spectrometry, thin-layer chromatography, etc.) may lack the sensitivity or specificity to detect low levels of xenobiotics or their metabolites, missing crucial information about exposure and effects (Qriouet et al., 2019). Traditional methods (UV-Vis spectroscopy, Fluorescence, Basic gas chromatography, etc.) struggle to decipher the complex interactions and effects of xenobiotic mixtures commonly found in environmental and occupational surroundings (Grocholska et al., 2022). Certain methods, especially those involving animal models or invasive techniques, pose ethical concerns or practical limitations in terms of scalability and relevance to human health.

Addressing these limitations requires integrating advanced omics approaches (genomics, proteomics, metabolomics), computational modelling, and systems biology to provide a more comprehensive understanding of xenobiotic pathways and their implications for health and the environment.

1.3 Role of Systems Biology and Integrative Omics in Advancing the Field

Systems biology and integrative omics have revolutionized the study of xenobiotic pathways by providing a holistic, data-driven approach. These methods allow for a more comprehensive understanding of how xenobiotics interact with biological systems (Shi et al., 2024).

Systems biology uses computational and mathematical models to map complex interactions between xenobiotics, enzymes, transporters, and cellular pathways (Rai et al., 2023). Unlike traditional static approaches, systems biology enables time-resolved analysis of xenobiotic metabolism, revealing how responses change over time. It connects molecular-level processes (gene expression) with higher-order physiological responses, improving predictions of xenobiotic toxicity and metabolism (Rai et al., 2023; Shi et al., 2024).

1.4. Integrative Omics: A Multi-Layered Approach

Omics technologies provide high-throughput data that enhance our understanding of xenobiotic metabolism and toxicity. Genomics identifies genetic variations influencing xenobiotic metabolism, like polymorphisms in cytochrome P450 enzymes (Abdelmonem et al., 2024). Transcriptomics reveals changes in gene expression patterns in response to xenobiotic exposure, help identify stress responses and adaptive mechanisms (Yu et al., 2022a). Proteomics examines changes in protein levels and modifications, offer insights into enzyme activity and signalling cascades involved in xenobiotic metabolism (Xie et al., 2022). Metabolomics captures real-time metabolic profiles, help detect xenobiotic metabolites, bioactivation pathways, and potential toxic intermediates (Fetse et al., 2024). Epigenomics studies shows xenobiotics inducing epigenetic modifications (DNA methylation, histone modifications) that may affect long-term gene expression and toxicity (Terrazas-Salgado et al., 2022).

Integration of multiple omics layers, help researchers to uncover novel pathways and interactions that would be missed using traditional reductionist methods. Omics-driven personalized risk assessment approaches could be executed that can enable precision toxicology, predicting individual responses to xenobiotics based on genetic and metabolic profiles (Boyce et al., 2023). Systems biology models combined with omics data improve predictions of xenobiotic toxicity, reducing reliance on animal models and improving regulatory assessments. Multi-omics analysis helps researchers discover early biomarkers of xenobiotic exposure and toxicity, aiding in early diagnosis and intervention (Capone et al., 2024).

Integration of systems biology with multi-omics technologies, researchers can move beyond traditional limitations to develop a predictive, systems-level understanding of xenobiotic metabolism. This approach enhances drug development, environmental toxicology, and precision medicine, ultimately improving human and environmental health.

1.5 Rationale, Need and Purpose of the Present Study

1.5.1 Rationale of the Chapter

Xenobiotic metabolism involves a cascade of biochemical reactions governed by complex and dynamic interactions across multiple biological systems. Traditional single analyses (genomics or metabolomics alone) often fail to capture the full scope of these interactions, limiting our understanding of how xenobiotics exert their effects on human health and the environment. With the emergence of high-throughput technologies, the integration of omics data has become a powerful tool to dissect the multifaceted nature of xenobiotic biotransformation, enabling a more systems-level perspective.

1.5.2 Need for the Present Study

Despite the availability of vast omics datasets, their fragmented use impedes comprehensive insight into xenobiotic metabolism. A consolidated, systems biology-based approach is illustrated in this chapter to unravel metabolic networks, regulatory pathways, and inter-individual variations in response to xenobiotic exposure. This need is amplified by the growing complexity of chemical exposures in modern life, identifying innovative analytical frameworks.

1.5.3 Objectives of the Chapter

- Highlight the significance of integrating genomics, transcriptomics, proteomics, and metabolomics in xenobiotic metabolism studies.
- Discuss current tools, platforms, and computational approaches enabling such integration.
- Demonstrate how systems biology enhances our understanding of xenobiotic effects, toxicity mechanisms, and personalized responses.
- Offer insights into future directions and challenges in applying omics integration for precision toxicology.

2. XENOBIOTIC-METABOLIZING PATHWAYS

Xenobiotic metabolism is a critical process that determines the fate of xenobiotic compounds (drugs, environmental pollutants, and dietary components) in living organisms. It primarily occurs in the liver and follows a structured pathway involving enzymatic modifications (Table 2) that enhance xenobiotic solubility and facilitate excretion (Rai et al., 2023). The metabolizing process can be divided into Phase I and Phase II reactions, regulated by enzymes like cytochrome P450s (and glutathione S-transferases) and transporters (ATP-binding cassette, Efflux proteins, Membrane proteins) and controlled by regulatory networks that respond dynamically to xenobiotic exposure (Capone et al., 2024). The regulatory networks associated with xenobiotics primarily involve nuclear receptors like aryl hydrocarbon receptor (AhR), constitutive androstane receptor (CAR), pregnane X receptor (PXR), and peroxisome proliferator-activated receptors (PPARs), which act as key sensors to detect and respond to xenobiotics by regulating the expression of genes involved in their metabolism and detoxification, often through pathways (Nrf2 signalling cascade and AhR linked pathway) (Shi et al., 2024).

Table 2. Phase I (oxidation, reduction, hydrolysis) and Phase II (conjugation) reactions metabolizing xenobiotics

Reaction Type	Enzymes Involved	Reaction Mechanism	Instances of Substrates	Products	Key Cofactors	References
Oxidation	Cytochrome P450 monooxygenases (CYP450s)	Addition of an oxygen atom to increase hydrophilicity	Benzopyrene, Acetaminophen, Codeine	Hydroxylated/metabolized forms	NADPH, O_2	Yang et al., 2024
	Flavin-containing monooxygenases (FMOs)	Oxidation of nitrogen, sulfur, phosphorus-containing compounds	Nicotine, Cimetidine, Methimazole	N-oxides, S-oxides, P-oxides	NADPH, O_2	Alipour et al., 2024
	Alcohol dehydrogenase (ADH)	Converts alcohols to aldehydes	Ethanol, Methanol	Acetaldehyde, Formaldehyde	NAD^+	Gyaneshwari, et al., 2023
	Aldehyde dehydrogenase (ALDH)	Converts aldehydes to carboxylic acids	Acetaldehyde	Acetic acid	NAD^+	Bojić et al., 2024
Reduction	Cytochrome P450 reductase	Reduction of nitro, azo, and carbonyl groups	Nitrobenzene, Prontosil (azo dyes)	Amines, Hydroxylamines	NADPH	Surendradoss et al., 2024
	NADPH-quinone oxidoreductase	Reduction of quinones to hydroquinones	Quinones (e.g., menadione)	Hydroquinones	NADPH	Penning et al., 2022
	Carbonyl reductase	Reduction of ketones and aldehydes to alcohols	Doxorubicin	Secondary alcohols	NADPH	Nagini et al., 2024

continued on following page

Table 2. Continued

Reaction Type	Enzymes Involved	Reaction Mechanism	Instances of Substrates	Products	Key Cofactors	References
Hydrolysis	Esterases	Cleavage of ester bonds	Aspirin, Procaine	Salicylic acid, PABA	H_2O	Farrukh et al., 2024
	Amidases	Cleavage of amide bonds	Lidocaine, Procainamide	Carboxylic acids, Amines	H_2O	Bisen et al., 2023
	Epoxide hydrolases (EH)	Converts epoxides to diols to prevent toxicity	Aflatoxin epoxide, Benzo[a]pyrene epoxide	Trans-dihydrodiols	H_2O	Bučko et al., 2023
Conjugation						
Glucuronidation	UDP-glucuronosyltransferases (UGTs)	Addition of glucuronic acid to hydroxyl, carboxyl, amino, or thiol groups	Morphine, Acetaminophen, Bilirubin	Glucuronide conjugates (e.g., Morphine-6-glucuronide)	UDP-glucuronic acid (UDPGA)	Dimunová et al., 2022
Sulfation	Sulfotransferases (SULTs)	Transfer of sulfate group ($-SO_3H$) to hydroxyl or amine groups	Acetaminophen, Estradiol, Dopamine	Sulphate conjugates (e.g., Acetaminophen sulphate)	3′-Phosphoadenosine-5′-phosphosulfate (PAPS)	Kurogi et al., 2024
Glutathione Conjugation	Glutathione S-transferases (GSTs)	Conjugation of glutathione (GSH) to electrophilic xenobiotics	Aflatoxin, NAPQI (Acetaminophen metabolite), Epoxides	Glutathione conjugates (detoxified metabolites)	Glutathione (GSH)	Xie et al., 2022

continued on following page

Table 2. Continued

Reaction Type	Enzymes Involved	Reaction Mechanism	Instances of Substrates	Products	Key Cofactors	References
Acetylation	N-acetyltransferases (NAT1, NAT2)	Transfer of acetyl group (-$COCH_3$) to amines or hydrazines	Isoniazid, Sulfamethazine	N-acetylated metabolites	Acetyl-CoA	Salazar-González et al., 2023
Methylation	Methyltransferases (COMT, TPMT, NNMT)	Transfer of methyl group (-CH_3) to hydroxyl, amine, or thiol groups	Dopamine, Thiopurines, Nicotine	Methylated metabolites (e.g., Metanephrine from Epinephrine)	S-adenosylmethionine (SAM)	Cannon et al., 2022
Amino Acid Conjugation	Acyl-CoA synthetase & Acyltransferase	Conjugation of xenobiotics to amino acids (glycine, glutamine, taurine)	Salicylic acid, Benzoic acid	Amino acid conjugates (e.g., Hippuric acid from benzoic acid)	Glycine, Glutamine, Taurine	Skonberg and Olsen, 2023

2.1 Metabolic Homeostasis

The dynamic balance of metabolites, proteins, gene transcripts, and regulatory molecules like microRNAs (miRNA), plays a crucial role in maintaining cellular function under normal and stressed conditions. Exposure to xenobiotics disrupts this balance, leading to measurable alterations across multiple biological systems. Metabolite profiles can reveal shifts in energy metabolism, oxidative stress, or detoxification pathways, serving as early indicators of xenobiotic-induced stress. Proteins involved in xenobiotic metabolism (cytochrome P450 enzymes) show altered expression patterns correlating with exposure levels and bioactivation of toxic compounds (Abdelmonem et al., 2024; Mokhosoev et al., 2024). Likewise, gene transcripts associated with inflammation, apoptosis, or xenobiotic processing pathways are often up- or down-regulated in response to chemical exposure. miRNAs, as post-transcriptional regulators, offer highly sensitive markers of toxicological responses and can reflect organ-specific damage, such as hepatotoxicity or nephrotoxicity (Durník et al., 2022; Singh et al., 2023a). The integration of these multi-omics signatures enables the prediction of adverse outcomes, even before clinical symptoms appear. Importantly, these molecular alterations can help identify target organ toxicity, providing a mechanistic understanding of xenobiotic effects. Metabolic homeostasis as a systems biology biomarker could offers a powerful tool for exposure assessment, risk prediction, and the development of personalized approaches in toxicology and environmental health monitoring.

2.1 Cytochrome P450 (CYP) Enzyme Family and Other Significant Enzymes

Cytochrome P450 enzymes (CYPs) play a critical role in the metabolism of xenobiotics, including drugs, environmental chemicals, and toxins. These heme-containing monooxygenases (enzymes) catalyse oxidation reactions that increase the solubility of hydrophobic compounds, facilitating their excretion. CYPs are primarily found in the liver (endoplasmic reticulum) but are also present in other tissues, contributing to both detoxification and bioactivation processes. Their activity significantly influences drug efficacy, toxicity, and individual variability in response to chemical exposures. CYP-mediated metabolism is significant for predicting drug interactions, assessing toxicological risks, and developing safer therapeutic agents in the context of personalized and precision medicine.

CYP enzymes are the most important Phase I enzymes, found mainly in the liver and also in intestines, lungs, and kidneys. One of the most abundant and significant CYP enzymes in the human liver and intestine is CYP3A4 (metabolizes ~50% of statins, benzodiazepines-based drugs) (Sayyed et al., 2022). It is also involved in metabolizing nearly 50% of clinically used drugs like midazolam (a benzodiazepine) and cyclosporine (an immunosuppressant) and CYP3A4 is inhibited by grapefruit juice, which can lead to increased drug toxicity (Dayyih et al., 2024). Similarly, CYP2D6 is responsible for metabolizing approximately 25% of drugs, including antidepressants, beta-blockers and opioids and plays role in converting codeine into its active form, morphine (Ghai et al., 2024). Genetic polymorphisms significantly influence CYP2D6 activity, leading to variability in drug response among individuals. Furthermore, CYP2C9 metabolizes NSAIDs, warfarin and CYP1A2 metabolizes caffeine, polycyclic aromatic hydrocarbons (Hua, 2024).

The other significant enzymes involved in xenobiotics metabolism involves flavin-containing monooxygenases (FMOs) that is involved in oxidation of nitrogen- and sulfur-containing compounds, aldehyde dehydrogenases (ALDHs) that detoxify aldehydes (ethanol metabolism), esterases (Carboxylesterases, Paraoxonases) catalyze hydrolysis of esters and amides and glutathione S-transferases (GSTs) that conjugate reactive metabolites to glutathione for detoxification (Candura et al., 2020).

2.2 Transporters and Their Role in Xenobiotic Excretion

After metabolism, xenobiotics and their metabolites must be transported out of cells for elimination. This process is mediated by transport proteins located in the liver, kidneys, intestines, and blood-brain barrier (Liu, 2019). The key xenobiotic transporters are ATP-Binding Cassette (ABC) transporters that pump drugs out of cells and are energy dependent like P-glycoprotein (P-gp, ABCB1) affecting drug absorption, multidrug resistance-associated proteins (MRPs, ABCCs) involved in transporting conjugated metabolites (glucuronides) and breast cancer resistance protein (BCRP, ABCG2) exporting anticancer drugs (Liu, 2019; Koehn, 2022).

Another class of transporters are SLC (solute carrier transporters), they facilitate passive or active uptake of xenobiotics into cells. For instance, organic anion transporters (OATs) that import anionic drugs into the kidney for excretion and Organic Cation Transporters (OCTs) that are involved in transportation of positively charged drugs (Talevi and Bellera, 2022). The other transporter types include hepatic transporters (remove xenobiotics into bile for faecal excretion), renal transporters (mediate drug excretion into urine) and blood-brain barrier transporters (protect the brain from toxic xenobiotics damage) (Durník et al., 2022).

2.3 Regulatory Networks and Feedback Mechanisms

Xenobiotic metabolism involves a complex network of pathways and enzymes that detoxify and eliminate foreign compounds, including drugs, environmental pollutants, and dietary chemicals (Singh et al., 2023a). This process is tightly regulated by intricate regulatory networks and feedback mechanisms to ensure a balanced response to xenobiotic exposure while preventing toxicity or metabolic overload (Singh et al., 2023a). The metabolism of xenobiotics occurs in three main phases: Phase I (functionalization), Phase II (conjugation), and Phase III (transport and excretion) (Sayyed et al., 2022). These phases are controlled by key regulatory pathways, including nuclear receptors, signalling molecules, and feedback loops that modulate enzyme expression and activity in response to xenobiotic burden (Luan et al., 2022). Some of the significant xenobiotic-responsive transcription factors include, Aryl Hydrocarbon Receptor (AhR) - regulates CYP1A1 and CYP1A2 in response to polycyclic aromatic hydrocarbons, Pregnane X Receptor (PXR) - regulates CYP3A4, P-gp, and UGTs in response to drugs and toxins, Constitutive Androstane Receptor (CAR), that Controls CYP2B6, UGTs, and SULTs, particularly for barbiturates and Nuclear Factor Erythroid 2-Related Factor 2 (Nrf2) – regulates antioxidant responses and GSTs to detoxify reactive xenobiotics (Gagliardi et al., 2023; Mokhosoev et al., 2024).

In Phase I, cytochrome P450 (CYP) enzymes catalyse oxidation reactions that introduce functional groups into xenobiotics, making them more reactive. However, excessive CYP activity can lead to an overload of reactive metabolites, causing oxidative stress and cellular damage (Dayyih et al., 2024). To counteract this, feedback mechanisms involving nuclear receptors like the pregnane X receptor (PXR), constitutive androstane receptor (CAR), and aryl hydrocarbon receptor (AhR) regulate CYP enzyme expression (Mahanayak, 2024). For instance, when high levels of reactive oxygen species (ROS) are generated due to excessive CYP activity, the nuclear factor erythroid 2-related factor 2 (Nrf2) is activated through phosphorylation (Sayyed et al., 2022). Nrf2 upregulates antioxidant enzymes and Phase II detoxification enzymes to neutralize ROS and prevent cellular damage (Mokhosoev et al., 2024). Additionally, CYP enzyme induction is self-regulated through negative feedback, when xenobiotic levels decrease, reducing the activation of nuclear receptors like PXR and slowing down CYP enzyme production (Garcia et al., 2018).

Phase II metabolism involves conjugation reactions that are catalysed by enzymes like glutathione S-transferases (GSTs), UDP-glucuronosyltransferases (UGTs), and sulfotransferases (SULTs), is also subject to feedback regulation (Sharma et al., 2024). These enzymes attach hydrophilic groups (H/OH) to xenobiotics, enhancing their solubility for excretion (sharma et al., 2024). However, an excessive demand for conjugation reactions can deplete cofactors like glutathione (GSH), UDP-glucuronic acid, and sulphate. For instance, when high levels of reactive metabolites deplete GSH, Nrf2 signalling is triggered to enhance the expression of GSTs and promote GSH biosynthesis (Panda et al., 2023). Similarly, the availability of sulphate and glucuronic acid controls the activity of SULTs and UGTs, respectively. If conjugation capacity is exceeded, unmetabolized xenobiotics accumulate, leading to feedback inhibition of Phase I enzymes to prevent further reactive metabolite formation (Yu et al., 2022b).

In Phase III, ATP-binding cassette (ABC) transporters like P-glycoprotein (P-gp), multidrug resistance-associated proteins (MRPs), and cancer resistance protein (CRP) facilitate xenobiotic excretion (Liu, 2019). Feedback mechanisms regulate transporter expression in response to xenobiotic burden. For instance, when intracellular xenobiotic levels rise, PXR and CAR induce the expression of P-gp and MRPs to enhance drug efflux (Koehn, 2022). Conversely, if excessive transporter activity depletes cellular ATP, feedback inhibition occurs to prevent energy exhaustion (Brouwer et al., 2022). Additionally, phosphorylation and ubiquitination modify transporter activity based on cellular conditions, ensuring a balance between xenobiotic removal and metabolic homeostasis

Disruptions in these regulatory pathways can lead to drug interactions, metabolic disorders, or increased susceptibility to environmental toxins, highlighting their importance in pharmacology, toxicology, and personalized medicine.

3. OMICS TECHNOLOGIES IN XENOBIOTIC METABOLISM

Omics technologies have revolutionized our understanding of xenobiotic metabolism, offering insights at various molecular levels. Genomic studies involve identifying genetic variations that influence how organisms metabolize xenobiotics (Abudahab et al., 2024). Researchers can pinpoint specific genes or alleles that encode enzymes responsible for metabolizing drugs, environmental toxins, or dietary compounds, by studying genomes. For instance, CYP450 genetic variations in cytochrome P450 (CYP450) enzymes, particularly CYP2D6, CYP3A4, and CYP1A2, can significantly influence the metabolism of drugs (Abdelmonem et al., 2024). Personalized medicine can be improved by identifying individuals with genetic polymorphisms that affect drug metabolism (Mokhosoev et al., 2024).

Transcriptomics focuses on RNA molecules, providing a view of gene expression patterns under different conditions. In the context of xenobiotic metabolism, transcriptomic studies reveal about the regulation of genes involved in detoxification pathways (Kleino et al., 2022). Changes in RNA levels can indicate adaptive responses to xenobiotics, shedding light on mechanisms of tolerance or susceptibility. For instance, liver enzyme induction on xenobiotics like alcohol or pharmaceuticals induce the expression of detoxifying enzymes (cytochrome P450 family) (Park et al., 2023). Transcriptomic analysis helps in understanding how the expression levels of these enzymes change in response to various compounds (Kleino et al., 2022). Moreover, the response to toxicants in lung cells, in cases of environmental toxicant exposure (cigarette smoke or air pollution) transcriptomics can reveal the altered expression of genes related to oxidative stress, inflammation, and xenobiotic metabolism, helping predict lung toxicity (Rahman et al., 2022).

Proteomics explores the entire complement of proteins expressed by an organism or tissue. In xenobiotic metabolism, proteomic analyses identify enzymes responsible for metabolizing foreign compounds (Miglani et al., 2022). Mapping protein interactions and enzyme activity helps understand how these proteins work together to detoxify or activate xenobiotics, influencing pharmacokinetics and toxicological outcomes (Rai et al., 2023). For instance, identification of drug-protein interaction approaches can identify novel protein targets for xenobiotics. A proteomic analysis may uncover new interactions between drug molecules and proteins like transporters or enzymes, improving understanding of drug absorption and efficacy (Singh et al., 2023b). Proteomics can also be used to study changes in the expression or activation of specific enzymes.

Metabolomics examines small molecules (metabolites) produced by cellular processes, offering a comprehensive view of metabolic outputs influenced by xenobiotics. Profiling of metabolites in biological samples, researchers can identify biomarkers of exposure, assess metabolic pathways affected by xenobiotics, and predict metabolic outcomes in response to environmental or therapeutic agents (Wright et al., 2023). Xenobiotics can alter normal metabolic pathways, and metabolomics can track these changes. Exposure to drugs or environmental pollutants disrupt the normal lipid metabolism pathways, which could be studied using high-resolution mass spectrometry (Liu et al., 2022). Metabolomics helps in identification of biomarkers that can predict drug responses or adverse effects. Metabolite profiles indicate whether a drug is being metabolized efficiently or if a patient may experience toxic effects due to impaired metabolism (Sayyed et al., 2022). It identifies microbial enzymes that can modify xenobiotics and affect drug bioavailability and efficacy. The gut microbiota has been shown to modify the efficacy and toxicity of certain drugs, like the conversion of levodopa (used for Parkinson's disease) to its active form in the gut (Pant et al., 2023). Some gut bacteria (*Lactobacillus, Bifidobacterium,* and *E. coli*) assist in detoxifying xenobiotics by breaking them down into less toxic metabolites, while others may activate pro-toxins (Khani et al., 2025). Studying microbiome shifts in response to exposure to environmental pollutants or drugs can provide insights into how xenobiotics are processed in the body.

These omics approaches collectively enhance our understanding of xenobiotic metabolism, offering insights into genetic predispositions, molecular mechanisms of detoxification, and microbial contributions, thereby advancing drug development, environmental risk assessment, and precision health strategies.

4. SYSTEMS BIOLOGY APPROACHES

Systems biology integrates computational and experimental techniques to study complex biological interactions holistically. In xenobiotic metabolism, systems biology approaches help in understanding metabolic pathways, predicting responses to foreign compounds, and developing strategies for personalized medicine and environmental toxicology (Del Giudice et al., 2024). Network-based modelling of xenobiotic pathways involves the construction and analysis of biological networks to elucidate the metabolism of foreign compounds (Mardinoglu and Palsson, 2025). These models depict the interactions among genes, proteins, and metabolites, offering insights into crucial regulatory points. The Human Liver Metabolic Network (HLMN) predicts hepatic drug processing, identifying drug-drug interactions and potentially toxic metabolites (Izat et al., 2025). Similarly, networks focusing on cytochrome P450 enzymes enable predictions of how genetic variations impact drug metabolism and individual drug responses, showcasing the utility of network models in pharmacogenomics and toxicology research (Fetse et al., 2024).

Dynamic modelling and simulation of metabolic flux analyse the flow of metabolites through biochemical pathways, offering insights into the kinetics of xenobiotic metabolism under varying conditions. Flux Balance Analysis (FBA) is a widely used approach to predict how different xenobiotics are processed in human cells by simulating metabolic fluxes through detoxification pathways (Chatterjee et al., 2024). Additionally, Physiologically Based Pharmacokinetic (PBPK) models simulate the absorption, distribution, metabolism, and excretion of drugs across different organs, aiding in dose optimization and risk assessment (Ozbek et al., 2024). These dynamic models are essential for understanding metabolic responses and improving drug safety evaluations.

Multi-omics data integration techniques (Table 5) combine genomic, transcriptomic, proteomic, and metabolomic datasets to provide a comprehensive understanding of xenobiotic metabolism (Shi et al., 2024). Establishing link between genetic variants with proteomic data, genomics-proteomics integration helps determine the influence of genetic polymorphism on enzyme activity and drug metabolism. Metabolomics-transcriptomics integration in toxicology enables the identification of early biomarkers of toxicity, improving drug safety assessments (Acharya and Mukhopadhyay, 2024). These multi-omics approaches enhance biomarker discovery, facilitate personalized medicine, and offer deeper insights into the regulatory mechanisms governing xenobiotic metabolism.

Artificial intelligence (AI) and machine learning (ML) play a crucial role in xenobiotic research by analysing large datasets to identify patterns in metabolism, predict drug interactions, and enhance drug design (Lettieri et al., 2024). Deep learning models trained on xenobiotic metabolism data can accurately predict how new drugs will be processed, reducing reliance on extensive *in-vitro* and *in-vivo* testing (Dudas and Miteva, 2024). Additionally, ML-based toxicity prediction utilizes chemical structure and biological response data to assess the toxicity of environmental contaminants and pharmaceuticals (Priyadarshini, 2024). These AI-driven approaches improve efficiency, accuracy, and safety in toxicological assessments and drug development.

Systems biology approaches provide powerful tools for understanding xenobiotic metabolism, integrating computational models, high-throughput data, and AI-driven predictions. These methods enhance drug development, toxicology research, and precision medicine by offering mechanistic insights and predictive capabilities.

5. APPLICATIONS OF INTEGRATIVE OMICS IN XENOBIOTIC METABOLISM

Integrative omics approaches combine genomics, transcriptomics, proteomics, metabolomics, and microbiomics to provide a comprehensive understanding of xenobiotic metabolism (Table 3). These methods have various applications in pharmacology, toxicology, and personalized medicine.

5.1 Drug Metabolism: Precision Medicine and Predicting Drug Efficacy/Toxicity

Omics technologies help identify genetic and molecular factors influencing drug metabolism, enabling precision medicine by predicting individual responses to drugs and minimizing adverse effects. Pharmacogenomics plays a crucial role in cancer therapy by assessing genetic variations in enzymes like cytochrome P450 (CYP2D6, CYP3A4), influencing the metabolism of chemotherapeutic agents like tamoxifen (Narendra et al., 2022). This profiling enables personalized dose adjustments, enhancing treatment efficacy while minimizing adverse effects. Conversely, metabolomics aids in identifying biomarkers for drug toxicity, exemplified in acetaminophen (paracetamol) use, where early detection of liver toxicity markers through metabolomic analysis enables timely interventions, promoting safer medication practices (Ratnasekhar et al., 2024). These approaches illustrate how genomic and metabolomic insights are transforming personalized medicine, optimizing therapeutic outcomes and patient safety in clinical settings.

5.2 Environmental Toxicology: Assessing Pollutant Impact and Bioremediation

Integrative omics methods provide valuable insights into how pollutants impact biological systems and support bioremediation efforts by identifying microorganisms capable of degrading toxic compounds (Mokrani et al., 2024). Transcriptomic analysis of fish exposed to heavy metals (Hg, As, Cd) reveals changes in gene expression, offering a means to assess environmental toxicity and ecosystem health (Lu et al., 2024). Similarly, microbiomic studies leverage metagenomic sequencing to identify bacterial strains in soil microbiomes that can break down oil spills, facilitating the development of effective microbial bioremediation strategies (Table 4) (Aakula et al., 2024). These approaches enhance our understanding of pollution's biological effects while advancing sustainable environmental restoration techniques.

5.3 Personalized Risk Assessment: Genetic and Epigenetic Variability in Xenobiotic Responses

Integration of genetic, epigenetic, and environmental data could help researchers to assess individual susceptibility to toxins and inform public health interventions (Motsinger-Reif et al., 2024). Epigenomic studies reveal that DNA methylation changes in inflammation-related genes contribute to differences in sensitivity to air pollution, explaining why some individuals are more prone to diseases like asthma (Abudahab et al., 2024). Similarly, genome-wide association studies (GWAS) identify genetic variants linked to pesticide metabolism, enabling the detection of agricultural labours at higher risk of pesticide-related illnesses (Table 4) (Mardinoglu and Palsson, 2025). These integrative approaches enhance our ability to predict health risks and develop targeted strategies for disease prevention and environmental safety.

Integrative omics approaches provide deep insights into xenobiotic metabolism, improving drug safety, environmental risk assessment, and personalized health strategies (Stanley, 2024). Researchers can develop targeted interventions and advance precision medicine and environmental health initiatives, analysing multi-omics data.

6. CASE STUDIES

Table 3. Insights into specific drugs or pollutants using integrative omics

Case Study	Target Drug/Pollutant	Omics Approaches Used	Key Findings	Implications	Reference
Multi-omics analysis of acetaminophen-induced liver toxicity	Acetaminophen (Paracetamol)	Transcriptomics, Proteomics, Metabolomics	Identified oxidative stress markers, mitochondrial dysfunction, and metabolic pathway alterations in hepatocytes	Improved understanding of acetaminophen hepatotoxicity, potential biomarkers for early detection	Gaither et al., 2025
Integrative omics for benzene-induced hematotoxicity	Benzene	Epigenomics, Transcriptomics, Metabolomics	DNA methylation changes, dysregulated hematopoiesis, and altered metabolite profiles in exposed workers	Insight into benzene-induced leukemia risk and personalized exposure assessments	Fetes et al., 2024
Omics-based evaluation of endocrine-disrupting chemicals (EDCs)	Bisphenol A (BPA)	Epigenomics, Proteomics, Metabolomics	Identified changes in hormone receptor expression, metabolic pathways, and epigenetic modifications	Highlights long-term risks of BPA exposure, guiding regulatory policies	Pecori Giraldi et al., 2024
Systems biology approach for drug-induced cardiotoxicity	Doxorubicin	Transcriptomics, Metabolomics, Lipidomics	Mitochondrial lipid metabolism disruption and oxidative damage in cardiomyocytes	Potential cardioprotective interventions in chemotherapy	Chatterjee et al., 2022
Multi-omics profiling of arsenic exposure effects	Arsenic	Genomics, Epigenomics, Proteomics	Altered gene expression, histone modifications, and protein dysregulation linked to cancer	Understanding arsenic-related diseases, risk assessment strategies	Bhardwaj et al., 2021
Metabolomics-driven insights into glyphosate toxicity	Glyphosate (herbicide)	Metabolomics, Proteomics	Disrupted amino acid metabolism, oxidative stress response in exposed organisms	Environmental safety assessments and regulatory frameworks	Yu et al., 2022b
Integrative omics for opioid addiction mechanisms	Fentanyl	Transcriptomics, Proteomics, Epigenomics	Epigenetic changes in brain reward pathways, altered neurotransmitter-related proteins	Target identification for opioid addiction treatments	Alipour et al., 2024

continued on following page

Table 3. Continued

Case Study	Target Drug/Pollutant	Omics Approaches Used	Key Findings	Implications	Reference
Systems pharmacology approach to statin-induced myopathy	Statins (e.g., Atorvastatin)	Proteomics, Metabolomics, Lipidomics	Muscle cell energy metabolism disturbances, oxidative stress markers	Biomarkers for predicting statin-induced adverse effects	Shreenidhi et al., 2024
Integrative Omics Analysis of Herbicide Toxicity	Formulated Herbicide	Transcriptomics, Proteomics	Identified reproductive toxicity mechanisms in *Folsomia candida*, including oxidative stress and mitochondrial dysfunction.	Enhanced understanding of herbicide-induced toxicity pathways, supporting environmental risk assessments.	Park et al., 2023
Multi-Omics Data Integration in Toxicology	Various Environmental Chemicals	Transcriptomics, Proteomics, Metabolomics	Demonstrated that single-omics approaches are insufficient for systemic toxicity understanding; multi-omics integration provides comprehensive insights into toxicity pathways.	Supports the adoption of integrative omics in toxicological studies for better risk assessment.	Liu et al., 2022
Integrative Omics in Drug Discovery	Various Drugs	Genomics, Transcriptomics, Proteomics, Metabolomics	Highlighted the application of integrative omics in understanding disease mechanisms, identifying therapeutic targets, and facilitating drug discovery.	Promotes the use of multi-omics approaches to enhance drug development processes.	Narendra et al., 2022

Table 4. Instances of microbiome-host interactions in xenobiotic metabolism

Xenobiotic Class	Instance Compound	Microbial Action	Host Consequence	References
Drugs	Acetaminophen	Sulphate depletion by gut microbes reduces detoxification	Increased hepatotoxicity due to decreased sulfation	Huang et al., 2024
Irinotecan (CPT-11)	β-glucuronidases reactivate drug from its conjugated form	Increased intestinal toxicity, limiting chemotherapy efficacy	Relevant in cancer treatment	Xu et al., 2024
Digoxin	Reduction by *Eggerthella lenta* lowers drug bioavailability	Decreased therapeutic effect in heart failure patients	Microbial impact on cardiotonic drugs	Mousa et al., 2023
Dietary Compounds	Isoflavones (Soya)	Bacterial metabolism produces equol, an active estrogenic metabolite	Potential benefits in hormone-related conditions (e.g., menopause)	Gong et al., 2023
Red Meat (L-carnitine)	Conversion to TMA, further metabolized to TMAO by liver	Associated with increased cardiovascular risk	TMAO linked to atherosclerosis	Gaither et al., 2025
Environmental Pollutants	Polycyclic Aromatic Hydrocarbons (PAHs)	Bacterial biotransformation to hydroxylated metabolites	Potentially increased carcinogenicity or detoxification	Khmaissa et al., 2024
Pesticides	Organophosphates	Microbial hydrolysis of ester bonds	Reduced toxicity or persistence in the gut	Mahanayak, 2024
Artificial Sweeteners	Aspartame, Saccharin	Gut microbiota-dependent metabolism alters glucose metabolism	Possible impact on insulin sensitivity and metabolic disorders	Del Pozo et al., 2022
Probiotics & Xenobiotic Detox	Lactobacillus spp.	Bile salt hydrolase activity affects drug absorption	Alters bioavailability of statins and other drugs	Das et al., 2024

Table 5. Data Integration Platforms in Systems Biology for Xenobiotics

Platform	Type	Developer(s)	Features	Use in Xenobiotics	Website
Ingenuity Pathway Analysis (IPA)	Commercial	QIAGEN Digital Insights	• Multi-omics integration • Pathway & toxicity analysis • Upstream regulator prediction	Identifies biological pathways, regulators, and toxicity effects of xenobiotics	https://www.qiagen.com/ipa
MetaboAnalyst	Open-source	Xia Lab, McGill University	• Metabolomics & statistical analysis • Pathway enrichment • Network-based analysis	Analyzes metabolic signatures from xenobiotic exposure	https://www.metaboanalyst.ca
Cytoscape	Open-source	Institute for Systems Biology + UCSD + collaborators	• Network visualization • Plugin support (e.g., Metscape) • Gene-metabolite integration	Visualization of xenobiotic-perturbed biological networks	https://cytoscape.org
KNIME Analytics Platform	Open-source	KNIME AG	• Workflow-based analytics • Bio- & chemo-informatics tools • Modular interface	Combines chemical, genomic, and toxicological data for xenobiotic assessment	https://www.knime.com
ToxCast / Tox21 Dashboard	Open Access	US EPA & NIH	• High-throughput screening (HTS) • Toxicity pathway mapping • Predictive toxicology	Provides mechanistic and predictive data for xenobiotic toxicity	https://www.epa.gov/chemical-research/toxcast-dashboard

continued on following page

Table 5. Continued

Platform	Type	Developer(s)	Features	Use in Xenobiotics	Website
BioMart / Ensembl BioMart	Open-source	EMBL-EBI / Ensembl Project	• Cross-species gene queries • Genomic annotations • Batch data retrieval	Identifies xenobiotic-responsive genes and functional annotations	https://www.ensembl.org/biomart
OmicsNet	Open-source	Xia Lab, McGill University	• 3D network visualization • Multi-omics integration • Web interface	Builds interaction networks involving xenobiotic-affected entities	https://www.omicsnet.ca
Reactome	Open-source	OICR + EBI + Collaborators	• Pathway browsing • Multi-species support • Drug/pathway linking	Maps xenobiotic interactions with cellular signaling pathways	https://reactome.org
PathVisio	Open-source	Netherlands Bioinformatics Centre (NBIC)	• Custom pathway creation • Data visualization • WikiPathways integration	Used to model metabolic and signaling pathways affected by xenobiotics	https://www.pathvisio.org
OpenTox	Open-source	OpenTox Consortium	• Predictive modelling • Toxicological ontologies • REST APIs	Integrates chemoinformatics and bioinformatics for xenobiotic profiling	https://www.opentox.net

continued on following page

Table 5. Continued

Platform	Type	Developer(s)	Features	Use in Xenobiotics	Website
ChemRICH	Open Access	Fiehn Lab, UC Davis	• Chemical similarity clustering • Non-pathway enrichment • Metabolite annotation	Identifies clusters of chemically similar xenobiotic metabolites	http://chemrich.fiehnlab.ucdavis.edu
AOP-Wiki (Adverse Outcome Pathway)	Open-source	OECD + AOP Knowledge Base Network	• AOP frameworks • Molecular-to-phenotypic events • Regulatory relevance	Models how xenobiotics lead to toxicity through key biological events	https://aopwiki.org
Precision Medicine Analytics Platform (PMAP)	Institutional / Research	Johns Hopkins University	• Clinical + omics integration • Real-time data analytics • Focus on individualized treatment	Used to study xenobiotic impacts on personalized patient pathways and drug response	https://ictr.johnshopkins.edu/pmap

Foot Notes:

• PMAP (Johns Hopkins): Offers a secure, HIPAA-compliant environment for analysing patient-level omics data along with environmental exposures (including xenobiotics).

• Interoperability: Many of the platforms above can be integrated through workflow managers like Galaxy, KNIME, or APIs.

• Regulatory Relevance: AOP-Wiki, OpenTox, and Tox21 have strong ties to regulatory toxicology and risk assessment.

7. CHALLENGES AND FUTURE PERSPECTIVES

Xenobiotic metabolism involves the biotransformation of foreign compounds, like drugs, pollutants, and dietary chemicals, into more easily excretable forms. The complexity of this process necessitates a multi-omics approach, integrating genomics, transcriptomics, proteomics, metabolomics, and epigenomics, to entirely understand individual and population-wide variations in xenobiotic responses. However, this integration presents several challenges and future opportunities, as outlined below.

7.1 Technical and Computational Challenges in Multi-Omics Integration

The integration of multiple omics layers in xenobiotic metabolism is technically demanding. Omics technologies generate diverse data types with varying formats, scales, and quality levels, posing challenges for integration and analysis. For instance, RNA sequencing in transcriptomics produces high-dimensional count data, while metabolomics yields continuous concentration values, making cross-omics comparisons complex (Park et al., 2022). The absence of standardized workflows for data preprocessing, normalization, and integration further complicates reproducibility, limiting the reliability of multi-omics studies. Establishing uniform protocols and analytical frameworks is crucial for improving data harmonization and ensuring the consistency of omics-based research.

Multi-omics studies generate vast datasets with millions of features, leading to significant computational challenges and high processing costs. The high-dimensional nature of these data increases the complexity of statistical analyses, raising the risk of overfitting in machine learning models and reducing predictive accuracy (Lettieri et al., 2024). Efficient data reduction techniques, advanced computational frameworks, and robust statistical approaches are essential to manage the dimensionality and ensure reliable insights from multi-omics research.

Xenobiotic metabolism is governed by a complex network of enzymes, transporters, and regulatory elements, making it challenging to capture interactions across multiple biological layers (Bojić et al., 2024). Existing multi-omics integration methods often struggle to model the intricate cross-talk between genomics, transcriptomics, proteomics, and metabolomics, limiting the accuracy of pathway analyses (Shi et al., 2024). Advancing computational models and network-based approaches is crucial for improving our understanding of these dynamic interactions and enhancing predictions in toxicology and drug metabolism.

Integrating multi-omics data requires advanced computational tools, like multi-block principal component analysis and deep learning, which often demand extensive parameter tuning and optimization (Dudas and Miteva, 2024). However, the complexity of these methods limits their accessibility and interpretability, highlighting the need for more efficient machine learning models capable of selecting relevant cross-omics features (Rahman et al., 2022). Developing algorithms that balance computational efficiency with biological interpretability will be crucial for improving multi-omics data integration and facilitating meaningful discoveries in systems biology.

7.2 Ethical and Data-Sharing Concerns in Systems Biology Research

Integrating omics data from diverse populations raises ethical, legal, and social concerns. Ensuring compliance with regulations like GDPR and HIPAA while maintaining data accessibility for research presents a major challenge (Herath et al., 2024). Robust encryption, secure data-sharing frameworks, and federated learning approaches are essential to protect patient privacy while enabling scientific advancements in personalized medicine and public health.

Patients and participants often have concerns about the ownership of their omics data and how it is utilized, especially as such data can have long-term implications for their health (Mohr et al., 2024). To address these concerns, dynamic consent models are necessary, allowing participants to adjust their data-sharing preferences over time. These models provide greater transparency and control for individuals, ensuring that their rights are respected while supporting the responsible use of omics data in research (Gupta and Kumar, 2023).

Many multi-omics datasets are biased towards Western populations, limiting the generalizability of findings to diverse ethnic groups and potentially exacerbating health disparities. To address this issue, ethical frameworks should be implemented to promote greater diversity in omics research, ensuring that findings are inclusive and applicable to a wider range of populations. This would help in developing equitable healthcare applications that benefit individuals from all backgrounds, leading to more accurate and effective treatments for everyone.

7.3 Socio-Economic and Ethical Challenges

The application of xenobiotics in pesticides, industrial chemicals, and pharmaceuticals raises critical socio-economic and ethical concerns, particularly in developing regions. One of the foremost challenges is affordability. The safe use, monitoring, and regulation of xenobiotics often require sophisticated technologies and testing protocols, which are costly and largely inaccessible to small-scale farmers and under-resourced communities. As a result, cheaper and potentially more hazardous chemicals continue to be used, posing serious risks to human and environmental health. Compounding this issue is the lack of adequate farmer training. Many agricultural workers lack the necessary education or support to understand the risks associated with xenobiotics, proper usage protocols, or safe disposal methods. This knowledge gap leads to unsafe practices that increase exposure and environmental contamination. Furthermore, long-term environmental monitoring systems are either weak or absent in many regions, hindering the ability to track bioaccumulation, resistance development, or ecosystem disruptions caused by persistent xenobiotics and their metabolites. Ethically, this raises concerns about environmental justice, as marginalized communities often bear a disproportionate burden of chemical exposure. Environmental risks associated with xenobiotic metabolism include the formation of toxic byproducts, bioaccumulation in food chains, and the disruption of microbial and aquatic ecosystems. These risks necessitate transparent regulatory policies, equitable access to safer alternatives, and participatory decision-making that includes farmers, scientists, and policymakers.

7.4 The Future Role of AI and Machine Learning in Predictive Modelling

AI and machine learning (ML) are transforming xenobiotic metabolism studies and predicted AI-driven models have the potential to enhance predictive toxicology by forecasting how individuals metabolize drugs based on their multi-omics profiles, enabling personalized treatment strategies (Lettieri et al., 2024). Computational techniques, like deep learning, can uncover novel drug metabolism pathways, offering valuable insights into the interactions between drugs and the human body (Dudas and Miteva, 2024). These advancements promise to improve drug safety, optimize therapeutic efficacy, and reduce adverse drug reactions by tailoring interventions to individual metabolic profiles.

Machine learning (ML) algorithms are increasingly used to integrate omics and clinical data, enabling the prediction of drug toxicity risks and improving patient safety. Through incorporating pharmacogenomic insights, AI models can identify specific patient subgroups that are more likely to experience adverse drug reactions, allowing for more tailored and effective treatment strategies (Herath et al., 2024). These advancements hold the potential to revolutionize personalized medicine, minimizing harmful side effects and optimizing therapeutic outcomes for individuals based on their unique genetic and clinical profiles.

AI techniques (causal modelling and Bayesian networks) offer powerful tools for uncovering regulatory relationships in xenobiotic metabolism by identifying the interactions between genes, enzymes, and environmental factors (Priya et al., 2024). These models enhance our understanding of gene-environment interactions, allowing for more precise insights into how environmental exposures influence biological pathways and contribute to disease (Edo et al., 2024). AI-driven approaches provide valuable knowledge that could inform strategies for personalized medicine and environmental health interventions.

To overcome data limitations in multi-omics research, techniques like transfer learning and federated learning enable models to learn from decentralized datasets without the need for direct data sharing, ensuring privacy and data security. Additionally, self-supervised AI methods can extract meaningful insights from small-scale multi-omics datasets, allowing researchers to make progress even when large, comprehensive datasets are unavailable. These approaches help maximize the value of limited data, enhancing the scalability and effectiveness of omics-based research.

7.5 Towards a Personalized and System-Wide Approach to Xenobiotic Metabolism

Precision pharmacology leverages multi-omics-guided drug dosing strategies to optimize therapeutic efficacy while minimizing toxicity, ensuring that patients receive the most appropriate treatment for their individual profiles (Singh et al., 2023b). Pharmaco-omics tools are particularly valuable in predicting how specific genetic variants influence drug metabolism, allowing for more personalized and effective drug regimens (Khalil et al., 2024). Incorporating genetic, transcriptomic, proteomic, and metabolomic data, these altogether enhance the ability to tailor treatments based on an individual's unique biological makeup, leading to better outcomes and reduced adverse effects.

Integration of omics data with digital health technologies, like wearable sensors and electronic health records (EHRs), enables real-time monitoring of drug metabolism, enhancing personalized treatment strategies (Acharya and Mukhopadhyay, 2024). Through combining these data sources, healthcare providers can track biomarker changes in real-time, allowing for more timely adjustments in drug dosing and therapy. Additionally, AI-powered apps can offer personalized recommendations based on dynamic biomarker data, providing patients with tailored insights and optimizing health outcomes through continuous, data-driven decision-making (Ratnasekhar et al., 2024).

The gut microbiota plays a crucial role in xenobiotic metabolism, making metagenomic profiling essential for personalized medicine, as it helps predict how individuals process various compounds (Pant et al., 2023). Additionally, environmental exposures like diet and pollutants significantly influence metabolic processes and health outcomes, highlighting the need to incorporate these factors into predictive models for comprehensive risk assessments (De Filippis et al., 2024). Considering both microbiome composition and environmental influences, we can better understand individual responses to drugs and toxins, leading to more accurate and personalized healthcare strategies.

The future of personalized medicine relies on multi-scale models that combine molecular omics data with whole-body physiology to make accurate, system-wide predictions of drug responses. These integrated models could revolutionize how we predict individual reactions to treatments, offering tailored therapeutic strategies. Additionally, advancements in digital twins, AI-based simulations of individual metabolic profiles, hold great potential to transform drug development by enabling virtual testing of drugs on personalized models, improving treatment outcomes, and accelerating the discovery of safe and effective therapies.

Despite significant advancements, integrating multi-omics data in xenobiotic metabolism faces technical, computational, ethical, and scalability challenges. Addressing these issues will require novel AI techniques, better data-sharing policies, and a more holistic approach that considers environmental and microbiome factors. The future of xenobiotic metabolism research lies in moving towards precision medicine, where personalized drug metabolism predictions improve treatment outcomes and reduce adverse effects.

8. CONCLUSION

The integration of multi-omics approaches in understanding xenobiotic metabolism has provided unprecedented insights into how foreign compounds are processed in biological systems. Through systems biology frameworks, researchers have been able to dissect the intricate interactions between genes, proteins, metabolites, and environmental factors that influence the metabolism of drugs, pollutants, and dietary xenobiotics. This holistic approach has not only enhanced our fundamental understanding of xenobiotic metabolism but also holds transformative implications for human health, precision medicine, drug development, and environmental safety.

8.1 Summary of Insights Gained From Omics Integration and Systems Biology

Multi-omics integration, encompassing genomics, transcriptomics, proteomics, metabolomics, epigenomics, and microbiomics, has revealed complex regulatory networks that govern xenobiotic metabolism. Genomic and transcriptomic studies have identified key genetic variants and gene expression changes associated with variations in metabolic enzyme activity. Proteomics has provided insights into post-translational modifications and enzyme abundance, while metabolomics has enabled real-time tracking of metabolic byproducts, allowing researchers to map detailed biochemical pathways. Epigenomic studies have further demonstrated how environmental exposures and lifestyle factors influence gene regulation, altering xenobiotic metabolism across different life stages and disease conditions.

Systems biology has played a crucial role in integrating these diverse datasets, moving beyond reductionist approaches to construct comprehensive models of metabolic pathways. Network-based approaches have uncovered regulatory hubs that coordinate drug metabolism, helping to predict individual variability in drug response and toxicity. Advanced computational models, including AI-driven predictive analytics, have further improved our ability to analyse high-dimensional data, allowing for the identification of novel biomarkers for xenobiotic metabolism efficiency and susceptibility to adverse drug reactions.

One of the most significant findings from omics integration is the role of the gut microbiome in xenobiotic metabolism. Metagenomic studies have shown that gut microbial enzymes contribute significantly to the biotransformation of drugs, pollutants, and dietary compounds, influencing drug efficacy and toxicity. These discoveries underscore the importance of a system-wide approach that considers not only host genetics but also microbiome interactions in xenobiotic metabolism research.

8.2 Implications for Human Health, Drug Development, and Environmental Safety

The advancements in omics-driven xenobiotic metabolism research have far-reaching implications across multiple domains, particularly in human health, pharmaceutical development, and environmental toxicology. One of the most direct benefits of multi-omics research is the ability to personalize drug treatments based on an individual's metabolic profile. Pharmacogenomics, combined with proteomics and metabolomics, allows for tailored drug dosing strategies that minimize adverse effects and optimize therapeutic efficacy. This is particularly important in oncology, psychiatry, and cardiology, where inter-individual differences in drug metabolism can significantly impact treatment outcomes.

The pharmaceutical industry is increasingly leveraging multi-omics approaches to enhance drug discovery and development. AI-powered systems biology models are being used to simulate metabolic pathways, enabling the design of safer and more effective drugs. Additionally, omics-based biomarkers are being used to identify high-risk populations and guide regulatory decisions on drug approvals.

Beyond pharmaceuticals, omics integration has crucial implications for assessing the impact of environmental pollutants on human health. Exposure to industrial chemicals, pesticides, and air pollutants can disrupt metabolic pathways, leading to long-term health risks. Multi-omics studies help elucidate the mechanisms of toxicity, enabling the development of better risk assessment models and targeted interventions to mitigate environmental exposure effects.

Furthermore, understanding microbial-mediated xenobiotic metabolism is essential in biodegradation and bioremediation strategies, where engineered microbial communities can be used to detoxify pollutants in contaminated ecosystems.

8.3 Final Thoughts

The integration of multi-omics approaches into xenobiotic metabolism research represents a paradigm shift in how we study drug metabolism, toxicity, and environmental interactions. Through systems biology perspectives, researchers are moving towards a more predictive, personalized, and system-wide approach to understanding xenobiotic metabolism. Future advancements in AI-driven analytics, improved data-sharing frameworks, and deeper integration of microbiome research will further refine our ability to optimize drug therapies, reduce adverse effects, and protect public health and the environment. The continued evolution of omics technologies promises a future where xenobiotic metabolism is understood at an unprecedented level of detail, ultimately driving innovations in medicine, biotechnology, and toxicology.

REFERENCES

Aakula, M., Kedare, M. M., Satyam, S., Patra, S., & Singha, S. (2024). Unraveling Microbial Dynamics in Hydrocarbon Contaminated Sites: A Comparative Metagenomic Perspective. *Available at SSRN* 5035502. DOI: 10.2139/ssrn.5035502

Abdelmonem, B. H., Abdelaal, N. M., Anwer, E. K., Rashwan, A. A., Hussein, M. A., Ahmed, Y. F., Khashana, R., Hanna, M. M., & Abdelnaser, A. (2024). Decoding the role of CYP450 enzymes in metabolism and disease: A comprehensive review. *Biomedicines, 12*(7), 1467. DOI: 10.3390/biomedicines12071467 PMID: 39062040

Abudahab, S., Kronfol, M. M., Dozmorov, M. G., Campbell, T., Jahr, F. M., Nguyen, J., AlAzzeh, O., Al Saeedy, D. Y., Victor, A., Lee, S., Malay, S., Lapato, D. M., Halquist, M. S., McRae, M. P., Deshpande, L. S., Slattum, P. W., Price, E. T., & McClay, J. L. (2024). Genome-wide analysis of hepatic DNA methylation reveals impact of epigenetic aging on xenobiotic metabolism and transport genes in an aged mouse model. *GeroScience, 46*(6), 1–14. DOI: 10.1007/s11357-024-01137-9 PMID: 38558216

Acharya, D., & Mukhopadhyay, A. (2024). A comprehensive review of machine learning techniques for multi-omics data integration: Challenges and applications in precision oncology. *Briefings in Functional Genomics, 23*(5), elae013. Advance online publication. DOI: 10.1093/bfgp/elae013 PMID: 38600757

Alipour, M., Moghanibashi, M., Naeimi, S., & Mohamadynejad, P. (2024). Integrative bioinformatics analysis reveals ECM and nicotine-related genes in both LUAD and LUSC, but different lung fibrosis-related genes are involved in LUAD and LUSC. *Nucleosides, Nucleotides & Nucleic Acids, 43*(9), 1–20. DOI: 10.1080/15257770.2023.2300982 PMID: 38198447

Beigh, S. (2024). A Phytochemicals Approach towards the Role of Dioxins in Disease Progression Targeting Various Pathways: Insights. *Ind. J. Pharm. Edu. Res, 58*(3s), s732–s756. DOI: 10.5530/ijper.58.3s.76

Bernardo, J., & Valentão, P. (2024). Herb-drug interactions: A short review on central and peripheral nervous system drugs. *Phytotherapy Research, 38*(4), 1903–1931. DOI: 10.1002/ptr.8120 PMID: 38358734

Bhardwaj, A., Sharma, R. K., & Singh, G. B. (2021). Contagious Progression and Distribution of Arsenic in India: A Key Towards Bioremediation. *Nature Environment & Pollution Technology, 20*(2). Advance online publication. DOI: 10.46488/NEPT.2021.v20i02.037

Bisen, A. C., Sanap, S. N., Agrawal, S., Biswas, A., & Bhatta, R. S. (2023). Chemical metabolite synthesis and profiling: Mimicking in vivo biotransformation reaction. *Bioorganic Chemistry, 106722*, 106722. Advance online publication. DOI: 10.1016/j.bioorg.2023.106722

Bojić, M., Debeljak, Ž., & Guengerich, F. P. (2024). Principles of Xenobiotic Metabolism (Biotransformation). In *Pharmacogenomics in Clinical Practice* (pp. 13–33). Springer International Publishing. DOI: 10.1007/978-3-031-45903-0_2

Boyce, M., Favela, K. A., Bonzo, J. A., Chao, A., Lizarraga, L. E., Moody, L. R., Owens, E. O., Patlewicz, G., Shah, I., Sobus, J. R., Thomas, R. S., Williams, A. J., Yau, A., & Wambaugh, J. F. (2023). Identifying xenobiotic metabolites with *in-silico* prediction tools and LCMS suspect screening analysis. *Frontiers in Toxicology*, *5*, 1051483. DOI: 10.3389/ftox.2023.1051483 PMID: 36742129

Brouwer, K. L., Evers, R., Hayden, E., Hu, S., Li, C. Y., Meyer zu Schwabedissen, H. E., Neuhoff, S., Oswald, S., Piquette-Miller, M., Saran, C., Sjöstedt, N., Sprowl, J. A., Stahl, S. H., & Yue, W. (2022). Regulation of drug transport proteins—From mechanisms to clinical impact: A white paper on behalf of the international transporter consortium. *Clinical Pharmacology and Therapeutics*, *112*(3), 461–484. DOI: 10.1002/cpt.2605 PMID: 35390174

Bučko, M., Kaniaková, K., Hronská, H., Gemeiner, P., & Rosenberg, M. (2023). Epoxide hydrolases: Multipotential biocatalysts. *International Journal of Molecular Sciences*, *24*(8), 7334. DOI: 10.3390/ijms24087334 PMID: 37108499

Candura, S. M., Manzo, L., Castoldi, A. F., & Costa, L. G. (2020). Metabolism and toxicity of occupational neurotoxicants: genetic, physiological, and environmental determinants. In *Occupational neurotoxicology* (pp. 21–48). CRC Press. DOI: 10.1201/9780429281044-2

Cannon, J. R., Vachaspati, P., & Yuan, Y. (2022). A Comprehensive Picture of Biotransformation in Drug Discovery. *Drug Metabolism Handbook: Concepts and Applications in Cancer Research*, *1*, 41–101. DOI: 10.1002/9781119851042.ch4

Capone, P., Chiarella, P., & Sisto, R. (2024). Advanced technologies in genomic toxicology: Current trend and future directions. *Current Opinion in Toxicology*, *37*, 100444. DOI: 10.1016/j.cotox.2023.100444

Cassotta, M., Cianciosi, D., Elexpuru-Zabaleta, M., Pascual, I. E., Cano, S. S., Giampieri, F., & Battino, M. (2024). Human-based new approach methodologies to accelerate advances in nutrition research. *Food Frontiers*, *5*(3), 1031–1062. DOI: 10.1002/fft2.369

Chatterjee, G., Negi, S., Basu, S., Faintuch, J., O'donovan, A., & Shukla, P. (2022). Microbiome systems biology advancements for natural well-being. *The Science of the Total Environment, 838*, 155915. DOI: 10.1016/j.scitotenv.2022.155915 PMID: 35568180

Das, P., Banka, R., Ghosh, J., Singh, K., Choudhury, S. R., & Koner, S. (2024). Synergism of Diet, Genetics, and Microbiome on Health. In *Nutrition Controversies and Advances in Autoimmune Disease* (pp. 131–189). IGI Global. DOI: 10.4018/979-8-3693-5528-2.ch006

Dayyih, W. A., Al-Ani, I., Hailat, M., Alarman, S. M., Zakaraya, Z., Assab, M. A., & Alkhader, E. (2024). Review of grapefruit juice-drugs interactions mediated by intestinal CYP3A4 inhibition. *Journal of Applied Pharmaceutical Science, 14*(5), 59-68. DOI: 10.7324/JAPS.2024.160197

De Almeida, A. J. P. O., de Oliveira, J. C. P. L., da Silva Pontes, L. V., de Souza Júnior, J. F., Gonçalves, T. A. F., Dantas, S. H., de Almeida Feitosa, M. S., Silva, A. O., & de Medeiros, I. A. (2022). ROS: Basic concepts, sources, cellular signaling, and its implications in aging pathways. *Oxidative Medicine and Cellular Longevity, 2022*(1), 1225578. DOI: 10.1155/2022/1225578 PMID: 36312897

De Filippis, F., Valentino, V., Sequino, G., Borriello, G., Riccardi, M. G., Pierri, B., Cerino, P., Pizzolante, A., Pasolli, E., Esposito, M., Limone, A., & Ercolini, D. (2024). Exposure to environmental pollutants selects for xenobiotic-degrading functions in the human gut microbiome. *Nature Communications, 15*(1), 4482. DOI: 10.1038/s41467-024-48739-7 PMID: 38802370

Del Giudice, G., Serra, A., Pavel, A., Torres Maia, M., Saarimäki, L. A., Fratello, M., Federico, A., Alenius, H., Fadeel, B., & Greco, D. (2024). A network toxicology approach for mechanistic modelling of nanomaterial hazard and adverse outcomes. *Advancement of Science, 11*(32), 2400389. DOI: 10.1002/advs.202400389 PMID: 38923832

Del Pozo, S., Gómez-Martínez, S., Díaz, L. E., Nova, E., Urrialde, R., & Marcos, A. (2022). Potential effects of sucralose and saccharin on gut microbiota: A review. *Nutrients, 14*(8), 1682. DOI: 10.3390/nu14081682 PMID: 35458244

Dharmarathne, G., Kazi, S., King, S., & Jayasinghe, T. N. (2024). The Bidirectional Relationship Between Cardiovascular Medications and Oral and Gut Microbiome Health: A Comprehensive Review. *Microorganisms, 12*(11), 2246. DOI: 10.3390/microorganisms12112246 PMID: 39597635

Dimunová, D., Matoušková, P., Podlipná, R., Boušová, I., & Skálová, L. (2022). The role of UDP-glycosyltransferases in xenobioticresistance. *Drug Metabolism Reviews*, *54*(3), 282–298. DOI: 10.1080/03602532.2022.2083632 PMID: 35635097

Dudas, B., & Miteva, M. A. (2024). Computational and artificial intelligence-based approaches for drug metabolism and transport prediction. *Trends in Pharmacological Sciences*, *45*(1), 39–55. Advance online publication. DOI: 10.1016/j.tips.2023.11.001 PMID: 38072723

Durník, R., Šindlerová, L., Babica, P., & Jurček, O. (2022). Bile acids transporters of enterohepatic circulation for targeted drug delivery. *Molecules (Basel, Switzerland)*, *27*(9), 2961. DOI: 10.3390/molecules27092961 PMID: 35566302

Edo, G. I., Samuel, P. O., Oloni, G. O., Ezekiel, G. O., Ikpekoro, V. O., Obasohan, P., Ongulu, J., Otunuya, C. F., Opiti, A. R., Ajakaye, R. S., Essaghah, A. E. A., & Agbo, J. J. (2024). Environmental persistence, bioaccumulation, and ecotoxicology of heavy metals. *Chemistry and Ecology*, *40*(3), 322–349. DOI: 10.1080/02757540.2024.2306839

Farrukh, M., Shahzadi, S., & Irfan, M. (2024). Drug Metabolism: Phase I and Phase II Metabolic Pathways. In *Drug Metabolism and Pharmacokinetics*. IntechOpen. DOI: 10.5772/intechopen.112854

Fetse, J., Olawode, E. O., & Deb, S. (2024). Personalized Medicine Approach to Proteomics and Metabolomics of Cytochrome P450 Enzymes: A Narrative Review. *European Journal of Drug Metabolism and Pharmacokinetics*, *49*(6), 661–676. DOI: 10.1007/s13318-024-00912-5 PMID: 39269556

Gagliardi, A., Bajraktari-Sylejmani, G., Barocelli, E., Weiss, J., & Rigalli, J. P. (2023). Extracellular vesicles as surrogates for drug metabolism and clearance: Promise vs. reality. *Life (Chicago, Ill.)*, *13*(8), 1745. DOI: 10.3390/life13081745 PMID: 37629602

Gaither, K. A., Yue, G., Singh, D. K., Trudeau, J., Ponraj, K., Davydova, N. Y., Lazarus, P., Davydov, D. R., & Prasad, B. (2025). Effects of Chronic Alcohol Intake on the Composition of the Ensemble of Drug-Metabolizing Enzymes and Transporters in the Human Liver. *Journal of Xenobiotics*, *15*(1), 20. DOI: 10.3390/jox15010020 PMID: 39997363

Garcia, M., Thirouard, L., Sedès, L., Monrose, M., Holota, H., Caira, F., Volle, D. H., & Beaudoin, C. (2018). Nuclear receptor metabolism of bile acids and xenobiotics: A coordinated detoxification system with impact on health and diseases. *International Journal of Molecular Sciences*, *19*(11), 3630. DOI: 10.3390/ijms19113630 PMID: 30453651

Ghai, R., Mittal, A., Pandey, D., Alam, M. S., Kaushik, S., Ishtiyaq, P., Kaushik, Y., & Mishra, S. K. (2024). Role of Personalized Medicine in Clinical Practice: An Overview of Current and Future Perspectives. *Biomedical & Pharmacology Journal, 17*(4), 2111–2133. DOI: 10.13005/bpj/3011

Gong, Y., Lv, J., Pang, X., Zhang, S., Zhang, G., Liu, L., Wang, Y., & Li, C. (2023). Advances in the metabolic mechanism and functional characteristics of equol. *Foods, 12*(12), 2334. DOI: 10.3390/foods12122334 PMID: 37372545

Grocholska, P., Popiel, D., Walter, M., Biernat, M., Cebrat, M., Kuczer, M., Modzel, M., Bąchor, R., & Kluczyk, A. (2022). Citius, Altius, Fortius—Advanced Mass Spectrometry in Service of Forensic Analysis. *Chemosensors (Basel, Switzerland), 10*(8), 324. DOI: 10.3390/chemosensors10080324

Gupta, G., Maurya, S., Jha, P. N., & Chauhan, P. S. (2024). Valorization of Mushroom Spent Mushroom Substrate: A Sustainable Approach to Remediation of Xenobiotic Compounds-A Comprehensive Review. *Groundwater for Sustainable Development, 101290*. Advance online publication. DOI: 10.1016/j.gsd.2024.101290

Gupta, N. S., & Kumar, P. (2023). Perspective of artificial intelligence in healthcare data management: A journey towards precision medicine. *Computers in Biology and Medicine, 162*, 107051. DOI: 10.1016/j.compbiomed.2023.107051 PMID: 37271113

Gyaneshwari, U., Swati, K., Singh, A. K., Prakash, A., Pal, P., Kumari, B., & Pandey, B. (2023). Alcohol Dehydrogenase: Structural and Functional Diversity. In *Integrative Approaches to Biotechnology* (pp. 249-265). CRC Press. DOI: 10.1201/9781003324706-21

Hart, X. M., Gründer, G., Ansermot, N., Conca, A., Corruble, E., Crettol, S., Cumming, P., Frajerman, A., Hefner, G., Howes, O., Jukic, M. M., Kim, E., Kim, S., Maniscalco, I., Moriguchi, S., Müller, D. J., Nakajima, S., Osugo, M., Paulzen, M., & Eap, C. B. (2024). Optimisation of pharmacotherapy in psychiatry through therapeutic drug monitoring, molecular brain imaging and pharmacogenetic tests: Focus on antipsychotics. *The World Journal of Biological Psychiatry, 25*(9), 451–536. DOI: 10.1080/15622975.2024.2366235 PMID: 38913780

Herath, H. M. S. S., Herath, H. M. K. K. M. B., Madhusanka, B. G. D. A., & Guruge, L. G. P. K. (2024). Data protection challenges in the processing of sensitive data. In *Data Protection: The Wake of AI and Machine Learning* (pp. 155–179). Springer Nature Switzerland. DOI: 10.1007/978-3-031-76473-8_8

Himmel, L. E., Wilson, K. L., Santagostino, S. F., & Bolon, B. (2022). Genetically Engineered Animal Models in Toxicologic Research. In *Haschek and Rousseaux's Handbook of Toxicologic Pathology* (pp. 859–924). Academic Press. DOI: 10.1016/B978-0-12-821044-4.00024-8

Hua, Z. L. (2024). Elucidating the Role of Cytochrome p450 Enzymes in Drug Metabolism and Interactions. *Clinical Journal for Medicine, Health and Pharmacy, 2*(3), 1-10. http://cjmhp.com/index.php/journal/article/view/2.3.01

Huang, Y., Zhang, Y., Wu, K., Tan, X., Lan, T., & Wang, G. (2024). Role of Gut Microecology in the Pathogenesis of Drug-Induced Liver Injury and Emerging Therapeutic Strategies. *Molecules (Basel, Switzerland), 29*(11), 2663. DOI: 10.3390/molecules29112663 PMID: 38893536

Izat, N., Bolleddula, J., Carione, P., Huertas Valentin, L., Jones, R. S., Kulkarni, P., Moss, D., Peterkin, V. C., Tian, D. D., Treyer, A., Venkatakrishnan, K., Zientek, M. A., Barber, J., Houston, J. B., Galetin, A., & Scotcher, D. (2025). Establishing a physiologically based pharmacokinetic framework for aldehyde oxidase and dual aldehyde oxidase-CYP substrates. *CPT: Pharmacometrics & Systems Pharmacology, 14*(1), 164–178. DOI: 10.1002/psp4.13255 PMID: 39444174

Khalil, S. M., MacKenzie, K. R., Maletic-Savatic, M., & Li, F. (2024). Metabolic bioactivation of antidepressants: Advance and underlying hepatotoxicity. *Drug Metabolism Reviews, 56*(2), 97–126. DOI: 10.1080/03602532.2024.2313967 PMID: 38311829

Khani, N., Soleimani, R. A., & Rad, A. H. (2025). Potential of Postbiotics for the Biodegradation of Xenobiotics: A Review. *Current Nutrition and Food Science, 21*(6), 653–670. Advance online publication. DOI: 10.2174/0115734013325225241211033631

Khmaissa, M., Zouari-Mechichi, H., Sciara, G., Record, E., & Mechichi, T. (2024). Pollution from livestock farming antibiotics an emerging environmental and human health concern: A Review. *Journal of Hazardous Materials Advances, 100410*, 100410. Advance online publication. DOI: 10.1016/j.hazadv.2024.100410

Kleino, I., Frolovaitė, P., Suomi, T., & Elo, L. L. (2022). Computational solutions for spatial transcriptomics. *Computational and Structural Biotechnology Journal, 20*, 4870–4884. DOI: 10.1016/j.csbj.2022.08.043 PMID: 36147664

Koehn, L. M. (2022). ABC Transporters: An Overview. In Talevi, A. (Ed.), *The ADME Encyclopedia*. Springer., DOI: 10.1007/978-3-030-84860-6_76

Kurogi, K., Suiko, M., & Sakakibara, Y. (2024). Evolution and multiple functions of sulfonation and cytosolic sulfotransferases across species. *Bioscience, Biotechnology, and Biochemistry*, *88*(4), 368–380. DOI: 10.1093/bbb/zbae008 PMID: 38271594

Lettieri, M., Rodda, M., & Carlucci, V. (2024). Machine Learning in Early Prediction of Metabolism of Drugs. In *Computational Toxicology: Methods and Protocols* (pp. 275–291). Springer US., DOI: 10.1007/978-1-0716-4003-6_13

Li, S., Jiang, Z., & Wei, S. (2024). Interaction of heavy metals and polycyclic aromatic hydrocarbons in soil-crop systems: The effects and mechanisms. *Environmental Research*, *120035*, 120035. Advance online publication. DOI: 10.1016/j.envres.2024.120035 PMID: 39313170

Li, Y. (2025). Cellular Antioxidants and Phase 2 Proteins. *Molecular Basis of Oxidative Stress: Chemistry, Toxicology, Disease Pathogenesis. Diagnostics and Therapeutics*, 113–127. DOI: 10.1002/9781119790419.ch5

Liu, L., Wu, Q., Miao, X., Fan, T., Meng, Z., Chen, X., & Zhu, W. (2022). Study on toxicity effects of environmental pollutants based on metabolomics: A review. *Chemosphere*, *286*, 131815. DOI: 10.1016/j.chemosphere.2021.131815 PMID: 34375834

Liu, X. (2019). ABC Family Transporters. In Liu, X., & Pan, G. (Eds.), *Drug Transporters in Drug Disposition, Effects and Toxicity. Advances in Experimental Medicine and Biology* (Vol. 1141). Springer. DOI: 10.1007/978-981-13-7647-4_2

Lu, X., Zhang, L., Lin, G. M., Lu, J. G., & Cui, Z. B. (2024). Analysis of Differential Gene Expression under Acute Lead or Mercury Exposure in Larval Zebrafish Using RNA-Seq. *Animals (Basel)*, *14*(19), 2877. DOI: 10.3390/ani14192877 PMID: 39409826

Luan, Z. L., Zhang, C., Ming, W. H., Huang, Y. Z., Guan, Y. F., & Zhang, X. Y. (2022). Nuclear receptors in renal health and disease. *EBioMedicine*, *76*, 103855. Advance online publication. DOI: 10.1016/j.ebiom.2022.103855 PMID: 35123268

Mahanayak, B. (2024). Biotransformation reactions of xenobiotics: Mechanisms and implications for environmental and human health. *World Journal of Biology Pharmacy and Health Sciences*, *19*(1), 158–164. DOI: 10.30574/wjbphs.2024.19.1.0406

Makmor Bakry, M., Huri, Z. H., Suppiah, V., Toh, G. T., Chua, E. W., Tan, S. L. J., & Yow, H. Y. (2024). Interplay Between Genetic Variants and Morphine: Toward Personalized Medicine in Cancer Pain Management. In: *Interdisciplinary Cancer Research*. Springer, Cham. DOI: 10.1007/16833_2024_333

Mardinoglu, A., & Palsson, B. Ø. (2025). Genome-scale models in human metabologenomics. *Nature Reviews. Genetics, 26*(2), 123–140. DOI: 10.1038/s41576-024-00768-0 PMID: 39300314

Miglani, R., Parveen, N., Kumar, A., Ansari, M. A., Khanna, S., Rawat, G., Panda, A. K., Bisht, S. S., Upadhyay, J., & Ansari, M. N. (2022). Degradation of xenobiotic pollutants: An environmentally sustainable approach. *Metabolites, 12*(9), 818. DOI: 10.3390/metabo12090818 PMID: 36144222

Mohr, A. E., Ortega-Santos, C. P., Whisner, C. M., Klein-Seetharaman, J., & Jasbi, P. (2024). Navigating challenges and opportunities in multi-omics integration for personalized healthcare. *Biomedicines, 12*(7), 1496. DOI: 10.3390/biomedicines12071496 PMID: 39062068

Mokhosoev, I. M., Astakhov, D. V., Terentiev, A. A., & Moldogazieva, N. T. (2024). Human Cytochrome P450 Cancer-Related Metabolic Activities and Gene Polymorphisms: A Review. *Cells, 13*(23), 1958. DOI: 10.3390/cells13231958 PMID: 39682707

Mokrani, S., Houali, K., Yadav, K. K., Arabi, A. I. A., Eltayeb, L. B., AwjanAlreshidi, M., Benguerba, Y., Cabral-Pinto, M. M. S., & Nabti, E. (2024). Bioremediation techniques for soil organic pollution: Mechanisms, microorganisms, and technologies-A comprehensive review. *Ecological Engineering, 207*, 107338. DOI: 10.1016/j.ecoleng.2024.107338

Motsinger-Reif, A. A., Reif, D. M., Akhtari, F. S., House, J. S., Campbell, C. R., Messier, K. P., Fargo, D. C., Bowen, T. A., Nadadur, S. S., Schmitt, C. P., Pettibone, K. G., Balshaw, D. M., Lawler, C. P., Newton, S. A., Collman, G. W., Miller, A. K., Merrick, B. A., Cui, Y., Anchang, B., & Woychik, R. (2024). Gene-environment interactions within a precision environmental health framework. *Cell Genomics, 4*(7), 100591. Advance online publication. DOI: 10.1016/j.xgen.2024.100591 PMID: 38925123

Mousa, S., Sarfraz, M., & Mousa, W. K. (2023). The interplay between gut microbiota and oral medications and its impact on advancing precision medicine. *Metabolites, 13*(5), 674. DOI: 10.3390/metabo13050674 PMID: 37233715

Nagini, S., Kallamadi, P. R., Tanagala, K. K. K., & Reddy, G. B. (2024). Aldo-keto reductases: Role in cancer development and theranostics. *Oncology Research, 32*(8), 1287–1308. DOI: 10.32604/or.2024.049918 PMID: 39055885

Narendra, G., Choudhary, S., Raju, B., Verma, H., & Silakari, O. (2022). Role of genetic polymorphisms in drug-metabolizing enzyme-mediated toxicity and pharmacokinetic resistance to anti-cancer agents: A review on the pharmacogenomics aspect. *Clinical Pharmacokinetics*, *61*(11), 1495–1517. DOI: 10.1007/s40262-022-01174-7 PMID: 36180817

Ouma, R. B., Ngari, S. M., & Kibet, J. K. (2024). A review of the current trends in computational approaches in drug design and metabolism. *Discover Public Health*, *21*(1), 108. DOI: 10.1186/s12982-024-00229-3

Ozbek, O., Genc, D. E., & Ulgen, O., K. (. (2024). Advances in Physiologically Based Pharmacokinetic (PBPK) Modeling of Nanomaterials. *ACS Pharmacology & Translational Science*, *7*(8), 2251–2279. DOI: 10.1021/acsptsci.4c00250 PMID: 39144562

Panda, C., Komarnytsky, S., Fleming, M. N., Marsh, C., Barron, K., Le Brun-Blashka, S., & Metzger, B. (2023). Guided Metabolic Detoxification program supports phase II detoxification enzymes and antioxidant balance in healthy participants. *Nutrients*, *15*(9), 2209. DOI: 10.3390/nu15092209 PMID: 37432335

Panebianco, C., Andriulli, A., & Pazienza, V. (2018). Pharmacomicrobiomics: Exploiting the drug-microbiota interactions in anticancer therapies. *Microbiome*, *6*(1), 1–13. DOI: 10.1186/s40168-018-0483-7 PMID: 29789015

Pant, A., Maiti, T. K., Mahajan, D., & Das, B. (2023). Human gut microbiota and drug metabolism. *Microbial Ecology*, *86*(1), 97–111. DOI: 10.1007/s00248-022-02081-x PMID: 35869999

Park, H. E., Jo, S. H., Lee, R. H., Macks, C. P., Ku, T., Park, J., Lee, C. W., Hur, J. K., & Sohn, C. H. (2023). Spatial transcriptomics: Technical aspects of recent developments and their applications in neuroscience and cancer research. *Advancement of Science*, *10*(16), 2206939. DOI: 10.1002/advs.202206939 PMID: 37026425

Pecori Giraldi, F., Ferraù, F., Ragonese, M., & Cannavò, S. (2024). Endocrine disruptors, aryl hydrocarbon receptor and cortisol secretion. *Journal of Endocrinological Investigation*, *47*(10), 1–13. DOI: 10.1007/s40618-024-02371-w PMID: 38637430

Penning, T. M., Su, A. L., & El-Bayoumy, K. (2022). Nitroreduction: A critical metabolic pathway for drugs, environmental pollutants, and explosives. *Chemical Research in Toxicology*, *35*(10), 1747–1765. DOI: 10.1021/acs.chemrestox.2c00175 PMID: 36044734

Priya, A. K., Muruganandam, M., Kumar, A., Senthilkumar, N., Shkir, M., Pandit, B., Imran, M., Prakash, C., & Ubaidullah, M. (2024). Recent advances in microbial-assisted degradation and remediation of xenobiotic contaminants; challenges and future prospects. *Journal of Water Process Engineering*, *60*, 105106. DOI: 10.1016/j.jwpe.2024.105106

Priyadarshini, B. I.B. Indira Priyadarshini. (2024). Deep Learning for Predictive Toxicology Assessment Early Detection of Adverse Drug Reactions. *Power System Technology*, *48*(1), 680–697. DOI: 10.52783/pst.322

Qriouet, Z., Qmichou, Z., Bouchoutrouch, N., Mahi, H., Cherrah, Y., & Sefrioui, H. (2019). Analytical methods used for the detection and quantification of benzodiazepines. *Journal of Analytical Methods in Chemistry*, *2019*(1), 2035492. DOI: 10.1155/2019/2035492 PMID: 31583157

Rahman, M., Irmler, M., Introna, M., Beckers, J., Palmberg, L., Johanson, G., Upadhyay, S., & Ganguly, K. (2022). Insight into the pulmonary molecular toxicity of heated tobacco products using human bronchial and alveolar mucosa models at air–liquid interface. *Scientific Reports*, *12*(1), 16396. DOI: 10.1038/s41598-022-20657-y PMID: 36180488

Rai, M., Paudel, N., Sakhrie, M., Gemmati, D., Khan, I. A., Tisato, V., Kanase, A., Schulz, A., & Singh, A. V. (2023). Perspective on quantitative structure–toxicity relationship (QSTR) models to predict hepatic biotransformation of xenobiotics. *Livers*, *3*(3), 448–462. DOI: 10.3390/livers3030032

Ratnasekhar, C. H., Rathor, P., Rakwal, P., Verma, A. K., & Khan, S. (2024). Analytical platforms in metabolomics of health and disease. In *Comprehensive Analytical Chemistry* (Vol. 104, pp. 1–20). Elsevier. DOI: 10.1016/bs.coac.2023.09.007

Rodríguez, A. T. (2024). Clinically important pharmacokinetic drug-drug interactions with antibacterial agents. *Revista Española de Quimioterapia*, *37*(4), 299–322. DOI: 10.37201/req/037.2024 PMID: 38840420

Salazar-González, R. A., Doll, M. A., & Hein, D. W. (2023). N-acetyltransferase 2 genetic polymorphism modifies genotoxic and oxidative damage from new psychoactive substances. *Archives of Toxicology*, *97*(1), 189–199. DOI: 10.1007/s00204-022-03383-2 PMID: 36138126

Sayyed, Y., Rehman, K., Akash, M. S. H., Kamran, S. H., & Badran, M. (2022). Xenobiotics and drug-metabolizing enzymes: Challenges and strategies. In *Biochemistry of Drug Metabolizing Enzymes* (pp. 305–321). Academic Press., DOI: 10.1016/B978-0-323-95120-3.00007-5

Sharma, P., Siwan, D., & Rudrapal, M. (2024). Introductory Chapter: Pharmacokinetics and Drug Metabolism with Special Reference to Herbal Formulations. In *Drug Metabolism and Pharmacokinetics*. IntechOpen. DOI: 10.5772/intechopen.112889

Shi, C., Cheng, L., Yu, Y., Chen, S., Dai, Y., Yang, J., Zhang, H., Chen, J., & Geng, N. (2024). Multi-omics integration analysis: Tools and applications in environmental toxicology. *Environmental Pollution, 124675*, 124675. Advance online publication. DOI: 10.1016/j.envpol.2024.124675 PMID: 39103035

Shi, Y. S., Zhao, Y., Li, X. N., Li, M. Z., & Li, J. L. (2023). Xenobiotic-sensing nuclear receptors as targets for phthalates-induced lung injury and antagonism of lycopene. *Chemosphere, 312*, 137265. DOI: 10.1016/j.chemosphere.2022.137265 PMID: 36403809

Shi, Z., & Han, S. (2025). Personalized statin therapy: Targeting metabolic processes to modulate the therapeutic and adverse effects of statins. *Heliyon, 11*(1), e41629. Advance online publication. DOI: 10.1016/j.heliyon.2025.e41629 PMID: 39866414

Show, S., & Halder, G. (2024). Biodegradation of Anti-Inflammatory, Non-Steroidal, Pharmaceutical Active Compounds. In *Biodegradation of Toxic and Hazardous Chemicals* (pp. 14–29). CRC Press. DOI: 10.1201/9781003391487-2

Shreenidhi, K. S., Vigneshwar, R., Sv, S. R., Maline, M., Roy, S., & Geetha, V. (2024). A Study on Toxicity Mechanisms of Xenobiotics Using Network Pharmacology Approach. *Current Trends in Biotechnology and Pharmacy, 18*(4s), 138–151. DOI: 10.5530/ctbp.2024.4s.11

Singh, M., Mishra, R. C., Shah, I., Wadhwa, V., & Mor, V. (2023a). Xenobiotics: Sources, Pathways, Degradation, and Risk Associated with Major Emphasis on Pharmaceutical Compounds. In *Xenobiotics in Urban Ecosystems: Sources, Distribution and Health Impacts* (pp. 87–106). Springer International Publishing. DOI: 10.1007/978-3-031-35775-6_5

Singh, S., Sarma, D. K., Verma, V., Nagpal, R., & Kumar, M. (2023b). Unveiling the future of metabolic medicine: Omics technologies driving personalized solutions for precision treatment of metabolic disorders. *Biochemical and Biophysical Research Communications, 682*, 1–20. Advance online publication. DOI: 10.1016/j.bbrc.2023.09.064 PMID: 37788525

Skonberg, C., & Olsen, J. (2023). A review of the synthesis, bioanalysis, and chemical reactivity of xenobiotic acyl-coenzyme a thioesters. *Medicinal Chemistry Research, 32*(9), 2001–2015. DOI: 10.1007/s00044-023-03129-4

Stanley, L. A. (2024). Drug metabolism. In *Pharmacognosy* (pp. 597–624). Academic Press. DOI: 10.1016/B978-0-443-18657-8.00029-3

Surendradoss, J., Varghese, A., & Deb, S. (2023). Drug metabolism: Detoxification and xenobiotic biotransformation. In *Biologically Active Small Molecules* (pp. 287–332). Apple Academic Press. DOI: 10.1201/9781003283119-17

Talevi, A., & Bellera, C. L. (2022). Organic anion transporters and organic anion transporting polypeptides. In *The ADME Encyclopedia: A Comprehensive Guide on Biopharmacy and Pharmacokinetics* (pp. 739–745). Springer International Publishing. DOI: 10.1007/978-3-030-84860-6_84

Terrazas-Salgado, L., García-Gasca, A., Betancourt-Lozano, M., Llera-Herrera, R., Alvarado-Cruz, I., & Yáñez-Rivera, B. (2022). Epigenetic transgenerational modifications induced by xenobiotic exposure in zebrafish. *Frontiers in Cell and Developmental Biology*, *10*, 832982. DOI: 10.3389/fcell.2022.832982 PMID: 35281093

Vicidomini, C., Palumbo, R., Moccia, M., & Roviello, G. N. (2024). Oxidative Processes and Xenobiotic Metabolism in Plants: Mechanisms of Defense and Potential Therapeutic Implications. *Journal of Xenobiotics*, *14*(4), 1541–1569. DOI: 10.3390/jox14040084 PMID: 39449425

Wright, A. T., Hudson, L. A., & Garcia, W. L. (2023). Activity-Based Protein Profiling–Enabling Phenotyping of Host-Associated and Environmental Microbiomes. *Israel Journal of Chemistry*, *63*(3-4), e202200099. DOI: 10.1002/ijch.202200099

Xie, M. Z., Liu, J. L., Gao, Q. Z., Bo, D. Y., Wang, L., Zhou, X. C., Zhao, M. M., Zhang, Y. C., Zhang, Y. J., Zhao, G. A., & Jiao, L. Y. (2022). Proteomics-based evaluation of the mechanism underlying vascular injury via DNA interstrand crosslinks, glutathione perturbation, mitogen-activated protein kinase, and Wnt and ErbB signaling pathways induced by crotonaldehyde. *Clinical Proteomics*, *19*(1), 33. DOI: 10.1186/s12014-022-09369-7 PMID: 36002804

Xu, S., Lan, H., Huang, C., Ge, X., & Zhu, J. (2024). Mechanisms and emerging strategies for irinotecan-induced diarrhea. *European Journal of Pharmacology*, *176614*, 176614. Advance online publication. DOI: 10.1016/j.ejphar.2024.176614 PMID: 38677535

Yang, H., Yu, F., Qian, Z., Huang, T., Peng, T., & Hu, Z. (2024). Cytochrome P450 for environmental remediation: Catalytic mechanism, engineering strategies and future prospects. *World Journal of Microbiology & Biotechnology*, *40*(1), 33. DOI: 10.1007/s11274-023-03823-w PMID: 38057619

Yu, F., Liu, Y., Zhang, R., Zhu, L., Zhang, T., & Shi, Y. (2022a). Recent advances in circadian-regulated pharmacokinetics and its implications for chronotherapy. *Biochemical Pharmacology, 203*, 115185. DOI: 10.1016/j.bcp.2022.115185 PMID: 35902039

Yu, W., Zhang, Y., & Sang, W. (2022b). Integration of transcriptomic and metabolomic reveals metabolic pathway alteration in earthworms (*Eisenia fetida*) under copper exposure. *Comparative Biochemistry and Physiology. Toxicology & Pharmacology : CBP*, *260*, 109400. DOI: 10.1016/j.cbpc.2022.109400 PMID: 35753647

Chapter 3

Systems Biology and Integrative Omics Decoding Xenobiotic Metabolism in Environmental Carcinogenesis:
Xenobiotic Metabolism in Carcinogenesis

Wael Mohamed El-Sayed
https://orcid.org/0000-0002-3622-1417
Ain Shams University, Cairo, Egypt

Yaser Mahmoud Hassan
http://orcid.org/0009-0008-0061-739X
Ain Shams University, Cairo, Egypt

Hafsa Abdellah Gwidah
Tanta University, Tanta, Egypt

Abdulrahman Khalid Shalaby
https://orcid.org/0009-0001-8672-854X
Ain Shams University, Cairo, Egypt

Mahmoud Salah Mahmoud
Ain Shams University, Cairo, Egypt

Mohamed Mohseen Waly
https://orcid.org/0009-0002-6529-6570
Helwan University, Cairo, Egypt

Ahmed Samy Mohamed
Ain Shams University, Cairo, Egypt

Youssef Mohamed Hassan
Ain Shams University, Cairo, Egypt

Majdeldin Ehab Abdelgilil
Ain Shams University, Cairo, Egypt

DOI: 10.4018/979-8-3373-2165-3.ch003

ABSTRACT

This chapter explores how xenobiotics contribute to cancer development through interactions with DNA and disruption of metabolic processes. It highlights the role of drug-metabolizing enzymes in cancer risk. The chapter emphasizes the importance of an integrated approach, combining genetic, environmental, and metabolic factors for cancer prevention. The emerging field of cancer exposomics is discussed, with a focus on how environmental exposures, such as pollution and diet, alter molecular pathways involved in inflammation, oxidative stress, and cancer cell proliferation. The role of the gut microbiome in metabolizing xenobiotics is explored, as well as the potential for therapies like probiotics, prebiotics, and fecal microbiota transplantation to reduce cancer risk. Additionally, epigenetic changes are examined in the context of cancer susceptibility and detoxification. The chapter concludes with a discussion of how systems biology, omics technologies, and epigenetics offer new opportunities for personalized cancer prevention and treatment strategies.

INTRODUCTION

Cancer remains one of the most pressing public health challenges globally, and growing evidence implicates chronic environmental exposures in its development. While genetics plays a crucial role in cancer susceptibility, it is now clear that xenobiotics—foreign chemical substances originating from industrial pollutants, pesticides, pharmaceuticals, and dietary sources—significantly influence disease onset and progression. Despite this, the molecular mechanisms through which xenobiotics contribute to carcinogenesis are not fully understood, and their role is often underestimated in traditional cancer research.

Increasing environmental exposure to xenobiotics—such as heavy metals, pesticides, and endocrine-disrupting chemicals—has been implicated in the rising incidence of various cancers. These exposures disrupt normal metabolic processes and epigenetic regulation, leading to increased cancer susceptibility. Understanding the mechanisms by which xenobiotics contribute to cancer risk is crucial for developing targeted therapeutic strategies aimed at mitigating these effects. Particularly, xenobiotic-induced metabolic and epigenetic disruptions may play a critical role in cancer complications such as metastasis, underscoring the urgency of therapeutic interventions that address these underlying mechanisms.

This chapter addresses an urgent need to examine how xenobiotics interact with metabolic and genetic systems to disrupt cellular homeostasis, promote DNA damage, and drive epigenetic alterations that increase cancer risk. It comes at a critical time when the fields of systems biology, exposomics, and integrative omics are converging to provide more holistic and mechanistic insights into environmental carcinogenesis.

By synthesizing current evidence, this chapter aims to highlight the clinical and societal relevance of decoding xenobiotic metabolism within the context of cancer risk and chemoprevention. It explores how gene-environment interactions, metabolic pathways, and microbiome dynamics shape individual responses to toxic exposures, offering potential avenues for biomarker discovery, targeted interventions, and personalized medicine. Ultimately, these insights hold transformative potential for advancing cancer prevention strategies and guiding the development of future therapies tailored to environmentally driven carcinogenic processes.

1. SYNOPSIS OF XENOBIOTICS METABOLISM AND CANCER

The human body is continually exposed to xenobiotics—foreign substances from environmental, dietary, and pharmaceutical sources. How these compounds are metabolized plays a pivotal role in determining whether they are detoxified or transformed into harmful agents. While some undergo harmless excretion, others are metabolically activated into carcinogens capable of damaging DNA and other cellular components. These interactions can accumulate over time, contributing to carcinogenesis.

Understanding xenobiotic metabolism is essential for evaluating cancer risk. Metabolic processes are influenced not only by chemical structure but also by genetic variability and environmental factors. This section explores how xenobiotics are processed in the body and how their metabolic fate can influence cancer development, with a focus on the integrative role of environmental, genetic, and lifestyle factors.

1.1. Introduction to Xenobiotics

Xenobiotics include any compounds not naturally produced by the human body. These substances may originate from air pollutants, industrial chemicals, pesticides, food additives, and pharmaceuticals. For instance, tobacco smoke contains numerous xenobiotics, including carcinogens such as benzo[a]pyrene, a polycyclic aromatic hydrocarbon (PAH). When metabolized, benzo[a]pyrene can form reactive intermediates that bind to DNA and potentially lead to cancer (He & Feng, 2015). Other xenobiotics include foodborne toxins and persistent agricultural chemicals like DDT, which, although banned in many countries, remains in the environment. DDT is metabolized into compounds capable of binding DNA and contributing to cancers in the lung, liver, and other organs (Moon et al., 2006). Heavy metals such as arsenic—a well-documented carcinogen (Goode et al., 2011)—and synthetic compounds in cosmetics, plastics, and industrial waste also fall under this category. The toxicological impact of xenobiotics depends on their chemical properties, metabolic fate, and individual genetic susceptibility.

1.2. Xenobiotics Metabolism and Procarcinogen Activation

The body metabolizes xenobiotics through a two-phase enzymatic system that modifies their structure for detoxification or, in some cases, activation into more harmful forms. Phase I metabolism involves oxidation, reduction, or hydrolysis reactions that introduce or expose functional groups. The cytochrome P450 (CYP) family, especially hepatic enzymes, plays a pivotal role. For instance, CYP1A1 breaks down benzo[a]pyrene into reactive intermediates that can form DNA adducts, thereby initiating carcinogenesis (Guengerich, 2006). Although Phase I can detoxify certain substances, it may also activate procarcinogens—compounds that become carcinogenic only after metabolic conversion. A classic example is aflatoxin B1 (AFB1), a dietary contaminant that is metabolized into DNA-binding intermediates associated with cancer (Phillips, 1999).

Other procarcinogens include benzo[a]pyrene and nitrosamines, which are activated by CYP enzymes. Benzo[a]pyrene, found in tobacco smoke, grilled foods, and pollutants, becomes a potent DNA-reactive carcinogen after metabolic activation (Williams & Phillips, 2000). Similarly, nitrosamines from processed meats and tobacco undergo CYP-mediated bioactivation, producing mutagenic compounds linked to stomach, liver, and lung cancers (He & Feng, 2015; Mokhosoev et al., 2024).

Phase II metabolism follows, where the reactive intermediates are conjugated with molecules like glucuronic acid, sulfate, or glutathione. These reactions increase the water solubility of the compounds, promoting their excretion via urine or bile. Enzymes such as UDP-glucuronosyltransferases (UDPGTs) and glutathione S-transferases (GSTs) are central to this detoxification phase. However, in rare cases, Phase II can also generate toxic intermediates that form DNA adducts or induce oxidative stress (Clerici et al., 2014). Understanding the dual roles of xenobiotic-metabolizing enzymes—both in detoxification and procarcinogen activation—is essential to identifying environmental and dietary cancer risk factors (Figure 1).

Figure 1. Xenobiotic metabolism occurs in two phases. Phase I, mediated by cytochrome P450 enzymes, introduces functional groups through oxidation, reduction, or hydrolysis, activating pro-carcinogens like benzo[a]pyrene, aflatoxin B1, and nitrosamines into DNA-reactive intermediates. Phase II involves conjugation with glucuronic acid, sulfate, or glutathione to enhance solubility and facilitate excretion, with key enzymes like UDP-glucuronosyltransferases and glutathione S-transferases. While Phase II generally detoxifies, some reactions can produce reactive species, influencing cancer risk from environmental and dietary exposures.

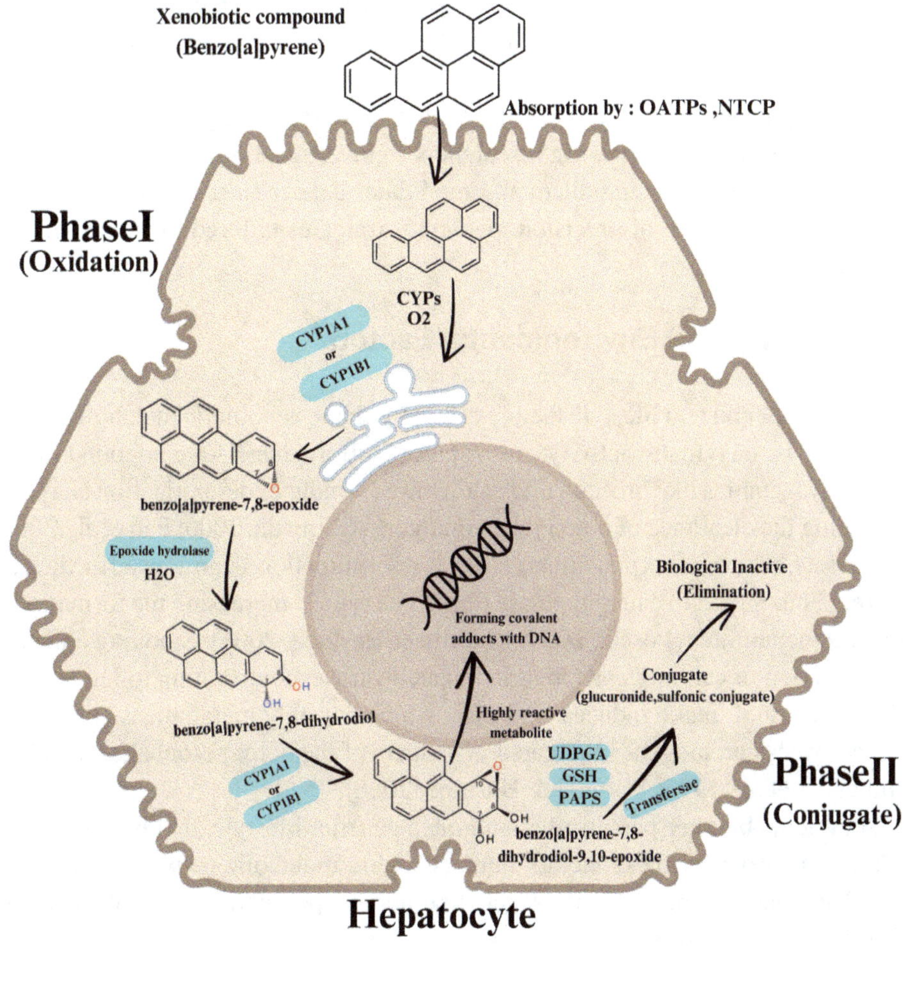

1.3. Genetic Variations in Xenobiotic-Metabolizing Enzymes

Genetic polymorphisms in xenobiotic-metabolizing enzymes significantly affect how individuals process foreign compounds. Variations in genes encoding CYP1A1 and CYP2E1 may enhance or reduce enzyme activity, thereby altering cancer susceptibility. For instance, certain CYP1A1 polymorphisms are associated with increased activation of tobacco-related carcinogens and a heightened risk of lung cancer (Masson et al., 2005; C. S. Yang, 2015). Similarly, polymorphisms in Phase II enzymes such as GSTs may impair the detoxification of reactive intermediates, increasing cancer risk when individuals are exposed to environmental toxins (Lauby-Secretan et al., 2016).

Recent progress in systems biology enables integration of genomic, proteomic, and metabolomic data, allowing researchers to investigate how genetic variability influences xenobiotic metabolism and modulates cancer risk. This approach supports the development of precision medicine strategies tailored to an individual's genetic profile.

1.4. Lifestyle and Environmental Factors

Environmental and lifestyle factors critically shape xenobiotic metabolism. Diet can modulate enzymatic activity; for instance, sulforaphane—a compound in cruciferous vegetables like broccoli and cauliflower—induces detoxification enzymes, enhancing the clearance of potential carcinogens (Shimada, 2006; Fan et al., 2007). Conversely, behaviors such as smoking, alcohol consumption, or prolonged medication use (e.g., omeprazole) can upregulate Phase I enzymes, increasing the formation of harmful metabolites (Poschl, 2004; Boffetta & Hashibe, 2006). Smoking enhances the activation of carcinogens found in tobacco smoke, contributing to lung cancer. Chronic alcohol intake induces CYP2E1, which not only metabolizes ethanol but also activates carcinogens implicated in cancers of the colon, esophagus, and liver (Anderson et al., 1995; Boffetta & Hashibe, 2006).

A systems biology perspective integrates genetic, lifestyle, and environmental data to uncover how these factors interact within metabolic networks. This integrated approach enables identification of vulnerable populations and informs more effective, targeted prevention strategies.

Conclusion

Xenobiotic metabolism plays a central role in determining cancer risk. While Phase I and Phase II pathways generally aid in detoxification, they can also generate reactive intermediates capable of initiating cancer. Genetic differences in enzyme expression, coupled with environmental and lifestyle exposures, further modulate these effects. Through systems biology and integrative omics, researchers can comprehensively assess the interactions between xenobiotics, genetics, and environmental factors. This insight is pivotal for advancing cancer prevention, personalized therapies, and public health strategies.

Key Takeaways

- Xenobiotics are foreign substances (e.g., pollutants, tobacco, pesticides) that may increase cancer risk through DNA and protein interactions.
- Phase I metabolism (e.g., CYP enzymes) can activate procarcinogens such as benzo[a]pyrene and aflatoxin B1.
- Phase II metabolism typically detoxifies these intermediates but may also yield harmful byproducts in rare cases.
- Genetic polymorphisms in metabolic enzymes (e.g., CYP1A1, GSTs) influence how individuals process xenobiotics, affecting cancer risk.
- Lifestyle and environmental exposures (e.g., smoking, diet, alcohol) alter enzyme activity and influence carcinogen activation or detoxification.
- Systems biology and omics offer a powerful framework to understand xenobiotic metabolism and enable personalized cancer prevention.

2. SYSTEMS BIOLOGY IN CANCER EXPOSOMICS

Cancer exposomics involves the comprehensive study of environmental factors—such as pollution, tobacco smoke, occupational chemicals, and diet—and their interactions with biological systems that contribute to cancer development. This approach emphasizes the importance of understanding how environmental exposures influence the molecular processes involved in cancer initiation and progression. In cancer research, systems biology is invaluable for understanding how these environmental exposures interact with host factors to drive cancer development. By integrating multi-omics data, systems biology helps unravel the complex molecular networks that govern cancer initiation and progression, providing insights that are not apparent when studying individual components in isolation (Mathis et al., 2015).

2.1. Mapping Exposures to Molecular Pathways

Environmental exposures, such as pollution, tobacco smoke, and occupational chemicals, can significantly alter biological processes and molecular pathways, potentially leading to cancer. Systems biology approaches have been pivotal in linking these environmental exposures to the molecular mechanisms driving cancer biology. These methods provide insight into how environmental factors influence cancer initiation and progression by connecting them to specific molecular pathways (Mathis et al., 2015).

A key aspect of systems biology in cancer exposomics involves the use of computational models to understand how environmental toxins, such as air pollution and tobacco smoke, trigger biological pathways. These models help researchers outline the sequence of cellular events initiated by the body's response to these toxins. By identifying genes, proteins, and metabolic pathways activated or suppressed by environmental exposures, computational models enable researchers to correlate these molecular changes with cancer development (J. N. Smith et al., 2022). For instance, exposure to cigarette smoke has been shown to activate transcription factors like AP-1 and NFE2L2, which play a role in signaling the oxidative stress response. In response to cigarette smoke, the proteins KEAP1 and Bach1 are normally responsible for suppressing NFE2L2. This inhibition leads to the activation of detoxification genes, including those involved in CYP450 metabolism, which is crucial for the breakdown of xenobiotics (Mathis et al., 2015).

Beyond oxidative stress, cigarette smoke also affects inflammatory pathways, altering key pathways like the interferon gamma-dependent pathway and inhibiting NF-κB. Chronic inflammation, a common feature of diseases like chronic obstructive pulmonary disease (COPD), leads to increased production of reactive nitrogen and oxygen species (RNOS). These species are implicated in lung cancer development (Parris et al., 2019). Moreover, the activation of the NF-κB signaling pathway is linked to enhanced cancer cell invasion, migration, and proliferation—processes that contribute to cancer progression and metastasis (Neagu et al., 2024).

Environmental exposures also influence cellular proliferation pathways. For example, following exposure to cigarette smoke, there is an increase in the activity of EGF receptor (EGFR) family members and their ligands, which activate signaling pathways like MAPK, PI3K, and RAS—well-known drivers of cancer cell growth (Mathis et al., 2015). Similarly, other xenobiotics, such as Bisphenol A (BPA), activate the Wnt/β-catenin pathway, enhancing both cancer cell proliferation and aggressiveness (Neagu et al., 2024). These pathways contribute to genetic instability, DNA damage, and aberrant DNA methylation, further advancing cancer progression (Neagu et al., 2024).

Environmental exposures can also modulate immune system responses, with significant implications for cancer development. For instance, research has shown that the lung microbiome can activate γδ T-cells, producing IL-17—a cytokine that contributes to inflammation and tumor proliferation in the lungs. Chronic inflammation, resulting from environmental exposures, is closely linked to increased cellular proliferation, metastasis, and chemotherapy resistance in lung tumors (Parris et al., 2019). This highlights the complex interplay between the immune system, inflammation, and cancer, with environmental factors playing a pivotal role in shaping these responses (Figure 2).

Figure 2. A circular systems biology framework illustrating how environmental exposures, such as cigarette smoke (CS), particulate matter (PM2.5), bisphenol A (BPA), and industrial xenobiotics, interact with cellular sensors (e.g., KEAP1, EGFR, AHR) to activate signaling pathways. These pathways, including oxidative stress (via NFE2L2), inflammation (via NF-κB and IL-17), and cell proliferation (via MAPK, PI3K, Wnt/β-catenin), drive oncogenic processes like DNA damage, genomic instability, DNA methylation alterations, immune modulation, tumor growth, metastasis, and therapy resistance. The systems biology hub integrates multi-omics data using computational models to identify exposure-specific networks and predict links between environmental factors and cancer. The closed-loop design emphasizes the ongoing impact of environmental exposure on sustained oncogenic signaling.

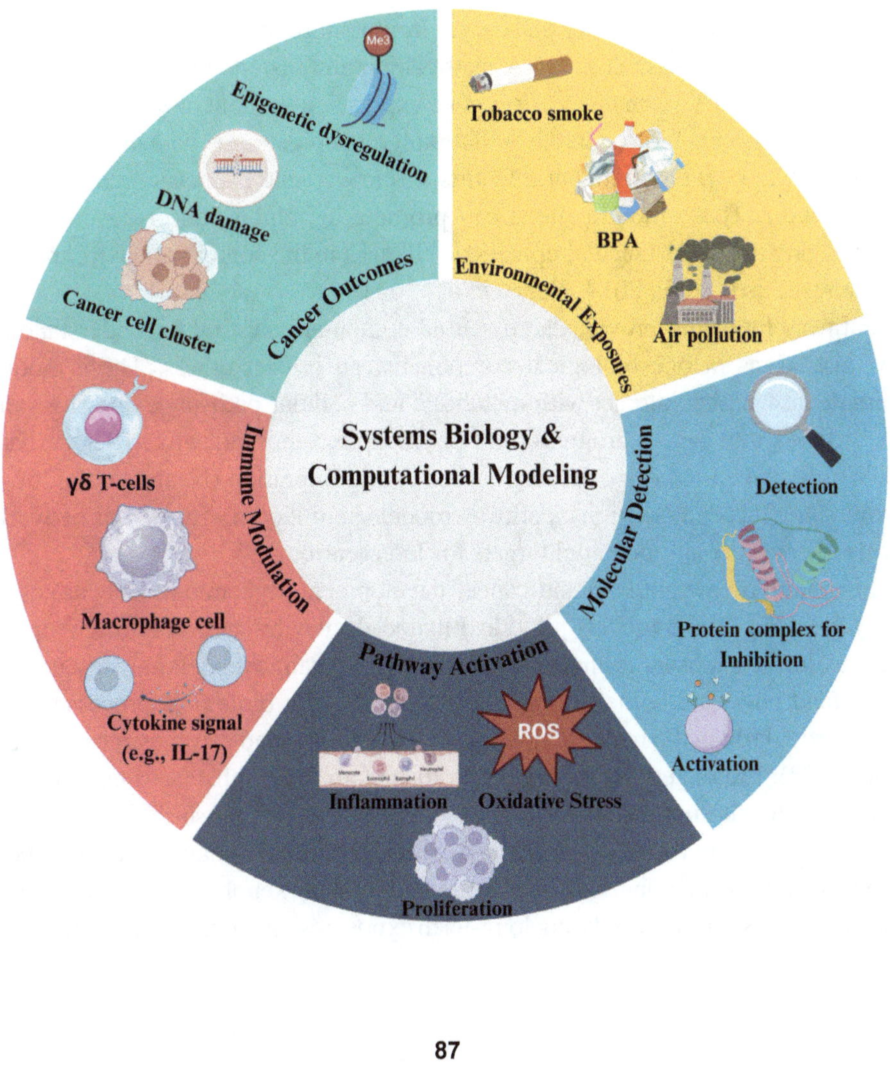

2.2. Key Tools and Techniques in Systems Biology

Recent advances in technology have allowed researchers to uncover the molecular impacts of environmental exposures that may otherwise be difficult to detect using traditional methods. Key techniques in systems biology, such as gene expression profiling, epigenomics, and pathway modeling, are essential for understanding how xenobiotics affect biological systems and contribute to cancer development.

Gene expression profiling is one critical tool, enabling researchers to monitor the expression levels of thousands of genes simultaneously. This technique helps reveal how environmental exposures influence cellular activity and gene expression. By comparing gene expression before and after exposure to carcinogens, researchers can identify genes associated with cancer development. For instance, large-scale studies of gene expression have provided valuable insights into lung cancer and COPD, linking environmental exposures to altered gene expression patterns (Parris et al., 2019).

Epigenomics, which focuses on how environmental exposures can induce changes in the epigenome—such as DNA methylation and histone modifications—also plays a key role. These changes affect gene expression without altering the genetic code itself. Systems biology models that integrate epigenomic data are crucial for understanding how environmental factors influence gene expression and contribute to cancer. These modifications can promote or inhibit cancer development, emphasizing the importance of epigenetic changes in the context of environmental exposures (Parris et al., 2019; Neagu et al., 2024).

Pathway modeling provides an essential computational tool for understanding how alterations in one biological component can impact others. These models simulate how toxins interact with metabolic and cellular pathways, offering valuable insights into cancer progression. For example, xenobiotics like BPA activate the Wnt/β-catenin pathway, driving cancer cell proliferation (Neagu et al., 2024). By mapping these interactions, pathway models help identify molecular networks involved in cancer and potential targets for intervention.

In xenobiotic metabolism and cancer development, dynamic models are especially valuable. These models provide a nuanced view by incorporating temporal changes during exposure to environmental toxins. Dynamic models help researchers understand how environmental exposures interact with biological processes over time, particularly in the realm of xenobiotic metabolism and carcinogenesis (Lapin et al., 2022). Prolonged or cumulative exposures to toxic substances can increase cancer risk by altering metabolic pathways and cellular responses.

Time-dependent feedback loops are a critical feature of dynamic models. These loops illustrate how feedback mechanisms evolve during xenobiotic metabolism and cancer progression. By simulating long-term exposures, dynamic models show how detoxification pathways adapt to environmental stress, emphasizing the increasing cancer risk linked to cumulative exposures (Smith et al., 2022). These models offer critical insights into the temporal nature of toxic exposure and its cumulative effects on cancer risk.

CYP enzymes play a central role in metabolizing many carcinogens, including polycyclic aromatic hydrocarbons (PAHs) found in tobacco smoke. Enzymes like CYP1A1 and CYP2C19 are involved in bioactivating carcinogens like Benzo[a]pyrene (BaP), converting them into reactive metabolites that can damage DNA (Smith et al., 2022). However, enzymes like CYP3A4 also play a protective role by helping detoxify BaP. The dual roles of enzymes like CYP1A1—participating in both bioactivation and detoxification—make them crucial for understanding cancer risk, particularly in the context of environmental exposures (Smith et al., 2022).

PAH metabolism is often studied to understand the long-term effects of repeated exposure to carcinogens like those found in tobacco smoke. Systems biology tools enable researchers to simulate how genetic variations in detoxifying enzymes, such as CYP450, influence cancer risk in smokers, crucial for assessing individual susceptibility to cancer following environmental toxin exposure (Smith et al., 2022).

Competitive metabolism is another important consideration in xenobiotic metabolism. Studies have shown that PAHs in mixtures can compete for the same metabolic pathways, potentially altering the bioactivation of carcinogens. For example, BaP can inhibit the metabolism of another carcinogen, DBC, highlighting the complexity of interactions among environmental toxins (Smith et al., 2022). This underscores the importance of considering the interplay between various toxins when assessing cancer risk.

Physiologically based pharmacokinetic (PBPK) models provide insights into how competitive metabolism affects the internal dosimetry of chemicals. These models are valuable for predicting how mixtures of chemicals interact within the body and evaluating the potential risks posed by environmental toxins (Smith et al., 2022). PBPK models help refine our understanding of exposure risks by simulating the behavior of multiple toxins within biological systems.

Case Studies: Applications of Systems Biology in Environmental Carcinogenesis

Case studies demonstrate the power of systems biology in understanding the intricate interactions between environmental toxins and cancer biology. By integrating multiple layers of biological data, systems biology enables researchers to explore how environmental exposures contribute to cancer initiation and progression. Two key case studies—tobacco smoke and arsenic exposure—illustrate how these approaches enhance our understanding of carcinogenesis.

Case Study 1: Tobacco Smoke and Lung Cancer

Systems biology plays a pivotal role in uncovering how the toxic chemicals in tobacco affect cellular processes, particularly through their interactions with the p53 tumor suppressor gene. Tobacco smoke contains a variety of carcinogens, including PAHs and N-nitrosamines, metabolized into reactive forms capable of damaging DNA (Gibbons et al., 2014). This damage initiates mutations in critical genes, setting the stage for lung cancer development.

One of the most frequently mutated genes in lung cancer is p53, a key player in regulating the cell cycle and apoptosis. In smokers, lung adenocarcinoma patients exhibit a significantly higher mutational burden, with mutations in the p53 gene being particularly prevalent (Gibbons et al., 2014). Smoking-induced mutations in p53 impair the cell's ability to respond to DNA damage, increasing the likelihood of lung cancer (Rossman, 2003).

Tobacco smoke exposure also triggers various cellular mechanisms contributing to cancer progression. DNA adduct formation, resulting from carcinogen exposure, leads to oncogenic mutations, a key step in lung cancer development (Gibbons et al., 2014). Chronic tobacco smoke exposure induces oxidative stress, inflammation, and epigenetic alterations, which collectively fuel carcinogenesis (Vineis et al., 2010). These findings highlight the multifaceted nature of tobacco-related cancer and demonstrate how systems biology can help unravel these complex molecular interactions.

Case Study 2: Arsenic and Skin Cancer

Systems biology is equally valuable for understanding the effects of arsenic exposure, which is linked to skin cancer. Arsenic induces both genotoxic and non-genotoxic effects. Genotoxic effects include oxidative DNA damage, chromosome aberrations, and micronuclei formation, while non-genotoxic effects involve immune response modulation and cell cycle progression alterations (Rossman, 2003). Integrating these biological effects provides a more comprehensive view of arsenic's role in carcinogenesis.

Arsenic exposure activates cellular pathways that influence cell survival and proliferation, both crucial for cancer development. For example, arsenic exposure leads to EGFR phosphorylation and MAPK signaling pathway activation (Rossman, 2003). These changes promote keratinocyte transformation, leading to skin cancer development. Systems biology approaches help map these interactions, offering insights into the molecular mechanisms driving arsenic-induced skin cancer.

Both case studies highlight the potential of integrating systems biology with omics technologies and dynamic modeling to explore complex relationships between environmental exposures and cancer. These tools allow researchers to identify key molecular events and disrupted pathways, informing public health strategies aimed at reducing cancer risks from environmental toxins.

Key Takeaways

- Cancer Exposomics studies the impact of environmental factors (e.g., pollution, tobacco smoke, diet) on cancer development, using systems biology to understand molecular interactions driving cancer progression.
- Mapping Exposures to Molecular Pathways involves using computational models to link environmental toxins (e.g., tobacco smoke, air pollution) to altered biological pathways, such as oxidative stress, inflammation, and cellular proliferation, contributing to cancer.
- Key Tools in Systems Biology include gene expression profiling, epigenomics, and pathway modeling. These tools help identify how environmental exposures affect gene expression and contribute to cancer, highlighting the role of epigenetic changes and dynamic models in understanding long-term exposures.
- Case Studies:
  - Tobacco Smoke and Lung Cancer: Tobacco carcinogens induce DNA damage and mutations in the p53 gene, contributing to lung cancer through oxidative stress, inflammation, and epigenetic alterations.
  - Arsenic and Skin Cancer: Arsenic activates pathways like EGFR and MAPK, promoting cell transformation and skin cancer development. Systems biology helps map these interactions, offering insights into cancer mechanisms.
- Systems Biology enhances understanding of environmental carcinogenesis by integrating data from omics technologies, enabling the identification of disrupted pathways and informing targeted prevention strategies.

3. INTEGRATIVE OMICS: A MULTI-LAYERED APPROACH

Integrative omics integrates multiple biological data layers—genomics, proteomics, metabolomics, and transcriptomics—to offer a comprehensive view of how environmental exposures, such as xenobiotics, influence disease mechanisms, particularly in cancer research. Advances in these technologies have significantly enhanced our understanding of molecular interactions driving disease and are already being applied in clinical settings, especially for personalized medicine. However, the complexity of human diseases, like cancer, cannot be fully captured by any single technology. Therefore, integrating data across these omics layers is essential for a holistic understanding of biological processes and disease mechanisms (Bersanelli et al., 2016; Karczewski & Snyder, 2018).

3.1 What is Integrative Omics?

Integrative omics is a systems biology approach that merges multiple omics data layers to create a more comprehensive picture of biological responses, especially in complex diseases like cancer (Hasin et al., 2017). Genomics focuses on mutations and structural variations in the genome that drive cancer progression (Heo et al., 2021). Proteomics examines the entire set of proteins expressed in cells, shedding light on how environmental exposures affect protein function (Pool et al., 2017). Metabolomics studies small molecules and metabolic pathways, crucial for understanding how environmental toxins are processed in the body (Table 1), and whether they disrupt cellular metabolism, leading to cancer (Pinu et al., 2019). By integrating these diverse omics technologies, researchers can gain a system-level understanding of cancer mechanisms, enhancing biomarker discovery and the development of precision medicine (Subramanian et al., 2020).

Table 1. The Integrative Omics Approaches

Omics Layer	Focus	Role in Cancer Research	References
Genomics	- Study of the genome, including gene sequences, mutations, and structural variations.	- Identifies mutations driving tumor development and progression.	(Athreya et al., 2018)
Proteomics	- Study of the entire set of proteins, including their structure, function, and interactions.	- Reveals how environmental exposures (e.g., xenobiotics) influence protein function.	(Mertins et al., 2016)
	- Study of small molecules (metabolites) and their role in biochemical pathways.	- Investigates how environmental toxins disrupt cellular metabolism and promote cancer.	(Pinu et al., 2019; Ogunjobi et al., 2024)

3.2 Linking Xenobiotic Exposure to Cancer Using Integrative Omics

Environmental toxins, such as industrial chemicals, pollutants, and dietary carcinogens, interact with the genome, proteome, and metabolome, triggering or accelerating carcinogenesis. Integrating genomic, proteomic, and metabolomic data allows researchers to map how these toxins disrupt molecular pathways, facilitating early cancer detection and risk assessment (Jiang et al., 2016). For instance, PAHs, found in tobacco smoke and air pollution, have been studied using integrative omics. Genomic and metabolomic data have identified specific metabolic byproducts linked to PAH exposure and lung cancer risk, offering potential early biomarkers for lung cancer detection (D. Li et al., 2019).

Similarly, BPA, an endocrine-disrupting chemical, has been linked to hormone-related cancers such as breast cancer. Proteomic studies have shown that BPA alters estrogen receptor signaling, and by integrating these findings with metabolomic analyses, researchers can uncover how BPA-driven protein modifications disrupt metabolic pathways, promoting estrogen-driven breast cancer (Yang et al., 2023). Table 2 provides a comprehensive overview of key carcinogens studied through integrative omics approaches, highlighting the potential of this methodology for advancing cancer research (Figure 3).

Table 2. Linking Xenobiotic Exposure to Cancer Using Integrative Omics

Xenobiotic	Cancer Type	Key Findings	References
Polycyclic Aromatic Hydrocarbons (PAHs)	Lung Cancer	- Integrative omics identified metabolic byproducts correlating with PAH exposure and lung cancer risk.	(D. Li et al., 2019)
Bisphenol A (BPA)	Breast Cancer	- Proteomic studies revealed BPA alters estrogen receptor signaling and protein expression.	(Yang et al., 2023)
Aflatoxin	Liver Cancer (HCC)	- Multi-omics approaches integrated genomic analysis of the APRT gene with metabolomic profiling to identify early markers of liver cancer.	(Chen et al., 2022)
Arsenic	Bladder Cancer	- Genomic and proteomic studies showed arsenic exposure leads to DNA damage and altered protein expression in bladder cells.	(Mertins et al., 2016)
Cadmium	Prostate Cancer	- Metabolomic and proteomic analyses revealed cadmium disrupts zinc homeostasis and promotes prostate cancer progression.	(Ledda, 2018)
Formaldehyde	Nasopharyngeal Cancer	- Integrative omics identified formaldehyde-induced DNA-protein crosslinks and metabolic disruptions in nasopharyngeal cells.	(Merk & Speit, 1998)
Dioxins	Endometrial Cancer	- Multi-omics studies linked dioxin exposure to altered estrogen signaling and metabolic pathways in endometrial tissue.	(Kogevinas, 2001)
Heterocyclic Amines (HCAs)	Colorectal Cancer	- Integrative omics revealed HCAs from cooked meat are metabolized into genotoxic compounds, increasing colorectal cancer risk.	(Ollberding et al., 2012)
Pesticides (e.g., DDT)	Breast Cancer	- Proteomic and metabolomic studies showed DDT exposure alters hormone-related pathways and promotes breast cancer.	(Winz et al., 2023)
Asbestos	Mesothelioma	- Genomic and proteomic analyses identified asbestos-induced mutations in tumor suppressor genes and altered protein expression.	(Carbone et al., 2019)
Radon	Lung Cancer	- Multi-omics approaches revealed radon exposure leads to oxidative stress and DNA damage in lung cells.	(Taş et al., 2024)
Phthalates	Testicular Cancer	- Metabolomic and proteomic studies linked phthalate exposure to disruptions in testosterone production and testicular cancer risk.	(W. Wang et al., 2024)

Figure 3. Illustrates how environmental toxicants, such as PAHs, BPA, and pesticides, interact with the genome, proteome, and metabolome, leading to DNA mutations, disruption of protein pathways, and metabolic imbalances. By integrating multi-omics data, researchers can identify early biomarkers and molecular mechanisms that link these exposures to cancer development.

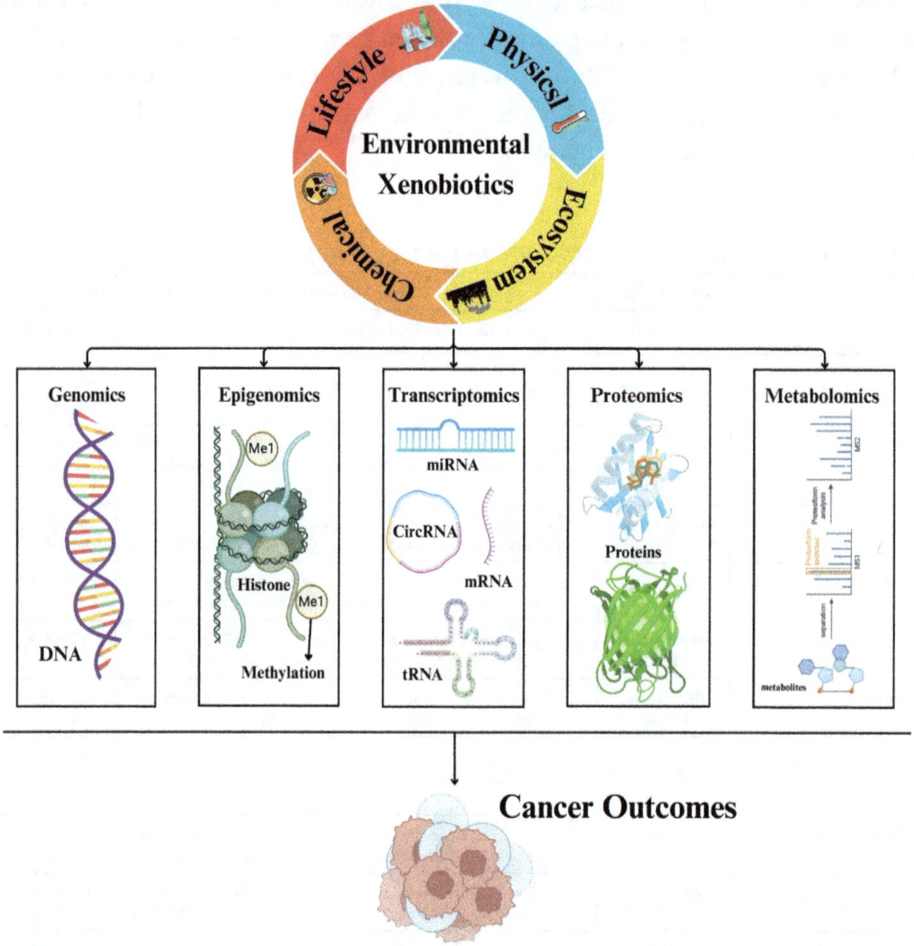

3.3 Identification of Exposure Biomarkers

One of the most promising applications of integrative omics in cancer research is the identification of biomarkers that signal exposure to environmental toxins, potentially enabling early cancer detection before clinical symptoms appear. By combining genomics, proteomics, and metabolomics, researchers can identify biomarkers that reflect both exposure and biological responses at multiple molecular levels (Ludovini et al., 2017). For example, genetic variations in the CYP450 enzyme family affect the metabolism of PAHs and influence cancer risk, making these polymorphisms valuable biomarkers for assessing susceptibility to cancer (Cheng et al., 2022).

Proteomic studies have identified changes in protein expression, such as alterations in p53 protein levels due to heavy metals like arsenic and cadmium. These changes can serve as biomarkers for early-stage cancer detection. Additionally, small-molecule metabolic changes, such as shifts in lipid metabolism due to BPA exposure or bile acid metabolism disruptions from pesticide exposure, can also indicate the onset of xenobiotic-induced carcinogenesis (W. Wang et al., 2024).

3.4 Early Cancer Detection

Traditional cancer detection methods often identify cancer at advanced stages, limiting treatment options and survival rates. Integrative omics offers an alternative by enabling the detection of early molecular alterations linked to carcinogenesis, well before clinical symptoms appear. By integrating genomics, proteomics, and metabolomics, researchers can uncover biomarkers that indicate pre-cancerous conditions, allowing for earlier interventions and better patient outcomes (Xu et al., 2022).

For example, aflatoxin exposure, a major risk factor for hepatocellular carcinoma (HCC), can be detected early through multi-omics approaches. Integrating genomic analysis of the APRT gene with metabolomic profiling of detoxification metabolites allows researchers to identify early molecular markers of liver cancer, facilitating earlier intervention (Chen et al., 2022).

3.5 How Integrative Omics Reveals Mechanisms of Carcinogenesis

Beyond identifying biomarkers, integrative omics provides valuable insights into the molecular mechanisms through which environmental toxins drive cancer. By combining genomic, proteomic, and metabolomic data, researchers can uncover how xenobiotics affect cellular pathways involved in DNA repair, apoptosis, cell-cycle regulation, and immune response—key mechanisms in cancer initiation and progression (Annalora et al., 2024).

For instance, studies on BaP have shown how BaP interacts with the p53 tumor suppressor gene, disrupting DNA repair mechanisms and increasing mutation rates, ultimately contributing to lung cancer. Integrating genomic, proteomic, and metabolomic data has helped researchers map the pathways through which BaP induces mutations, alters protein expression, and disrupts metabolic processes, fueling carcinogenesis in lung cells (Taş et al., 2024).

3.6 Future Directions of Integrative Omics in Cancer Research

As technologies continue to evolve, the potential for integrative omics to revolutionize cancer research is expanding rapidly. Emerging techniques, such as single-cell omics, longitudinal multi-omics studies, and AI-driven data analysis, will further enhance our ability to predict cancer risk, detect cancer earlier, and tailor interventions to individual patients (Table 3).

Table 3. Approaches of Integrative Omics Applications in Cancer Research

Application	Description	Key Findings	References
Biomarker Discovery	- Identifies molecular signatures of xenobiotic exposure and early cancer.	- Genomic, proteomic, and metabolomic biomarkers enable early detection.	(Ludovini et al., 2017; Cheng et al., 2022; W. Wang et al., 2024)
Early Cancer Detection	- Detects molecular alterations before clinical symptoms appear.	- Multi-omics approaches identify early markers for liver and breast cancer.	(Chen et al., 2022; Winz et al., 2023)
Mechanisms of Carcinogenesis	- Elucidates how xenobiotics disrupt cellular pathways leading to cancer.	- Integrative omics maps the progression from exposure to carcinogenesis.	(Annalora et al., 2024; Taş et al., 2024)
Future Directions	- Emerging technologies (e.g., single-cell omics, AI) enhance cancer research.	- Enables personalized risk assessment, early detection, and prevention.	(Uyar et al., 2021; Aguilar & Colacino, 2024; Yang et al., 2024)

Single-cell omics offers insights into tumor heterogeneity by tracking molecular changes at the individual cell level, while longitudinal studies will allow researchers to monitor how cumulative exposure to environmental toxins influences cancer development over time (Aguilar & Colacino, 2024; Yang et al., 2024). AI and machine learning algorithms will optimize the analysis of multi-omics data, helping to identify hidden relationships between environmental exposures and cancer-related molecular changes, which will improve risk prediction and intervention strategies (Uyar et al., 2021; Ogunjobi et al., 2024).

As integrative omics technologies continue to evolve, their applications in cancer prevention, early detection, and precision medicine will transform our approach to cancer risk and treatment, paving the way for more personalized and effective strategies (Raufaste-Cazavieille et al., 2022).

Key Takeaways

- Integrative Omics combines multiple biological data layers (genomics, transcriptomics, proteomics, metabolomics) to offer a comprehensive view of how environmental exposures impact disease, especially cancer. Each omics technology contributes uniquely to our understanding of cellular pathways and disease mechanisms.
- Components of Integrative Omics:
    - Genomics: Studies mutations and structural variations in the genome, driving cancer progression.
    - Proteomics: Examines protein function and how environmental exposures affect protein signaling.
    - Metabolomics: Investigates small molecules and metabolic pathways, crucial for understanding how environmental toxins are processed by the body.
- Linking Xenobiotic Exposure to Cancer: Integrative omics reveals how environmental toxins (e.g., PAHs, BPA) interact with the genome, proteome, and metabolome, accelerating carcinogenesis. Integrating genomic, proteomic, and metabolomic data helps identify biomarkers for early cancer detection.
- Identification of Exposure Biomarkers: Integrating omics helps discover biomarkers that reflect environmental toxin exposure and early biological responses. These biomarkers can enable earlier detection of cancer before clinical symptoms appear.
- Early Cancer Detection: Traditional cancer detection often occurs at advanced stages. Integrative omics offers an alternative by identifying early molecular changes linked to carcinogenesis, providing tools for earlier interventions and better outcomes.
- Mechanisms of Carcinogenesis: Integrative omics helps elucidate how environmental toxins (e.g., Benzo(a)pyrene) affect DNA repair, apoptosis, cell-cycle regulation, and immune responses, shedding light on cancer initiation and progression.
- Future Directions:
    - Single-Cell Omics: Allows tracking molecular changes at the individual cell level, aiding in the understanding of tumor heterogeneity.
    - Longitudinal Multi-Omics: Studies how cumulative exposure to toxins influences cancer development over time.
    - AI and Machine Learning: Will enhance multi-omics data analysis, improving risk prediction, early detection, and personalized intervention strategies.

Integrative omics is poised to revolutionize cancer research by enabling personalized medicine, improving early detection, and enhancing cancer prevention strategies.

4. MECHANISMS LINKING XENOBIOTIC METABOLISM TO CARCINOGENESIS

Environmental pollutants, including pharmaceuticals, microplastics, endocrine-disrupting chemicals (EDCs), and heavy metals, interfere with metabolic pathways, disrupting cellular homeostasis and contributing to diseases like cancer. One significant consequence of xenobiotic exposure is the generation of ROS, which play a central role in carcinogenesis.

4.1 ROS and the Pathogenesis of Cancer

ROS are essential for normal cellular function but can be harmful when in excess. Environmental factors like smoking, radiation, and air pollution disrupt the balance between ROS and antioxidants, causing oxidative stress (Bhattacharyya et al., 2014). Excessive ROS lead to DNA mutations, inflammation, and dysregulated growth factors, all of which contribute to tumorigenesis (Pizzino et al., 2017).

For instance, in colorectal cancer (CRC), ROS-induced mutations in tumor suppressor genes like p53 and APC have been well documented (Lei et al., 2021; Hahm et al., 2022). The mutation of p53, a tumor suppressor gene, is a common result of ROS, contributing to genomic instability in CRC (Tomonaga et al., 2021). Elevated levels of oxidative markers, such as 8-oxoguanine, have been linked to CRC progression and are often detectable in patient urine (Obtulowicz et al., 2010).

4.2 The Role of mTORC2 in Cancer

The mTORC2 protein complex plays a pivotal role in regulating cell growth, metabolism, survival, and apoptosis, making it a critical player in the development of HCC. One of its core subunits, Rictor, has been shown to interact with the tumor suppressor protein p53 (wild-type p53), inactivating its tumor-suppressive functions. This interaction disrupts p53's ability to initiate apoptosis and maintain genomic integrity, allowing hepatocytes to escape programmed cell death and accumulate mutations that fuel tumorigenesis.

Remarkably, chromosomal gains of RICTOR have been identified in approximately 25% of HCC cases, a significantly higher frequency than observed in other cancers (Villanueva et al., 2008; Kim et al., 2017). This frequent amplification underscores Rictor's crucial role in driving HCC pathogenesis. In the early stages of carcinogenesis, Rictor is predominantly localized in the nucleus, where it binds to p53^wt. This binding inhibits p53's transcriptional activity, impairing its ability to induce cell cycle arrest or apoptosis in response to DNA damage. As a result, hepatocytes bypass these protective mechanisms, survive with accumulating genetic mutations, and continue proliferating.

As HCC progresses, Rictor translocates to the cytoplasm, where it facilitates a range of processes essential for tumor progression. This includes promoting metastasis through reorganization of the cytoskeleton, enhancing cellular motility, and increasing the phosphorylation of AKT—an essential step in driving pro-survival and proliferative signaling pathways (Sarbassov et al., 2005; Feng, 2010). The movement of Rictor from the nucleus to the cytoplasm highlights its dual functionality in both the initiation and the advancement of cancer, reinforcing its potential as a therapeutic target.

4.3 Inflammatory Pathways and Cancer

Environmental pollutants like tobacco smoke and industrial chemicals activate inflammatory pathways such as NF-κB and MAPK, both of which drive carcinogenesis by promoting cell survival, proliferation, and resistance to apoptosis. For example, NF-κB activation has been linked to chemotherapy resistance by enhancing survival signaling pathways (Vasan et al., 2019).

A prominent example is tobacco smoke, which induces both direct DNA damage and chronic inflammation, synergistically promoting lung carcinogenesis. ROS and reactive nitrogen species in tobacco smoke oxidize DNA, causing mutations like 8-oxo-7,8-dihydro-2'-deoxyguanosine (Dizdaroglu, 2015; Cadet et al., 2017). This oxidative damage overwhelms base excision repair pathways, increasing genomic instability (Hayes et al., 2005; Foronjy et al., 2006; Birben et al., 2012). Inflammatory pathways like NF-κB and STAT3 are activated, amplifying oxidative stress and contributing to carcinogenesis (Huynh, 2017; Kawanishi et al., 2017; Kay et al., 2019).

4.4 Xenobiotics and Cell Cycle Regulation

Xenobiotics interfere with key regulators of the cell cycle, which contributes to genomic instability and cancer development. Tumor suppressor p53 is crucial for halting the cell cycle or inducing apoptosis in response to DNA damage, but certain xenobiotics inhibit p53's function, allowing damaged cells to proliferate (Creamer et al., 2020).

Chemotherapy drugs like vincristine, for instance, induces p53 activation in cancer cells, leading to the activation of p53-dependent pathways that promote cell cycle arrest and apoptosis in response to DNA damage (Zhu et al., 2024). Xenobiotics can also disrupt the balance of cyclin-dependent kinases (CDKs) and the retinoblastoma (Rb) protein, leading to uncontrolled cell cycle progression (Li et al., 2022). Under normal conditions, Rb binds to and inhibits E2F transcription factors, preventing the cell from progressing through the G1-S phase checkpoint. However, xenobiotics can interfere with this process, either by activating CDKs or by inactivating Rb, leading to the uncontrolled progression of cells through the cell cycle even in the presence of DNA damage. This dysregulation further destabilizes the genome and enhances the likelihood of mutations and chromosomal abnormalities (Li et al., 2022).

Moreover, xenobiotics can inhibit apoptotic pathways by modulating BCL-2 family proteins, allowing genetically altered cells to evade cell death (Zhu et al., 2024).

4.5 Environmental Pollutants and Cellular Signaling

Environmental pollutants disrupt cellular signaling pathways such as Ras/Raf/Mek/Erk and PI3K/Akt/mTOR, which regulate cell survival, growth, and apoptosis. These disruptions activate oncogenes and suppress tumor suppressor pathways, promoting tumorigenesis. For example, the activation of TrkA receptors can trigger Ras/MAPK and PI3K/Akt signaling pathways, both of which contribute to cellular transformation (Islam et al., 2020). Similarly, the phosphorylation of Akt and ERK1/2 supports cancer cell survival, contributing to tumorigenesis and resistance to therapy (Zemskov et al., 2021).

4.6 Real-World Examples of Xenobiotic-Induced Carcinogenesis

Environmental pollutants and industrial chemicals have been implicated in carcinogenesis through various mechanisms. Real-world examples illustrate the broad range of carcinogenic effects that result from prolonged exposure to xenobiotics.

4.6.1 Benzene and PCBs: Industrial Carcinogens

Exposure to industrial pollutants like benzene and polychlorinated biphenyls (PCBs) has been linked to leukemia and lymphoma. Benzene, a volatile organic compound found in industrial emissions and fuel combustion, is classified as a Group 1 carcinogen by the International Agency for Research on Cancer (IARC). Its strong association with acute myeloid leukemia (AML) is attributed to its ability to induce oxidative DNA damage, impair genomic repair mechanisms, and drive mutations in tumor suppressor genes, promoting leukemogenesis (Howarth & Eiser, 2023).

Similarly, PCBs—once widely used as electrical insulators—cause chromosomal instability and immune dysfunction, both of which are key factors in the development of non-Hodgkin lymphoma. PCBs interfere with endocrine signaling and activate inflammatory pathways, promoting tumor survival and proliferation.

By inhibiting apoptosis, PCBs allow genetically damaged cells to evade cell death, further contributing to carcinogenesis (Koual et al., 2020).

4.6.2 Aflatoxin B1: Hepatocellular Carcinogenesis

AFB1, a potent carcinogen produced by the fungus *Aspergillus flavus*, is a significant environmental contaminant commonly found in crops such as peanuts and corn. Chronic exposure to AFB1 is strongly associated with HCC. The carcinogenic effects of AFB1 occur primarily through the formation of DNA adducts, which induce mutations in TP53 (Ally et al., 2017; Eisenstein, 2022).

4.6.3 Asbestos and Inflammation in Mesothelioma Pathogenesis

Asbestos exposure causes necrosis in mesothelial cells, triggering the release of high mobility group box 1 (HMGB1), a protein that plays a central role in sustaining inflammation and activating immune responses (Yang et al., 2010). HMGB1 acts as a damage-associated molecular pattern molecule, recruiting macrophages to the site of injury. Once activated, macrophages initiate the NLRP3 inflammasome, leading to the secretion of pro-inflammatory cytokines like IL-1β and TNF-α (Hillegass et al., 2013). This chronic inflammatory environment results in continuous DNA damage, particularly double-strand breaks, which accelerates tumorigenesis.

The link between asbestos exposure and mesothelioma is further compounded in individuals with germline mutations in the BAP1 gene, a tumor suppressor that maintains genomic stability. In these individuals, the persistent inflammation induced by asbestos fibers leads to malignant transformation, as DNA damage is not adequately repaired, fostering mesothelioma development (Huang et al., 2011; Carbone et al., 2019). Notably, targeting the inflammatory pathways activated by asbestos—such as inhibiting the NLRP3 inflammasome or blocking HMGB1—has shown promise in preclinical models for reducing inflammation and tumor growth (Dostert et al., 2008; Pellegrini et al., 2017).

4.6.4 Vinyl Chloride and Cancer

Vinyl chloride (VC), a chemical used in the production of polyvinyl chloride, is classified as a Group 1 carcinogen by IARC due to its established link to liver cancers, including HCC and hepatic angiosarcoma (Towle et al., 2021). The carcinogenic effects of VC are largely attributed to its metabolites, such as chloroethylene oxide, which form DNA adducts and cause mutations in TP53. These mutations impair apoptosis and allow mutant cells to survive and proliferate (Mastrangelo et al., 2004).

4.6.5 Arsenic-Induced Cancer

Long-term exposure to arsenic activates NF-κB, a key transcription factor that promotes inflammation, cell survival, and proliferation—each of which contributes to carcinogenesis (Yu et al., 2020). Additionally, arsenic activates the MAPK signaling pathway, including ERK, JNK, and p38 cascades, which promote cellular proliferation and resistance to apoptosis (Guo et al., 2024). These alterations are linked to several cancers including bladder, lung, and skin cancers.

4.7 Future Directions for Cancer Prevention

Our growing understanding of how xenobiotics contribute to cancer at the molecular level presents new opportunities for cancer prevention. One promising approach is using biomarkers for early detection, which can identify individuals at higher genetic risk for exposure to specific carcinogens. This could guide personalized health interventions, such as dietary or pharmaceutical agents that modulate detoxification enzymes to reduce the impact of environmental toxins.

For instance, sulforaphane, found in cruciferous vegetables, activates the Nrf2 pathway to upregulate phase II detoxification enzymes, improving the body's ability to neutralize carcinogens before they cause DNA damage (Hao et al., 2020). Similarly, targeting inflammatory pathways like NF-κB with bioactive proteins such as lactoferrin shows promise in preventing inflammation-related carcinogenesis (Aoyama et al., 2021).

Integrating genetic screening, biomarker identification, and precision medicine offers great potential for personalized cancer prevention strategies. Ultimately, reducing exposure to carcinogens, alongside advances in molecular diagnostics and targeted therapies, will be key to mitigating the cancer burden from environmental toxins.

Key Takeaways

- Xenobiotics, including pharmaceuticals and heavy metals, disrupt metabolic pathways and generate ROS, contributing to cancer development.
- ROS, while essential for normal cell function, cause DNA mutations, cell damage, and inflammation, playing a role in cancers like colorectal cancer.
- mTORC2, through its subunit Rictor, promotes HCC by inactivating p53 and facilitating tumor progression, making it a potential therapeutic target.
- Environmental pollutants like tobacco smoke activate inflammatory pathways (NF-κB, MAPK), promoting cancer cell survival, proliferation, and resistance to treatment.

- Xenobiotics disrupt cell cycle regulators (p53, CDKs, Rb), causing genomic instability and allowing damaged cells to proliferate, contributing to cancer.
- Pollutants interfere with cellular signaling (e.g., Ras/Raf, PI3K/Akt), activating oncogenes and suppressing tumor suppressors, promoting cancer progression.
- Benzene and PCBs cause leukemia and lymphoma through oxidative DNA damage and immune dysfunction.
- Aflatoxin B1 causes liver cancer by forming DNA adducts and mutating tumor suppressor genes.
- Asbestos causes mesothelioma through inflammation and DNA damage.
- Vinyl chloride induces liver cancer by forming DNA adducts and impairing apoptosis.
- Arsenic activates NF-κB and MAPK pathways, contributing to bladder, lung, and skin cancers.
- Understanding xenobiotic-induced carcinogenesis could improve cancer prevention through genetic screening, targeted interventions, and reducing carcinogen exposure.

5. ADVANCED COMPUTATIONAL APPROACHES IN CANCER EXPOSOMICS

Cancer exposomics explores how environmental factors interact with the genome to influence cancer risk and progression (Bucher et al., 2023). This requires integrating vast, multi-dimensional data from genomics, transcriptomics, proteomics, and metabolomics. The central challenge lies in analyzing these complex datasets to uncover actionable patterns that inform research and patient care.

5.1. Machine Learning and Multi-Omics in Cancer Research

Machine learning (ML) models—such as support vector machines, deep learning, and random forests—are pivotal in deciphering complex cancer data (Cesario et al., 2021). They detect hidden patterns and associations that traditional methods often miss, illuminating how environmental exposures affect molecular processes. Spatial multi-omics enhances this by localizing omics data within the tumor microenvironment, allowing researchers to map intercellular communication and signaling pathways critical to tumor progression (Sun et al., 2023). This targeted approach improves understanding of cancer heterogeneity and supports the development of precision therapies (see Figure 4).

Figure 4. Depicts the role of multi-omics data integration in advancing precision medicine for cancer. The process begins with biological sample collection from cancer patients and healthy individuals, followed by data acquisition using high-throughput technologies. Multi-omics approaches, including genomics, epigenomics, transcriptomics, proteomics, metabolomics, and microbiome profiling, provide a comprehensive view of cancer biology. Computational techniques, including correlation-based analyses, machine learning (ML), and graph neural networks (GNNs), are applied to integrate and analyze these datasets. This integration enables cancer subtype classification, personalized treatment strategies, survival analysis, identification of therapeutic targets, and biomarker discovery for early diagnosis and disease monitoring. Ultimately, multi-omics integration transforms cancer research, improving prognostics and therapeutic development to enhance patient outcomes.

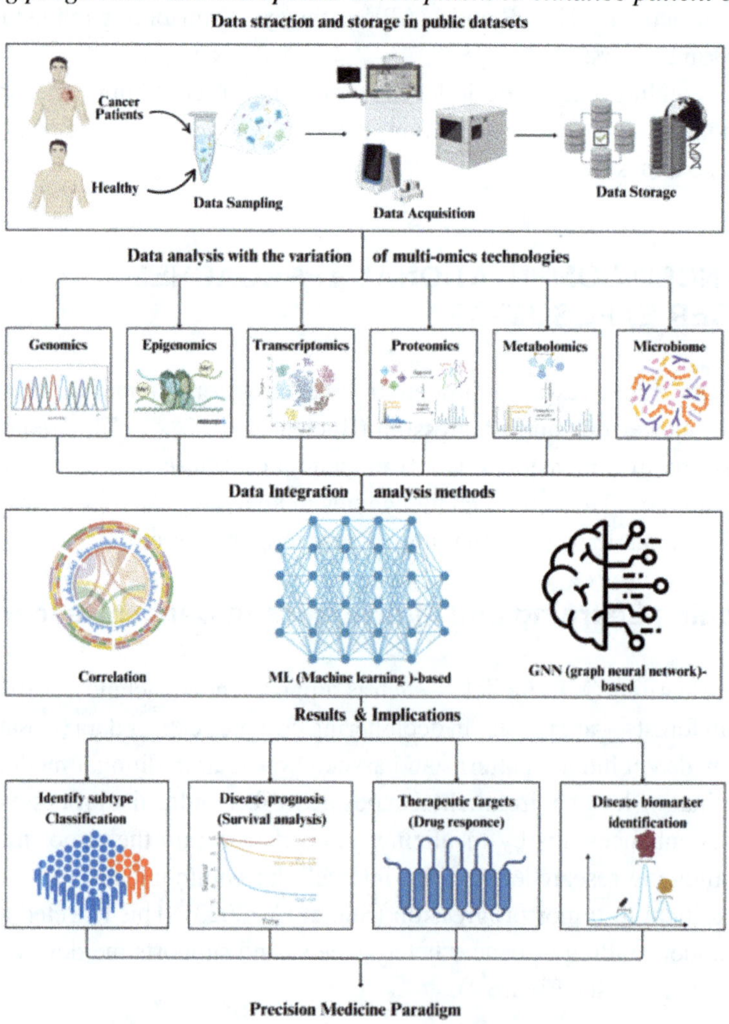

5.2. High-Performance Computing and Cancer Research

High-performance computing (HPC) accelerates the analysis of massive multi-omics datasets. Platforms like the Data Science and Informatics Core for Cancer Research (DSICCR) support seamless integration from molecular to population-level data (Cai et al., 2024; F. Wang et al., 2024). The Exascale Computing Project's CANDLE (Cancer Distributed Learning Environment) exemplifies this progress, using deep learning to derive insights from large-scale patient data, with applications in surveillance, personalized treatment, and drug discovery (Cai et al., 2022; Leng et al., 2022).

5.3. Challenges in High-Performance Data Analysis

Despite progress, several hurdles remain. A lack of data standardization—across genomic, transcriptomic, and imaging datasets—impedes integration. Inconsistent formats and variable quality delay analysis and compromise reproducibility. Missing data in longitudinal studies further reduces model accuracy, while privacy concerns and the high cost of large-scale HPC hinder clinical translation (Cai et al., 2022, 2024).

5.4. Future Directions: Federated Learning, Explainable AI, and Real-Time Hypothesis Testing

Emerging tools offer solutions to these barriers. Federated learning enables collaborative ML model training without sharing sensitive patient data, addressing privacy concerns (Sheller et al., 2020). Explainable AI (XAI) enhances clinical trust by making AI predictions more transparent and interpretable. Additionally, real-time hypothesis testing, powered by high-speed computing, allows models to evolve with incoming data—accelerating discovery and adaptive research in cancer biology (Truhn et al., 2024). Continued investment in standardization, privacy-respecting platforms, and explainable computational frameworks will unlock new opportunities in precision oncology and improve patient outcomes.

Key Takeaways

- Exposomics connects environmental exposures with cancer risk through multi-omics analysis.
- Machine learning and spatial multi-omics reveal critical patterns in tumor biology.
- HPC platforms like CANDLE enable scalable cancer modeling and personalized medicine.

- Integration challenges include data inconsistency, missing values, privacy risks, and cost.
- Federated learning, XAI, and real-time modeling are poised to overcome current limitations.
- Future progress depends on balancing technological innovation with accessibility and ethical data use.

6. FUTURE DIRECTIONS AND IMPLICATIONS FOR CANCER PREVENTION AND TREATMENT

As global cancer incidence rises, the urgency to understand and mitigate carcinogenic risks intensifies. Chronic exposure to xenobiotics—environmental pollutants, industrial chemicals, tobacco smoke, and contaminated food—plays a significant role in cancer development. Future prevention efforts must merge molecular science with public health by focusing on genetic screening, biomarker discovery, detoxification, and policy reform (Nogacka et al., 2019).

6.1 Genetic Risk Assessment and Personalized Prevention

Genetic predispositions significantly influence individual responses to carcinogens. Variants in detoxification enzymes (e.g., CYP450, GSTs, UDPGTs) or DNA repair genes (e.g., BRCA1/2, TP53) can impair the body's ability to eliminate or repair damage caused by xenobiotics, increasing cancer risk (Reszka et al., 2006; Maksymchuk & Kashuba, 2019).

Personalized prevention—combining genetic screening with lifestyle and dietary modifications—holds promise. Nutrigenomics, for instance, links diet to gene expression. Bioactive compounds like polyphenols, curcumin, and sulforaphane may bolster cellular defenses and offset environmental damage (Wen & Han, 2021).

6.2 Biomarkers for Early Detection and Risk Assessment

Biomarkers enable early identification of exposure effects and cancer risk. DNA adducts, oxidative stress indicators (e.g., 8-OHdG), and metabolomic shifts provide measurable insights into early carcinogenesis (Berrandou et al., 2019; Singh et al., 2023). Validating these biomarkers in population studies and integrating them into routine screenings can improve early detection and treatment outcomes (Lee et al., 2022; Wang et al., 2023).

6.3 Detoxification Enzymes and Chemopreventive Agents

The body's detoxification system is pivotal in neutralizing xenobiotics. Phase I enzymes (e.g., CYP1A1, CYP2E1, CYP3A4) initiate detoxification but may generate reactive intermediates. Phases II and III—mediated by GSTs, UDPGTs, and ABC transporters—conjugate and expel these intermediates, reducing DNA damage (Li et al., 2017).

Chemopreventive agents such as resveratrol, sulforaphane, and epigallocatechin gallate enhance detoxification and reduce inflammation, offering potential cancer-preventive effects (Table 4). Select synthetic agents, like selective estrogen receptor modulators and nonsteroidal anti-inflammatory drugs, have also shown efficacy in specific cancer types (Kim et al., 2024).

Table 4. Detoxification Enzymes and Chemopreventive Agents

	Enzymes Involved	Function	Chemopreventive Agents	References
	- Cytochrome P450 enzymes (CYP1A1, CYP2E1, CYP3A4).	- Oxidize, reduce, or hydrolyze xenobiotics into more water-soluble forms.	- Resveratrol, indole-3-carbinol, epigallocatechin gallate.	(Li et al., 2017)
	- Glutathione S-transferases (GSTs), UDP-glucuronosyltransferases (UGTs), sulfotransferases (SULTs).	- Conjugate toxic intermediates with molecules like glutathione, sulfate, or glucuronic acid.	- Synthetic chemopreventive agents (e.g., NSAIDs, SERMs).	(Ruiz-Saavedra et al., 2022)
	- ATP-binding cassette (ABC) transporters.	- Actively remove detoxified carcinogens from cells.		(Bhagyaraj et al., 2019)

6.4 Policy and Public Health Interventions

Regulatory measures remain central to reducing exposure to carcinogens. Policies targeting industrial pollutants, pesticides (e.g., glyphosate, atrazine), and tobacco are essential. For example, laws aimed at controlling industrial emissions such as benzene, formaldehyde, and dioxins should be strengthened to reduce carcinogenic exposure in both occupational and public environments. Similarly, pesticide restrictions are crucial, with the phasing out of harmful chemicals like glyphosate, atrazine, and organophosphates, which have been linked to an increased cancer risk. Public health interventions—including taxation, emission controls, and awareness campaigns—can lower exposure risks and empower healthier lifestyle choices (Bhagyaraj et al., 2019).

6.5 Future Research Directions

Advancing cancer prevention requires a deeper understanding of the intricate interplay between genetic, environmental, and molecular factors. Emerging fields like toxicology and exposomics offer comprehensive approaches for exploring how environmental exposures contribute to carcinogenesis. Future research should focus on the following areas: discovering new biomarkers and treatment targets through the integration of multi-omics techniques (genomics, epigenomics, proteomics, and metabolomics); developing personalized cancer prevention strategies based on individual environmental and genetic risk factors; and investigating immune system modification as a potential means to prevent xenobiotic-induced carcinogenesis (Albuquerque et al., 2021).

Collectively, these strategies provide a clear roadmap for clinicians, public health professionals, and policymakers to implement preventive and therapeutic measures against xenobiotic-induced carcinogenesis—emphasizing the need for integrative, personalized, and policy-driven approaches in cancer control.

Key Takeaways

- Environmental carcinogens significantly influence cancer risk; prevention requires integrating molecular research, screening, and public policy.
- Genetic screening identifies at-risk individuals; nutrigenomics enables personalized interventions.
- Biomarkers aid in early detection; metabolomics offers non-invasive monitoring.
- Detoxification enzymes and chemopreventive agents mitigate carcinogenic effects.
- Stronger environmental policies and public health initiatives can reduce exposure.
- Future research should explore personalized prevention and immune modulation using systems biology tools.

7. ROLE OF THE GUT MICROBIOME IN XENOBIOTIC METABOLISM

The gut microbiome—a complex ecosystem of bacteria, fungi, and viruses in the gastrointestinal tract—plays a vital role in health by influencing digestion, immune responses, and metabolism. One of its most intriguing functions is its interaction with xenobiotics, or foreign compounds such as pharmaceuticals, dietary elements, and environmental toxins.

7.1 The Composition and Role of the Gut Microbiome

Dominated by the phyla Firmicutes and Bacteroidetes, the gut microbiota also includes Actinobacteria, Proteobacteria, and Verrucomicrobia. Its composition is shaped by diet, genetics, and environment, beginning at birth and stabilizing by age three. The microbiome plays several essential roles in maintaining health, including protecting against harmful pathogens, interacting with gut-associated lymphoid tissue (GALT) to modulate immune responses, and maintaining the structural integrity of the gut mucosal barrier. These microbes aid in nutrient extraction and synthesis, particularly of vitamins, amino acids, and short-chain fatty acids (SCFAs), which influence energy metabolism and immune regulation (Khosravi & Mazmanian, 2013; Sender et al., 2016).

From birth, the microbiome begins its development, with the mode of delivery (vaginal or caesarean) significantly influencing early microbial colonization. Breastfeeding further shapes microbiome development, as human milk contains oligosaccharides that promote the growth of beneficial bacteria like *Bifidobacterium*. By the age of three, the microbiome stabilizes into an adult-like configuration, although it remains adaptable to dietary changes, medication use, and environmental influences (Sender et al., 2016; Senghor et al., 2018). The composition of the microbiome is highly individualized and shaped by factors such as genetics, diet, age, geography, and lifestyle.

Dysbiosis—an imbalance in microbial composition—is linked to diseases such as obesity, diabetes, inflammatory bowel disease, and even cancer. This imbalance can disrupt xenobiotic metabolism, increasing toxicity and disease risk (Gholami et al., 2023).

7.1.1 The Gut Microbiome and Xenobiotics: Metabolic Interactions

The gut microbiome can both detoxify and activate xenobiotics through microbial enzymes that mediate reactions such as hydrolysis, reduction, and deconjugation. For instance, sulfasalazine is activated into its therapeutic form, 5-aminosalicylic acid, by gut bacteria (Wilson & Nicholson, 2017; Lima et al., 2024). Conversely, the bacterium *Eggerthella lenta* can inactivate digoxin, and others can convert harmless compounds into toxic or carcinogenic forms—e.g., cyclamate into cyclohexylamine (Haiser et al., 2013).

Polyphenols in fruits and vegetables are transformed by gut microbes into anti-inflammatory metabolites. However, certain environmental pollutants such as polycyclic aromatic hydrocarbons (PAHs) and artificial additives can be bioactivated into harmful carcinogenic compounds (Table 5), highlighting the dual role of the microbiome in modulating xenobiotic effects (Pant et al., 2023).

Table 5. Gut Microbiome Interactions with Xenobiotics

Xenobiotic Type	Microbiome Interaction	Outcome	References
Pharmaceuticals	- Converts pro-drug sulfasalazine into active 5-aminosalicylic acid. - Inactivates cardiac glycoside digoxin via *Eggerthella lenta.*	- Treats inflammatory bowel disease. - Reduces drug efficacy.	(Wilson & Nicholson, 2017; Wang et al., 2022; Lima et al., 2024)
Dietary Components	- Metabolizes polyphenols into bioactive compounds. - Converts cyclamate (artificial sweetener) into cyclohexylamine.	- Exerts antioxidant and anti-inflammatory effects. - Potential carcinogenic effects.	(Haiser et al., 2013)
Environmental Toxins	- Metabolizes PAHs and particulate matter into reactive intermediates.	- May contribute to carcinogenesis or gut dysbiosis.	(Pant et al., 2023; Emanowicz et al., 2024)
	- Detoxifies BPA into less harmful metabolites.	- Reduces toxicity.	

7.1.2 The Microbiome mediates Environmental Exposures and Host Metabolism

The microbiome acts as a mediator between environmental exposures and host metabolism. Heavy metals like cadmium, lead, and arsenic disrupt microbial diversity by reducing the abundance of beneficial bacteria such as *Lactobacillus* and *Bifidobacterium*, while promoting the growth of opportunistic pathogens. This impairs intestinal integrity, promoting systemic inflammation, and affecting the body's immune responses (X. Li et al., 2019; Rezazadegan et al., 2025). While some pollutants are detoxified, others—such as PAHs in grilled meats—are activated into carcinogenic forms via microbial enzymes, increasing cancer risk (Pant et al., 2023; Emanowicz et al., 2024).

7.2. Microbial Enzymes in Xenobiotic Activation and Detoxification

Microbial enzymes such as azoreductases, β-glucuronidases, and nitroreductases can activate procarcinogens into DNA-damaging agents (Figure 5). For example, heterocyclic amines (HCAs) like PhIP, found in cooked meat, are converted by gut bacteria into mutagenic intermediates linked to colorectal cancer. Individuals with higher levels of HCA-metabolizing microbes, such as *E. coli* and *Bacteroides* spp., may face elevated cancer risk (Garcia et al., 2022; Roje et al., 2024).

Figure 5. Illustrates the gut microbiome's role in PhIP metabolism. The liver detoxifies PhIP by conjugating it with glucuronic acid to form PhIP-glucuronide for excretion. In the intestine, gut bacteria express β-glucuronidase (B-GUS) to deconjugate PhIP-glucuronide, releasing free PhIP and counteracting liver detoxification. Additionally, certain bacteria convert glycerol into 3-hydroxypropionaldehyde (3-HPA), which can form acrolein, potentially converting PhIP into its reactive metabolite PhIP-M1. This figure highlights the gut microbiome's impact on the bioactivity and toxicity of PhIP.

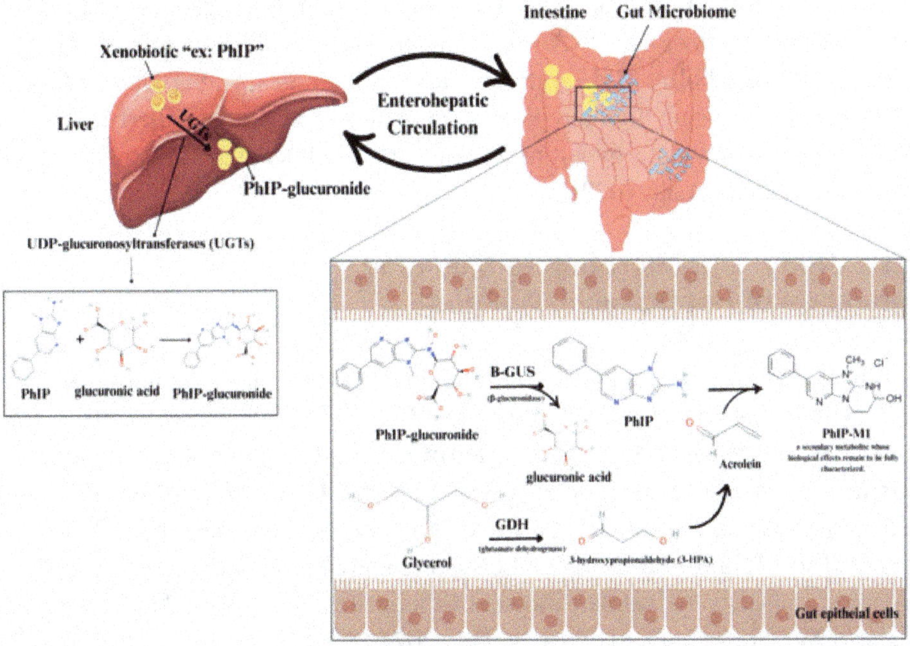

7.2.1 Activation of Procarcinogens by the Gut Microbiome (Table 6)

Table 6. Microbial Enzymes in Xenobiotic Activation and Detoxification

Process	Enzymes Involved	Examples of Xenobiotics	Outcome	Cancer Pathways Impacted	References
Activation	Azoreductases, Cytochrome P450	Aromatic amines, PAHs, HCAs	Converts procarcinogens into reactive, mutagenic forms.	Initiates mutations, activates Wnt/β-catenin pathway, DNA adduct formation	(Garcia et al., 2022; Hillege et al., 2024)
	Hydrolases, Transferases, Lyases	Phthalates, Estrogen derivatives	Converts toxic substances into less harmful metabolites	Reduces DNA damage, inhibits estrogen receptor signaling pathways	(Chiu et al., 2020; Eslami-S et al., 2020)

The gut microbiome plays a pivotal role in modulating the effects of procarcinogens. Microbial enzymes such as azoreductases, β-glucuronidases, nitroreductases, and CYP450-like enzymes catalyze key reactions including reduction, hydrolysis, and oxidation. While these reactions can aid detoxification, they can also transform otherwise inert dietary and environmental compounds into reactive, mutagenic metabolites (Hillege et al., 2024; Roje et al., 2024).

Notably, compounds like aromatic amines, PAHs, and heterocyclic amines (HCAs)—commonly found in tobacco smoke, charred meats, and air pollutants—are known procarcinogens that undergo microbial activation. Bacterial nitroreductases convert aromatic amines into DNA-reactive intermediates, while microbial CYP450-like enzymes metabolize PAHs into epoxides capable of forming DNA adducts. HCAs, produced during high-temperature cooking of meat, are similarly activated into genotoxic compounds by gut microbes, particularly contributing to colorectal cancer risk (Garcia et al., 2022).

Case Study: Gut Microbiome-Mediated Activation of Heterocyclic Amines

A well-characterized example is the microbial metabolism of 2-amino-1-methyl-6-phenylimidazo[4,5-b]pyridine (PhIP), an HCA formed during meat grilling or frying. Once in the colon, PhIP is converted by bacterial enzymes into DNA-reactive intermediates that promote mutagenesis. Elevated levels of PhIP-metabolizing microbes—such as *Escherichia coli* and *Bacteroides* spp.—have been linked to increased susceptibility to colorectal cancer (Figure 5). This underscores the microbiome's capacity to modulate dietary carcinogen metabolism and influence host cancer risk (Garcia et al., 2022; Roje et al., 2024).

7.2.2 Detoxification Mechanisms of Xenobiotics by the Gut Microbiome

Beyond activating procarcinogens, the gut microbiome plays a vital role in detoxifying xenobiotics encountered through diet, environmental exposure, and pharmaceuticals. Microbial enzymes such as hydrolases, transferases, and lyases catalyze reactions that convert harmful substances into less toxic, more excretable forms, thereby mitigating cellular damage and disease risk.

7.2.2.1 Aliphatic Hydrocarbons and Phthalates

Microbial metabolism is particularly important for breaking down aliphatic hydrocarbons—commonly found in petroleum products—and phthalates, which are widely used industrial plasticizers and endocrine disruptors. Bacterial esterases convert phthalates into monoester derivatives, which are more readily excreted and less toxic. Additionally, probiotic interventions have shown promise in restoring microbial balance disrupted by phthalate exposure (Chiu et al., 2020).

7.2.2.2 Estrogen Derivatives

Gut microbes can influence estrogen metabolism through the activity of β-glucuronidases and sulfatases, which deconjugate estrogens normally destined for excretion. This deconjugation promotes estrogen reabsorption and prolongs hormonal activity, contributing to estrogen-dependent cancers such as breast and endometrial cancer (Eslami-S et al., 2020).

Case Study: The Role of Lactobacilli in Estrogen Metabolism and Cancer Prevention

Lactobacillus species have demonstrated protective roles in modulating estrogen metabolism. By inhibiting microbial β-glucuronidase activity, *Lactobacillus reuteri* reduces estrogen reabsorption and may lower cancer risk. The collective microbial influence on estrogen dynamics, known as the "estrobolome," underscores the microbiome's role in hormonal cancer prevention (Eslami-S et al., 2020).

7.2.3 Probiotic Interventions and Dietary Factors

Probiotic-rich diets, particularly those containing *Lactobacillus* species, are associated with decreased β-glucuronidase activity and improved estrogen detoxification. Consumption of fermented dairy products, such as those containing *Lactobacillus casei*, has been inversely linked with the incidence of estrogen-related cancers, reinforcing the preventive potential of microbiota-focused dietary interventions (Thu et al., 2023).

7.3 Diet, Xenobiotics, and the Gut Microbiome (Table 7)

Table 7. Diet, Xenobiotics, and the Gut Microbiome

Dietary Component	Effect on Gut Microbiome	Health Implications	References
Fiber	- Increases beneficial bacteria (e.g., *Bifidobacterium*, *Lactobacillus*). - Enhances gut barrier function.	- Produces SCFAs (anti-inflammatory, anti-carcinogenic). - Reduces colorectal cancer risk.	(David et al., 2014; Louis et al., 2014; O'Keefe, 2016)
Saturated Fats	- Promotes pathogenic bacteria (e.g., *Bacteroides*).	- Increases secondary bile acids, inflammation, and cancer risk.	(Schwabe & Jobin, 2013; O'Keefe, 2016)
Omega-3 Fatty Acids	- Promotes beneficial microbial communities.	- Reduces inflammation and chronic disease risk.	
Plant-Based Proteins	- Associated with a favorable microbial profile.	- Reduces pro-inflammatory cytokines	(O'Keefe, 2016)
Red Meat	- Increases *Bacteroides*, decreases *Bifidobacterium*.	- Contributes to pro-inflammatory environment and colorectal cancer risk.	(O'Keefe, 2016)
Food Additives	- Alters microbial composition (e.g., emulsifiers, artificial sweeteners).	- Promotes inflammation and metabolic dysfunction.	(Chiu et al., 2020)

Diet is a major determinant of gut microbiome composition and function, directly influencing the host's ability to metabolize xenobiotics. Dietary patterns can either promote a resilient, health-supportive microbiota or contribute to dysbiosis and chronic disease risk, including cancer (David et al., 2014; O'Keefe, 2016).

7.3.1 Dietary Influence on Microbial Composition and Function

The Western diet—rich in processed foods, refined sugars, and saturated fats—is associated with a less diverse, more pro-inflammatory microbiome. In contrast, plant-based diets encourage the growth of beneficial microbes, enhancing gut barrier integrity and immune function (Louis et al., 2014; Sonnenburg & Bäckhed, 2016).

Fiber, indigestible to human enzymes but fermentable by microbes, is a cornerstone of a microbiota-friendly diet. Fermentation produces SCFAs such as butyrate and propionate, which are anti-inflammatory and protective against cancer. High-fiber diets increase populations of beneficial bacteria like *Bifidobacterium* and *Lactobacillus,* which enhance immune function and reduce inflammation (Louis et al., 2014; O'Keefe, 2016). Butyrate has well-established anti-carcinogenic effects—it supports gut barrier integrity, induces apoptosis in cancer cells, inhibits proliferation, and modulates inflammation, all of which are crucial for colorectal cancer prevention (David et al., 2014; Louis et al., 2014; Sonnenburg & Bäckhed, 2016).

Dietary fats also shape microbial composition. While omega-3 fatty acids support microbial diversity and anti-inflammatory pathways, high intake of saturated fats fosters pathogenic bacteria that produce harmful metabolites like secondary bile acids and trimethylamine N-oxide—both implicated in carcinogenesis (Schwabe & Jobin, 2013).

Protein source matters as well: plant-based proteins are linked with favorable microbial profiles, whereas high red meat consumption correlates with increased heme iron and pro-inflammatory metabolites, elevating colorectal cancer risk (O'Keefe, 2016).

Finally, diet interacts with xenobiotics such as food additives, pesticides, and antibiotics. These agents can disrupt microbial balance, lower diversity, and promote inflammation. Antibiotics, for instance, reduce microbial diversity and contribute to antibiotic resistance, while artificial sweeteners and emulsifiers may impair metabolic health (Sonnenburg & Bäckhed, 2016; Chiu et al., 2020).

7.3.2 Protective Effects of Dietary Components

Cruciferous vegetables like broccoli and Brussels sprouts contain glucosinolates, which gut microbes convert into bioactive isothiocyanates (Table 8). These compounds exert strong chemoprotective effects by inducing phase II detoxification enzymes, inhibiting histone deacetylases, and reducing tumor growth (Kensler et al., 2012). The microbiota plays a key role in mediating these conversions, reinforcing the functional relationship between diet and microbial metabolism (Schwabe & Jobin, 2013).

Table 8. Protective Effects of Dietary Components

Dietary Component	Mechanism	Health Benefits	References
Fiber	- Fermented by gut bacteria to produce SCFAs (e.g., butyrate).	- Anti-carcinogenic, enhances gut barrier function, reduces inflammation.	(Louis et al., 2014; O'Keefe, 2016; Sonnenburg & Bäckhed, 2016)
Cruciferous Vegetables	- Glucosinolates metabolized into isothiocyanates.	- Induces phase II detoxification enzymes, inhibits tumor growth.	(Kensler et al., 2012; Schwabe & Jobin, 2013)
Polyphenols	- Metabolized into bioactive compounds by gut bacteria.	- Modulates immune responses, reduces oxidative stress.	(Louis et al., 2014)
Indoles	- Derived from tryptophan metabolism by gut bacteria.	- Enhances gut barrier function, reduces inflammation, protects against cancer.	(Schwabe & Jobin, 2013)

Similarly, dietary polyphenols—from berries and tea—are metabolized by gut microbes into active compounds that reduce oxidative stress, modulate immune responses, and counteract inflammation and tumorigenesis (Louis et al., 2014). Indoles, produced via microbial tryptophan metabolism, also contribute to intestinal health by strengthening barrier integrity and suppressing pro-inflammatory signaling (Schwabe & Jobin, 2013).

7.3.3 High-Fat Diets and Increased Cancer Risk

In contrast, high-fat diets—particularly those rich in saturated fats—have been consistently associated with gut dysbiosis and elevated cancer risk. These diets favor the growth of pathogenic microbes and the production of harmful metabolites, including secondary bile acids like deoxycholic and lithocholic acid, which promote inflammation, DNA damage, and cell proliferation (Louis et al., 2014; O'Keefe, 2016).

Moreover, high-fat diets influence xenobiotic metabolism by increasing the microbial activation of dietary carcinogens such as PAHs and HCAs, commonly found in processed meats. These xenobiotic metabolites induce genotoxic stress, particularly in the colon, compounding cancer risk (Schwabe & Jobin, 2013).

Animal studies corroborate this association: high-fat diets have been shown to enrich inflammation-associated genera such as *Alistipes* and *Bilophila* while depleting SCFA-producing bacteria (David et al., 2014). The resulting shift increases secondary bile acids and decreases SCFA levels, fostering a carcinogenic gut environment. Notably, a study in *Cell* demonstrated that the cancer-promoting effects of a high-fat diet were microbiome-dependent (Table 9); antibiotic treatment mitigated tumor formation, emphasizing the gut microbiota's central role (Sonnenburg & Bäckhed, 2016).

Table 9. High-Fat Diets and Cancer Risk

Aspect	Details	References
Microbial Changes	- Increases *Bacteroides*, decreases *Bifidobacterium*. - Promotes pathogenic bacteria (e.g., *Alistipes, Bilophila*).	(David et al., 2014; Louis et al., 2014; O'Keefe, 2016)
Metabolic Effects	- Elevates secondary bile acids (e.g., deoxycholic acid). - Reduces SCFA production	(Louis et al., 2014)
Cancer Risk	- Increases DNA damage, inflammation, and colorectal cancer risk.	(Schwabe & Jobin, 2013; David et al., 2014; Sonnenburg & Bäckhed, 2016)

7.4 Environmental Toxins and the Gut Microbiome

Beyond diet, environmental toxins are potent disruptors of the gut microbiome and can contribute significantly to disease risk. Pollutants such as air particulates, pesticides, and synthetic chemicals alter microbial composition and function, driving dysbiosis that predisposes individuals to cancer and other chronic conditions (Jin et al., 2017).

7.4.1 Impact of Environmental Pollutants on the Gut Microbiome

Particulate matter (PM2.5; particles less than 2.5 μm), a major air pollutant, can translocate from the lungs to the gut, disrupting microbial diversity and promoting inflammation. Studies in mice show PM2.5 exposure reduces beneficial bacteria like *Lactobacillus* and *Bifidobacterium*, while increasing pathogenic *Clostridium.* These shifts are linked to gut barrier dysfunction and systemic inflammation, both key contributors to carcinogenesis. Interestingly, altering the microbiome with antibiotics mitigated this risk, highlighting microbial involvement (Kish et al., 2013; Singh et al., 2022).

Other pollutants such as glyphosate (herbicide) and BPA (plasticizer) similarly disrupt the microbiota. Glyphosate suppresses beneficial species, while BPA increases gut permeability and inflammatory signaling—both mechanisms implicated in cancer progression (Jin et al., 2017).

7.4.2 Persistent Organic Pollutants (POPs) and Microbial Dysbiosis

Persistent organic pollutants (POPs) such as dioxins and PCBs accumulate in the food chain and resist degradation, exerting long-term toxic effects. These chemicals disrupt microbial communities, often reducing diversity and enriching pro-inflammatory taxa. In mouse studies, dioxin exposure diminished *Lactobacillus* and *Bifidobacterium* while promoting *Clostridium*, leading to gut barrier compromise and systemic inflammation—conditions associated with liver and endometrial cancers (Jin et al., 2017; Singh et al., 2022). These findings underscore the microbiome's role as a mediator of environmental toxin effects and highlight a pressing need for deeper mechanistic insight and potential interventions.

7.4.3 Cigarette Smoke and the Gut Microbiome

Cigarette smoke, containing over 7,000 chemicals—many of them carcinogenic—affects not only respiratory health but also the gut microbiome. Smoking has been associated with decreased levels of beneficial bacteria such as *Lactobacillus* and *Bifidobacterium*, and an increased abundance of pro-inflammatory taxa like *Clostridium*. These microbial shifts contribute to gut barrier disruption, systemic inflammation, and increased cancer susceptibility. Studies have shown that smokers exhibit reduced microbial diversity and an enrichment of pathogenic bacteria compared to non-smokers (Biedermann et al., 2013; Lee et al., 2018). Encouragingly, smoking cessation has been shown to partially restore microbial composition, indicating the potential reversibility of tobacco-induced dysbiosis.

Beyond altering composition, the gut microbiome also mediates the metabolism of tobacco carcinogens. Nitrosamines—tobacco-specific carcinogens—can be transformed by gut bacteria into reactive intermediates capable of inducing DNA damage and promoting tumor development. Experimental models reveal that antibiotic-mediated depletion of gut microbiota diminishes colorectal cancer risk linked to nitrosamine exposure, underscoring the microbiome's role in tobacco-related carcinogenesis (Lee et al., 2018; see Table 10).

Table 10. The Environmental Toxins and Their Effects on the Gut Microbiome

	Effects on Gut Microbiome	Health Implications	Cancer Risk	References
Air Pollution (PM2.5)	Decreases microbial diversity; reduces Lactobacillus and Bifidobacterium.	Increases gut permeability and systemic inflammation.	PM2.5 disrupts the microbiome, leading to chronic inflammation, which is linked to lung cancer and colorectal cancer through the gut-lung axis.	(Kish et al., 2013; Salim et al., 2014; Singh et al., 2022)
Pesticides (Glyphosate)	Reduces Lactobacillus and Bifidobacterium; increases Clostridium.	Increases gut permeability and systemic inflammation.	Glyphosate-induced dysbiosis can enhance inflammation and promote carcinogenesis, contributing to leukemia and non-Hodgkin lymphoma.	(Jin et al., 2017; Singh et al., 2022)
Industrial Chemicals (BPA)	Alters gut microbiome composition; reduces beneficial bacteria.	Increases gut permeability and systemic inflammation.	BPA-induced microbial changes and inflammation can disrupt endocrine signaling, leading to breast cancer and prostate cancer.	(Singh et al., 2022)

continued on following page

Table 10. Continued

	Effects on Gut Microbiome	Health Implications	Cancer Risk	References
Dioxins	Reduces Lactobacillus and Bifidobacterium; increases Clostridium.	Increases gut permeability and systemic inflammation.	Dioxins alter gut microbiota, promote chronic inflammation, and are associated with endometrial cancer via disrupted immune responses.	(Singh et al., 2022; Kish et al., 2013)
PCBs	Alters gut microbiome composition, promoting pathogenic bacteria.	Promotes inflammatory pathways linked to liver cancer.	PCBs disrupt the gut microbiome, leading to immune dysregulation, which increases risk of liver cancer and non-Hodgkin lymphoma.	(Jin et al., 2017)
Cigarette Smoke	Decreases Lactobacillus and Bifidobacterium; increases Clostridium.	Increases gut permeability and systemic inflammation.	Cigarette smoke promotes inflammation, oxidative stress, and DNA damage, leading to lung cancer and bladder cancer.	(Biedermann et al., 2013; S. Lee et al., 2018)

7.5 Therapeutic Potential: Modulating the Gut Microbiome for Cancer Prevention

The gut microbiome plays a pivotal role in maintaining host health, with growing evidence linking its composition and activity to cancer prevention and treatment outcomes. Emerging therapeutic strategies—including probiotics, prebiotics, and FMT—aim to restore or enhance microbial balance, reduce inflammation, and promote xenobiotic detoxification (Wong & Yu, 2019).

7.5.1 Probiotics and Cancer Prevention

Probiotics are live microorganisms that, when consumed in sufficient amounts, offer health benefits—including cancer risk reduction. Species such as *Lactobacillus* and *Bifidobacterium* enhance detoxification pathways, modulate immune responses, and fortify the intestinal barrier (Ishikawa et al., 2005).

Probiotic strains can bind, degrade, or transform dietary carcinogens such as HCAs and PAHs, reducing their toxicity and bioavailability (Rafter, 2003). They also promote the activity of detoxification enzymes such as GSTs and cytochrome P450s, which facilitate xenobiotic metabolism and excretion.

Immunomodulatory effects are also critical. Probiotics affect immune function by stimulating GALT to produce anti-inflammatory cytokines and reduces pro-inflammatory cytokines. *Bifidobacterium infantis*, for example, reduces levels of IL-6 and TNF-α—both implicated in tumor development (Zitvogel et al., 2018). Probiotics also enhance intestinal barrier integrity by stimulating tight junction proteins and mucin production, limiting pathogen translocation and chronic inflammation (see Table 11).

Table 11. Probiotics and Cancer Prevention

Aspect	Details	Health Implications	References
Probiotic Strains	- *Lactobacillus* and *Bifidobacterium* sp.	- Enhance detoxification pathways, modulate immune responses, reduce inflammation.	(Ishikawa et al., 2005; Zitvogel et al., 2018)
Mechanisms of Action	- Bind and degrade carcinogens (e.g., HCAs, PAHs). - Enhance detoxification enzymes (e.g., GSTs, cytochrome P450). - Stimulate anti-inflammatory cytokines and immune cells (e.g., NK cells). - Strengthen intestinal epithelial barrier.	- Reduce bioavailability and toxicity of carcinogens. - Facilitate excretion of harmful compounds. - Reduce pro-inflammatory cytokines (e.g., IL-6, TNF-α). - Prevent translocation of pathogenic bacteria and endotoxins.	(Rafter, 2003; Cummings & Macfarlane, 2002; Zitvogel et al., 2018)
Clinical Evidence	- Probiotic supplementation reduces colorectal adenoma recurrence.	- 45% reduction in adenoma recurrence with *Lactobacillus acidophilus* and *Bifidobacterium lactis*.	(Heavey & Rowland, 2004)

Meta-analyses of clinical trials underscore their value: supplementation with *Lactobacillus acidophilus* and *Bifidobacterium lactis* has been associated with up to a 45% reduction in colorectal adenoma recurrence—a key precursor to colorectal cancer (Heavey & Rowland, 2004).

7.5.2 Prebiotics and Xenobiotic Detoxification

Prebiotics are non-digestible dietary fibers that selectively stimulate the growth of beneficial microbes. Compounds such as inulin, fructooligosaccharides (FOS), and galactooligosaccharides (GOS) promote the expansion of *Lactobacillus* and *Bifidobacterium*, enhancing the detoxification of environmental toxins and dietary carcinogens (Suez et al., 2018).

A central mechanism by which prebiotics exert their anti-cancer effects is through increased production of SCFAs, particularly butyrate. Butyrate supports intestinal health, induces apoptosis in cancer cells, and inhibits histone deacetylases (HDACs), which are involved in tumor progression (Cummings & Macfarlane, 2002).

Prebiotics also reduce the prevalence of microbial taxa that convert xenobiotics into genotoxic intermediates. Prebiotic supplementation has been shown to decrease the metabolism of PAHs into reactive genotoxic and carcinogenic intermediates (Wong & Yu, 2019). In clinical trials, inulin supplementation has been shown to lower pro-inflammatory cytokines and fecal bile acids, while enhancing anti-inflammatory mediators like IL-10—shaping a more protective colonic environment (Ishikawa et al., 2005; see Table 12).

Table 12. Prebiotics and Xenobiotic Detoxification

Aspect	Details	Health Implications	Cancer Risk	References
Prebiotic Types	Inulin, fructooligosaccharides (FOS), galactooligosaccharides (GOS).	Promote growth of beneficial bacteria like Lactobacillus and Bifidobacterium.	These prebiotics enhance detoxification, reducing carcinogen absorption and promoting gut health, thereby reducing colorectal cancer risk.	(Suez et al., 2018)
	Serve as substrates for SCFA production (e.g., butyrate, acetate).	SCFAs, particularly butyrate, modulate inflammation and cell proliferation.	Butyrate induces apoptosis in cancer cells and inhibits histone deacetylases (HDACs), reducing DNA damage and carcinogenesis, particularly in colorectal cancer.	(Cummings & Macfarlane, 2002; Wong & Yu, 2019)
Clinical Evidence	Prebiotic supplementation reduces fecal bile acids; increases fecal SCFA concentrations.	Supports cancer prevention by reducing toxic bile acids and promoting beneficial microbial activities.	By enhancing the microbiome and reducing oxidative stress, prebiotics contribute to cancer prevention, particularly in the colon.	(Heavey & Rowland, 2004)

7.5.3 Fecal Microbiota Transplantation (FMT) in Cancer Therapy

FMT, the transfer of stool from a healthy donor into a recipient's gut, is gaining attention as a means of restoring microbial balance in cancer patients. Dysbiosis—commonly seen in patients undergoing chemotherapy or radiation—impairs immune surveillance and worsens treatment responses (DeFilipp et al., 2019).

FMT has been shown to reestablish microbial diversity and restore populations of anti-inflammatory species such as *Faecalibacterium prausnitzii*, which support gut integrity. In addition, certain bacteria introduced via FMT, such as *Eubacterium limosum*, can metabolize chemotherapeutic drugs into their active forms, enhancing efficacy (Zitvogel et al., 2018).

Clinical trials demonstrate FMT's potential to mitigate gastrointestinal side effects like mucositis and diarrhea. In hematopoietic stem cell transplant patients, FMT significantly reduced chemotherapy-induced diarrhea (Suez et al., 2018). Most notably, a groundbreaking study found that FMT could overcome resistance to immune checkpoint inhibitors (ICIs) in metastatic melanoma patients. Transplanting microbiota from ICI-responsive donors restored treatment sensitivity in previously unresponsive patients, achieving a 30% clinical response rate—a major advancement in cancer immunotherapy (Zitvogel et al., 2018).

7.6 Future Directions: Gut Microbiome Research in Cancer Exposomics

With advances in sequencing and bioinformatics, microbiome research has become integral to cancer exposomics. This section explores future directions, emphasizing multi-omics integration, personalized interventions, and current research challenges.

7.6.1 Integrating Microbiome Data into Multi-Omics Approaches

Combining microbiome data with genomics, proteomics, and metabolomics offers a comprehensive view of host–microbe interactions in cancer. Microbial metabolites like butyrate can modulate gene expression through HDAC inhibition, affecting cancer-related pathways and epigenetic regulation. Additionally, microbial enzymes metabolize dietary components into bioactive compounds, which can influence host proteomics and metabolomics. Gut microbes also convert dietary and host compounds—such as bile acids—into metabolites that influence cancer risk.

Importantly, distinct microbial signatures have been associated with various cancers. For example, *Fusobacterium nucleatum* is linked to colorectal cancer, while *Porphyromonas gingivalis* has been implicated in pancreatic cancer. When integrated with host omics data, such signatures could improve early detection and non-invasive diagnostics through stool or saliva sampling.

7.6.2 Personalized Microbiome Interventions

The individuality of the gut microbiome, shaped by genetics, diet, and environment, supports the need for personalized approaches in cancer prevention and therapy. FMT, personalized probiotics, and prebiotics are being explored to modulate microbial communities and improve outcomes.

For example, tailored probiotic formulations containing *Lactobacillus* or *Bifidobacterium* strains may reduce inflammation and enhance immune responses in colorectal cancer. Similarly, personalized prebiotics like inulin can promote beneficial bacteria and SCFA production, contributing to anti-cancer effects.

7.6.3 Challenges, Limitations, and Opportunities in Microbiome Research

Microbiome research faces challenges, including variability across individuals and difficulties in establishing causality. Most studies are correlative, highlighting the need for mechanistic and longitudinal investigations.

Future research should leverage single-cell microbiome analysis and AI-based tools to interpret complex datasets. These approaches can uncover hidden patterns, improve predictive models, and advance microbiome-targeted strategies for cancer prevention and treatment.

Key Takeaways

- The gut microbiome metabolizes xenobiotics like drugs, food components, and pollutants, influencing cancer risk through detoxification or activation of harmful compounds.
- Microbial enzymes can activate procarcinogens such as PAHs and HCAs or detoxify harmful substances, affecting DNA integrity and cancer development.
- Environmental toxins including heavy metals, pesticides, BPA, air pollution, and cigarette smoke disrupt microbial diversity and promote inflammation-linked cancer.
- Diet strongly shapes microbiome composition; fiber-rich, plant-based diets support beneficial bacteria and SCFA production, while high-fat and processed diets promote dysbiosis and carcinogenesis.
- Omega-3 fatty acids and plant proteins support microbial health, whereas saturated fats and animal proteins are associated with inflammatory microbes and increased colorectal cancer risk.
- Certain foods like cruciferous vegetables, polyphenols, and prebiotic fibers enhance detoxification and reduce inflammation via microbiome-derived metabolites like butyrate.
- Probiotics such as *Lactobacillus* and *Bifidobacterium* improve immune function, bind carcinogens, and reduce inflammation and tumor risk.
- Prebiotics like inulin and FOS support beneficial microbes, reduce carcinogen metabolism, and increase SCFA production with anti-cancer effects.
- FMT restores microbial diversity, alleviates chemotherapy side effects, and enhances immunotherapy response in some cancer patients.
- Integrating microbiome data with genomics, proteomics, and metabolomics reveals new biomarkers and therapeutic targets for early cancer detection and prevention.
- Personalized microbiome interventions, including tailored probiotics and prebiotics, offer targeted strategies for cancer prevention and improved treatment outcomes.
- Major research challenges include variability in microbial communities and difficulties proving causality in microbiome-cancer links.
- Future studies should employ longitudinal designs, single-cell analysis, and AI tools to better understand microbiome roles in cancer and develop precise interventions.

8. EPIGENETIC REGULATION IN XENOBIOTIC METABOLISM AND CANCER

Epigenetic regulation—through mechanisms like DNA methylation, histone modification, and non-coding RNAs—modulates gene expression without altering DNA sequences. These changes are highly responsive to environmental exposures, including xenobiotics, and play a pivotal role in both detoxification and carcinogenesis. Increasing evidence links xenobiotic-induced epigenetic alterations to cancer development, drug resistance, and impaired metabolic pathways.

8.1 Understanding Epigenetics and Xenobiotic-Induced Epigenetic Alterations in Cancer

Epigenetics refers to changes in gene expression that do not involve modifications to the DNA sequence itself. These changes encompass DNA methylation, histone modifications, and the regulation of gene expression by non-coding RNAs that can cause multidrug resistance (MDR), silencing of tumor suppressor genes, and cancer (Figure 6). Environmental exposures, including dietary toxins and pollutants, can induce epigenetic modifications that disrupt gene expression and cellular detoxification processes (Gibney & Nolan, 2010). Xenobiotics may promote cancer through the epigenetic silencing of tumor suppressor genes or the activation of oncogenes, often contributing to chemoresistance (Table 13). These changes particularly affect genes encoding phase I (e.g., CYP450s) and phase II (e.g., GSTs) metabolizing enzymes (Hahm et al., 2022; Zhang et al., 2024).

Table 13. Epigenetic Mechanisms and Their Role in Xenobiotic Metabolism and Cancer

Epigenetic Mechanism	Description	Role in Xenobiotic Metabolism	Role in Cancer Development	References
DNA Methylation	Addition of a methyl group to cytosine residues, often leading to gene silencing.	Alters expression of genes encoding xenobiotic-metabolizing enzymes (e.g., CYP1A1, GSTP1).	Hypermethylation of tumor suppressor genes (e.g., p16, BRCA1) silences these genes, leading to uncontrolled cell proliferation and tumorigenesis.	(Kulis & Esteller, 2010; Tamási et al., 2011)
Histone	Chemical changes to histone proteins (e.g., acetylation, methylation).	Regulates the expression of detoxification enzymes (e.g., GSTP1, UGT1A1).	Aberrant histone modifications can silence tumor suppressors or activate oncogenes. Histone deacetylation is linked to aggressive cancer progression (e.g., liver and lung cancer).	(Bannister & Kouzarides, 2011; Schnekenburger et al., 2014)
Non-Coding RNAs	miRNAs and lncRNAs regulate gene expression post-transcriptionally.	miRNAs (e.g., miR-21, miR-34) regulate enzymes involved in xenobiotic metabolism, influencing detoxification.	Dysregulation of miRNAs and lncRNAs can promote cancer by altering pathways that control cell growth, apoptosis, and DNA repair. For instance, miR-21 is involved in reducing the expression of tumor suppressors.	(Iorio & Croce, 2012; Dong et al., 2020)

Figure 6. Illustrates the gut microbiome's role in PhIP metabolism. The liver detoxifies PhIP by conjugating it with glucuronic acid via UDP-glucuronosyltransferases (UDPGTs), forming PhIP-glucuronide for excretion. In the intestine, gut bacteria express β-glucuronidase (B-GUS), which deconjugates PhIP-glucuronide, releasing free PhIP and counteracting the liver's detoxification. Certain bacteria also metabolize glycerol into 3-hydroxypropionaldehyde (3-HPA), which can form acrolein, potentially converting PhIP into its carcinogenic metabolite PhIP-M1. This figure highlights the interaction between gut microbiota and host metabolism in influencing the toxicity of PhIP.

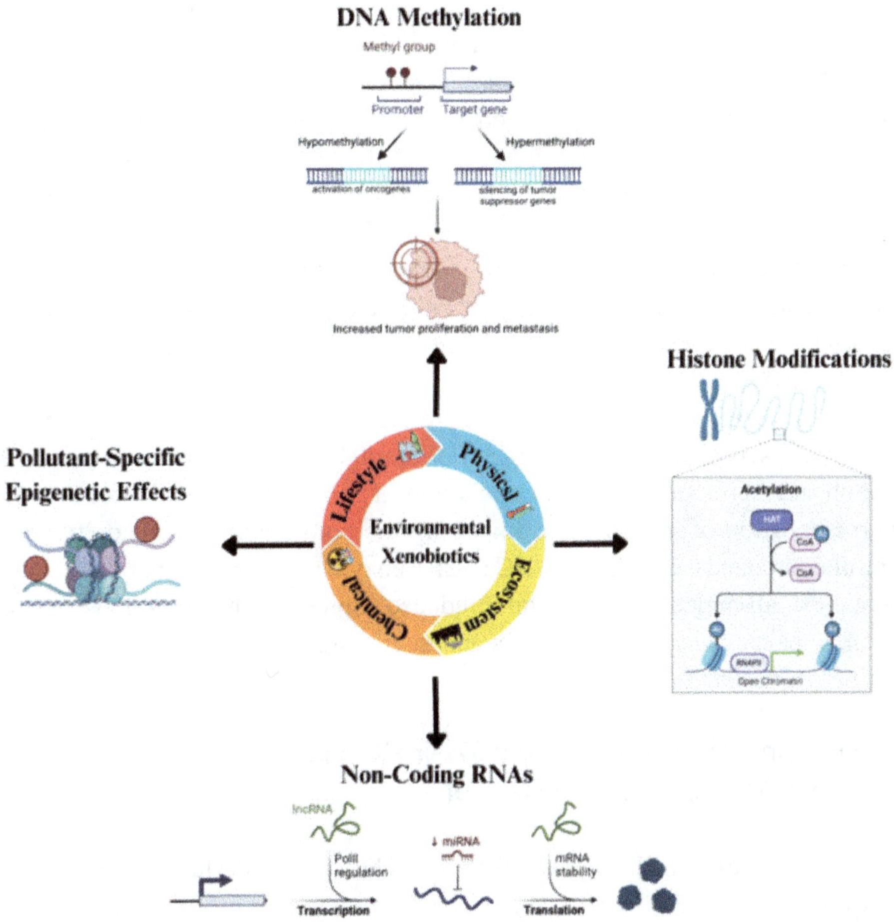

8.1.1 DNA Methylation and Its Role in Cancer and Xenobiotic Metabolism

DNA methylation involves the addition of a methyl group to the 5' position of cytosine residues, particularly within gene promoter regions, leading to gene silencing. Abnormal DNA methylation, such as hypermethylation of tumor suppressor gene promoters, disrupts normal cell growth regulation, leading to uncontrolled proliferation and increased genetic instability. This process is critically implicated in both cancer progression and xenobiotic metabolism (Kulis & Esteller, 2010; Toraño et al., 2016).

Xenobiotics can alter DNA methylation patterns, disrupting detoxification pathways and increasing susceptibility to carcinogens. For instance, in colorectal cancer, hypermethylation of the *hMLH1* promoter inhibits mismatch repair, increasing genomic instability and resistance to platinum-based therapies (Mansoori et al., 2017). Conversely, hypomethylation of oncogenes like *CD24* in breast cancer has been linked to increased tumor proliferation and metastasis (Zhang et al., 2019). Demethylating agents such as 5-aza-2'-deoxycytidine (decitabine, DAC) have shown potential in reversing hypermethylation and restoring chemosensitivity to cisplatin and 5-fluorouracil in resistant cancers (Mansoori et al., 2017; Patnaik & Anupriya, 2019).

DNA methylation also regulates the expression of phase I xenobiotic-metabolizing enzymes, such as CYP450 enzymes. For example, the CYP1A1 enzyme, which metabolizes PAHs found in tobacco smoke and air pollution, can be silenced through hypermethylation of its promoter, impairing the body's ability to detoxify these harmful compounds. Similarly, the CYP2E1 enzyme, which metabolizes alcohol and other small molecules, can exhibit reduced expression due to promoter methylation, impairing alcohol metabolism and increasing the risk of liver damage and other health issues (Tekpli et al., 2012).

8.1.2 Histone Modifications and Their Role in Xenobiotic Metabolism and Cancer

Histone modifications—including acetylation, methylation, and phosphorylation—are crucial for regulating gene expression and chromatin architecture. Xenobiotic exposure can induce these changes, leading to chromatin remodeling and silencing of tumor suppressor genes. Acetylation generally promotes gene transcription by loosening chromatin structure, while methylation can either activate or repress gene expression depending on the specific modification context (Tamási et al., 2011; Geissler et al., 2024).

In phase I enzymes such as the CYP450 family, xenobiotics can trigger histone acetylation or methylation, enhancing the transcription of genes involved in metabolizing toxins. Conversely, histone deacetylation or repressive methylation patterns can suppress these enzymes, weakening the body's detoxification capabilities. Similarly, phase II enzymes like GSTs and UDPGTs are also regulated through histone modifications. For instance, reduced acetylation at the GSTP1 promoter impairs its expression and may heighten cancer susceptibility (Schnekenburger et al., 2014; Rahbar et al., 2022).

Histone deacetylase inhibitors (HDACi), including Vorinostat and CUDC-101, can reverse these epigenetic alterations by restoring acetylation and reactivating silenced pro-apoptotic genes. CUDC-101, a dual HDAC/kinase inhibitor, has shown potential in resensitizing resistant cancers by targeting both epigenetic and signaling mechanisms (Shimizu et al., 2014; Goey et al., 2016).

8.1.2.1 Histone Acetylation

Histone acetylation, mediated by histone acetyltransferases (HATs), relaxes chromatin structure and promotes transcription by neutralizing histone charges and enhancing transcription factor access. This modification upregulates phase II detoxification enzymes like UDPGTs, with increased acetylation at their promoters linked to elevated expression in response to xenobiotic stimuli (Eberharter & Becker, 2002; Bannister & Kouzarides, 2011).

8.1.2.2 Histone Methylation

Histone methylation, by methyltransferases, can activate or repress gene transcription depending on the residue modified. For instance, H3K4 methylation activates, while H3K9 methylation silences gene expression. These patterns regulate detoxifying enzymes like GSTs, affecting the body's ability to eliminate toxic compounds (Bannister & Kouzarides, 2011; Zou & Mallampalli, 2014).

8.1.2.3 Histone Phosphorylation

Histone phosphorylation involves the addition of phosphate groups to serine, threonine, or tyrosine residues and plays a role in chromatin remodeling, DNA repair, and stress responses. Though less understood, it is crucial for cellular defense and homeostasis under xenobiotic stress (Bannister & Kouzarides, 2011).

8.1.3 Non-Coding RNAs

Non-coding RNAs, such as miRNAs and lncRNAs, modulate gene expression post-transcriptionally. Dysregulation of miRNAs affects apoptosis, proliferation, and drug resistance. For instance, miR-27b-3p downregulation in breast cancer reduces tamoxifen sensitivity (Zhu et al., 2016), while miR-508-5p inhibition in gastric cancer increases ABCB1 expression, enhancing drug efflux (Shang et al., 2014).

Environmental toxins like TCDD can induce epigenetic changes, such as DNA hypermethylation and histone modifications, leading to silencing of tumor suppressors like p16INK4A and promoting cancer progression (Goodman et al., 2022; Singh, 2024). Therapeutic strategies targeting oncogenic miRNAs (e.g., miR-21) or restoring tumor-suppressive miRNAs (e.g., miR-34a) show promise in overcoming multidrug resistance (Si et al., 2019).

8.2 Environmental Pollutants and Their Epigenetic Effects

Environmental pollutants, particularly endocrine-disrupting chemicals (EDCs) like bisphenol A (BPA), exert epigenetic effects that contribute to carcinogenesis. BPA increases histone acetylation at promoters of carcinogenic genes (e.g., *HOXC6*, *HOXB9*) in breast cancer cells, enhancing estrogen receptor signaling—a key driver in hormone-dependent cancers (Bhan et al., 2014; Deb et al., 2016). Acting as an estrogen mimic, BPA binds to estrogen receptors and disrupts normal gene regulation (Kuiper et al., 1997; Delfosse et al., 2012). It also upregulates EZH2, a histone methyltransferase linked to aggressive breast cancer (Bhan et al., 2014; Deb et al., 2016). Animal studies show that prenatal BPA exposure induces persistent epigenetic changes in breast tissue, increasing cancer susceptibility (Ho et al., 2006; Altamirano et al., 2017).

Pollutants also affect the expression of xenobiotic-metabolizing enzymes, such as CYP450s, GSTs, and UDPGTs, thereby altering detoxification capacity (see Table 14).

Table 14. Environmental Exposures and Their Epigenetic Effects on Xenobiotic Metabolism

	Epigenetic Effect	Impact on Xenobiotic Metabolism	Cancer Risk	References
Dietary Factors	Alcohol: Alters DNA methylation and histone modifications of detoxification genes. High-fat diets: Dysregulates lipid metabolism genes via epigenetic changes.	Alcohol: Reduces expression of ADH1B and CYP2E1, impairing alcohol metabolism. High-fat diets: Impair detoxification pathways.	Alcohol consumption increases the risk of liver, esophageal, and breast cancers. High-fat diets promote obesity-related cancers (e.g., colorectal, pancreatic).	(Singh & Li, 2012)
Pollutants and Chemicals	Arsenic: Hypermethylation of GSTP1 and p16 genes. Cadmium: Alters histone modifications, silencing CYP450 genes.	Reduces detoxification capacity, leading to toxin accumulation.	Arsenic is linked to bladder and lung cancers. Cadmium is a risk factor for lung cancer and prostate cancer.	(Pal & Firdous, 2024; Singh, 2024)
Air Pollutants	PAHs: Induce DNA methylation of CYP1A1 and histone deacetylation of NQO1.	Disrupts detoxification of PAHs, leading to reactive metabolite accumulation.	PAHs are a major risk factor for lung cancer.	(Mandal et al., 2023; A. Zhang et al., 2024)
Tobacco Smoke	Hypermethylation of CYP1A1 and GSTP1 promoters.	Reduces detoxification of PAHs and other carcinogens.	Tobacco smoke is a leading cause of lung and bladder cancers.	(Roje et al., 2024; Zhang et al., 2024)
Pesticides and Herbicides	DDT: Silences CYP450 genes via DNA methylation. Glyphosate: Alters histone modifications, downregulating GST genes.	Impairs detoxification of pesticides and other xenobiotics.	DDT exposure is linked to non-Hodgkin lymphoma, while glyphosate exposure increases the risk of leukemia.	(Pelkonen et al., 2023)
Radiation	UV radiation: Silences CYP450 genes via DNA methylation. Ionizing radiation: Alters histone modifications, downregulating NQO1.	Impairs detoxification of reactive metabolites.	UV radiation is a primary cause of melanoma, while ionizing radiation increases leukemia risk.	(Katiyar et al., 2012)

8.2.1 Dietary Factors

Dietary habits, such as alcohol consumption and high-fat diets, influence xenobiotic metabolism via epigenetic changes. Alcohol alters the methylation and histone modification of detox genes like *ADH1B* and *CYP2E1*, contributing to cancers of the liver, esophagus, and breast by silencing tumor suppressors and activating oncogenes (Singh & Li, 2012; Singh, 2024). High-fat diets similarly affect epigenetic regulation of lipid and detox pathways, promoting inflammation and obesity-related cancers like colorectal and pancreatic cancer.

8.2.2 Pollutants and Chemicals

Heavy metals such as arsenic and cadmium induce harmful epigenetic changes. Arsenic causes hypermethylation of the *GSTP1* gene, impairing detoxification and increasing bladder cancer risk. Cadmium alters histone modifications, repressing *CYP450* genes and elevating lung cancer risk (Pal & Firdous, 2024; Singh et al., 2024).

8.2.3 Air Pollutants

Airborne pollutants, especially particulate matter and PAHs like benzo[a]pyrene, modulate xenobiotic metabolism. PAHs initially induce *CYP1A1* expression, but chronic exposure leads to its methylation and silencing, disrupting detox pathways. These pollutants also downregulate *NQO1*, reducing protection against reactive metabolites (Mandal et al., 2023).

8.2.4 Tobacco Smoke and Cytochrome P450 Enzymes

Tobacco smoke, responsible for 71% of global lung cancer deaths (Heppel et al., 2009), contains nitrosamines (e.g., NNK) and PAHs metabolized by CYP2A6 and CYP2A13 into DNA-damaging intermediates (Hecht, 2012; Stepanov et al., 2013; Goyal et al., 2023). Smoking also induces hypermethylation of *CYP1A1* (reducing its ability to metabolize PAHs), and *GSTP1*, and silences tumor suppressors like *p16* and *FHIT*, increasing cancer risk (Thum et al., 2006; A. Zhang et al., 2024).

8.2.5 Pesticides and Herbicides

Pesticides like DDT and herbicides such as glyphosate epigenetically silence detox genes. DDT inhibits *CYP450s*, elevating non-Hodgkin lymphoma risk. Glyphosate alters histone modifications and downregulates *GSTs*, contributing to leukemogenesis through dysregulated proliferation and survival (Pelkonen et al., 2023).

8.2.6 Radiation

Radiation, including UV and ionizing forms, triggers epigenetic alterations. UV radiation silences *CYP450* genes via DNA methylation, promoting melanoma. Ionizing radiation affects histone modifications, downregulating *NQO1* and other detox enzymes, weakening oxidative stress defenses and increasing leukemia risk through tumor suppressor silencing (Katiyar et al., 2012).

8.3 Environmental Chemicals and Epigenetic Reprogramming

Environmental chemicals, particularly endocrine-disrupting compounds (EDCs) like bisphenol A (BPA), are known to induce epigenetic reprogramming—long-lasting changes in gene expression that can persist across generations. These alterations can disrupt normal detoxification pathways, interfere with hormonal signaling, and heighten cancer susceptibility.

BPA, a prevalent EDC found in plastics and food packaging, has been linked to aberrant DNA methylation patterns, including hypermethylation of tumor suppressor genes (e.g., *BRCA1*) and hypomethylation of oncogenes (e.g., *MYC*), contributing to tumor initiation and progression (Jadhav et al., 2017; Qin et al., 2021). Additionally, BPA exposure can synergize with polycyclic aromatic hydrocarbons (PAHs), further compounding DNA damage and carcinogenic potential.

Other ubiquitous chemicals, such as phthalates (in plastics and cosmetics) and PAHs (from tobacco smoke and air pollution), similarly modulate epigenetic machinery. Phthalates alter DNA methylation and histone modifications in hormone-regulating genes, dampening detoxifying enzymes like UDP-glucuronosyltransferases (Singh & Li, 2012). PAHs influence methylation of key detoxification genes (*CYP1A1*, *GSTP1*), impairing xenobiotic clearance and increasing cancer risk (Baccarelli & Bollati, 2009).

Alarmingly, these epigenetic modifications can be heritable. Animal models show that exposure to EDCs during development causes persistent changes in the germline, affecting gene expression and health outcomes across multiple generations (F1–F4) (Korolenko et al., 2023).

8.3.1 Dioxins and Their Carcinogenic Mechanisms

Dioxins, particularly TCDD, are persistent organic pollutants (POPs) with potent carcinogenic effects. Classified as Group 1 carcinogens by the IARC, they have been implicated in cancers such as non-Hodgkin lymphoma and soft tissue sarcoma, with elevated risks observed in populations exposed to Agent Orange (Vuong, 2022).

Dioxins exert toxicity primarily via the aryl hydrocarbon receptor (AhR). Upon activation, the AhR-ARNT complex translocates to the nucleus, modulating genes involved in xenobiotic metabolism, including *CYP1A1*, *CYP1B1*, and *GSTs*. However, prolonged dioxin exposure also induces epigenetic silencing—such as histone deacetylation and promoter hypermethylation—of these same detoxification genes (Kogevinas, 2001; Vuong, 2022). This paradox impairs detoxification, increasing toxicant bioaccumulation and cancer risk.

Additionally, AhR signaling interacts with NF-κB, promoting chronic inflammation, another key driver of carcinogenesis. Dioxins' lipophilic nature facilitates accumulation in adipose tissue, enabling sustained molecular disruption.

8.4 Potential for Therapeutic Targeting of Epigenetic Changes

Given the role of epigenetic reprogramming in cancer induced by environmental chemicals, epigenetic therapy represents a promising strategy to reverse aberrant gene expression. These therapies aim to reactivate silenced tumor suppressors, restore detoxification enzymes, and suppress oncogenes, using two main drug classes: DNA methyltransferase inhibitors (DNMTi) and histone deacetylase inhibitors (HDACi).

8.4.1 DNMT Inhibitors

DNMT inhibitors counter DNA hypermethylation by preventing methyl group addition to gene promoters. Agents like 5-azacytidine (Vidaza) and 5-aza-2′-deoxycytidine (Decitabine), approved for myelodysplastic syndromes and AML, restore expression of silenced tumor suppressors such as *p16* and *BRCA1* (Giri & Aittokallio, 2019). These compounds also reactivate detoxification-related genes like *CYP1A1*, improving xenobiotic metabolism.

8.4.2 HDAC Inhibitors

HDAC inhibitors promote chromatin relaxation by increasing histone acetylation, thereby enabling transcription of previously silenced genes. Vorinostat and Romidepsin, FDA-approved for cutaneous and peripheral T-cell lymphomas, re-establish expression of detoxification genes such as *GSTP1* and *UDPGT1A1*, enhancing the body's capacity to neutralize carcinogens (Xu et al., 2007).

8.4.3 Future Directions

Next-generation epigenetic therapies aim for greater specificity and lower toxicity by targeting distinct molecular signatures. Combination strategies—integrating epigenetic drugs with immunotherapies (e.g., PD-1 inhibitors) or chemotherapy—are showing promise. For instance, DNMT inhibitors can boost MHC gene expression, improving immune detection of tumors (Hu et al., 2021; Liu et al., 2022).

Identifying biomarkers that predict response to DNMTi and HDACi is also a priority. Recent advances highlight specific methylation profiles and histone signatures as potential tools for personalized therapy (Dai et al., 2024; Gao et al., 2024), paving the way for precision oncology in populations exposed to environmental carcinogens.

8.5 Challenges in Applying Systems Biology to Environmental Toxicology

Despite its transformative potential, the application of systems biology in environmental toxicology presents several challenges. One key limitation is the integration of heterogeneous data types—such as genomic, transcriptomic, proteomic, and metabolomic datasets—which requires sophisticated computational tools and interdisciplinary expertise. Furthermore, environmental exposures often involve complex mixtures of chemicals at low doses over long periods, making it difficult to model precise cause-effect relationships.

Another challenge is the limited availability of standardized, high-quality omics data from human populations exposed to environmental pollutants, which hampers reproducibility and cross-study comparisons. The inclusion of potential biases, such as batch effects, confounding variables, and normalization issues in the data, poses additional complications. These biases can distort results and impact the credibility of findings, making it crucial to implement stringent quality control measures. Furthermore, the dynamic nature of biological systems and inter-individual variability, including genetic background and microbiome composition, adds layers of complexity to data interpretation.

Addressing these issues requires investment in data standardization, development of robust computational models, and cross-disciplinary collaborations between toxicologists, systems biologists, bioinformaticians, and experts in quality control. By addressing these challenges, the full potential of systems biology in environmental toxicology research can be realized.

Key takeaways

- Epigenetic Regulation: DNA methylation, histone modifications, and non-coding RNAs play a critical role in xenobiotic metabolism and cancer development.
- Xenobiotic Exposure and Cancer: Environmental pollutants like BPA, phthalates, and dioxins can trigger epigenetic changes that affect cancer progression, chemoresistance, and multidrug resistance, often through silencing tumor suppressor genes.
- DNA Methylation and Detoxification: Epigenetic modifications, especially DNA methylation, can silence key detoxifying enzymes (e.g., cytochrome P450 enzymes), increasing susceptibility to carcinogens.
- Histone Modifications and Cancer: Histone acetylation, methylation, and phosphorylation influence the expression of enzymes involved in xenobiotic metabolism and contribute to cancer progression by altering gene expression.

- Non-coding RNAs in Drug Resistance: miRNAs and lncRNAs regulate drug resistance by modulating genes involved in apoptosis, proliferation, and drug efflux.
- Environmental Pollutants and Transgenerational Effects: Chemicals like dioxins, phthalates, and BPA induce epigenetic changes that impair detoxification, increase cancer risk, and can cause transgenerational effects.
- Dioxins, BPA, and Carcinogenesis: DNA methylation and histone modifications induced by exposure to chemicals like dioxins and BPA can disrupt detoxification pathways, activate oncogenes, and promote carcinogenesis.
- Epigenetic Therapy: DNMT inhibitors (e.g., decitabine) and HDAC inhibitors (e.g., vorinostat) offer promising strategies to reverse harmful epigenetic changes, restore detoxification functions, and reduce cancer risk.
- Future Directions in Therapy: Future epigenetic therapies will focus on developing targeted, less toxic treatments and combining them with chemotherapy or immunotherapy for better efficacy.
- Personalizing Treatments with Biomarkers: Identifying biomarkers for epigenetic alterations will enable personalized treatment approaches, maximizing efficacy while minimizing side effects.

CONCLUSIONS

Environmental pollutants play a significant role in shaping the epigenome and increasing cancer susceptibility through mechanisms such as DNA methylation, histone modifications, and gene silencing. The impact of pollutants—including endocrine-disrupting chemicals, heavy metals, and tobacco smoke—underscores the need for continued research into how these environmental exposures reprogram gene expression and interfere with detoxification pathways. Furthermore, the promising therapeutic strategies based on epigenetic targeting—such as the use of DNMT and HDAC inhibitors—offer potential solutions to reverse these harmful changes and restore normal cellular function.

Despite these advancements, challenges remain in applying systems biology to environmental toxicology, particularly in the integration of diverse data types and the need for robust computational models. Addressing these challenges will be critical to fully realizing the potential of systems biology in identifying novel biomarkers, developing targeted therapies, and improving public health strategies.

This chapter highlights the urgent need to address the role of xenobiotics in cancer risk, particularly through their impact on metabolic and epigenetic processes. By focusing on xenobiotic-induced metabolic reprogramming and gene-environment interactions, we can lay the foundation for more personalized, effective approaches to cancer treatment. Future research should prioritize the development of interventions that target these molecular disruptions, ultimately enhancing therapeutic efficacy and informing cancer prevention strategies.

The ongoing exploration of environmental carcinogenesis through epigenetic mechanisms reinforces the importance of integrating exposomic insights with precision medicine. As we deepen our understanding of how environmental factors contribute to cancer development, we move closer to realizing the full potential of preventative and personalized therapeutic approaches.

LIST OF ABBREVIATIONS

AFB1	Aflatoxin B1
AhR	Aryl hydrocarbon receptor
AML	Acute myeloid leukemia
APC	Adenomatous polyposis coli
AP-1	Activator protein 1
APRT	Adenine phosphoribosyltransferase
ASL	Hepatic angiosarcoma
BaP	Benzo[a]pyrene
BAP1	BRCA1-associated protein 1
BPA	Bisphenol A
BRAF	B-Raf proto-oncogene
CD24	Cluster of differentiation 24
CDKs	Cyclin-dependent kinases
COPD	Chronic obstructive pulmonary disease
CRC	Colorectal cancer
CTCL	Cutaneous T-cell lymphoma
CYP	Cytochrome P450
DAC	5-Aza-2'-deoxycytidine (Decitabine)
DBC	Dibenz[a,h]anthracene
DDT	Dichlorodiphenyltrichloroethane
DNMT	DNA methyltransferase
E2F	E2F transcription factor
EDCs	Endocrine-disrupting chemicals
EGFR	Epidermal growth factor receptor
ERK	Extracellular signal-regulated kinase
FMT	Fecal microbiota transplantation
GALT	Gut-associated lymphoid tissue
GSTs	Glutathione S-transferases

HATs	Histone acetyltransferases
HCC	Hepatocellular carcinoma
HCAs	Heterocyclic amines
HDACs	Histone deacetylases
HMGB1	High mobility group box 1
ICIs	Immune checkpoint inhibitors
IARC	International Agency for Research on Cancer
lncRNAs	Long non-coding RNAs
MAPK	Mitogen-activated protein kinase
MDR	Multidrug resistance
miRNAs	MicroRNAs
MLH1	MutL homolog 1
mTORC2	Mammalian target of rapamycin complex 2
NATs	N-acetyltransferases
NF-κB	Nuclear factor kappa-light-chain-enhancer of activated B cells
NFE2L2	Nuclear factor erythroid 2-related factor 2
NLRP3	NLR family pyrin domain containing 3
NNK	4-(Methylnitrosamino)-1-(3-pyridyl)-1-butanone
NQO1	NAD(P)H quinone dehydrogenase 1
PAHs	Polycyclic aromatic hydrocarbons
PCBs	Polychlorinated biphenyls
PBPK	Physiologically based pharmacokinetic
PI3K	Phosphatidylinositol 3-kinase
PM2.5	Particulate matter (2.5 micrometers or less)
POPs	Persistent organic pollutants
Rb	Retinoblastoma protein
RICTOR	Rapamycin-insensitive companion of mTOR
ROS	Reactive oxygen species
SCFAs	Short-chain fatty acids
TCDD	2,3,7,8-Tetrachlorodibenzo-p-dioxin
TNF-α	Tumor necrosis factor-alpha
TP53	Tumor protein p53
TSNA	Tobacco-specific nitrosamines
UDPGTs	UDP-glucuronosyltransferases
VC	Vinyl chloride
XAI	Explainable artificial intelligence

REFERENCES

Aguilar, D.Jr, & Colacino, J. A. (2024). Single cell approaches to understand environmental impacts on aggressive breast cancers. *Current Opinion in Toxicology, 37*, 100459. DOI: 10.1016/j.cotox.2024.100459

Albuquerque, C., Manguinhas, R., Costa, J. G., Gil, N., Codony-Servat, J., Castro, M., Miranda, J. P., Fernandes, A. S., Rosell, R., & Oliveira, N. G. (2021). A narrative review of the migration and invasion features of non-small cell lung cancer cells upon xenobiotic exposure: Insights from in vitro studies. *Translational Lung Cancer Research, 10*(6), 2698–2714. DOI: 10.21037/tlcr-21-121 PMID: 34295671

Ally, A., Balasundaram, M., Carlsen, R., Chuah, E., Clarke, A., Dhalla, N., Holt, R. A., Jones, S. J. M., Lee, D., Ma, Y., Marra, M. A., Mayo, M., Moore, R. A., Mungall, A. J., Schein, J. E., Sipahimalani, P., Tam, A., Thiessen, N., Cheung, D., & Laird, P. W. (2017). Comprehensive and Integrative Genomic Characterization of Hepatocellular Carcinoma. *Cell, 169*(7), 1327–1341.e23. DOI: 10.1016/j.cell.2017.05.046 PMID: 28622513

Altamirano, G. A., Ramos, J. G., Gomez, A. L., Luque, E. H., Muñoz-de-Toro, M., & Kass, L. (2017). Perinatal exposure to bisphenol A modifies the transcriptional regulation of the β-Casein gene during secretory activation of the rat mammary gland. *Molecular and Cellular Endocrinology, 439*, 407–418. DOI: 10.1016/j.mce.2016.09.032 PMID: 27697584

Anderson, L. M., Chhabra, S. K., Nerurkar, P. V., Souliotis, V. L., & Kyrtopoulos, S. A. (1995). Alcohol-related cancer risk: A toxico kinetic hypothesis. *Alcohol (Fayetteville, N.Y.), 12*(2), 97–104. DOI: 10.1016/0741-8329(94)00089-1 PMID: 7772272

Annalora, A. J., Coburn, J. L., Jozic, A., Iversen, P. L., & Marcus, C. B. (2024). Global transcriptome modulation by xenobiotics: The role of alternative splicing in adaptive responses to chemical exposures. *Human Genomics, 18*(1), 127. DOI: 10.1186/s40246-024-00694-6 PMID: 39558396

Aoyama, Y., Naiki-Ito, A., Xiaochen, K., Komura, M., Kato, H., Nagayasu, Y., Inaguma, S., Tsuda, H., Tomita, M., Matsuo, Y., Takiguchi, S., & Takahashi, S. (2021). Lactoferrin Prevents Hepatic Injury and Fibrosis via the Inhibition of NF-κB Signaling in a Rat Non-Alcoholic Steatohepatitis Model. *Nutrients, 14*(1), 42. DOI: 10.3390/nu14010042 PMID: 35010924

Athreya, A., Iyer, R., Neavin, D., Wang, L., Weinshilboum, R., Kaddurah-Daouk, R., Rush, J., Frye, M., & Bobo, W. (2018). Augmentation of Physician Assessments with Multi-Omics Enhances Predictability of Drug Response: A Case Study of Major Depressive Disorder. *IEEE Computational Intelligence Magazine, 13*(3), 20–31. DOI: 10.1109/MCI.2018.2840660 PMID: 30467458

Baccarelli, A., & Bollati, V. (2009). Epigenetics and environmental chemicals. *Current Opinion in Pediatrics, 21*(2), 243–251. DOI: 10.1097/MOP.0b013e32832925cc PMID: 19663042

Bannister, A. J., & Kouzarides, T. (2011). Regulation of chromatin by histone modifications. *Cell Research, 21*(3), 381–395. DOI: 10.1038/cr.2011.22 PMID: 21321607

Berrandou, T., Mulot, C., Cordina-Duverger, E., Arveux, P., Laurent-Puig, P., Truong, T., & Guénel, P. (2019). Association of breast cancer risk with polymorphisms in genes involved in the metabolism of xenobiotics and interaction with tobacco smoking: A gene-set analysis. *International Journal of Cancer, 144*(8), 1896–1908. DOI: 10.1002/ijc.31917 PMID: 30303517

Bersanelli, M., Mosca, E., Remondini, D., Giampieri, E., Sala, C., Castellani, G., & Milanesi, L. (2016). Methods for the integration of multi-omics data: Mathematical aspects. *BMC Bioinformatics, 17*(S2), S15. DOI: 10.1186/s12859-015-0857-9 PMID: 26821531

Bhagyaraj, E., Ahuja, N., Kumar, S., Tiwari, D., Gupta, S., Nanduri, R., & Gupta, P. (2019). TGF-β induced chemoresistance in liver cancer is modulated by xenobiotic nuclear receptor PXR. *Cell Cycle (Georgetown, Tex.), 18*(24), 3589–3602. DOI: 10.1080/15384101.2019.1693120 PMID: 31739702

Bhan, A., Hussain, I., Ansari, K. I., Bobzean, S. A. M., Perrotti, L. I., & Mandal, S. S. (2014). Histone Methyltransferase EZH2 Is Transcriptionally Induced by Estradiol as Well as Estrogenic Endocrine Disruptors Bisphenol-A and Diethylstilbestrol. *Journal of Molecular Biology, 426*(20), 3426–3441. DOI: 10.1016/j.jmb.2014.07.025 PMID: 25088689

Bhattacharyya, A., Chattopadhyay, R., Mitra, S., & Crowe, S. E. (2014). Oxidative Stress: An Essential Factor in the Pathogenesis of Gastrointestinal Mucosal Diseases. *Physiological Reviews, 94*(2), 329–354. DOI: 10.1152/physrev.00040.2012 PMID: 24692350

Biedermann, L., Zeitz, J., Mwinyi, J., Sutter-Minder, E., Rehman, A., Ott, S. J., Steurer-Stey, C., Frei, A., Frei, P., Scharl, M., Loessner, M. J., Vavricka, S. R., Fried, M., Schreiber, S., Schuppler, M., & Rogler, G. (2013). Smoking Cessation Induces Profound Changes in the Composition of the Intestinal Microbiota in Humans. *PLoS One*, *8*(3), e59260. DOI: 10.1371/journal.pone.0059260 PMID: 23516617

Birben, E., Sahiner, U. M., Sackesen, C., Erzurum, S., & Kalayci, O. (2012). Oxidative Stress and Antioxidant Defense. *The World Allergy Organization Journal*, *5*(1), 9–19. DOI: 10.1097/WOX.0b013e3182439613 PMID: 23268465

Boffetta, P., & Hashibe, M. (2006). Alcohol and cancer. *The Lancet. Oncology*, *7*(2), 149–156. DOI: 10.1016/S1470-2045(06)70577-0 PMID: 16455479

Bucher, M. L., Anderson, F. L., Lai, Y., Dicent, J., Miller, G. W., & Zota, A. R. (2023). Exposomics as a tool to investigate differences in health and disease by sex and gender. *Exposome*, *3*(1), osad003. Advance online publication. DOI: 10.1093/exposome/osad003 PMID: 37122372

Cadet, J., Davies, K. J. A., Medeiros, M. H., Di Mascio, P., & Wagner, J. R. (2017). Formation and repair of oxidatively generated damage in cellular DNA. *Free Radical Biology & Medicine*, *107*, 13–34. DOI: 10.1016/j.freeradbiomed.2016.12.049 PMID: 28057600

Cai, Z., Apolinário, S., Baião, A. R., Pacini, C., Sousa, M. D., Vinga, S., Reddel, R. R., Robinson, P. J., Garnett, M. J., Zhong, Q., & Gonçalves, E. (2024). Synthetic augmentation of cancer cell line multi-omic datasets using unsupervised deep learning. *Nature Communications*, *15*(1), 10390. DOI: 10.1038/s41467-024-54771-4 PMID: 39614072

Cai, Z., Poulos, R. C., Liu, J., & Zhong, Q. (2022). Machine learning for multi-omics data integration in cancer. *iScience*, *25*(2), 103798. DOI: 10.1016/j.isci.2022.103798 PMID: 35169688

Carbone, M., Adusumilli, P. S., Alexander, H. R.Jr, Baas, P., Bardelli, F., Bononi, A., Bueno, R., Felley-Bosco, E., Galateau-Salle, F., Jablons, D., Mansfield, A. S., Minaai, M., De Perrot, M., Pesavento, P., Rusch, V., Severson, D. T., Taioli, E., Tsao, A., Woodard, G., & Pass, H. I. (2019). Mesothelioma: Scientific clues for prevention, diagnosis, and therapy. *CA: a Cancer Journal for Clinicians*, *69*(5), 402–429. DOI: 10.3322/caac.21572 PMID: 31283845

Cesario, A., D'Oria, M., Calvani, R., Picca, A., Pietragalla, A., Lorusso, D., Daniele, G., Lohmeyer, F. M., Boldrini, L., Valentini, V., Bernabei, R., Auffray, C., & Scambia, G. (2021). The Role of Artificial Intelligence in Managing Multimorbidity and Cancer. *Journal of Personalized Medicine, 11*(4), 314. DOI: 10.3390/jpm11040314 PMID: 33921621

Chen, F., Wang, J., Wu, Y., Gao, Q., & Zhang, S. (2022). Potential Biomarkers for Liver Cancer Diagnosis Based on Multi-Omics Strategy. *Frontiers in Oncology, 12*, 822449. DOI: 10.3389/fonc.2022.822449 PMID: 35186756

Cheng, T., Gamage, S. M. K., Lu, C.-T., Aktar, S., Gopalan, V., & Lam, A. K. (2022). Polymorphisms in PAH metabolising enzyme CYP1A1 in colorectal cancer and their clinicopathological correlations. *Pathology, Research and Practice, 231*, 153801. DOI: 10.1016/j.prp.2022.153801 PMID: 35180652

Chiu, K., Warner, G., Nowak, R. A., Flaws, J. A., & Mei, W. (2020). The Impact of Environmental Chemicals on the Gut Microbiome. *Toxicological Sciences, 176*(2), 253–284. DOI: 10.1093/toxsci/kfaa065 PMID: 32392306

Clerici, M., Colombo, G., Secundo, F., Gagliano, N., Colombo, R., Portinaro, N., Giustarini, D., Milzani, A., Rossi, R., & Dalle-Donne, I. (2014). Cigarette smoke induces alterations in the drug-binding properties of human serum albumin. *Blood Cells, Molecules & Diseases, 52*(4), 166–174. DOI: 10.1016/j.bcmd.2013.12.001 PMID: 24388826

Creamer, B. A., Sloan, S. N. B., Dennis, J. F., Rogers, R., Spencer, S., McCuen, A., Persaud, P., & Staudinger, J. L. (2020). Associations between Pregnane X Receptor and Breast Cancer Growth and Progression. *Cells, 9*(10), 2295. DOI: 10.3390/cells9102295 PMID: 33076284

Cummings, J. H., & Macfarlane, G. T. (2002). Gastrointestinal effects of prebiotics. *British Journal of Nutrition, 87*(S2), S145–S151. DOI: 10.1079/BJN/2002530 PMID: 12088511

Dai, W., Qiao, X., Fang, Y., Guo, R., Bai, P., Liu, S., Li, T., Jiang, Y., Wei, S., Na, Z., Xiao, X., & Li, D. (2024). Epigenetics-targeted drugs: Current paradigms and future challenges. *Signal Transduction and Targeted Therapy, 9*(1), 332. DOI: 10.1038/s41392-024-02039-0 PMID: 39592582

David, L. A., Maurice, C. F., Carmody, R. N., Gootenberg, D. B., Button, J. E., Wolfe, B. E., Ling, A. V., Devlin, A. S., Varma, Y., Fischbach, M. A., Biddinger, S. B., Dutton, R. J., & Turnbaugh, P. J. (2014). Diet rapidly and reproducibly alters the human gut microbiome. *Nature, 505*(7484), 559–563. DOI: 10.1038/nature12820 PMID: 24336217

Deb, P., Bhan, A., Hussain, I., Ansari, K. I., Bobzean, S. A., Pandita, T. K., Perrotti, L. I., & Mandal, S. S. (2016). Endocrine disrupting chemical, bisphenol-A, induces breast cancer associated gene HOXB9 expression in vitro and in vivo. *Gene, 590*(2), 234–243. DOI: 10.1016/j.gene.2016.05.009 PMID: 27182052

DeFilipp, Z., Bloom, P. P., Torres Soto, M., Mansour, M. K., Sater, M. R. A., Huntley, M. H., Turbett, S., Chung, R. T., Chen, Y.-B., & Hohmann, E. L. (2019). Drug-Resistant *E. coli* Bacteremia Transmitted by Fecal Microbiota Transplant. *The New England Journal of Medicine, 381*(21), 2043–2050. DOI: 10.1056/NEJMoa1910437 PMID: 31665575

Delfosse, V., Grimaldi, M., Pons, J.-L., Boulahtouf, A., Le Maire, A., Cavailles, V., Labesse, G., Bourguet, W., & Balaguer, P. (2012). Structural and mechanistic insights into bisphenols action provide guidelines for risk assessment and discovery of bisphenol A substitutes. *Proceedings of the National Academy of Sciences of the United States of America, 109*(37), 14930–14935. DOI: 10.1073/pnas.1203574109 PMID: 22927406

Dizdaroglu, M. (2015). Oxidatively induced DNA damage and its repair in cancer. *Mutation Research/Reviews in Mutation Research, 763*, 212–245. DOI: 10.1016/j.mrrev.2014.11.002 PMID: 25795122

Dong, Y., Xiao, Y., Shi, Q., & Jiang, C. (2020). Dysregulated lncRNA-miRNA-mRNA Network Reveals Patient Survival-Associated Modules and RNA Binding Proteins in Invasive Breast Carcinoma. *Frontiers in Genetics, 10*, 1284. DOI: 10.3389/fgene.2019.01284 PMID: 32010179

Dostert, C., Pétrilli, V., Van Bruggen, R., Steele, C., Mossman, B. T., & Tschopp, J. (2008). Innate Immune Activation Through Nalp3 Inflammasome Sensing of Asbestos and Silica. *Science, 320*(5876), 674–677. DOI: 10.1126/science.1156995 PMID: 18403674

Eberharter, A., & Becker, P. B. (2002). Histone acetylation: A switch between repressive and permissive chromatin: Second in review series on chromatin dynamics. *EMBO Reports, 3*(3), 224–229. DOI: 10.1093/embo-reports/kvf053 PMID: 11882541

Eisenstein, M. (2022). p53: An anticancer protein's chequered past and promising future. *Nature, 603*(7899), S1–S1. DOI: 10.1038/d41586-022-00565-x PMID: 35236979

Emanowicz, P., Średnicka, P., Wójcicki, M., Roszko, M., & Juszczuk-Kubiak, E. (2024). Mitigating Dietary Bisphenol Exposure Through the Gut Microbiota: The Role of Next-Generation Probiotics in Bacterial Detoxification. *Nutrients, 16*(21), 3757. DOI: 10.3390/nu16213757 PMID: 39519589

Eslami-S, Z., Majidzadeh-A, K., Halvaei, S., Babapirali, F., & Esmaeili, R. (2020). Microbiome and Breast Cancer: New Role for an Ancient Population. *Frontiers in Oncology, 10*, 120. DOI: 10.3389/fonc.2020.00120 PMID: 32117767

Fan, C., Jin, M., Chen, K., Zhang, Y., Zhang, S., & Liu, B. (2007). Case-only study of interactions between metabolic enzymes and smoking in colorectal cancer. *BMC Cancer, 7*(1), 115. DOI: 10.1186/1471-2407-7-115 PMID: 17603900

Feng, Z. (2010). P53 Regulation of the IGF-1/AKT/mTOR Pathways and the Endosomal Compartment. *Cold Spring Harbor Perspectives in Biology, 2*(2), a001057–a001057. DOI: 10.1101/cshperspect.a001057 PMID: 20182617

Foronjy, R. F., Mirochnitchenko, O., Propokenko, O., Lemaitre, V., Jia, Y., Inouye, M., Okada, Y., & D'Armiento, J. M. (2006). Superoxide Dismutase Expression Attenuates Cigarette Smoke– or Elastase-generated Emphysema in Mice. *American Journal of Respiratory and Critical Care Medicine, 173*(6), 623–631. DOI: 10.1164/rccm.200506-850OC PMID: 16387805

Gao, J., Shi, W., Wang, J., Guan, C., Dong, Q., Sheng, J., Zou, X., Xu, Z., Ge, Y., Yang, C., Li, J., Bao, H., Zhong, X., & Cui, Y. (2024). Research progress and applications of epigenetic biomarkers in cancer. *Frontiers in Pharmacology, 15*, 1308309. DOI: 10.3389/fphar.2024.1308309 PMID: 38681199

Garcia, W. L., Miller, C. J., Lomas, G. X., Gaither, K. A., Tyrrell, K. J., Smith, J. N., Brandvold, K. R., & Wright, A. T. (2022). Profiling How the Gut Microbiome Modulates Host Xenobiotic Metabolism in Response to Benzo[*a*]pyrene and 1-Nitropyrene Exposure. *Chemical Research in Toxicology, 35*(4), 585–596. DOI: 10.1021/acs.chemrestox.1c00360 PMID: 35347982

Geissler, F., Nesic, K., Kondrashova, O., Dobrovic, A., Swisher, E. M., Scott, C. L., & Wakefield, J., M. (. (2024). The role of aberrant DNA methylation in cancer initiation and clinical impacts. *Therapeutic Advances in Medical Oncology, 16*, 17588359231220511. DOI: 10.1177/17588359231220511 PMID: 38293277

Gholami, H., Chmiel, J. A., Burton, J. P., & Maleki Vareki, S. (2023). The Role of Microbiota-Derived Vitamins in Immune Homeostasis and Enhancing Cancer Immunotherapy. *Cancers (Basel), 15*(4), 1300. DOI: 10.3390/cancers15041300 PMID: 36831641

Gibbons, D. L., Byers, L. A., & Kurie, J. M. (2014). Smoking, p53 Mutation, and Lung Cancer. *Molecular Cancer Research, 12*(1), 3–13. DOI: 10.1158/1541-7786.MCR-13-0539 PMID: 24442106

Gibney, E. R., & Nolan, C. M. (2010). Epigenetics and gene expression. *Heredity, 105*(1), 4–13. DOI: 10.1038/hdy.2010.54 PMID: 20461105

Giri, A. K., & Aittokallio, T. (2019). DNMT Inhibitors Increase Methylation in the Cancer Genome. *Frontiers in Pharmacology, 10*, 385. DOI: 10.3389/fphar.2019.00385 PMID: 31068808

Goey, A. K., Sissung, T. M., Peer, C. J., & Figg, W. D. (2016). Pharmacogenomics and Histone Deacetylase Inhibitors. *Pharmacogenomics, 17*(16), 1807–1815. DOI: 10.2217/pgs-2016-0113 PMID: 27767376

Goode, E. L., White, K. L., Vierkant, R. A., Phelan, C. M., Cunningham, J. M., Schildkraut, J. M., Berchuck, A., Larson, M. C., Fridley, B. L., Olson, J. E., Webb, P. M., Chen, X., Beesley, J., Chenevix-Trench, G., & Sellers, T. A.Ovarian Cancer Association Consortium. (2011). Xenobiotic-Metabolizing gene polymorphisms and ovarian cancer risk. *Molecular Carcinogenesis, 50*(5), 397–402. DOI: 10.1002/mc.20714 PMID: 21480392

Goodman, S., Chappell, G., Guyton, K. Z., Pogribny, I. P., & Rusyn, I. (2022). Epigenetic alterations induced by genotoxic occupational and environmental human chemical carcinogens: An update of a systematic literature review. *Mutation Research/Reviews in Mutation Research, 789*, 108408. DOI: 10.1016/j.mrrev.2021.108408 PMID: 35690411

Goyal, N., Do, C., Sridhar, J., Shaik, S., Thompson, A., Perry, T., Carter, L., & Foroozesh, M. (2023). Design, Synthesis, and Biological Studies of Flavone-Based Esters and Acids as Potential P450 2A6 Inhibitors. *Chemical Research in Toxicology, 36*(12), 1973–1979. DOI: 10.1021/acs.chemrestox.3c00249 PMID: 37963190

Guengerich, F. P. (2006). Cytochrome P450s and other enzymes in drug metabolism and toxicity. *The AAPS Journal, 8*(1), E101–E111. DOI: 10.1208/aapsj080112 PMID: 16584116

Guo, Q., Jin, Y., Chen, X., Ye, X., Shen, X., Lin, M., Zeng, C., Zhou, T., & Zhang, J. (2024). NF-κB in biology and targeted therapy: New insights and translational implications. *Signal Transduction and Targeted Therapy, 9*(1), 53. DOI: 10.1038/s41392-024-01757-9 PMID: 38433280

Hahm, J. Y., Park, J., Jang, E.-S., & Chi, S. W. (2022). 8-Oxoguanine: From oxidative damage to epigenetic and epitranscriptional modification. *Experimental & Molecular Medicine, 54*(10), 1626–1642. DOI: 10.1038/s12276-022-00822-z PMID: 36266447

Haiser, H. J., Gootenberg, D. B., Chatman, K., Sirasani, G., Balskus, E. P., & Turnbaugh, P. J. (2013). Predicting and Manipulating Cardiac Drug Inactivation by the Human Gut Bacterium *Eggerthella lenta*. *Science, 341*(6143), 295–298. DOI: 10.1126/science.1235872 PMID: 23869020

Hao, Q., Wang, M., Sun, N., Zhu, C., Lin, Y., Li, C., Liu, F., & Zhu, W. (2020). Sulforaphane suppresses carcinogenesis of colorectal cancer through the ERK/Nrf2-UDP glucuronosyltransferase 1A metabolic axis activation. *Oncology Reports*. Advance online publication. DOI: 10.3892/or.2020.7495 PMID: 32323779

Hasin, Y., Seldin, M., & Lusis, A. (2017). Multi-omics approaches to disease. *Genome Biology, 18*(1), 83. DOI: 10.1186/s13059-017-1215-1 PMID: 28476144

Hayes, J. D., Flanagan, J. U., & Jowsey, I. R. (2005). Glutathione transferases. *Annual Review of Pharmacology and Toxicology, 45*(1), 51–88. DOI: 10.1146/annurev.pharmtox.45.120403.095857 PMID: 15822171

He, X., & Feng, S. (2015). Role of Metabolic Enzymes P450 (CYP) on Activating Procarcinogen and their Polymorphisms on the Risk of Cancers. *Current Drug Metabolism, 16*(10), 850–863. DOI: 10.2174/1389200216101512101645 01 PMID: 26652254

Heavey, P. M., & Rowland, I. R. (2004). Gastrointestinal cancer. *Best Practice & Research. Clinical Gastroenterology, 18*(2), 323–336. DOI: 10.1016/j.bpg.2003.10.003 PMID: 15123073

Hecht, S. S. (2012). Lung carcinogenesis by tobacco smoke. *International Journal of Cancer, 131*(12), 2724–2732. DOI: 10.1002/ijc.27816 PMID: 22945513

Heo, Y. J., Hwa, C., Lee, G.-H., Park, J.-M., & An, J.-Y. (2021). Integrative Multi-Omics Approaches in Cancer Research: From Biological Networks to Clinical Subtypes. *Molecules and Cells, 44*(7), 433–443. DOI: 10.14348/molcells.2021.0042 PMID: 34238766

Heppel, C. W., Heling, A.-K., & Richter, E. (2009). Ultrasensitive method for the determination of 4-hydroxy-1-(3-pyridyl)-1-butanone-releasing DNA adducts by gas chromatography–high resolution mass spectrometry in mucosal biopsies of the lower esophagus. *Analytical and Bioanalytical Chemistry, 393*(5), 1525–1530. DOI: 10.1007/s00216-008-2566-y PMID: 19104779

Hillegass, J. M., Miller, J. M., MacPherson, M. B., Westbom, C. M., Sayan, M., Thompson, J. K., Macura, S. L., Perkins, T. N., Beuschel, S. L., Alexeeva, V., Pass, H. I., Steele, C., Mossman, B. T., & Shukla, A. (2013). Asbestos and erionite prime and activate the NLRP3 inflammasome that stimulates autocrine cytokine release in human mesothelial cells. *Particle and Fibre Toxicology*, *10*(1), 39. DOI: 10.1186/1743-8977-10-39 PMID: 23937860

Hillege, L. E., Stevens, M. A. M., Kristen, P. A. J., De Vos-Geelen, J., Penders, J., Redinbo, M. R., & Smidt, M. L. (2024). The role of gut microbial β-glucuronidases in carcinogenesis and cancer treatment: A scoping review. *Journal of Cancer Research and Clinical Oncology*, *150*(11), 495. DOI: 10.1007/s00432-024-06028-2 PMID: 39537966

Ho, S.-M., Tang, W.-Y., Belmonte De Frausto, J., & Prins, G. S. (2006). Developmental Exposure to Estradiol and Bisphenol A Increases Susceptibility to Prostate Carcinogenesis and Epigenetically Regulates Phosphodiesterase Type 4 Variant 4. *Cancer Research*, *66*(11), 5624–5632. DOI: 10.1158/0008-5472.CAN-06-0516 PMID: 16740699

Howarth, M. V., & Eiser, A. R. (2023). Environmentally Mediated Health Disparities. *The American Journal of Medicine*, *136*(6), 518–522. DOI: 10.1016/j.amjmed.2023.02.008 PMID: 36828212

Hu, C., Liu, X., Zeng, Y., Liu, J., & Wu, F. (2021). DNA methyltransferase inhibitors combination therapy for the treatment of solid tumor: Mechanism and clinical application. *Clinical Epigenetics*, *13*(1), 166. DOI: 10.1186/s13148-021-01154-x PMID: 34452630

Huang, S. X. L., Jaurand, M.-C., Kamp, D. W., Whysner, J., & Hei, T. K. (2011). Role of Mutagenicity in Asbestos Fiber-Induced Carcinogenicity and Other Diseases. *Journal of Toxicology and Environmental Health. Part B, Critical Reviews*, *14*(1–4), 179–245. DOI: 10.1080/10937404.2011.556051 PMID: 21534089

Huynh, K. (2017). Targeting inflammatory pathways to treat atherosclerosis and cancer. *Nature Reviews. Cardiology*, *14*(11), 629–629. DOI: 10.1038/nrcardio.2017.152 PMID: 28905870

Iorio, M. V., & Croce, C. M. (2012). Causes and Consequences of MicroRNA Dysregulation. *Cancer Journal (Sudbury, Mass.)*, *18*(3), 215–222. DOI: 10.1097/PPO.0b013e318250c001 PMID: 22647357

Ishikawa, H., Akedo, I., Otani, T., Suzuki, T., Nakamura, T., Takeyama, I., Ishiguro, S., Miyaoka, E., Sobue, T., & Kakizoe, T. (2005). Randomized trial of dietary fiber andLactobacillus casei administration for prevention of colorectal tumors. *International Journal ofCancer, 116*(5), 762–767. DOI: 10.1002/ijc.21115 PMID: 15828052

Islam, T., Majumder, M., Kalita, B., Bhattacharjee, A., Mukhopadhyay, R., & Mukherjee, A. K. (2020). Transcriptomic, proteomic, and biochemical analyses reveal a novel neuritogenesis mechanism of *Naja naja* venom α-elapitoxin post binding to TrkA receptor of rat pheochromocytoma cells. *Journal of Neurochemistry, 155*(6), 612–637. DOI: 10.1111/jnc.15153 PMID: 33460153

Jadhav, R., Santucci-Pereira, J., Wang, Y., Liu, J., Nguyen, T., Wang, J., Jenkins, S., Russo, J., Huang, T., Jin, V., & Lamartiniere, C. (2017). DNA Methylation Targets Influenced by Bisphenol A and/or Genistein Are Associated with Survival Outcomes in Breast Cancer Patients. *Genes, 8*(5), 144. DOI: 10.3390/genes8050144 PMID: 28505145

Jiang, G., Zhang, S., Yazdanparast, A., Li, M., Pawar, A. V., Liu, Y., Inavolu, S. M., & Cheng, L. (2016). Comprehensive comparison of molecular portraits between cell lines and tumors in breast cancer. *BMC Genomics, 17*(S7), 525. DOI: 10.1186/s12864-016-2911-z PMID: 27556158

Jin, Y., Wu, S., Zeng, Z., & Fu, Z. (2017). Effects of environmental pollutants on gut microbiota. *Environmental Pollution, 222*, 1–9. DOI: 10.1016/j.envpol.2016.11.045 PMID: 28086130

Karczewski, K. J., & Snyder, M. P. (2018). Integrative omics for health and disease. *Nature Reviews. Genetics, 19*(5), 299–310. DOI: 10.1038/nrg.2018.4 PMID: 29479082

Katiyar, S. K., Singh, T., Prasad, R., Sun, Q., & Vaid, M. (2012). Epigenetic Alterations in Ultraviolet Radiation-Induced Skin Carcinogenesis: Interaction of Bioactive Dietary Components on Epigenetic Targets†. *Photochemistry and Photobiology, 88*(5), 1066–1074. DOI: 10.1111/j.1751-1097.2011.01020.x PMID: 22017262

Kawanishi, S., Ohnishi, S., Ma, N., Hiraku, Y., & Murata, M. (2017). Crosstalk between DNA Damage and Inflammation in the Multiple Steps of Carcinogenesis. *International Journal of Molecular Sciences, 18*(8), 1808. DOI: 10.3390/ijms18081808 PMID: 28825631

Kay, J., Thadhani, E., Samson, L., & Engelward, B. (2019). Inflammation-induced DNA damage, mutations and cancer. *DNA Repair, 83*, 102673. DOI: 10.1016/j.dnarep.2019.102673 PMID: 31387777

Kensler, T. W., Ng, D., Carmella, S. G., Chen, M., Jacobson, L. P., Muñoz, A., Egner, P. A., Chen, J. G., Qian, G. S., Chen, T. Y., Fahey, J. W., Talalay, P., Groopman, J. D., Yuan, J.-M., & Hecht, S. S. (2012). Modulation of the metabolism of airborne pollutants by glucoraphanin-rich and sulforaphane-rich broccoli sprout beverages in Qidong, China. *Carcinogenesis, 33*(1), 101–107. DOI: 10.1093/carcin/bgr229 PMID: 22045030

Khosravi, A., & Mazmanian, S. K. (2013). Disruption of the gut microbiome as a risk factor for microbial infections. *Current Opinion in Microbiology, 16*(2), 221–227. DOI: 10.1016/j.mib.2013.03.009 PMID: 23597788

Kim, K.-H., Lee, S. J., Kim, J., & Moon, Y. (2024). Leveraging Xenobiotic-Responsive Cancer Stemness in Cell Line-Based Tumoroids for Evaluating Chemoresistance: A Proof-of-Concept Study on Environmental Susceptibility. *International Journal of Molecular Sciences, 25*(21), 11383. DOI: 10.3390/ijms252111383 PMID: 39518936

Kim, S. T., Kim, S. Y., Klempner, S. J., Yoon, J., Kim, N., Ahn, S., Bang, H., Kim, K.-M., Park, W., Park, S. H., Park, J. O., Park, Y. S., Lim, H. Y., Lee, S. H., Park, K., Kang, W. K., & Lee, J. (2017). Rapamycin-insensitive companion of mTOR (RICTOR) amplification defines a subset of advanced gastric cancer and is sensitive to AZD2014-mediated mTORC1/2 inhibition. *Annals of Oncology : Official Journal of the European Society for Medical Oncology, 28*(3), 547–554. DOI: 10.1093/annonc/mdw669 PMID: 28028034

Kish, L., Hotte, N., Kaplan, G. G., Vincent, R., Tso, R., Gänzle, M., Rioux, K. P., Thiesen, A., Barkema, H. W., Wine, E., & Madsen, K. L. (2013). Environmental Particulate Matter Induces Murine Intestinal Inflammatory Responses and Alters the Gut Microbiome. *PLoS One, 8*(4), e62220. DOI: 10.1371/journal.pone.0062220 PMID: 23638009

Kogevinas, M. (2001). Human health effects of dioxins: Cancer, reproductive and endocrine system effects. *Human Reproduction Update, 7*(3), 331–339. DOI: 10.1093/humupd/7.3.331 PMID: 11392380

Korolenko, A. A., Noll, S. E., & Skinner, M. K. (2023). Epigenetic Inheritance and Transgenerational EnvironmentalJustice. *The Yale Journal of Biology and Medicine, 96*(2), 241–250. DOI: 10.59249/FKWS5176 PMID: 37396986

Koual, M., Tomkiewicz, C., Cano-Sancho, G., Antignac, J.-P., Bats, A.-S., & Coumoul, X. (2020). Environmental chemicals, breast cancer progression and drug resistance. *Environmental Health : A Global Access Science Source, 19*(1), 117. DOI: 10.1186/s12940-020-00670-2 PMID: 33203443

Kuiper, G. G. J. M., Carlsson, B., Grandien, K., Enmark, E., Häggblad, J., Nilsson, S., & Gustafsson, J.-Å. (1997). Comparison of the Ligand Binding Specificity and Transcript Tissue Distribution of Estrogen Receptors α and β. *Endocrinology, 138*(3), 863–870. DOI: 10.1210/endo.138.3.4979 PMID: 9048584

Kulis, M., & Esteller, M. (2010). DNA Methylation and Cancer. In *Advances in Genetics* (Vol. 70, pp. 27–56). Elsevier., DOI: 10.1016/B978-0-12-380866-0.60002-2

Lapin, A., Perfahl, H., Jain, H. V., & Reuss, M. (2022). Integrating a dynamic central metabolism model of cancer cells with a hybrid 3D multiscale model for vascular hepatocellular carcinoma growth. *Scientific Reports, 12*(1), 12373. DOI: 10.1038/s41598-022-15767-6 PMID: 35858953

Lauby-Secretan, B., Scoccianti, C., Loomis, D., Grosse, Y., Bianchini, F., & Straif, K. (2016). Body Fatness and Cancer—Viewpoint of the IARC Working Group. *The New England Journal of Medicine, 375*(8), 794–798. DOI: 10.1056/NEJMsr1606602 PMID: 27557308

Ledda, C. (2018). Cadmium exposure and prostate cancer insights mechanisms and perspectives. *Frontiers in Bioscience, 23*(9), 1687–1700. DOI: 10.2741/4667 PMID: 29293457

Lee, D. G., Schuetz, J. M., Lai, A. S., Burstyn, I., Brooks-Wilson, A., Aronson, K. J., & Spinelli, J. J. (2022). Interactions between exposure to polycyclic aromatic hydrocarbons and xenobiotic metabolism genes, and risk of breast cancer. *Breast Cancer (Tokyo, Japan), 29*(1), 38–49. DOI: 10.1007/s12282-021-01279-0 PMID: 34351578

Lee, S., Yun, Y., Kim, S., Lee, E.-J., Chang, Y., Ryu, S., Shin, H., Kim, H.-L., Kim, H.-N., & Lee, J. (2018). Association between Cigarette Smoking Status and Composition of Gut Microbiota: Population-Based Cross-Sectional Study. *Journal of Clinical Medicine, 7*(9), 282. DOI: 10.3390/jcm7090282 PMID: 30223529

Lei, L., Yang, J., Zhang, J., & Zhang, G. (2021). The lipid peroxidation product EKODE exacerbates colonic inflammation and colon tumorigenesis. *Redox Biology, 42*, 101880. DOI: 10.1016/j.redox.2021.101880 PMID: 33541845

Leng, D., Zheng, L., Wen, Y., Zhang, Y., Wu, L., Wang, J., Wang, M., Zhang, Z., He, S., & Bo, X. (2022). A benchmark study of deep learning-based multi-omics data fusion methods for cancer. *Genome Biology, 23*(1), 171. DOI: 10.1186/s13059-022-02739-2 PMID: 35945544

Li, D., Yun, Y., & Gao, R. (2019). Oxygenated Polycyclic aromatic hydrocarbons (Oxy-PAHs) facilitate lung cancer metastasis by epigenetically regulating the epithelial-to-mesenchymal transition (EMT). *Environmental Pollution, 255*, 113261. DOI: 10.1016/j.envpol.2019.113261 PMID: 31580991

Li, X., Brejnrod, A. D., Ernst, M., Rykær, M., Herschend, J., Olsen, N. M. C., Dorrestein, P. C., Rensing, C., & Sørensen, S. J. (2019). Heavy metal exposure causes changes in the metabolic health-associated gut microbiome and metabolites. *Environment International, 126*, 454–467. DOI: 10.1016/j.envint.2019.02.048 PMID: 30844581

Li, Y., Steppi, A., Zhou, Y., Mao, F., Miller, P. C., He, M. M., Zhao, T., Sun, Q., & Zhang, J. (2017). Tumoral expression of drug and xenobiotic metabolizing enzymes in breast cancer patients of different ethnicities with implications to personalized medicine. *Scientific Reports, 7*(1), 4747. DOI: 10.1038/s41598-017-04250-2 PMID: 28684774

Li, Z., Kwon, S. M., Li, D., Li, L., Peng, X., Zhang, J., Sueyoshi, T., Raufman, J.-P., Negishi, M., Wang, X. W., & Wang, H. (2022). Human constitutive androstane receptor represses liver cancer development and hepatoma cell proliferation by inhibiting erythropoietin signaling. *The Journal of Biological Chemistry, 298*(5), 101885. DOI: 10.1016/j.jbc.2022.101885 PMID: 35367211

Lima, S. F., Pires, S., Rupert, A., Oguntunmibi, S., Jin, W.-B., Marderstein, A., Funez-dePagnier, G., Maldarelli, G., Viladomiu, M., Putzel, G., Yang, W., Tran, N., Xiang, G., Grier, A., Guo, C.-J., Lukin, D., Mandl, L. A., Scherl, E. J., & Longman, R. S. (2024). The gut microbiome regulates the clinical efficacy of sulfasalazine therapy for IBD-associated spondyloarthritis. *Cell Reports Medicine, 5*(3), 101431. DOI: 10.1016/j.xcrm.2024.101431 PMID: 38378002

Liu, Z., Ren, Y., Weng, S., Xu, H., Li, L., & Han, X. (2022). A New Trend in Cancer Treatment: The Combination of Epigenetics and Immunotherapy. *Frontiers in Immunology, 13*, 809761. DOI: 10.3389/fimmu.2022.809761 PMID: 35140720

Louis, P., Hold, G. L., & Flint, H. J. (2014). The gut microbiota, bacterial metabolites and colorectal cancer. *Nature Reviews. Microbiology, 12*(10), 661–672. DOI: 10.1038/nrmicro3344 PMID: 25198138

Ludovini, V., Chiari, R., Tomassoni, L., Antonini, C., Baldelli, E., Baglivo, S., Siggillino, A., Tofanetti, F. R., Bellezza, G., Hodge, K. A., Petricoin, E., Pierobon, M., Crinò, L., & Bianconi, F. (2017). Reverse phase protein array (RPPA) combined with computational analysis to unravel relevant prognostic factors in non- small cell lung cancer (NSCLC): A pilot study. *Oncotarget*, *8*(47), 83343–83353. DOI: 10.18632/oncotarget.18480 PMID: 29137348

Maksymchuk, O., & Kashuba, V. (2019). Dietary lipids and environmental xenobiotics as risk factors for prostate cancer: The role of cytochrome P450. *Pharmacological Reports*, *71*(5), 826–832. DOI: 10.1016/j.pharep.2019.04.011 PMID: 31382168

Mandal, A., Biswas, N., & Alam, M. N. (2023). Implications of xenobiotic-response element(s) and aryl hydrocarbon receptor in health and diseases. *Human Cell*, *36*(5), 1638–1655. DOI: 10.1007/s13577-023-00931-5 PMID: 37329424

Mansoori, B., Mohammadi, A., Davudian, S., Shirjang, S., & Baradaran, B. (2017). The Different Mechanisms of Cancer Drug Resistance: A Brief Review. *Advanced Pharmaceutical Bulletin*, *7*(3), 339–348. DOI: 10.15171/apb.2017.041 PMID: 29071215

Masson, L. F., Sharp, L., Cotton, S. C., & Little, J. (2005). Cytochrome P-450 1A1 Gene Polymorphisms and Risk of Breast Cancer: A HuGE Review. *American Journal of Epidemiology*, *161*(10), 901–915. DOI: 10.1093/aje/kwi121 PMID: 15870154

Mastrangelo, G., Fedeli, U., Fadda, E., Valentini, F., Agnesi, R., Magarotto, G., Marchì, T., Buda, A., Pinzani, M., & Martines, D. (2004). Increased Risk of Hepatocellular Carcinoma and Liver Cirrhosis in Vinyl Chloride Workers: Synergistic Effect of Occupational Exposure with Alcohol Intake. *Environmental Health Perspectives*, *112*(11), 1188–1192. DOI: 10.1289/ehp.6972 PMID: 15289165

Mathis, C., Gebel, S., Poussin, C., Belcastro, V., Sewer, A., Weisensee, D., Hengstermann, A., Ansari, S., Wagner, S., Peitsch, M. C., & Hoeng, J. (2015). A Systems Biology Approach Reveals the Dose- and Time-Dependent Effect of Primary Human Airway Epithelium Tissue Culture after Exposure to Cigarette Smoke in Vitro. *Bioinformatics and Biology Insights, 9. Bioinformatics and Biology Insights, S19908*, BBI.S19908. Advance online publication. DOI: 10.4137/BBI.S19908 PMID: 25788831

Merk, O., & Speit, G. (1998). Significance of formaldehyde-induced DNA–protein crosslinks for mutagenesis. *Environmental and Molecular Mutagenesis*, *32*(3), 260–268. DOI: 10.1002/(SICI)1098-2280(1998)32:3<260::AID-EM9>3.0.CO;2-M PMID: 9814441

Mertins, P., Mani, D. R., Ruggles, K. V., Gillette, M. A., Clauser, K. R., Wang, P., Wang, X., Qiao, J. W., Cao, S., Petralia, F., Kawaler, E., Mundt, F., Krug, K., Tu, Z., Lei, J. T., Gatza, M. L., Wilkerson, M., Perou, C. M., Yellapantula, V., & Carr, S. A. (2016). Proteogenomics connects somatic mutations to signalling in breast cancer. *Nature*, *534*(7605), 55–62. DOI: 10.1038/nature18003 PMID: 27251275

Mokhosoev, I. M., Astakhov, D. V., Terentiev, A. A., & Moldogazieva, N. T. (2024). Human Cytochrome P450 Cancer-Related Metabolic Activities and Gene Polymorphisms: A Review. *Cells*, *13*(23), 1958. DOI: 10.3390/cells13231958 PMID: 39682707

Moon, Y. J., Wang, X., & Morris, M. E. (2006). Dietary flavonoids: Effects on xenobiotic and carcinogen metabolism. *Toxicology In Vitro*, *20*(2), 187–210. DOI: 10.1016/j.tiv.2005.06.048 PMID: 16289744

Neagu, A.-N., Jayaweera, T., Corrice, L., Johnson, K., & Darie, C. (2024). Breast Cancer Exposomics. *Life (Chicago, Ill.)*, *14*(3), 402. DOI: 10.3390/life14030402 PMID: 38541726

Nogacka, A., Gómez-Martín, M., Suárez, A., González-Bernardo, O., De Los Reyes-Gavilán, C., & González, S. (2019). Xenobiotics Formed during Food Processing: Their Relation with the Intestinal Microbiota and Colorectal Cancer. *International Journal of Molecular Sciences*, *20*(8), 2051. DOI: 10.3390/ijms20082051 PMID: 31027304

O'Keefe, S. J. D. (2016). Diet, microorganisms and their metabolites, and colon cancer. *Nature Reviews. Gastroenterology & Hepatology*, *13*(12), 691–706. DOI: 10.1038/nrgastro.2016.165 PMID: 27848961

Obtulowicz, T., Swoboda, M., Speina, E., Gackowski, D., Rozalski, R., Siomek, A., Janik, J., Janowska, B., Ciesla, J. M., Jawien, A., Banaszkiewicz, Z., Guz, J., Dziaman, T., Szpila, A., Olinski, R., & Tudek, B. (2010). Oxidative stress and 8-oxoguanine repair are enhanced in colon adenoma and carcinoma patients. *Mutagenesis*, *25*(5), 463–471. DOI: 10.1093/mutage/geq028 PMID: 20534734

Ogunjobi, T. T., Ohaeri, P. N., Akintola, O. T., Atanda, D. O., Orji, F. P., Adebayo, J. O., Abdul, S. O., Eji, C. A., Asebebe, A. B., Shodipe, O. O., & Adedeji, O. O. (2024). *Bioinformatics Applications in Chronic Diseases: A Comprehensive Review of Genomic, Transcriptomics, Proteomic, Metabolomics, and Machine Learning Approaches*. Medinformatics., DOI: 10.47852/bonviewMEDIN42022335

Ollberding, N. J., Wilkens, L. R., Henderson, B. E., Kolonel, L. N., & Le Marchand, L. (2012). Meat consumption, heterocyclic amines and colorectal cancer risk: The Multiethnic Cohort Study. *International Journal of Cancer, 131*(7). Advance online publication. DOI: 10.1002/ijc.27546 PMID: 22438055

Pal, S., & Firdous, S. M. (2024). Unraveling the role of heavy metals xenobiotics in cancer: A critical review. *Discover. Oncology, 15*(1), 615. DOI: 10.1007/s12672-024-01417-y PMID: 39495398

Pant, A., Maiti, T. K., Mahajan, D., & Das, B. (2023). Human Gut Microbiota and Drug Metabolism. *Microbial Ecology, 86*(1), 97–111. DOI: 10.1007/s00248-022-02081-x PMID: 35869999

Parris, B. A., O'Farrell, H. E., Fong, K. M., & Yang, I. A. (2019). Chronic obstructive pulmonary disease (COPD) and lung cancer: Common pathways for pathogenesis. *Journal of Thoracic Disease, 11*(S17), S2155–S2172. DOI: 10.21037/jtd.2019.10.54 PMID: 31737343

Patnaik, S., & Anupriya, . (2019). Drugs Targeting Epigenetic Modifications and Plausible Therapeutic Strategies Against Colorectal Cancer. *Frontiers in Pharmacology, 10*, 588. DOI: 10.3389/fphar.2019.00588 PMID: 31244652

Pelkonen, O., Abass, K., Parra Morte, J. M., Panzarea, M., Testai, E., Rudaz, S., Louisse, J., Gundert-Remy, U., Wolterink, G., Jean-Lou Cm, D., Coecke, S., & Bernasconi, C. (2023). Metabolites in the regulatory risk assessment of pesticides in the EU. *Frontiers in Toxicology, 5*, 1304885. DOI: 10.3389/ftox.2023.1304885 PMID: 38188093

Pellegrini, L., Xue, J., Larson, D., Pastorino, S., Jube, S., Forest, K. H., Saad-Jube, Z. S., Napolitano, A., Pagano, I., Negi, V. S., Bianchi, M. E., Morris, P., Pass, H. I., Gaudino, G., Carbone, M., & Yang, H. (2017). HMGB1 targeting by ethyl pyruvate suppresses malignant phenotype of human mesothelioma. *Oncotarget, 8*(14), 22649–22661. DOI: 10.18632/oncotarget.15152 PMID: 28186988

Phillips, D. H. (1999). Polycyclic aromatic hydrocarbons in the diet. *Mutation Research/Genetic Toxicology and Environmental Mutagenesis, 443*(1–2), 139–147. DOI: 10.1016/S1383-5742(99)00016-2 PMID: 10415437

Pinu, F. R., Beale, D. J., Paten, A. M., Kouremenos, K., Swarup, S., Schirra, H. J., & Wishart, D. (2019). Systems Biology and Multi-Omics Integration: Viewpoints from the Metabolomics Research Community. *Metabolites, 9*(4), 76. DOI: 10.3390/metabo9040076 PMID: 31003499

Pizzino, G., Irrera, N., Cucinotta, M., Pallio, G., Mannino, F., Arcoraci, V., Squadrito, F., Altavilla, D., & Bitto, A. (2017). Oxidative Stress: Harms and Benefits for Human Health. *Oxidative Medicine and Cellular Longevity, 2017*(1), 8416763. DOI: 10.1155/2017/8416763 PMID: 28819546

Pool, M., De Boer, H. R., Hooge, M. N. L., Van Vugt, M. A. T. M., & De Vries, E. G. E. (2017). Harnessing Integrative Omics to Facilitate Molecular Imaging of the Human Epidermal Growth Factor Receptor Family for Precision Medicine. *Theranostics, 7*(7), 2111–2133. DOI: 10.7150/thno.17934 PMID: 28638489

Poschl, G. (2004). ALCOHOL AND CANCER. *Alcohol and Alcoholism, 39*(3), 155–165. DOI: 10.1093/alcalc/agh057 PMID: 15082451

Qin, T., Zhang, X., Guo, T., Yang, T., Gao, Y., Hao, W., & Xiao, X. (2021). Epigenetic Alteration Shaped by the Environmental Chemical Bisphenol A. *Frontiers in Genetics, 11*, 618966. DOI: 10.3389/fgene.2020.618966 PMID: 33505438

Rafter, J. (2003). Probiotics and colon cancer. *Best Practice & Research. Clinical Gastroenterology, 17*(5), 849–859. DOI: 10.1016/S1521-6918(03)00056-8 PMID: 14507593

Rahbar, M. H., Samms-Vaughan, M., Kim, S., Saroukhani, S., Bressler, J., Hessabi, M., Grove, M. L., Shakspeare-Pellington, S., & Loveland, K. A. (2022). Detoxification Role of Metabolic Glutathione S-Transferase (GST) Genes in Blood Lead Concentrations of Jamaican Children with and without Autism Spectrum Disorder. *Genes, 13*(6), 975. DOI: 10.3390/genes13060975 PMID: 35741737

Raufaste-Cazavieille, V., Santiago, R., & Droit, A. (2022). Multi-omics analysis: Paving the path toward achieving precision medicine in cancer treatment and immuno-oncology. *Frontiers in Molecular Biosciences, 9*, 962743. DOI: 10.3389/fmolb.2022.962743 PMID: 36304921

Reszka, E., Wasowicz, W., & Gromadzinska, J. (n.d.). *Genetic polymorphism of xenobiotic metabolising enzymes, diet and cancer susceptibility.* DOI: 10.1079/BJN20061878

Rezazadegan, M., Forootani, B., Hoveyda, Y., Rezazadegan, N., & Amani, R. (2025). Major heavy metals and human gut microbiota composition: A systematic review with nutritional approach. *Journal of Health, Population and Nutrition, 44*(1), 21. DOI: 10.1186/s41043-025-00750-4 PMID: 39871318

Roje, B., Zhang, B., Mastrorilli, E., Kovačić, A., Sušak, L., Ljubenkov, I., Ćosić, E., Vilović, K., Meštrović, A., Vukovac, E. L., Bučević-Popović, V., Puljiz, Ž., Karaman, I., Terzić, J., & Zimmermann, M. (2024). Gut microbiota carcinogen metabolism causes distal tissue tumours. *Nature*, *632*(8027), 1137–1144. DOI: 10.1038/s41586-024-07754-w PMID: 39085612

Rossman, T. (2003). Mechanism of arsenic carcinogenesis: An integrated approach. *Mutation Research. Fundamental and Molecular Mechanisms of Mutagenesis*, *533*(1–2), 37–65. DOI: 10.1016/j.mrfmmm.2003.07.009 PMID: 14643412

Ruiz-Saavedra, S., Zapico, A., Del Rey, C. G., Gonzalez, C., Suárez, A., Díaz, Y., De Los Reyes-Gavilán, C. G., & González, S. (2022). Dietary Xenobiotics Derived from Food Processing: Association with Fecal Mutagenicity and Gut Mucosal Damage. *Nutrients*, *14*(17), 3482. DOI: 10.3390/nu14173482 PMID: 36079735

Salim, S. Y., Kaplan, G. G., & Madsen, K. L. (2014). Air pollution effects on the gut microbiota: A link between exposure and inflammatory disease. *Gut Microbes*, *5*(2), 215–219. DOI: 10.4161/gmic.27251 PMID: 24637593

Sarbassov, D. D., Guertin, D. A., Ali, S. M., & Sabatini, D. M. (2005). Phosphorylation and Regulation of Akt/PKB by the Rictor-mTOR Complex. *Science*, *307*(5712), 1098–1101. DOI: 10.1126/science.1106148 PMID: 15718470

Schnekenburger, M., Karius, T., & Diederich, M. (2014). Regulation of epigenetic traits of the glutathione S-transferase P1 gene: From detoxification toward cancer prevention and diagnosis. *Frontiers in Pharmacology*, *5*. Advance online publication. DOI: 10.3389/fphar.2014.00170 PMID: 25076909

Schwabe, R. F., & Jobin, C. (2013). The microbiome and cancer. *Nature Reviews. Cancer*, *13*(11), 800–812. DOI: 10.1038/nrc3610 PMID: 24132111

Sender, R., Fuchs, S., & Milo, R. (2016). Revised Estimates for the Number of Human and Bacteria Cells in the Body. *PLoS Biology*, *14*(8), e1002533. DOI: 10.1371/journal.pbio.1002533 PMID: 27541692

Senghor, B., Sokhna, C., Ruimy, R., & Lagier, J.-C. (2018). Gut microbiota diversity according to dietary habits and geographical provenance. *Human Microbiome Journal*, *7–8*, 1–9. DOI: 10.1016/j.humic.2018.01.001

Shang, Y., Zhang, Z., Liu, Z., Feng, B., Ren, G., Li, K., Zhou, L., Sun, Y., Li, M., Zhou, J., An, Y., Wu, K., Nie, Y., & Fan, D. (2014). miR-508-5p regulates multidrug resistance of gastric cancer by targeting ABCB1 and ZNRD1. *Oncogene*, *33*(25), 3267–3276. DOI: 10.1038/onc.2013.297 PMID: 23893241

Sheller, M. J., Edwards, B., Reina, G. A., Martin, J., Pati, S., Kotrotsou, A., Milchenko, M., Xu, W., Marcus, D., Colen, R. R., & Bakas, S. (2020). Federated learning in medicine: Facilitating multi-institutional collaborations without sharing patient data. *Scientific Reports*, *10*(1), 12598. DOI: 10.1038/s41598-020-69250-1 PMID: 32724046

Shimada, T. (2006). Xenobiotic-Metabolizing Enzymes Involved in Activation and Detoxification of Carcinogenic Polycyclic Aromatic Hydrocarbons. *Drug Metabolism and Pharmacokinetics*, *21*(4), 257–276. DOI: 10.2133/dmpk.21.257 PMID: 16946553

Shimizu, T., LoRusso, P. M., Papadopoulos, K. P., Patnaik, A., Beeram, M., Smith, L. S., Rasco, D. W., Mays, T. A., Chambers, G., Ma, A., Wang, J., Laliberte, R., Voi, M., & Tolcher, A. W. (2014). Phase I First-in-Human Study of CUDC-101, a Multitargeted Inhibitor of HDACs, EGFR, and HER2 in Patients with Advanced Solid Tumors. *Clinical Cancer Research*, *20*(19), 5032–5040. DOI: 10.1158/1078-0432.CCR-14-0570 PMID: 25107918

Si, W., Shen, J., Zheng, H., & Fan, W. (2019). The role and mechanisms of action of microRNAs in cancer drug resistance. *Clinical Epigenetics*, *11*(1), 25. DOI: 10.1186/s13148-018-0587-8 PMID: 30744689

Singh, D. D. (2024). Epigenetic Mechanisms of Endocrine-Disrupting Chemicals in Breast Cancer and Their Impact on Dietary Intake. *Journal of Xenobiotics*, *15*(1), 1. DOI: 10.3390/jox15010001 PMID: 39846533

Singh, L. K., Kumar, A., Siddiqi, N. J., & Sharma, B. (2024). Heavy metals altered the xenobiotic metabolism of rats by targeting the GST enzyme: An in vitro and in silico study. *Toxicology*, *509*, 153946. DOI: 10.1016/j.tox.2024.153946 PMID: 39270966

Singh, R. D., Avadhesh, A., Sharma, G., Dholariya, S., Shah, R. B., Goyal, B., & Gupta, S. C. (2023). Potential of Cytochrome P450, a Family of Xenobiotic Metabolizing Enzymes, in Cancer Therapy. *Antioxidants & Redox Signaling*, *38*(10–12), 853–876. DOI: 10.1089/ars.2022.0116 PMID: 36242099

Singh, S., & Li, S. S.-L. (2012). Epigenetic Effects of Environmental Chemicals Bisphenol A and Phthalates. *International Journal of Molecular Sciences*, *13*(8), 10143–10153. DOI: 10.3390/ijms130810143 PMID: 22949852

Singh, S., Sharma, P., Pal, N., Kumawat, M., Shubham, S., Sarma, D. K., Tiwari, R. R., Kumar, M., & Nagpal, R. (2022). Impact of Environmental Pollutants on Gut Microbiome and Mental Health via the Gut–Brain Axis. *Microorganisms*, *10*(7), 1457. DOI: 10.3390/microorganisms10071457 PMID: 35889175

Smith, J. N., Gaither, K. A., & Pande, P. (2022). Competitive Metabolism of Polycyclic Aromatic Hydrocarbons (PAHs): An Assessment Using In Vitro Metabolism and Physiologically Based Pharmacokinetic (PBPK) Modeling. *International Journal of Environmental Research and Public Health, 19*(14), 8266. DOI: 10.3390/ijerph19148266 PMID: 35886113

Sonnenburg, J. L., & Bäckhed, F. (2016). Diet–microbiota interactions as moderators of human metabolism. *Nature, 535*(7610), 56–64. DOI: 10.1038/nature18846 PMID: 27383980

Stepanov, I., Muzic, J., Le, C. T., Sebero, E., Villalta, P., Ma, B., Jensen, J., Hatsukami, D., & Hecht, S. S. (2013). Analysis of 4-Hydroxy-1-(3-pyridyl)-1-butanone (HPB)-Releasing DNA Adducts in Human Exfoliated Oral Mucosa Cells by Liquid Chromatography–Electrospray Ionization–Tandem Mass Spectrometry. *Chemical Research in Toxicology, 26*(1), 37–45. DOI: 10.1021/tx300282k PMID: 23252610

Subramanian, I., Verma, S., Kumar, S., Jere, A., & Anamika, K. (2020). Multi-omics Data Integration, Interpretation, and Its Application. *Bioinformatics and Biology Insights, 14*, 117793221989905. DOI: 10.1177/1177932219899051 PMID: 32076369

Suez, J., Zmora, N., Zilberman-Schapira, G., Mor, U., Dori-Bachash, M., Bashiardes, S., Zur, M., Regev-Lehavi, D., Ben-Zeev Brik, R., Federici, S., Horn, M., Cohen, Y., Moor, A. E., Zeevi, D., Korem, T., Kotler, E., Harmelin, A., Itzkovitz, S., Maharshak, N., & Elinav, E. (2018). Post-Antibiotic Gut Mucosal Microbiome Reconstitution Is Impaired by Probiotics and Improved by Autologous FMT. *Cell, 174*(6), 1406–1423.e16. DOI: 10.1016/j.cell.2018.08.047 PMID: 30193113

Sun, C., Wang, A., Zhou, Y., Chen, P., Wang, X., Huang, J., Gao, J., Wang, X., Shu, L., Lu, J., Dai, W., Bu, Z., Ji, J., & He, J. (2023). Spatially resolved multi-omics highlights cell-specific metabolic remodeling and interactions in gastric cancer. *Nature Communications, 14*(1), 2692. DOI: 10.1038/s41467-023-38360-5 PMID: 37164975

Tamási, V., Monostory, K., Prough, R. A., & Falus, A. (2011). Role of xenobiotic metabolism in cancer: Involvement of transcriptional and miRNA regulation of P450s. *Cellular and Molecular Life Sciences : CMLS, 68*(7), 1131–1146. DOI: 10.1007/s00018-010-0600-7 PMID: 21184128

Taş, İ., Varlı, M., Pulat, S., Sim, H. B., Kim, J.-J., & Kim, H. (2024). TDO2 inhibition counters Benzo[a]pyrene-induced immune evasion and suppresses tumorigenesis in lung adenocarcinoma. *Cancer & Metabolism, 12*(1), 36. DOI: 10.1186/s40170-024-00365-z PMID: 39593177

Tekpli, X., Zienoldiny, S., Skaug, V., Stangeland, L., Haugen, A., & Mollerup, S. (2012). DNA methylation of the CYP1A1 enhancer is associated with smoking-induced genetic alterations in human lung. *International Journal of Cancer, 131*(7), 1509–1516. DOI: 10.1002/ijc.27421 PMID: 22213191

Thu, M. S., Ondee, T., Nopsopon, T., Farzana, I. A. K., Fothergill, J. L., Hirankarn, N., Campbell, B. J., & Pongpirul, K. (2023). Effect of Probiotics in Breast Cancer: A Systematic Review and Meta-Analysis. *Biology (Basel), 12*(2), 280. DOI: 10.3390/biology12020280 PMID: 36829557

Thum, T., Erpenbeck, V. J., Moeller, J., Hohlfeld, J. M., Krug, N., & Borlak, J. (2006). Expression of Xenobiotic Metabolizing Enzymes in Different Lung Compartments of Smokers and Nonsmokers. *Environmental Health Perspectives, 114*(11), 1655–1661. DOI: 10.1289/ehp.8861 PMID: 17107849

Tomonaga, T., Izumi, H., Yoshiura, Y., Nishida, C., Yatera, K., & Morimoto, Y. (2021). Examination of Surfactant Protein D as a Biomarker for Evaluating Pulmonary Toxicity of Nanomaterials in Rat. *International Journal of Molecular Sciences, 22*(9), 4635. DOI: 10.3390/ijms22094635 PMID: 33924924

Toraño, E. G., García, M. G., Fernández-Morera, J. L., Niño-García, P., & Fernández, A. F. (2016). The Impact of External Factors on the Epigenome: *In Utero* and over Lifetime. *BioMed Research International, 2016*, 1–17. DOI: 10.1155/2016/2568635 PMID: 27294112

Towle, K. M., Benson, S. M., Egnot, N. S., & Marsh, G. M. (2021). An Ecological Evaluation of Vinyl Chloride Exposure and Liver Cancer Incidence and Mortality in Texas. *Journal of Clinical and Translational Hepatology, 000*(000), 1–7. DOI: 10.14218/JCTH.2020.00073 PMID: 33604260

Truhn, D., Tayebi Arasteh, S., Saldanha, O. L., Müller-Franzes, G., Khader, F., Quirke, P., West, N. P., Gray, R., Hutchins, G. G. A., James, J. A., Loughrey, M. B., Salto-Tellez, M., Brenner, H., Brobeil, A., Yuan, T., Chang-Claude, J., Hoffmeister, M., Foersch, S., Han, T., & Kather, J. N. (2024). Encrypted federated learning for secure decentralized collaboration in cancer image analysis. *Medical Image Analysis, 92*, 103059. DOI: 10.1016/j.media.2023.103059 PMID: 38104402

Uyar, B., Ronen, J., Franke, V., Gargiulo, G., & Akalin, A. (2021). Multi-omics and deep learning provide a multifaceted view of cancer. *Bioinformatics (Oxford, England)*. Advance online publication. DOI: 10.1101/2021.09.29.462364

Vasan, N., Baselga, J., & Hyman, D. M. (2019). A view on drug resistance in cancer. *Nature, 575*(7782), 299–309. DOI: 10.1038/s41586-019-1730-1 PMID: 31723286

Villanueva, A., Chiang, D. Y., Newell, P., Peix, J., Thung, S., Alsinet, C., Tovar, V., Roayaie, S., Minguez, B., Sole, M., Battiston, C., Van Laarhoven, S., Fiel, M. I., Di Feo, A., Hoshida, Y., Yea, S., Toffanin, S., Ramos, A., Martignetti, J. A., & Llovet, J. M. (2008). Pivotal Role of mTOR Signaling in Hepatocellular Carcinoma. *Gastroenterology, 135*(6), 1972–1983.e11. DOI: 10.1053/j.gastro.2008.08.008 PMID: 18929564

Vineis, P., Schatzkin, A., & Potter, J. D. (2010). Models of carcinogenesis: An overview. *Carcinogenesis, 31*(10), 1703–1709. DOI: 10.1093/carcin/bgq087 PMID: 20430846

Vuong, T. P. (2022). Research on the Relationship between Exposure to Dioxins and Cancer Incidence in Vietnam. *Toxics, 10*(7), 384. DOI: 10.3390/toxics10070384 PMID: 35878289

Wang, F., Zhuang, Z., Gao, F., He, R., Zhang, S., Wang, L., Liu, J., & Li, Y. (2024). TMO-Net: An explainable pretrained multi-omics model for multi-task learning in oncology. *Genome Biology, 25*(1), 149. DOI: 10.1186/s13059-024-03293-9 PMID: 38845006

Wang, W., Rong, Z., Wang, G., Hou, Y., Yang, F., & Qiu, M. (2023). Cancer metabolites: Promising biomarkers for cancer liquid biopsy. *Biomarker Research, 11*(1), 66. DOI: 10.1186/s40364-023-00507-3 PMID: 37391812

Wang, W., Zhen, S., Ping, Y., Wang, L., & Zhang, Y. (2024). Metabolomic biomarkers in liquid biopsy: Accurate cancer diagnosis and prognosis monitoring. *Frontiers in Oncology, 14*, 1331215. DOI: 10.3389/fonc.2024.1331215 PMID: 38384814

Wang, X., Qi, Y., & Zheng, H. (2022). Dietary Polyphenol, Gut Microbiota, and Health Benefits. *Antioxidants, 11*(6), 1212. DOI: 10.3390/antiox11061212 PMID: 35740109

Wen, L., & Han, Z. (2021). Identification and validation of xenobiotic metabolism-associated prognostic signature based on five genes to evaluate immune microenvironment in colon cancer. *Journal of Gastrointestinal Oncology, 12*(6), 2788–2802. DOI: 10.21037/jgo-21-655 PMID: 35070407

Williams, J. A., & Phillips, D. H. (n.d.). *Mammary Expression of Xenobiotic Metabolizing Enzymes and Their Potential Role in Breast Cancer.*

Wilson, I. D., & Nicholson, J. K. (2017). Gut microbiome interactions with drug metabolism, efficacy, and toxicity. *Translational Research; the Journal of Laboratory and Clinical Medicine, 179*, 204–222. DOI: 10.1016/j.trsl.2016.08.002 PMID: 27591027

Winz, C., Zong, W., & Suh, N. (2023). Endocrine-disrupting compounds and metabolomic reprogramming in breast cancer. *Journal of Biochemical and Molecular Toxicology*, *37*(12), e23506. DOI: 10.1002/jbt.23506 PMID: 37598318

Wong, S. H., & Yu, J. (2019). Gut microbiota in colorectal cancer: Mechanisms of action and clinical applications. *Nature Reviews. Gastroenterology & Hepatology*, *16*(11), 690–704. DOI: 10.1038/s41575-019-0209-8 PMID: 31554963

Xu, M.-Q., Pan, F., Peng, L.-H., & Yang, Y.-S. (2024). Advances in the isolation, cultivation, and identification of gut microbes. *Military Medical Research*, *11*(1), 34. DOI: 10.1186/s40779-024-00534-7 PMID: 38831462

Xu, W. S., Parmigiani, R. B., & Marks, P. A. (2007). Histone deacetylase inhibitors: Molecular mechanisms of action. *Oncogene*, *26*(37), 5541–5552. DOI: 10.1038/sj.onc.1210620 PMID: 17694093

Xu, Y., Morales, A. J., Towlerton, A. M. H., Akilesh, S., Miller, C. P., Tykodi, S. S., & Warren, E. H. (2022). Integrated TCR repertoire analysis and single-cell transcriptomic profiling of tumor-infiltrating T cells in renal cell carcinoma identifies shared and tumor-restricted expanded clones with unique phenotypes. *Frontiers in Oncology*, *12*, 952252. DOI: 10.3389/fonc.2022.952252 PMID: 36185254

Yang, C. S. (2015). Influences of Dietary and Other Factors on Xenobiotic Metabolism and Carcinogenesis—A Review Article in Memory of Dr. Allan H. Conney (1930–2013). *Nutrition and Cancer*, *67*(8), 1209–1215. DOI: 10.1080/01635581.2015.1081010 PMID: 26474329

Yang, H., Rivera, Z., Jube, S., Nasu, M., Bertino, P., Goparaju, C., Franzoso, G., Lotze, M. T., Krausz, T., Pass, H. I., Bianchi, M. E., & Carbone, M. (2010). Programmed necrosis induced by asbestos in human mesothelial cells causes high-mobility group box 1 protein release and resultant inflammation. *Proceedings of the National Academy of Sciences of the United States of America*, *107*(28), 12611–12616. DOI: 10.1073/pnas.1006542107 PMID: 20616036

Yang, R., Lu, Y., Yin, N., & Faiola, F. (2023). Transcriptomic Integration Analyses Uncover Common Bisphenol A Effects Across Species and Tissues Primarily Mediated by Disruption of JUN/FOS, EGFR, ER, PPARG, and P53 Pathways. *Environmental Science & Technology*, *57*(48), 19156–19168. DOI: 10.1021/acs.est.3c02016 PMID: 37978927

Yang, Y., Chen, Y., Xu, S., Guo, X., Jia, G., Ping, J., Shu, X., Zhao, T., Yuan, F., Wang, G., Xie, Y., Ci, H., Liu, H., Qi, Y., Liu, Y., Liu, D., Li, W., Ye, F., Shu, X.-O., & Long, J. (2024). Integrating muti-omics data to identify tissue-specific DNA methylation biomarkers for cancer risk. *Nature Communications*, *15*(1), 6071. DOI: 10.1038/s41467-024-50404-y PMID: 39025880

Yu, H., Lin, L., Zhang, Z., Zhang, H., & Hu, H. (2020). Targeting NF-κB pathway for the therapy of diseases: Mechanism and clinical study. *Signal Transduction and Targeted Therapy*, *5*(1), 209. DOI: 10.1038/s41392-020-00312-6 PMID: 32958760

Zemskov, E. A., Wu, X., Aggarwal, S., Yegambaram, M., Gross, C., Lu, Q., Wang, H., Tang, H., Wang, T., & Black, S. M. (2021). Nitration of protein kinase G-Iα modulates cyclic nucleotide crosstalk via phosphodiesterase 3A: Implications for acute lung injury. *The Journal of Biological Chemistry*, *297*(2), 100946. DOI: 10.1016/j.jbc.2021.100946 PMID: 34252457

Zhang, A., Luo, X., Li, Y., Yan, L., Lai, X., Yang, Q., Zhao, Z., Huang, G., Li, Z., Wu, Q., & Wang, J. (2024). Epigenetic changes driven by environmental pollutants in lung carcinogenesis: A comprehensive review. *Frontiers in Public Health*, *12*, 1420933. DOI: 10.3389/fpubh.2024.1420933 PMID: 39440184

Zhang, P., Zheng, P., & Liu, Y. (2019). Amplification of the CD24 Gene Is an Independent Predictor for Poor Prognosis of Breast Cancer. *Frontiers in Genetics*, *10*, 560. DOI: 10.3389/fgene.2019.00560 PMID: 31244889

Zhu, J., Wu, Y., Ji, P., Qi, J., Yang, X., Pocha, C., Tustumi, F., & Biachi De Castria, T. (2024). Identification of a prognostic disulfidptosis-related gene signature in hepatocellular cancer. *Journal of Gastrointestinal Oncology*, *15*(4), 1647–1656. DOI: 10.21037/jgo-24-522 PMID: 39279954

Zhu, J., Zou, Z., Nie, P., Kou, X., Wu, B., Wang, S., Song, Z., & He, J. (2016). Downregulation of microRNA-27b-3p enhances tamoxifen resistance in breast cancer by increasing NR5A2 and CREB1 expression. *Cell Death & Disease*, *7*(11), e2454–e2454. DOI: 10.1038/cddis.2016.361 PMID: 27809310

Zitvogel, L., Ma, Y., Raoult, D., Kroemer, G., & Gajewski, T. F. (2018). The microbiome in cancer immunotherapy: Diagnostic tools and therapeutic strategies. *Science*, *359*(6382), 1366–1370. DOI: 10.1126/science.aar6918 PMID: 29567708

Zou, C., & Mallampalli, R. K. (2014). Regulation of histone modifying enzymes by the ubiquitin–proteasome system. *Biochimica et Biophysica Acta (BBA) -. Biochimica et Biophysica Acta. Molecular Cell Research*, *1843*(4), 694–702. DOI: 10.1016/j.bbamcr.2013.12.016 PMID: 24389248

Chapter 4
The Cancer Exposome: Gene-Environment Interactions (GxE) in Carcinogenesis

Divya A. P.
Sri Sathya Sai University for Human Excellence, Kalaburagi, India

Mahalakshmi K. M.
Sri Sathya Sai University for Human Excellence, Kalaburagi, India

Sai Priyanka J.
Sri Sathya Sai University for Human Excellence, Kalaburagi, India

Ramya Raghavan
https://orcid.org/0000-0002-9953-543X
Sri Sathya Sai University for Human Excellence, Kalaburagi, India

ABSTRACT

Gene-environment interactions play a crucial role in tumor initiation by influencing cellular and tissue plasticity. Environmental and internal factors influence carcinogenesis by acting on specific sensing genes and pathways, leading to epigenetic, genetic, and metabolic changes that shape the TME. Understanding the exposome can inform gene expression, epigenetic changes, and immune responses, particularly for the reproductive health and cancer prevention. The authors discuss the latest methodologies in exposome assessment, challenges in defining and measuring harmful environmental impacts. Exposome applications in public health policy face challenges and also opportunities in translating exposome research into actionable measures. Gene-environment interactions are shown by analyzing case studies, emerging debates in research, and clinical practice. This work highlights the transformative potential of exposome informed policies in addressing global

DOI: 10.4018/979-8-3373-2165-3.ch004

health challenges and reducing health disparities.

INTRODUCTION

Exposomics studies environmental, nongenetic determinants of human health. Exposome analysis is met with the complexity of exposures and interconnected etiological determinants of disease (Safarlou et al., 2024). Cancer, a global health challenge, emphasizes the need for a discovery-driven analysis of environmental risk factors. Cancers with multifactorial origin, show varying risk factors for population subgroups on incidence and mortality rates.

Environmental, social, chemical and biological factors shape the tumor micro-environment (TME) that drives carcinogenesis. The TME undergoes Epithelial-mesenchymal transition (EMT), and ECM remodeling (tissue morphogenesis) with abnormal cell growth and metabolism. Exposomics shows how environmental influences affect cellular and non-cellular components, including cancer-associated fibroblasts, extracellular matrix, endothelial and immune cells. These TME components are influenced by both internal (genetic, metabolic) and external (environmental, lifestyle) factors, towards immune escape, and resistance to treatment. However, some cancers show stronger associations with environmental factors, while others are more strongly linked to genetic predispositions (Biradar, Suresh, et al., 2025).

Gene-environment interactions (GxE) play a crucial role in tumor initiation by influencing cellular and tissue plasticity. Tumor-initiating plasticity is conceptualized as intrinsic responses of mutant epithelial cells to environmental changes, the reprogramming of non-neoplastic host cells. Exposomics enhances cancer biology by improving the understanding of how environmental exposures affect cellular and molecular processes. GxE can lead to pro-tumorigenic states in response to multiple environmental factors collectively known as the exposome. Epigenetic and metabolic changes in response to environment-sensing gene pathways. Phthalate exposure is linked to prostate cancer aggressiveness through the induction of microRNA-5010 and the Nrf2-EGR1-GDF15 signaling pathway (Tsai et al., 2025). Environmental carcinogens (e.g., benzo[a]pyrene, heavy metals, pesticides) induce DNA methylation changes, histone modifications, and alter sperm expression (Akhatova et al., 2025).

Epigenetic and metabolic changes can be transmitted across generations, priming offsprings for increased cancer susceptibility. Environment sensing genes involve cell surface receptors that bind to environmental cues (growth factors, cytokines), intracellular sensors for oxygen levels, DNA damage signaling pathways activated by environmental changes. Here we have some of the biomarkers of environment relevant to cancer biology (Table 1).

Telomeres

The NHANES blood levels data from 1999-2002, analyzing show C-reactive protein and γ-tocopherol, caffeine and fiber intake, are inversely related to telomere length. The individuals sex, race, and socioeconomic status have indirect effects mediated by C-reactive protein (Tedaldi et al., 2025). The critical role of histone phosphorylation in the DNA damage response, which is essential for maintaining genomic stability, DNA repair, signal transduction, and chromatin remodeling (Gong et al., 2025).

Aryl Hydrocarbon Receptor (AHR)

AHR can be activated by a diverse range of ligands, including synthetic and naturally derived molecules such as pollutants, phytochemicals, pharmaceuticals, and substances from amino acids and microorganisms. Aryl hydrocarbon receptor family senses environmental pollutants to regulate detoxification enzymes and act as a tumor suppressor. AHR represses oncogenic pathways by interacting with TGFβ and NRF2 in response to toxins like arsenic (Sahoo et al., 2025). The effects of AHR activation on the immune system are influenced by the type of AHR ligand and cell type, developmental stage, dosage, and timing of exposure.

Metabolic Disruptors: FTO Gene

The fat mass and obesity-associated protein (FTO) is involved in mRNA, m6A N6-methyladenosine demethylation. FTO could be associated with *H.pylori's* CagA, APOE, SERPINE1 mRNA. FTO is regulated by TTC7B, PI4KA, PKA1and RXRA. FTO gene variants can alter susceptibility to metabolic disruptors and in response to diet and physical activity (Somala et al., 2025). Metabolic disruptors can reprogram cellular metabolism, affecting pathways like glycolysis, amino acid, and nucleotide metabolism.

Energy and Nutrient Sensing Pathways

Genes and enzymes that sense cellular energy status (e.g., AMPK, mTOR, HIF pathways) are crucial in cancer. A bidirectional regulation between hypoxia-inducible factor-1 (HIF-1) and m6A modifications. Disruptions in these pathways, often triggered by metabolic changes or environmental exposures, drive m6A, FTO, HIF-1 axis, via complex RNA modification dynamics, and metabolic reprogramming (Benak et al., 2025).

Oxidative Stress in Gene-Environment Interactions

Genetic susceptibility (e.g., polymorphisms in metabolism or DNA repair genes) and environmental exposures determine the role of p53-binding protein 1 (53BP1) in regulating intracellular reactive oxygen species (ROS). Analysis of gene expression revealed that 53BP1 depletion led to increased NOX1 mRNA levels and decreased levels of metallothioneins (MT1F and MT2A) (Youn et al., 2025). High expression of H2AX mRNA and γ-H2AX protein in oropharyngeal squamous cell carcinoma in HPV-negative cases is fatal (Lyu et al., 2025).

Table 1. Biomarkers for Environmental Influences on Cancer

Biomarker	Environmental Influence	Pathways	Reference
Telomere Shortening	Stress, pollution, tobacco smoking, sleep	Genomic Instability	(Tedaldi et al., 2025)
AHR Activation (Aryl Hydrocarbon Receptor)	Dioxins, PCBs, diesel exhaust	Xenobiotic Response Pathways	(Sahoo et al., 2025)
Metabolic Disrupting Chemicals (Altered lactate, succinate, Aldehyde Dehydrogenase)	Hypoxia, urban pollution Alcohol, air pollutants	Cancer Stem-Like Cells Oncometabolites	(Tedaldi et al., 2025) (Weinberg et al., 2025)
Exosomal cargo, proteins, miRNAs	Stress, chemical exposure	Environmental Memory	(Abusara et al., 2025)
C-Reactive Protein (CRP)	Chronic inflammation, obesity, stress	Early Detection Biomarker	(Tedaldi et al., 2025)
HIF-1α, Nrf2 Activation	Hypoxia (pollution, poor air quality), Oxidative stress from chemicals or radiation	Low Oxygen Tension Cellular Antioxidant Response	(Benak et al., 2025) (Tsai et al., 2025)
Metallothionein (MT1, MT2)	Heavy metal exposure (cadmium, arsenic)	Protects Against Heavy Metal Toxicity	(Youn et al., 2025)
γ-H2AX (DNA double-strand breaks)	Ionizing radiation	DNA methylation patterns DNA Damage	(Lyu et al., 2025) (Ma et al., 2025)

Table 1 shows the increasing recognition of the importance of gene-environment interactions (GxE) in understanding cancer etiology. The nervous and immune systems adapt to environmental changes. The neuroimmune connectome serve as a framework for advancements in disease diagnosis, prediction, and personalized medicine (Wheeler & Quintana, 2025). Our study will critically examine the major debates and controversies surrounding the study of GxE in carcinogenesis and metastasis. The integration of environmental determinants of human health research is essential as exposome can influence gene expression, epigenetic modifications, and immune responses (Carra et al., 2025).

Figure 1. Array Of Environmental Exposures Individuals Encounter Over Their Lifetime

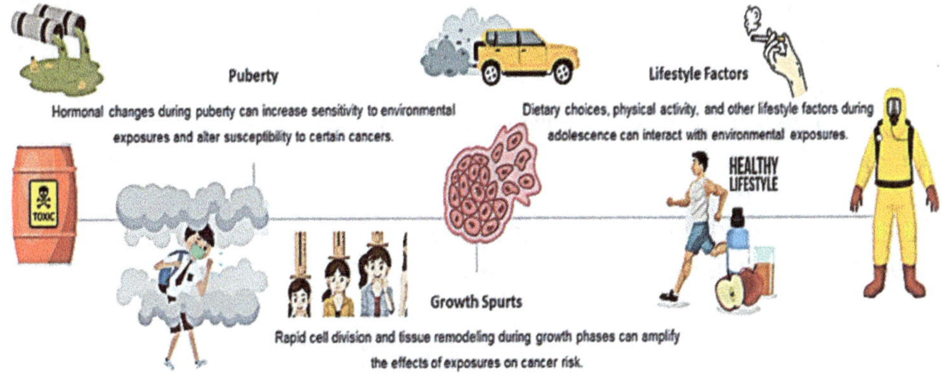

Challenges in Defining and Measuring Environmental Exposures

Despite the significant potential of exposomics, challenges currently hinder eradicating environmental influences on carcinogenesis. One major obstacle lies in accurately measuring the vast array of environmental exposures individuals encounter over their lifetimes. The dynamic and highly variable nature of an individual's exposome means that snapshot measurements taken at a single time. They are unlikely to provide a complete picture of all relevant exposures. Furthermore, the challenges of retrospectively assessing historical exposures, occurred decades prior to disease onset, remains a significant limitation.

There are several challenges when a mixture of environmental exposures modulates genes within the tumor microenvironment. These exposures influence gene expression, epigenetic states, and cellular interactions, affecting tumor development, progression, and the immune landscape. The complexity of multiple exposures, requires developing advanced analytical techniques, the availability of a wide range of chemical standards. Biomarker identification and quantification, needs innovative methods for prospective longitudinal studies and retrospective analyses that can capture the cumulative impact (Table 2). In this section we shall explore more on current limitations for comprehensive exposure assessment.

Complexity of Exposures

The traditional view of cancer as primarily driven by genetic mutations is being challenged by evidence of idiopathic oncogenic mutations in healthy tissues. Cancer cell identity is influenced by intrinsic and extrinsic factors, emphasizing the importance of nongenetic mechanisms in tumor initiation. Exposome studies face the difficulty in isolating specific causal agents within complex environmental mixtures.

Environmental factors as regulators and effectors of multistep carcinogenesis

Biomarkers for gene's sensing of the external exposome could be direct receptors binding to microbial products or inflammatory signals, byproducts of toxins. Biomarkers can work via signaling to have indirect downstream effects like hypoxia or altered growth factor signaling (Tsai et al., 2025).

Bioaccumulation and Latency of Disease Phenotypes

Gene-by-environment interactions can have chronic or latent disease phenotypes. Radiation influence carcinogenesis through somatic mutation, aberrant DNA methylation, and post-translational RNA modifications, affecting key oncoproteins and tumor suppressors over generations (Youn et al., 2025).

Latency is associated with cancer risks due to disinfection byproducts in drinking water. The time between exposure and cancer development can be decades. The primary source contaminants, including arsenic, asbestos, and radon, cancer risks. Furthermore, only in the recent years inorganic arsenic in drinking water as a known or suspected carcinogen (Sadee et al., 2025). Longitudinal studies are challenging in the investigations for nitrate exposure, and residential exposure to polychlorinated biphenyls (PCBs) and other chemicals (Tedaldi et al., 2025). Early risk biomarkers have shown agricultural chemicals and chlorination byproducts in drinking water correlates with an increased risk of bladder and rectal cancer (Weinberg et al., 2025). The impact of residential pesticide exposure was explored for 5-year survival of children when treated for acute lymphoblastic leukemia (ALL). It finds that exposure to rodenticides, particularly during pregnancy, is associated with an increased risk of mortality. ALL in children could be from several years of parental exposure, suggest the need for further research on environmental exposures during critical developmental periods (Desai et al., 2025). Many environmental exposures exert their effects through epigenetic modifications, which can have long-lasting transgenerational consequences.

Synergistic Effects

Scientific literature identifies multiple sources associated with cancer risk, identifying and characterizing exposome clusters encompass societal, social, built, and natural environmental (Telkmann et al., 2025). Critiques on the challenges in bringing diverse environmental chemical, physical, biological, lifestyle factors under a unified framework needs to be addressed.

The impact of indoor chemicals and air pollution from the use of indoor stoves or fireplaces has increased risks. Both breast and lung cancer links heavy metal toxicity from Superfund sites, elevated toenail metal levels, among non-Hispanic Black women (Madrigal et al., 2024). Regulatory agencies struggle to keep pace with increasing numbers of chemicals, complicated by confidential business clause or restrictions.

Exposures often combine and can have synergistic or antagonistic effects. The tumor microenvironment is a highly dynamic and heterogeneous exposures act on specific cell types within the immune cells, fibroblasts, endothelial cells (Ananthakumar et al., 2024). Complexity in considering all media (soil, water, air, food) and routes of entry (inhalation, ingestion, dermal absorption) makes accurate estimation challenging.

The microbiome, can act as an essential catalyst for multimorbidity, including cancers. Metagenomic evaluation is altered by an individual's diet, physical activity levels, and occupational exposures. Nutritionists' studies how dietary or nutraceuticals like saffron influence the microbiome and its impact on health, including cancer risk (Korrapati et al., 2024). Systemic metabolic or inflammatory status alter microbiome mechanisms of action associated with chemicals and contaminants. Many exposure assessments aren't updated regularly, potentially missing new risks or needed regulatory changes. Such limitations of retrospective studies demonstrate the need for improved longitudinal data collection.

Individual Variability

Genetic susceptibility, metabolism, and other individual factors play a crucial role in how exposures impact cancer risk. An exposome-wide analysis of all-cause mortality in the UK Biobank identified 25 independent environmental exposures associated with multimorbidity and major disease risk factors. While polygenic risk scores for 22 major diseases contributed less than 2 percentage points to mortality variation, the exposome accounted for an additional 17 percentage points, indicating a more substantial influence of environmental factors on mortality (Argentieri et al., 2025).

Significant geographic association between PM2.5 exposure and breast cancer risk has been observed across multiple cohorts, including the Sister Study and the NIH-AARP cohort (Madrigal et al., 2024). Findings indicate significant geographic variations in the association between PM2.5 and breast cancer risk, particularly among non-Hispanic Black women. Ongoing studies also explore the relationship between the use of hair products and the risk of hormone-related cancers, including breast, ovarian, and uterine cancer (Go et al., 2023) (Hou et al., 2025). The prevention strategies are tailored to both population and individual levels.

The changes induced by environmental factors include DNA methylation, histone modification, and noncoding RNA expression. The exposome accounts for a significant portion of mortality variation compared to polygenic risk scores (Argentieri et al., 2025). For example, smoking status emerged as a particularly potent environmental factor associated with 21 out of 25 age-related tested conditions. Thereby linking smoking to gene expression, epigenetic modifications, metabolic pathways, and immune responses. Understanding the mechanisms of carcinogenesis can aid in developing lifestyle modifications, exposure reduction preventive strategies. Precision medicine for specific genetic mutations or pathways involved in tumor development faces another significant hurdle in the difficulty in collecting and managing large and heterogeneous datasets. Establishing standard protocols for data access and sharing, as well as adopting semantic standards for data collection, storage, and analysis, are crucial.

Statistical and Methodological Hurdles

The limitations imposed by sample size requirements in detecting subtle GxE effects stem from population diversity. The concerns are around limited generalizability. Most studies focus on European populations, restricting understanding across different ethnic groups.

There are active temporal interactions between environmental exposures, microbiota, and immunity during carcinogenesis processes (Blériot et al., 2024). Critical windows in the embryonic or fetal period involve complex relationships, population stratification becomes a important confounding factor. The ethnic population parental interactions between environmental factors influences vary during cancer development in the offspring. The residential pesticide exposure during critical developmental periods affects 5-year survival rates in acute lymphoblastic leukemia children. Among the 837 children diagnosed with ALL, 108 (approximately 13%) died within 5 years of diagnosis. Parental diet, lifestyle, occupations also could have a notable association found between rodenticide exposure and increased mortality rates. Specifically, exposure to rodenticides was linked to a higher risk of death (hazard ratio of 1.70), with the strongest association observed when exposure occurred during pregnancy (hazard ratio of 1.90) (Desai et al., 2025). There is a risk of spurious associations if population structure isn't adequately controlled. The findings highlight the need for further research for diverse population to understand interaction variations across different genetic backgrounds. In particular paternal occupational exposure to rodenticides during pregnancy, may affect cancer outcomes in future generations.

Multiple Testing Issues

Analyzing the complex environment and cancer presents challenge on real-world chemical exposures and their effects. Pancreatic Ductal Adenocarcinoma (PDAC) is a highly aggressive cancer with poor survival rates due to late diagnosis and limited treatment options. The challenges of genome-wide interaction studies (GWIS) account for smoking, obesity, diabetes, diet, and alcohol consumption. The modifiable risk factors interact with genetic and metabolic profiles in the development of the disease (Lauri et al., 2025). To evaluate the false positives and the risk of false negatives, we need stringent statistical corrections. Statistical models revealed significant associations between chemical mixture exposure and hormones, highlighting an important gap in existing cancer research (Hou et al., 2025). Traditional statistical approaches, often designed for single exposure-outcome analyses. It may not be adequate for unraveling the exposome's intricate interactions and cumulative effects. Case-control studies are being conducted on various cancers, including non-Hodgkin's lymphoma and lung, bladder, colon, and other cancers. In particular studies on drinking water contaminants, airborne radon, and chlorinated hydrocarbons. Innovative exposure assessment methods, such as the CR-39 radon detector and the use of historical databases of water contaminants, are being developed to improve risk estimation (Hou et al., 2025). Extracting meaningful insights from these high-dimensional and heterogeneous datasets requires customized statistical methods and computational algorithms.

Environmental exposures such as outdoor air pollution factors that can contribute to cancer risk are mentioned explicitly as preventable risk factors. Hazard index measure exposures enhancing methods and tools to assess various environmental exposures accurately. Utilizing techniques such as PCA, K-means clustering, and map projection to create clusters of counties based on pollution data and calculated correlations with chronic disease prevalence. Significant associations were found between acetaldehyde and benzo(a)pyrene and chronic diseases such as hypertension, stroke, and diabetes mellitus. With aPEER producing over 68,000 interpretable maps that revealed distinct pollution-derived regions, findings demonstrated that pollutants could predict chronic disease geography. It is comparable or superior in accuracy to show social determinants of health and preventive healthcare models (Deonarine et al., 2025).

Establishing causal links between specific environmental exposures and cancer outcomes from observational exposomics data is difficult. For example, asthma and allergies, that need targeted interventions to mitigate these risks. Significant findings include long-term consumption of disinfection byproducts in drinking water and elevated risks of bladder and other cancers linked to arsenic exposure in drinking water supplies. Analytical techniques enhance the detection of polar organic pollutants, micro-nano plastics, and engineered nanomaterials in human exposure studies. Methods like ion chromatography and capillary electrophoresis coupled with mass spectrometry improve the mapping of the human physico-chemical exposome (Chetwynd et al., 2024). The assumptions and limitations of these models for biological interpretation still remains vague. This is due to the presence of numerous confounding factors and the need for advanced causal inference techniques.

Establishing Causality

Reports discuss the challenges of inferring causality from observational Endocrine-disrupting chemicals (EDCs) chemical studies. The association vs causality of industrial air pollution, emissions of carcinogenic chemicals, and the risk of postmenopausal breast cancer from the NIH-AARP Diet and Health Study was checked. A significant association between benzene emissions and breast cancer risk, particularly at a distance of 1 km from the source is reported. With a hazard ratio (HR) of 2.06 for the highest exposure quartile compared to non-exposed individuals, the data needs biomarkers to establish causality. The association between benzene emissions weakened with increasing distance, and the risk was more pronounced for invasive breast cancer rather than ductal carcinoma in situ. Additional elevated risks were noted for vinyl chloride at a distance of 5 km. The mechanisms behind these nongenetic alterations in cell identity, TME context-specific nature, remain inadequately understood. At the same time, suggestive associations were observed for other chemicals like asbestos, trichloroethylene, and styrene. Authors report that although these patterns were less clear and generally showed null associations for other chemicals (Madrigal et al., 2024). Exposome clusters are also influenced by contextual socioeconomic neighborhood, income, and deprivation, affecting response to cancer treatment. Understanding individual susceptibility to the harmful effects of tobacco products, identifies some individuals may be more vulnerable to the risks associated with tobacco exposure. Thus suggesting diversity in cell subpopulations with varying epigenetic and transcriptional patterns (Telkmann et al.,

2025). In the coming years the role of Mendelian randomization and other causal inference methods in this context maybe useful.

Figure 2. The Multifactorial Etiology Of Cancer Acknowledges Genetic and Environmental Factors

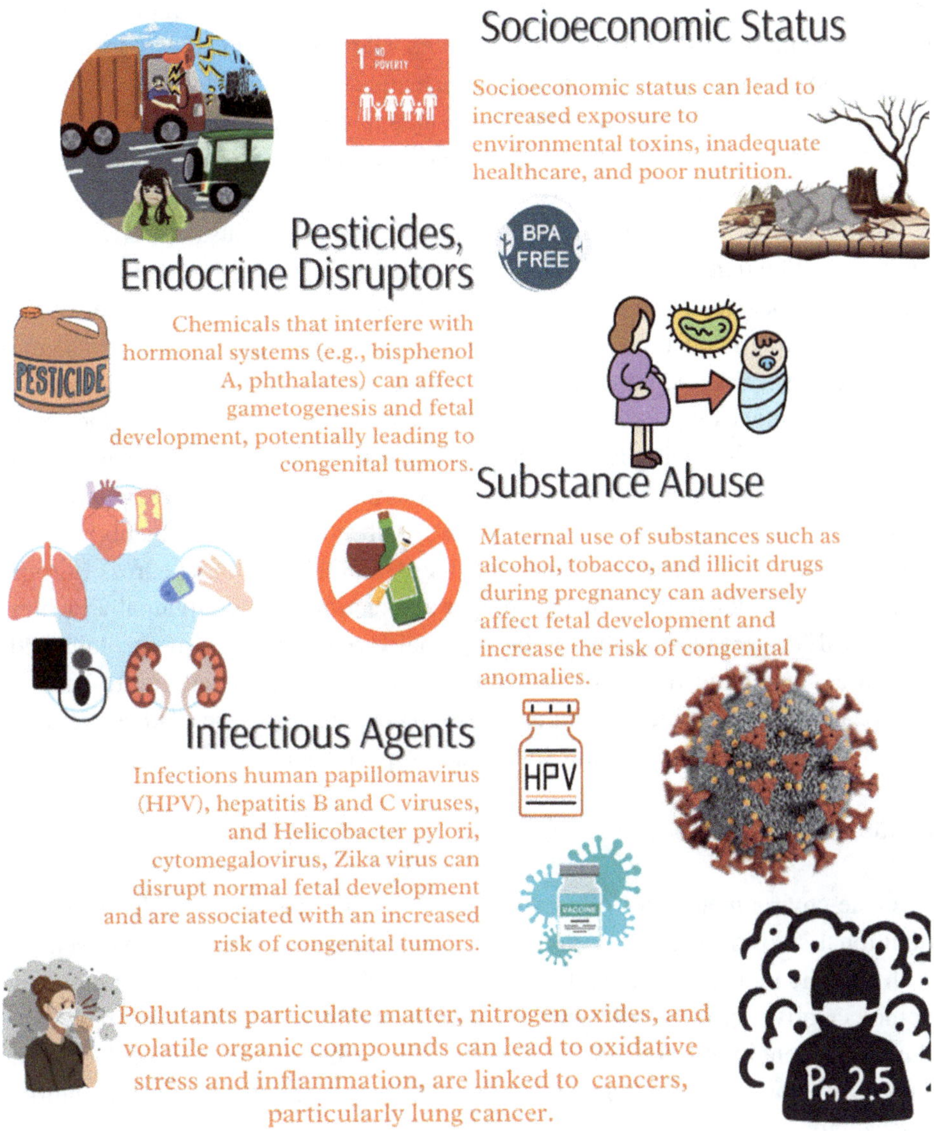

The exposome provides a framework for transitioning from candidate gene-environment studies to genome-wide interaction studies (GWISs). Untargeted environmental studies are termed exposome-wide association studies (ExWAS) or environment-wide association studies (EWAS/EnWAS). Gene-environment-wide interaction studies (GEWIS) aim to identify genetic loci with differential effects on phenotype stratified by environmental exposure levels. Analyzing the exposome, metabolome, methylome, and transcriptome would uncover the complex networks influencing tumor pathogenesis and outcomes. High-dimensional data from exposomics and advanced statistical and bioinformatics tools can aid in identifying key biomarkers that relate environmental exposures to disease outcomes. This insight allows for the development of preventive health strategies, before they lead to adverse health effects (Argentieri et al., 2025).

Genome-wide interaction studies face challenges with false positives due to multiple testing requirements. Techniques in multi-omics propose cumulative environmental exposures effects through epigenetic mechanisms. For example, studies have shown that exposure to pollutants like arsenic and benzene can lead to epigenetic changes that increase cancer risk. These changes can be transmitted across generations, suggesting various methods for studying the exposome's influence on neuroplasticity. Upcoming large-scale cohort studies, needs physiological sensors, neuroimaging, molecular biology, geospatial systems for evidence-based approaches. Significant variability in the urban exposome's socioeconomic determinants of health (SDOH), education, income vs unemployment. SDOH was found across Europe, with area-level indicators showing stronger associations than individual variables. EXPANSE Project research highlights regional variations in environmental health inequities, indicating the necessity for targeted interventions tailored to specific European contexts, particularly due to differing exposure patterns and temperature variability between Northern and Southern European countries (Saucy et al., 2024).

Statistical Power Issues

Gene-environment interaction studies require much larger sample sizes than traditional studies, leading to statistically underpowered research. Nano-sensors with specific biological recognition elements, such as DNA aptamers, antibodies, or molecularly imprinted polymers, can achieve highly targeted and trace detection. For carcinogens in complex environmental matrices, the appropriate model selection varies with communities and investigations. Debate continues over using additive versus multiplicative models for interaction effects.

Incorporating Epigenetic Modifications

The complex mechanisms of cancer epigenetics focus on the roles of DNA methylation, histone modifications, chromatin remodeling, and noncoding RNAs in influencing gene expression and cellular behavior. The potential of CRISPR-based epigenome editing and computational analysis is examined in cancer epigenetic research (Sherif et al., 2025).

Microbial metabolites can involve adding a methyl group to DNA, typically at CpG sites, which can silence gene expression. Environmental carcinogens such as pollutants and diet can alter DNA methylation patterns. Metabolites can influence gene expression and cellular behavior (Roje et al., 2024). Epigenetic modifications using short-chain fatty acids like butyrates as a therapeutic strategy for colorectal cancer (CRC). Histone Modification can affect gene expression by altering chromatin structure. Environmental exposures can lead to immunomodulatory histone modifications that have carcinogenic properties. Air pollution, encompassing both ambient air pollution and fine particulate matter (PM2.5), is repeatedly identified as a significant risk factor for several cancer types, including lung, bladder, breast, and prostate cancers. Diesel engine exhaust (DEE) is specifically associated with increased lung cancer risk. Moreover, specific air pollutants such as nitrogen oxides (NOx) are also linked to various health risks, including cancer. Environmental exposures, such as diet and pollutants, can lead to epigenetic modifications that influence gene expression and can be transmitted across generations. Noncoding RNAs can regulate gene expression and gene-environment interactions (GxE) in disease etiology. The current methodological approaches for studying gene-environment-epigenome interactions need to include the expression of noncoding RNAs.

Functional Validation Issues

Noncoding variants are genetic variants are in noncoding regions. This makes their biological significance harder to determine. Epigenetics findings from exposomic research can lead to developing preventive and treatment strategies for carcinogenesis, ultimately enhancing well-being and public health (Okwan-Duodu et al., 2024).

International organizations such as the World Health Organization (WHO) and the United Nations Environment Program (UNEP) play pivotal roles in shaping and implementing environmental health policies globally. A comprehensive approach is crucial for public health policies on a global scale. So, the emerging role of epigenetics in GxE needs interdisciplinary collaboration to discover mediating or modifying mechanistic genes. Functional validation of genes is critical in understanding the biological mechanisms underlying gene-environment interactions.

Tissue-specific and reversible nature of epigenetic changes adds complexity to the analysis and interpretation.

Challenges in Biological Relevance and Mechanisms

Translating genetic associations to functional mechanisms in the context of environmental exposures reveals that the exposome has a greater impact on lung, heart, and liver disease incidence. At the same time, polygenic risk scores are more significant for conditions like dementia and certain cancers. Data suggest distinct disease and mortality risk patterns shaped by environmental factors (Argentieri et al., 2025).

Understanding the mechanisms of cell, tissue, and organismal plasticity shaped by the exposome may offer new cancer prevention, detection, and intervention strategies.

Genetic vs. environmental contributions display breast, ovarian, prostate, and colorectal cancers, are primarily influenced by genetic factors, as indicated by polygenic risk scores, which account for a significant portion of the variation in these diseases (10.3–26.2%). Environmental contributions to cancer are higher for lung cancer and chronic obstructive pulmonary disease (COPD), wherein the exposome is more influential, explaining a larger proportion of the variation (Argentieri et al., 2025). Both mutagenic and non-mutagenic mechanisms by which various carcinogens, such as tobacco smoke, air pollutants, metals, diet, and alcohol, contribute to cancer development. Cancer cells are in a dynamic cell-state transition via the role of nongenetic plasticity, metabolic reprogramming, and gene expression changes. Molecular alterations identified through exposomics can serve as biomarkers for diagnosis, disease prediction, contributing to personalized medicine (França et al., 2024).

Pathway Complexity and Interconnectivity

Scientists are working on how specific GxE perturbations affect complex biological pathways involved in carcinogenesis and metastasis. Single cell omics literature critically evaluates the generalizability of GxE findings across different cancer types and subtypes. But, lack of standardized methods for integrating omics data creates analytical complexity. This highlights the importance of considering tumor heterogeneity in GxE research.

The evolving roles of tumor-associated macrophages in cancer emphasize their diverse functions and the interplay between inflammation and cancer over time. It proposes a new framework that incorporates temporal dynamics to better understand macrophage significance in the inflammatory processes related to cancer development and progression. The systems biology approaches to model these interactions can lead to personalized prevention strategies based on genetic profiles (Blériot et al., 2024).

Animal Models: Heterogeneity of Cancer

The vast amount of genetic and environmental data presents significant challenges in analysis and interpretation Animal models are the practical solution to overcome difficulties in incorporating gene-environment analyses limit result interpretation. The gut microbiota in the metabolism of carcinogens, specifically nitrosamines, impacts mouse tumor development. Depleting gut microbiota significantly reduces the severity and development of nitrosamine-induced urinary bladder cancer, indicating a link between microbial biotransformation and carcinogenesis. The metabolic activity of gut bacteria in converting carcinogens varies among individuals, suggesting personalized differences in cancer risk (Roje et al., 2024). Current advances link microbial dysbiosis to cancer, highlighting food borne effects on tumor microenvironments and immune modulation (Nagashri et al., 2024). Translating findings from in vitro and animal models to human populations should bypass the limitations of current model systems in recapitulating the complexity of human environments and genetic diversity. Thereby, exposome research effective public health interventions create policies addressing health disparities.

Debates in Translation to Public Health and Clinical Practice

Addressing Health Disparities is understanding of environmental exposures and their interactions with social determinants of health (SDOH). The integration of multimodal omics data with electronic health records has the potential to transform biomedical research and enhance understanding of health and disease. Translating exposome research into policy involves developing evidence-based guidelines and interventions. For instance, the Athlete project has developed approaches to summarize evidence on environmental factors affecting health outcomes, which can guide policy measures. These efforts are crucial for implementing public health interventions that address specific environmental exposures.

Cancer incidence patterns are shifting, with an increase awareness in early diagnoses. Specific cancer subtypes that were once geographically confined are now becoming globally prevalent, indicating a change in the environmental factors influencing cancer. The age-associated cancer subtypes in younger populations and fluctuating gender disparities in susceptibility across various malignancies has led multiomics approaches to study the exposome and its impact on cancer. The 2023 report by the American Cancer Society updates data on cancer disparities in the U.S., focusing on racial, ethnic, socioeconomic, and geographic factors that influence cancer occurrence and outcomes. Black and American Indian/Alaska Native populations experience disproportionately higher cancer mortality rates, with individuals having lower educational attainment facing significantly higher overall cancer mortality rates compared to those with higher education (Islami et al., 2024). Disparities in cancer mortality are more pronounced in nonmetropolitan areas compared to large metropolitan areas, with specific examples such as colorectal cancer mortality rates being notably higher in nonmetropolitan regions. The American Cancer Society report emphasizes that observed disparities in cancer mortality are linked to inequities in social determinants of health, highlighting the need for equitable policies and interventions to address these disparities effectively (Islami et al., 2024).

Incorporating GxE into Risk Prediction Models

Numerous carcinogens and pollutants in the air, water, and soil affect lifestyle factors such as diet and treatment response. Epidemiology studies the challenges of incorporating complex GxE into practical risk prediction tools. For instance, exposure to airborne pollutants has been linked to increased risks of breast, ovarian, and blood cancers. Data gave relation between area-level exposome factors and geographic disparities in aggressive prostate cancer in Pennsylvania. By linking cancer cases to various social determinants of health, that correlate with elevated odds, targeted interventions mitigate cancer burden in affected areas (Wiese et al., 2024). Key factors influencing cancer risk and survival identified include age, sex, housing status, employment status, and household income to poverty ratio. It finds that higher perceived social support and living with a spouse or partner are positively associated with breast and cervical cancer screening. Data in accounting for geographic differences in environmental exposures demonstrate less residential stability is linked to increased cervical cancer screening among younger females. The study suggests that enhancing social support networks could improve cancer control efforts (Baeker Bispo et al., 2025). Integrated environmental health impact assessments are necessary to address these challenges. There is also a need for policies that address intended impacts and consider unintended consequences, such as gentrification due to urban greenery enhancements. The clinical utility and predictive power of current GxE-based risk models desires machine learning, artificial intelligence or neuromorphic computing-based resources (GVS, Ananthakumar, et al., 2025).

Table 2. Biomarkers for Cancer Diagnostics and Therapies

Biomarker	Bioengineering Application	Cancer Therapy	Reference
Telomere Shortening γ-H2AX (DNA double-strand breaks)	Telomerase-based ATM/ATR inhibitors in radiotherapy gene therapy	Imetelstat (telomerase inhibitor) in breast cancer	(Tedaldi et al., 2025)
AHR Activation (Aryl Hydrocarbon Receptor)	AHR inhibitors; biosensor development	AHR antagonists for breast or liver cancer	(Sahoo et al., 2025)
Metabolic Disrupting Chemicals (Aldehyde Dehydrogenase)	Metabolic reprogramming	ALDH inhibitors in cancer stem cells IDH inhibitors in glioma and AML	(Tedaldi et al., 2025) (Weinberg et al., 2025)
Exosomal cargo, proteins, miRNAs	Targeted exosome therapy	Engineered exosomes for targeted delivery	(Abusara et al., 2025)
C-Reactive Protein (CRP)	Inflammatory biosensing	Anti-inflammatory regimens for colorectal cancer	(Tedaldi et al., 2025)
HIF-1α, Nrf2 Activation	Hypoxia-activated prodrugs	TH-302 (evofosfamide) in pancreatic cancer	(Benak et al., 2025) (Tsai et al., 2025)
Metallothionein (MT1, MT2)	Nrf2 pathway modulation Metal-responsive gene therapy tools	Nrf2 inhibitors Metal-chelating agents in chemo-resistant tumors	(Youn et al., 2025) (Lyu et al., 2025) (Ma et al., 2025)

Ethical and Social Issues in Targeted Prevention Strategies

Collection and use of genetic and environmental data raise significant privacy issues. Public health bodies can capture exposure timing and its effects during critical early stages.

The local bodies critically evaluate the ethical and practical considerations of implementing targeted public health strategies based on GxE profiles. The etiology of aggressive prostate cancer based on geospatial data, pinpoint geographic areas with elevated odds. Despite stable mutational landscapes, environmental exposures drive these changing incidence patterns. It also identifies associations between area-level exposome measures across SDOH domains. Debates over how to communicate findings to study participants and affected communities demonstrates the benefits and drawbacks of GxE approaches (Lakshmaiah et al., 2025).

The precision oncology assessment of exposures, chemicals, contaminants and lifestyle factors with exposure temporality helps understand the multifactorial etiology. The exposome research finding from Pennsylvania, stresses the importance of GxE understanding to inform personalized treatment strategies. Incorporating exposome-wide analyses in cancer epidemiology quantify the impact of environmental factors on cancer incidence alongside genetic predispositions (Wiese et al., 2024). Cancer therapies are often limited in efficacy due to an adaptive process that fosters drug resistance. Increasing use of geospatial data creates potential for individual re-identification which includes both genetic mutations and nongenetic plasticity (França et al., 2024).

FUTURE DIRECTIONS AND POTENTIAL SOLUTIONS

Advancements in exposure assessment technologies such as an air-liquid interface organ-level lung microfluidics platform analyze molecular mechanisms of cytotoxicity induced by cancer-causing fine particles. This methodology shows fine particulate matter exposure can cause carcinogenicity by activating 2532 genes and 25 signaling cascades, leading to cell differentiation, proliferation, and angiogenesis. Upcoming methods for translating research into assistive and augmentative health measures is through the integration and analysis of large datasets (GVS, Biradar, et al., 2025). There is essential for computational approaches to handle complex data integration. Machine learning for cancer risk prediction to identify and characterize germline-somatic interactions in cancer may significantly influence tumor heterogeneity, disease risk, and therapy response. Machine learning and network analysis algorithm designed to determine spatial relationships between chronic diseases and environmental pollutants (Deonarine et al., 2025).

Methodological Innovation

Nanomaterials like carbon nanotubes, graphene, and nanofibers possess unique structural and chemical properties that make them ideal for filtration applications, including high porosity, small and controllable pore sizes, and large surface areas for enhanced adsorption of pollutants. These advanced filters can effectively capture particulate matter that may carry carcinogenic substances and adsorb toxic chemicals from both air and water

The use of mass spectrometry in single-cell exposomics allows for detailed analysis of cellular dynamics, interactions, and responses to environmental stimuli. The risk of esophageal squamous cell carcinoma (ESCC) associated with serum circulating environmental chemical residues, specifically identifying 1H,1H,2H,2H-perfluorooctanesulfonic acid (6:2 FTS) as a risk factor linked to lipid metabolism-related chronic inflammation. Significant metabolic disruptions were found in ESCC cases, and a biomarker panel was developed to enhance early diagnosis and prevention of ESCC (Wang et al., 2025).

Nanotechnology

Integrating nanotechnology with other advanced analytical technologies further expands the capabilities of exposomics research. Notably, combining nanotechnology with high-resolution mass spectrometry (HRMS) offers a powerful platform for comprehensive chemical profiling of biological samples, enabling the detection and identification of a wide range of environmental exposures, including known and emerging carcinogens. High-resolution mass spectrometry (HRMS) profiles both targeted and untargeted chemical exposures in biological samples (Balcells et al., 2024). Heavy metals, defined as elements denser than water, are a significant global danger, with long-term exposure associated with increased cancer incidence rates. Of these, arsenic has the most substantial evidence for cancer risk, linked to cancers of the liver, lung, bladder, and kidney. The byproducts of chlorination in water treatment are associated with an increased risk of bladder and rectal cancer. Other contaminants include asbestos, radon, agricultural chemicals, and hazardous waste. For example, a study on breast cancer risk factors utilized liquid chromatography coupled with HRMS to analyze plasma samples for priority target analytes and over 94,000 untargeted features. Nanomaterials can be used to enhance sample preparation, improve ionization efficiency, and increase the sensitivity of HRMS, thereby allowing for the identification of novel exposure biomarkers and a deeper understanding of the complex chemical exposome. This integrated approach is crucial for advancing our knowledge of how environmental exposures contribute to cancer development (Zhi & Wang, 2024).

Multi-Omics Approaches

Advanced technologies, such as single-cell epigenomics, multi-omics approaches, spatial epigenomics, and long-read sequencing, enhance our understanding of tumor heterogeneity and evolution (Biradar, Suresh, et al., 2025). Recent findings suggest a phenotypes-first process, where nonheritable cellular variability generates novel traits later stabilized by genetic and epigenetic changes. Single-cell measurements indicate that phenotypes can precede genotypes, demonstrating that cancer evolution mirrors normal developmental plasticity and involves recombining different cellular developmental programs. Research in evolutionary biology supports the phenotypes-first approach, highlighting the role of developmental plasticity and recombination in developing novel traits in response to environmental challenges (Frank & Yanai, 2024). Molecular alterations identified through exposomics can serve as biomarkers for diagnosing diseases. Pancreatic ductal adenocarcinoma (PDAC) is a highly lethal cancer that is often asymptomatic in its early stages. Limitations of current biomarkers lead to a poor prognosis, with most patients succumbing within

6 months of diagnosis. The current blood-based biomarker, CA19-9, is not accurate for diagnosing PDAC, particularly in high-risk patient groups. A blood-based proteomic assay, multivariate index assays, and mass spectrometry (MS) applications facilitate the simultaneous analysis of endogenous metabolites and xenobiotics, predicting outcomes, enabling early detection, and facilitating personalized medicine approaches (Wan et al., 2025).

Synthetic Biology

Microbial profiling and manipulation strategies, such as probiotics, prebiotics, and fecal microbiota transplantation, are emerging as promising adjuncts in cancer prevention and therapy (Table 3). This includes the creation of highly sensitive and specific nucleic acid-based electrochemical nano biosensors for early detection of cancer and the development of portable, paper-based in vitro biosensing platforms for rapidly detecting pollutants like arsenic. Gene circuits or engineering principles can design living cells and cell-free systems to function as highly specific and sensitive detectors of analytes relevant to cancer and environmental health. For instance, bioengineered bacteria can be engineered to detect specific DNA sequences and mutations associated with tumors. Synthetic biomarkers, designed using inert carriers decorated with protein targets of tumor-associated enzymes, can amplify signs of early cancer, enabling detection at very small tumor volumes. These engineered biosensors offer high sensitivity, specificity, ease of use, on-site and real-time monitoring of environmental carcinogens (Biradar, Korrapati, et al., 2025).

Geographic Information Systems (GIS)

Geospatial science utilizes tools like geographic information systems (GIS) to analyze environmental features based on their locations, significantly enhancing cancer epidemiologic studies through large-scale environmental exposure assessments (VoPham et al., 2024). Geocoded exposure data is linked to specific geographic locations to assess exposure risks related to cancer. Chemical and nonchemical stressors or factors that should be included in exposome assessment. Global positioning and individual sensors and technologies are used to track location and collect data on particular behaviors and exposures. Algorithm to explore spatial relationships between 12 chronic diseases and 186 pollutants in the United States, producing 68,820 interpretable maps that reveal strong associations between specific pollutants and cancers (Deonarine et al., 2025). Opportunities for advancing geospatial science in cancer research include improving spatial and temporal data resolution, measuring climate change impacts, utilizing patient addresses in studies. Integrating internal exposome data with external exposure models, geospatial data allow personalized cancer screening and clinical decision-making.

Table 3. Examples of Clinical Trials based on Cancer Biomarkers Associated with Environmental Influences of Cancer Source: Clinicaltrials.Gov

Exposure	Biomarker	Cancer Therapy Example	Clinical Trial Number
Polycyclic Aromatic Hydrocarbons	DNA Adducts (BPDE-DNA Adducts)	PARP inhibitors in lung cancer HDAC inhibitors Vorinostat	NCT02498613
Industrial Pollutants, Tobacco Smoke, Heavy Metals	DNA Methylation Patterns (Hypermethylation of P16ink4a)	DNMT inhibitors 5-azacytidine for leukemia	NCT01462578
Hypoxia, Urban Pollution	Metabolomic Signatures (Altered Lactate, Succinate)	IDH inhibitors in glioma and AML	NCT01915498
Dioxins, PCBs, Diesel Exhaust	Ahr Activation (Aryl Hydrocarbon Receptor) Gene Expression Changes (CYP1A1 Upregulation)	AHR antagonists for breast or liver cancer CYP inhibitors or RNAi-based silencing in liver cancer	NCT04548814 NCT05375604 NCT05375604
Aflatoxin B1, Radiation, Benzene	Protein Biomarkers (P53 Mutation or Loss)	Gene therapy restoring wild-type p53 in HCC liver cancer	NCT02561546
Ionizing Radiation, Arsenic, Radon	Γ-H2AX (DNA Double-Strand Breaks)	HDR pathway ATM/ATR inhibitors in radiotherapy	NCT05917145
Chronic Infection, Asbestos, Diesel Exhaust	Inflammatory Cytokines (IL-6, TNF-A)	JAK/STAT inhibitors in inflammation-associated cancers	NCT02713386
Smoking, UV, ROS	Mitochondria DNA Mutations	Mitocans SynNotch CAR-T CAR-T + Vaccine	NCT06186401 NCT06253520

Regulatory Approaches

Recognizing the exposome's importance in human health has led to the development of various regulatory frameworks. The public health policies aim at mitigating the risks associated with environmental exposures. The public health exposome framework within a social-ecological context, highlight the need for community engagement and the integration of GIS for analytics. Individuals living with a spouse or partner only had higher odds of being screened for breast and colorectal cancer compared to those living without a spouse/partner or children. Less residential stability was linked to increased cervical cancer screening among younger females (ages 21-34), although it did not show a similar effect for breast or colorectal cancer screening. In the case of hepatocellular carcinoma, race and social determinants significantly influence curative treatment receipt and healthcare costs. The findings suggest that enhancing social support networks and can address the social needs of parents and caregivers. Therefore, public health professionals play a crucial role at the intersection of science and policy, particularly in environmental health (Baeker Bispo et al., 2025).

Urban Health Policies

The application of the exposome concept in urban health studies reflect multiple environmental co-exposures. The urban exposome assess the health impacts of urban design and planning. Compact high-density cities exhibit higher motorized traffic and NO2 exposure led surface urban heat island effects. Green low-density cities demonstrate a significantly lower surface urban heat island (SUHI) effect and lesser mortality rates. The analytical techniques, such as ion chromatography and capillary electrophoresis coupled with mass spectrometry, can enhance the detection of polar and ionic substances. The methods for characterizing particulate human exposure shows their applicability in large-scale biomonitoring programs (Chetwynd et al., 2024). So, the second generation of exposome research seeks to provide actionable knowledge for public health interventions but faces significant epistemological challenges. Despite the significant potential of exposome research data, barriers exist in exposome-informed policies across different international contexts. The authors advocate for greater reflexivity regarding the limitations and call for the integrative approach to public and environmental health (Iungman et al., 2024).

European Union (EU)

The EU has recognized the need for integrated and precautionary approaches to risk governance. Infections especially has systemic risks that are complex and interconnected. The European Union has made significant strides in incorporating exposome research into its public health frameworks. The HELIX project (The Human EarlyLife Exposome) is a notable example. HELIX portray the early life exposome by assessing exposure to various environmental hazards during pregnancy and childhood across multiple European cohorts. EU projects has generated comprehensive data sets that include geospatial exposure estimates, biomonitoring data, and child health outcomes, which are used to inform public health policies and interventions (Maitre et al., 2022).

U.S. Environmental Protection Agency (EPA

Air Quality Monitoring and continuous monitoring of air pollutants can help assess their impact on cancer risk, particularly in urban areas with high pollution levels. The U.S. Environmental Protection Agency (EPA) plays a significant role in integrating exposome data into public health policies. The EPA has developed frameworks for assessing health risks of environmental exposures, particularly focusing on vulnerable populations such as children. This includes considering exposures such as particulate matter, volatile organic compounds during all developmental life stages and integrating adverse health effects. Particulate matter less than 2.5 microns (PM2.5) increase the risks of nonalcoholic fatty liver disease (NAFLD) and hepatocellular carcinoma (HCC). The report emphasizes the need for equitable policies and interventions to address social determinants of health (SDOH) Pollution and disparities based on race, ethnicity, geography, sex reflect SDOH (VoPham et al., 2024). The Human Exposome Assessment Platform (HEAP) is an initiative that develops informatics platforms to analyze extensive datasets on environmental exposures and their health effects. Robotic approach also allows for the identification of exposure patterns and their associations with health outcomes, which can inform public health policies (Chandra et al., 2025).

In the United States, these policies have effectively reduced harmful health effects of pollutants by setting national standards for air and water quality. Environmental Health Policy Certificate aim to produce leaders who are fluent in both environmental health sciences and policy analysis. The COVID-19 pandemic highlighted the importance of understanding the exposome in managing infectious diseases. Exposome-based approaches were utilized to capture better the variability in SARSCoV2 spread and its associated exposures. This approach facilitated the identification of vulnerable populations and informed the deployment of nonpharmacological public health measures. The American Cancer Society's 2023 report updates data on cancer disparities in the U.S., based on race, ethnicity, socioeconomic status, and geographic location. It reveals that Black and American Indian/ Alaska Native populations face disproportionately higher cancer mortality rates, particularly influenced by educational attainment and living in nonmetropolitan areas. (Islami et al., 2024). By integrating individual and population characteristics with urban parameters, exposome studies have helped assess health disparities and improve public health.

The EPA's Center for Public Health and Environmental Assessment is actively involved in exposure science and cancer research. CPHEA supports national, regional, and local decision-making processes to safeguard human health and ecological integrity. The CPHEA's work emphasizes a One Health approach, among environmental, social, and economic systems.

One Health Approach

The integration of the exposome with the One Health approach, which considers the interconnectedness of human, animal, and environmental health, has provided a comprehensive framework for addressing public health challenges. One Health approach has been used to develop interventions that consider the broader environmental context, thereby enhancing the effectiveness of public health strategies.

Overarching Themes

Healthy People 2030 initiative focuses on reducing exposure to harmful pollutants in air, water, soil, food, and materials in homes and workplaces. There is a growing recognition of the need for holistic approaches considering the full spectrum of environmental influences on health. BreatheLife is an initiative by WHO and UNEP. The BreatheLife campaign aims to reduce air pollution for climate and health benefits. It engages countries, regions, and cities in commitments to improve air quality, impacting over 120 million people worldwide. Strategic Approach to International Chemicals Management (SAICM) has successfully phased out harmful substances like lead paint and mercury emissions, demonstrating effective international cooperation in chemical management (Non, 2025) There is a lack of standardized methods for detecting polar and ionic organic pollutants and characterizing particulate contaminants like micro-nano plastics and engineered nanomaterials (Chetwynd et al., 2024). Large international biomonitoring initiatives aim to map human exposure to environmental contaminants, but data is limited to a few contaminants due to methodological constraints.

One of the major challenges in policymaking is ensuring effective stakeholder participation. Advances in multi-omics technologies have improved the exploration of gene-environment interactions, but challenges such as dataset complexity, analytical limitations, and underrepresentation of non-European genetic ancestries hinder the generalizability of findings and exacerbate health disparities (Alemu et al., 2025). A large-scale, coordinated effort similar to the Human Genome Project is needed to realize the potential of exposome research fully. Interconnected challenges suggest the need for interdisciplinary collaboration, for longitudinal studies with updated the ethical considerations. Especially while dealing with the multicausal and nonlinear nature of relationships between environment and health. The integration of the exposome with the One Health and Planetary Health approaches represents another holistic framework for public health management. This integration emphasizes the interconnectedness of human, animal, and environmental health, fostering comprehensive strategies to address complex health challenges.

CONCLUSION

Environmental and internal factors influence carcinogenesis by acting on specific sensing genes and pathways, leading to epigenetic, genetic, and metabolic changes that shape the TME. These processes highlight the importance of gene-environment interactions and the central role of epigenetic regulation in cancer risk and progression. Understanding the exposome can inform gene expression, epigenetic changes, and immune responses, particularly for the reproductive health and cancer prevention (Wan et al., 2025).

Modulating the TME and its environment-sensing pathways is emerging as a promising strategy to combat cancer and other age-related diseases. Addressing the complex challenges inherent in studying the exposome and its relationship to cancer requires a unified and coordinated effort of researchers from various backgrounds.

REFERENCES

Abusara, O. H., Agha, A. S. A. A., & Bardaweel, S. K. (2025). Advancements and innovations in liquid biopsy through microfluidic technology for cancer diagnosis. *Analyst, 150*(9), 1711–1725. Advance online publication. DOI: 10.1039/D5AN00105F PMID: 40181713

Akhatova, A., Jones, C., Coward, K., & Yeste, M. (2025). How do lifestyle and environmental factors influence the sperm epigenome? Effects on sperm fertilising ability, embryo development, and offspring health. *Clinical Epigenetics, 17*(1), 1. Advance online publication. DOI: 10.1186/s13148-025-01815-1 PMID: 39819375

Alemu, R., Sharew, N. T., Arsano, Y. Y., Ahmed, M., Tekola-Ayele, F., Mersha, T. B., & Amare, A. T. (2025). Multi-omics approaches for understanding gene-environment interactions in noncommunicable diseases: Techniques, translation, and equity issues. *Human Genomics, 19*(1), 1. Advance online publication. DOI: 10.1186/s40246-025-00718-9 PMID: 39891174

Ananthakumar, B., Nanjundeshwara, N., Lakshmaiah, A., & Raghavan, R. (2024). Synthetic Gene Circuits as a Promising Approach in Cancer Immunotherapy. *Critical Developments in Cancer Immunotherapy*, 391–418. DOI: 10.4018/979-8-3693-3976-3.ch011

Argentieri, M. A., Amin, N., Nevado-Holgado, A. J., Sproviero, W., Collister, J. A., Keestra, S. M., Kuilman, M. M., Ginos, B. N. R., Ghanbari, M., Doherty, A., Hunter, D. J., Alvergne, A., & van Duijn, C. M. (2025). Integrating the environmental and genetic architectures of aging and mortality. *Nature Medicine, 31*(3), 1–10. DOI: 10.1038/s41591-024-03483-9 PMID: 39972219

Baeker Bispo, J., Lee, H., Jemal, A., & Islami, F. (2025). Associations of social support, living arrangements, and residential stability with cancer screening in the United States. *Cancer Causes & Control, 36*(2), 157–169. DOI: 10.1007/s10552-024-01913-0 PMID: 39422870

Balcells, C., Xu, Y., Gil-Solsona, R., Maitre, L., Gago-Ferrero, P., & Keun, H. C. (2024). Blurred lines: Crossing the boundaries between the chemical exposome and the metabolome. *Current Opinion in Chemical Biology, 78*, 102407. DOI: 10.1016/j.cbpa.2023.102407 PMID: 38086287

Benak, D., Alanova, P., Holzerova, K., Chalupova, M., Opletalova, B., Kolar, F., Pavlinkova, G., & Hlavackova, M. (2025). Epitranscriptomic regulation of HIF-1: Bidirectional regulatory pathways. *Molecular Medicine (Cambridge, Mass.), 31*(1), 1. Advance online publication. DOI: 10.1186/s10020-025-01149-x PMID: 40102715

Biradar, S., Korrapati, C., Krishna, R. J., & Nanjundeshwara, N. (2025). Spatial Omics and Gene Circuits: The Future in Cancer Biology. *Spatially Variable Genes in Cancer: Development, Progression, and Treatment Response*, 383–408. DOI: 10.4018/979-8-3693-7728-4.ch014

Biradar, S., Suresh, C., Nanjundeshwara, N., & Raghavan, R. (2025). Spatially Variable Genes. *Spatially Variable Genes in Cancer*, 1–28. DOI: 10.4018/979-8-3693-7728-4.ch001

Blériot, C., Dunsmore, G., Alonso-Curbelo, D., & Ginhoux, F. (2024). A temporal perspective for tumor-associated macrophage identities and functions. *Cancer Cell*, *42*(5), 747–758. DOI: 10.1016/j.ccell.2024.04.002 PMID: 38670090

Carra, D., Maas, S. C. E., Seoane, J. A., & Alonso-Curbelo, D. (2025). Exposomal determinants of non-genetic plasticity in tumor initiation. *Trends in Cancer*, *0*(0), 295–308. Advance online publication. DOI: 10.1016/j.trecan.2025.01.010 PMID: 40023688

Chandra, G. V. S. A., Biradar, S., & Raghavan, R. (2025). Recent Trends in Soft Robotics for Assistive Technologies. *Assistive Technology Solutions for Aging Adults and Individuals With Disabilities*, 119–144. DOI: 10.4018/979-8-3693-6308-9.ch006

Chetwynd, A. J., Louyer, M.-V., Mercier, F., Bessonneau, V., & David, A. (2024). Polar organic pollutants, micro-nano plastics and nanomaterials: Analytical techniques to reveal the still invisible human physico-chemical exposome. *Trends in Analytical Chemistry*, *177*, 117816. DOI: 10.1016/j.trac.2024.117816

Deonarine, A., Batwara, A., Wada, R., Sharma, P., Loscalzo, J., Ojikutu, B., & Hall, K. (2025). De Novo exposomic geospatial assembly of chronic disease regions with machine learning & network analysis. *EBioMedicine*, *112*, 105575. Advance online publication. DOI: 10.1016/j.ebiom.2025.105575 PMID: 39891994

Desai, S., Morimoto, L. M., Kang, A. Y., Miller, M. D., Wiemels, J. L., Winestone, L. E., & Metayer, C. (2025). Pre- and Postnatal Exposures to Residential Pesticides and Survival of Childhood Acute Lymphoblastic Leukemia. *Cancers (Basel)*, *17*(6), 6. Advance online publication. DOI: 10.3390/cancers17060978 PMID: 40149312

França, G. S., Baron, M., King, B. R., Bossowski, J. P., Bjornberg, A., Pour, M., Rao, A., Patel, A. S., Misirlioglu, S., Barkley, D., Tang, K. H., Dolgalev, I., Liberman, D. A., Avital, G., Kuperwaser, F., Chiodin, M., Levine, D. A., Papagiannakopoulos, T., Marusyk, A., & Yanai, I. (2024). Cellular adaptation to cancer therapy along a resistance continuum. *Nature*, *631*(8022), 876–883. DOI: 10.1038/s41586-024-07690-9 PMID: 38987605

Frank, S. A., & Yanai, I. (2024). The origin of novel traits in cancer. *Trends in Cancer*, *10*(10), 880–892. DOI: 10.1016/j.trecan.2024.07.005 PMID: 39112299

Go, Y.-M., Weinberg, J., Teeny, S., Cirillo, P. M., Krigbaum, N. Y., Singer, G., Tran, V., Cohn, B. A., & Jones, D. P. (2023). Exposome epidemiology for suspect environmental chemical exposures during pregnancy linked to subsequent breast cancer diagnosis. *Environment International*, *178*, 108112. DOI: 10.1016/j.envint.2023.108112 PMID: 37517180

Gong, P., Guo, Z., Wang, S., Gao, S., & Cao, Q. (2025). Histone Phosphorylation in DNA Damage Response. *International Journal of Molecular Sciences*, *26*(6), 6. Advance online publication. DOI: 10.3390/ijms26062405 PMID: 40141048

GVS, A. C., Ananthakumar, B., & Raghavan, R. (2025). Enhancing Assistive Technologies With Neuromorphic Computing. *Revolutionizing AI with Brain-Inspired Technology: Neuromorphic Computing*, 207–232. DOI: 10.4018/979-8-3693-6303-4.ch009

GVS, A. C., Biradar, S., & Raghavan, R. (2025). Neuroscience-Driven Solutions for Speech Impairment: Assistive Technologies for Speech Rehabilitation. *Advancing Medical Research Through Neuroscience*, 119–146. DOI: 10.4018/979-8-3693-5464-3.ch006

Hou, M., Tang, S., Zhang, F., Fu, S., Ding, H., Cha, Y., Ma, X., Shi, Y., & Cai, Y. (2025). Chemical exposure in females of childbearing age associated with sex hormones: Evidence from an untargeted exposomic approach. *Environment International*, *197*, 109362. DOI: 10.1016/j.envint.2025.109362 PMID: 40054345

Islami, F., Baeker Bispo, J., Lee, H., Wiese, D., Yabroff, K. R., Bandi, P., Sloan, K., Patel, A. V., Daniels, E. C., Kamal, A. H., Guerra, C. E., Dahut, W. L., & Jemal, A. (2024). American Cancer Society's report on the status of cancer disparities in the United States, 2023. *CA: a Cancer Journal for Clinicians*, *74*(2), 136–166. DOI: 10.3322/caac.21812 PMID: 37962495

Iungman, T., Khomenko, S., Barboza, E. P., Cirach, M., Gonçalves, K., Petrone, P., Erbertseder, T., Taubenböck, H., Chakraborty, T., & Nieuwenhuijsen, M. (2024). The impact of urban configuration types on urban heat islands, air pollution, CO2 emissions, and mortality in Europe: A data science approach. *The Lancet. Planetary Health*, *8*(7), e489–e505. DOI: 10.1016/S2542-5196(24)00120-7 PMID: 38969476

Korrapati, C., Yaraladdi, A. B., Vaddi, H., & Raghavan, R. (2024). Applications of the Saffron European Kitchen Spice Crocus sativus. *Therapeutic and Pharmacological Applications of Ethnobotany*, 98–127. DOI: 10.4018/979-8-3693-1986-4.ch005

Lakshmaiah, A., Korrapati, C., Suresh, C., & Raghavan, R. (2025). Synthetic Biology and AI. *Spatially Variable Genes in Cancer*, 265–290. DOI: 10.4018/979-8-3693-7728-4.ch010

Lauri, G., Mills, K., Majumder, S., & Capurso, G. (2025). The exposome as a target for primary prevention and a tool for early detection of pancreatic cancer. *Best Practice & Research. Clinical Gastroenterology*, *101991*, 101991. Advance online publication. DOI: 10.1016/j.bpg.2025.101991 PMID: 40210335

Lyu, S. I., Fretter, C., Eckel, H. N. C., Knipper, K., Schultheis, A. M., Büttner, R., Quaas, A., Klussmann, J. P., & Simon, A. G. (2025). High expression of H2AX/γ-H2AX is associated with distinct biological pathway alterations and shorter survival in oropharyngeal squamous cell carcinoma. *Oral Oncology*, *161*, 107171. DOI: 10.1016/j.oraloncology.2024.107171 PMID: 39756240

Ma, L., Zhang, Y., Xu, J., Yu, Y., Zhou, P., Liu, X., & Guan, H. (2025). Effects of Ionizing Radiation on DNA Methylation Patterns and Their Potential as Biomarkers. *International Journal of Molecular Sciences*, *26*(7), 7. Advance online publication. DOI: 10.3390/ijms26073342 PMID: 40244232

Madrigal, J. M., Pruitt, C. N., Fisher, J. A., Liao, L. M., Graubard, B. I., Gierach, G. L., Silverman, D. T., Ward, M. H., & Jones, R. R. (2024). Carcinogenic industrial air pollution and postmenopausal breast cancer risk in the National Institutes of Health AARP Diet and Health Study. *Environment International*, *191*, 108985. DOI: 10.1016/j.envint.2024.108985 PMID: 39226766

Maitre, L., Bustamante, M., Hernández-Ferrer, C., Thiel, D., Lau, C.-H. E., Siskos, A. P., Vives-Usano, M., Ruiz-Arenas, C., Pelegrí-Sisó, D., Robinson, O., Mason, D., Wright, J., Cadiou, S., Slama, R., Heude, B., Casas, M., Sunyer, J., Papadopoulou, E. Z., Gutzkow, K. B., & Vrijheid, M. (2022). Multi-omics signatures of the human early life exposome. *Nature Communications*, *13*(1), 7024. DOI: 10.1038/s41467-022-34422-2 PMID: 36411288

Nagashri, N., Archana, L., & Raghavan, R. (2024). Microbial Volatile Compounds (MVOCs) in Food Industries and Food Safety Applications. *Innovations, Securities, and Case Studies Across Healthcare, Business, and Technology*, 75–96. DOI: 10.4018/979-8-3693-1906-2.ch005

Non, A. L. (2025). The eighth annual US DOHAD meeting: Promising approaches in epigenetics research of early life exposures. *Epigenomics*, *17*(4), 209–211. DOI: 10.1080/17501911.2025.2459550 PMID: 39874076

Okwan-Duodu, D., Pandiri, A. R., & Adams, D. J. (2024). Not All Carcinogens Are Directly Mutagenic: A Holistic View of the Environmental Exposure–Cancer Connection. *Annual Review of Cancer Biology*. Advance online publication. DOI: 10.1146/annurev-cancerbio-060424-052905

Roje, B., Zhang, B., Mastrorilli, E., Kovačić, A., Sušak, L., Ljubenkov, I., Ćosić, E., Vilović, K., Meštrović, A., Vukovac, E. L., Bučević-Popović, V., Puljiz, Ž., Karaman, I., Terzić, J., & Zimmermann, M. (2024). Gut microbiota carcinogen metabolism causes distal tissue tumours. *Nature*, *632*(8027), 1137–1144. DOI: 10.1038/s41586-024-07754-w PMID: 39085612

Sadee, B. A., Zebari, S. M. S., Galali, Y., & Saleem, M. F. (2025). A review on arsenic contamination in drinking water: Sources, health impacts, and remediation approaches. *RSC Advances*, *15*(4), 2684–2703. DOI: 10.1039/D4RA08867K PMID: 39871983

Safarlou, C. W., Jongsma, K. R., & Vermeulen, R. (2024). Reconceptualizing and Defining Exposomics within Environmental Health: Expanding the Scope of Health Research. *Environmental Health Perspectives*, *132*(9), 095001. DOI: 10.1289/EHP14509 PMID: 39331035

Sahoo, R., Pattnaik, S., Mohanty, B., Mir, S. A., & Behera, B. (2025). Aryl hydrocarbon receptor (AHR) signalling: A double-edged sword guiding both cancer progression and cancer therapy. *Biochimica et Biophysica Acta (BBA) -. Biochimica et Biophysica Acta. G, General Subjects*, *1869*(6), 130805. DOI: 10.1016/j.bbagen.2025.130805 PMID: 40222634

Saucy, A., Coloma, F., Olmos, S., Åström, C., Blay, N., Boer, J. M. A., Dadvand, P., de Bont, J., de Cid, R., de Hoogh, K., Dimakopoulou, K., Gehring, U., Huss, A., Ibi, D., Katsouyanni, K., Koppelman, G., Ljungman, P., Melén, E., Nieuwenhuijsen, M., & Tonne, C. (2024). Socioeconomic Inequalities in the External Exposome in European Cohorts: The EXPANSE Project. *Environmental Science & Technology*, *58*(37), 16248–16257. DOI: 10.1021/acs.est.4c01509 PMID: 39237108

Sherif, Z. A., Ogunwobi, O. O., & Ressom, H. W. (2025). Mechanisms and technologies in cancer epigenetics. *Frontiers in Oncology*, *14*, 1513654. Advance online publication. DOI: 10.3389/fonc.2024.1513654 PMID: 39839798

Somala, C. S., Sathyapriya, S., Bharathkumar, N., Anand, T., Mathangi, D. C., & Saravanan, K. M. (2025). Therapeutic Potential of FTO Demethylase in Metabolism and Disease Pathways. *The Protein Journal*, *44*(1), 21–34. DOI: 10.1007/s10930-025-10250-3 PMID: 39923206

Tedaldi, A. M., Behrouzi, P., & Grootswagers, P. (2025). Diet, lifestyle and telomere length: Using Copula Graphical Models on NHANES data. *Aging (Albany NY), 17*(2), 329–356. DOI: 10.18632/aging.206194 PMID: 39883078

Telkmann, K., Gudi-Mindermann, H., Bogers, R., Ahrens, J., Tönnies, J., van Kamp, I., Vrijkotte, T., & Bolte, G. (2025). Identification of exposome clusters based on societal, social, built and natural environment – results of the ABCD cohort study. *Environment International, 197*, 109335. DOI: 10.1016/j.envint.2025.109335 PMID: 39983415

Tsai, Y.-S., Jou, Y.-C., Cheong, I. S., Tung, H.-T., Hsu, L.-N., Tsai, H.-T., & Tzai, T.-S. (2025). Phthalate exposure induces microRNA-5010/Nrf2-EGR1/GDF15 signaling expression in prostate cancer. *Ecotoxicology and Environmental Safety, 290*, 117759. DOI: 10.1016/j.ecoenv.2025.117759 PMID: 39837010

VoPham, T., White, A. J., & Jones, R. R.VoPham. (2024). Geospatial Science for the Environmental Epidemiology of Cancer in the Exposome Era. *Cancer Epidemiology, Biomarkers & Prevention, 33*(4), 451–460. DOI: 10.1158/1055-9965. EPI-23-1237 PMID: 38566558

Wan, M., Simonin, E. M., Johnson, M. M., Zhang, X., Lin, X., Gao, P., Patel, C. J., Yousuf, A., Snyder, M. P., Hong, X., Wang, X., Sampath, V., & Nadeau, K. C. (2025). Exposomics: A review of methodologies, applications, and future directions in molecular medicine. *EMBO Molecular Medicine, 17*(4), 1–10. DOI: 10.1038/s44321-025-00191-w PMID: 39870881

Wang, X., Guan, P., You, L., Qin, W., Li, Q., Wang, X., Chen, Q., Yu, D., Ye, Y., Wang, T., Liu, X., Fan, J., & Xu, G. (2025). Risk of serum circulating environmental chemical residues to esophageal squamous cell carcinoma: A nested case–control metabolome-wide association study. *Analytical and Bioanalytical Chemistry, 417*(13), 2783–2795. Advance online publication. DOI: 10.1007/s00216-025-05784-5 PMID: 39939416

Weinberg, B. A., Murphy, C. C., Freyer, D. R., Greathouse, K. L., Blancato, J. K., Stoffel, E. M., Drewes, J. L., Blaes, A., Salsman, J. M., You, Y. N., Arem, H., Mukherji, R., Kanth, P., Hu, X., Fabrizio, A., Hartley, M. L., Giannakis, M., & Marshall, J. L. (2025). Rethinking the rise of early-onset gastrointestinal cancers: A call to action. *JNCI Cancer Spectrum, 9*(1), pkaf002. Advance online publication. DOI: 10.1093/jncics/pkaf002 PMID: 39814070

Wheeler, M. A., & Quintana, F. J. (2025). The neuroimmune connectome in health and disease. *Nature, 638*(8050), 333–342. DOI: 10.1038/s41586-024-08474-x PMID: 39939792

Wiese, D., DuBois, T. D., Sorice, K. A., Fang, C. Y., Ragin, C., Daly, M., Reese, A. C., Henry, K. A., & Lynch, S. M. (2024). An exploratory analysis of the impact of area-level exposome on geographic disparities in aggressive prostate cancer. *Scientific Reports*, *14*(1), 16900. DOI: 10.1038/s41598-024-63726-0 PMID: 39075110

Youn, C. K., Koh, J. W., Lee, J.-H., & Park, S.-J. (2025). P53-binding Protein Inhibits Intracellular Reactive Oxygen Species by Increasing the Expression of Metallothioneins. *Anticancer Research*, *45*(4), 1535–1545. DOI: 10.21873/anticanres.17535 PMID: 40155029

Zhi, M.-X., & Wang, J.-S. (2024). [Advances in the applications of exposomics in the identification of environmental pollutants and their health hazards]. *Se Pu =. Se Pu = Chinese Journal of Chromatography*, *42*(2), 142–149. DOI: 10.3724/SP.J.1123.2023.12011 PMID: 38374594

Chapter 5

Insights on the Role of the Microbiome in Influencing Cancer Risk: How Ecological Exposures Affect Microbiome in Influencing Cancer Risk

Joyjyoti Das
https://orcid.org/0000-0001-6238-7667
Adamas University, Kolkata, India

Bandana Padhan
Adamas University, Kolkata, India

Anjali Sadhukhan
https://orcid.org/0009-0004-1540-2480
Adamas University, Kolkata, India

Ritika Halder
Adamas University, Kolkata, India

Swetashree Purohit
https://orcid.org/0000-0002-2738-0782
C.V. Raman Global University, India

Tania Aich
https://orcid.org/0009-0005-9203-6223
Adamas University, Kolkata, India

ABSTRACT

The microbiome refers to the complex community of microorganisms dwelling in and on the human body. Especially, the gut microbiota is involved in modulating a host of crucial physiological processes such as immunity development, anabolism, and nutrient uptake. Diverse ecological exposures ranging from environmental pollutants to dietary components and infectious agents may influence the microbiome to either promote carcinogenesis by inducing chronic inflammation and producing toxic metabolites or exert anticancer effects by boosting the host immune response. This chapter accounts for the various exposomes and their role in influencing microbiome-mediated cancer risk, the mechanisms involved, and the various novel

DOI: 10.4018/979-8-3373-2165-3.ch005

strategies that are being established by researchers for cancer prevention, early detection, and therapeutic interventions via the microbiome-alteration route. The role of advanced technologies such as metagenomics and NGS in enhancing the understanding of the microbiome-carcinogenesis crosstalk has also been discussed with the hope of fostering research in this domain.

1. INTRODUCTION

The human gut microbiota, a complex ecosystem of microorganisms, plays a fundamental role in human health by influencing various physiological processes, including digestion, immune system regulation, metabolic functions, and even mood and cognitive function (Hickman et al. 2024). Factors like diet, lifestyle, and antibiotic use significantly shape its composition, highlighting the importance of gut-friendly habits for overall well-being. The gut microbiota consists of a diverse community of microorganisms, including bacteria, viruses, fungi, and archaea. Furthermore, the gut microbiome supports immune system regulation by defending against harmful infections and promoting beneficial immune responses (Su and Liu 2021). Several factors can influence the diversity and stability of the gut microbiota, including diet, antibiotic use, stress, and lifestyle choices. Diet is a primary driver, with high-fat diets associated with reduced bacterial diversity and increased intestinal permeability (Hasan and Yang 2019). Antibiotic use can also disrupt the gut microbiota, leading to imbalances clinically termed as "Dysbiosis", while stress and mental health issues are linked to reduced diversity and altered microbiome composition. Geographical location, genetics, and other lifestyle factors also contribute to the variations in gut microbiota composition among individuals (Ren et al. 2023).

Cancer cases worldwide are soaring high, with an estimated 20 million new cases reported in 2022 and predictions of over 35 million by 2050, primarily driven by population growth, aging, and lifestyle risk factors such as tobacco, alcohol, and obesity (Bray et al. 2024). Traditional treatments such as surgery, radiotherapy, and chemotherapy primarily target cancer epithelial cells but do not sufficiently address the tumor microenvironment and its complex interactions, which play a crucial role in cancer progression (Charmsaz et al. 2019) . More importantly, the gut microbiota modulates responses to major anticancer therapies offering opportunities to improve therapeutic outcomes (Zhao et al. 2023a).

Gut dysbiosis, characterized by a less stable, diverse, and more pathogenic microbiota, contributes to pathological conditions, impacting cancer development and treatment. The disruption of the intestinal mucosal barrier may allow gut microbes to become intratumoral microbes, directly impacting cancer development (Zhao et al. 2023a). As shown in Figure 1, microbial diversity and load vary across different sections of the gastrointestinal tract.

Figure 1. Distribution of normal gut flora in different parts of intestine (Figure created in Biorender.com)

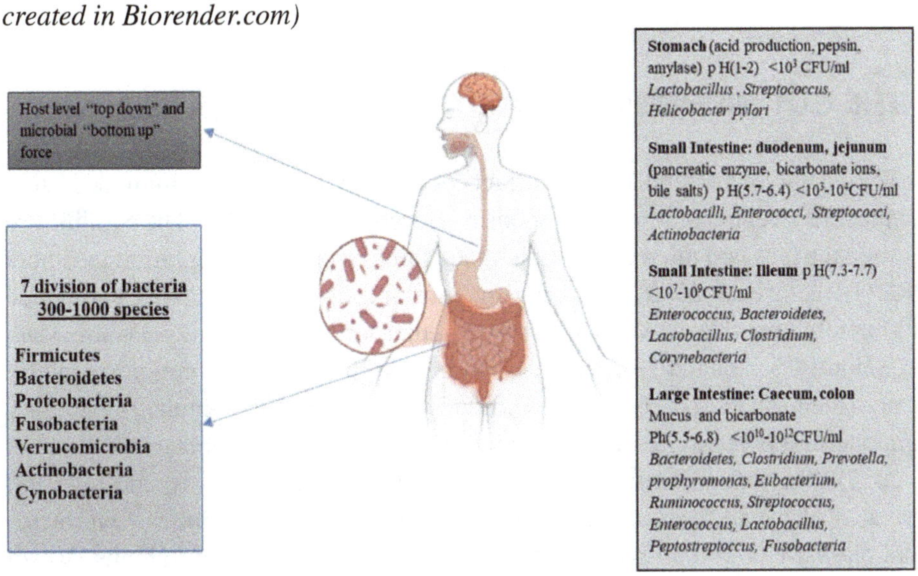

The human gut microbiome is a complex ecosystem comprising bacteria, archaea, eukarya, viruses, and parasites, with Firmicutes and Bacteroidetes as the predominant bacterial divisions (Zafar and Saier). These microbial communities are classified into Bacteroides, Prevotella, and Ruminococcus enterotypes, influenced by diet and impacting digestion, immune function, metabolism, and even mood (Khelaifia et al. 2016). Several key bacterial genera play significant roles in the gut ecosystem. Prevotella species, particularly *P. copri,* are associated with high-fiber diets and can be linked to both positive and adverse health conditions. Clostridium species are responsible for producing secondary bile acids and short-chain fatty acids like butyrate, which are crucial for gut health. Eubacterium species, including *E. rectale*, are also butyrate producers and contribute to bile acid and cholesterol transformations (Seekatz et al. 2022). *Ruminococcus gnavus* has been identified as a significant species that can be both beneficial and detrimental, depending on strain and niche (Crost et al. 2023). In addition to bacteria, archaea such as *Methanobrevibacter smithii*, a hydrogen-consuming methanogen, and the halophilic archaea *Haloferax alexandrinus* and *Haloferax massiliensis* are also found in the human gut (Khelaifia et al. 2016). This chapter delves into the complex interplay between the gut microbiome, dietary habits, and environmental influences in shaping cancer risk, with an emphasis on gastrointestinal cancers. Through the examination of case studies across various cancer types, it highlights how these interconnected factors contribute to carcinogenesis. A deeper understanding of these interactions is opening new avenues for cancer prevention, early diagnosis, and the development of targeted therapeutic strategies.

2. THE GUT MICROBIOTA AND ITS INFLUENCE ON IMMUNITY

The gut microbiota significantly influences the development of the immune system and the effectiveness of immune responses (Bosco and Noti 2021). The equilibrium between the host and microbes is maintained through pattern-recognition receptors (PRRs) (Zheng et al. 2020) . Furthermore, intestinal epithelial cells (IECs) produce anti-microbial peptides (AMPs), which are essential for innate immunity (Duarte-Mata and Salinas-Carmona 2023). The microbiota also influences the immune response through the formation of metabolites produced by the gut microbiome from dietary components, host products, or other microbial metabolites (Abdalkareem Jasim et al. 2022). Short-chain fatty acids (SCFAs), tryptophan metabolites, and bile acid derivatives have all been shown to possess immunoprotective abilities. Gut microbiota plays a vital role in promoting the maturation of the human immune system and maintaining immune system balance (Zhao et al. 2023b). Microbial dysbiosis in the gut is linked to abnormal production of inflammatory cytokines, affecting immune responses (Schirmer et al. 2016). Commensal microbes calibrate innate and adaptive immune responses, impacting the activation threshold for pathogenic stimulations, largely by producing small molecules that mediate host-microbial interactions (Schirmer et al. 2016). Immune dysregulation is linked to an increased risk of cancer due to immune surveillance failure (Matza Porges and Shamriz 2022). The immune system's critical role in identifying and eliminating tumors means that its dysregulation can increase cancer risk.

3. EXPOSOMES AFFECTING GUT MICROBIOTA: DIET, ANTIBIOTICS, AND ENVIRONMENTAL FACTORS

A healthy human gut microbiota consists primarily of benign bacterial species which defend human health by inhibiting potential harmful microorganisms from causing infections (Dahiya and Nigam 2023). The two main host physiological processes affected by gut microbiota composition include immune system response and medication breakdown which leads to multiple diseases affecting normal body operation. Understanding of how the environmental and lifestyle elements, together called as exposomes, alter gut microbiota is important because this knowledge is essential for human health.

3.1 The Impact of Diet on the Gut Microbiota Composition and Cancer Risk

3.1.1. Dietary Fiber and the Microbiome

A key component of the complex interaction between nutrition and the gut microbiota is dietary fiber, which has a major impact on the composition and function of the microbiota, which in turn has a major effect on host health. Dietary fiber, which is found in abundance in plant-based meals such as fruits, vegetables, whole grains, and legumes, serves as an essential prebiotic substrate that specifically nourishes good gut bacteria, promoting their development and metabolic activity (Turner and Lupton 2021; Munteanu and Schwartz 2024). Acetate, propionate, and butyrate are among the short-chain fatty acids (SCFAs) produced by this fermentation process, which is regulated by the gut flora (Lattimer and Haub 2010; den Besten et al. 2013; Munteanu and Schwartz 2024). These SCFAs are not just metabolic waste products; they are important signaling molecules that help the immune, neuroendocrine, and metabolic systems communicate extensively (den Besten et al. 2013; Gill et al. 2022; Munteanu and Schwartz 2024). As a result, they play crucial roles in controlling inflammation, maintaining energy homeostasis, and even affecting behavior and brain function (Zhang 2022; Munteanu and Schwartz 2024). In addition to its prebiotic action, dietary fiber supports gut health by increasing the number of bacteria that produce SCFA and fostering a microbial community structure that benefits host health (Fu et al. 2020; Munteanu and Schwartz 2024). The epidemiological connection between dietary fiber consumption and the risk of colorectal cancer is also emphasized in the literature (Zhou et al. 2021; Munteanu and Schwartz 2024). The reported inverse relationship between daily fiber intake and the risk of colorectal cancer (CRC) raises the possibility that the growing prevalence of this cancer is caused by a diet low in fiber, which is common in westernized nations (Hjorth et al. 2019; Munteanu and Schwartz 2024). Numerous processes underlie the preventive benefits of fiber, including the possible control of bile acid metabolism, which, if disturbed, may hasten the development of colon cancer.

3.1.2. Antioxidants and the Gut Microbiota

Humans' adequate diets and lifestyles impact their general health (Munteanu and Schwartz 2024). Micro-nutrients (vitamins, minerals, and bioactive compounds) play crucial roles in modulating different biochemical, metabolic, and signalling pathways. Most micronutrients function as antioxidant compounds to fight against nitric and oxidative stresses (Pisoschi and Pop 2015; Munteanu and Schwartz 2024). The antioxidant compounds consumed by humans include polyphenols, vitamins, selenium, and zinc. Their inadequate consumption has many harmful effects on immune function because of the link with the appearance of different diseases (Burk 2002; Prasad 2014; Fenech et al. 2018). Vegetables are rich in compounds with antioxidant characteristics, which may reduce the damaging impacts of the redox processes that every cell goes through as a result of its biochemical responses. Antioxidants are high electron density compounds that have the ability to neutralize free radicals by allowing them to give up one electron in order to quench the free radical (Lobo et al. 2010). Researchers have indicated that antioxidants, or free radical inhibitors, participate with free radical molecules in a series of chain reactions that result in the complex formation of blocker and free agent molecules that generate stable molecules.

3.2. The Impact of Antibiotics on the Gut Microbiota Composition and Cancer Risk

The gastrointestinal tract contains various microbial species which favor host health through metabolic activities. Antibiotic treatment results in severe damage to the natural microbiota living inside the gastrointestinal tract. The treatment changes a person's microbial diversity while transforming metabolic functions and generates antibiotic resistance. Antibiotics affect every type of microorganism therefore they reach and harm both pathogenic and beneficial intestinal flora. The wide-ranging mechanism of action from these drugs modifies the make-up of gut microbial populations. The host-microbe interactions deteriorate when people use antibiotics because the immune system equilibrium shatters and the gastrointestinal tract loses its ability to repel potential pathogenic strains (Dahiya and Nigam 2023). Multiple antibiotic usage alters microbiota equilibrium which causes dysbiosis with reduced beneficial flora and excess pathogenic bacteria (Gebrayel et al. 2022). Gut microbiota modifications are thought to significantly contribute to the emergence of different non-communicable diseases. The absence of proper dysbiosis control enables health conditions that should be treatable to become long-term illnesses with time. Dysbiosis functions as an established risk component which drives multiple illnesses affecting health including colitis and celiac disease together with irritable bowel syndrome (IBS) and inflammatory bowel disease (IBD) as well as leaky gut syndrome, liver disease, colorectal cancer, etc. The symptoms of dysbiosis become distinctive based on which gut bacteria are affected. Antibiotics significantly disrupt the gut microbiota by releasing chemicals that disturb the balance between normal gut bacteria and potentially harmful bacteria. This disruption can increase the risk of intestinal pathogen colonization (Dahiya and Nigam 2023). The effect of antibiotic treatments significantly alter the gut microbiota and its function (Table 1).

Table 1. List of antibiotics and their target pathogens which alters the host gut microbiota when used

Name of antibiotics	Target pathogen	Changes in host gut	References
Aminoglycoside; Macrolides; Lincosamide; Tetracycline; Rifamycin	Urinary tract infection, Gram-negative bacterial infections	Microbiome alterations weaken stress resistance; macrolides affect mucus production, ion movement, and inflammation.	(Kanoh and Rubin 2010; Ruiz et al. 2017; Xu and Li 2019; Patangia et al. 2022; Dahiya and Nigam 2023; Bui et al. 2025)
Beta-lactam and Glycopeptide (Amoxicillin, Cloxacillin, Ceftazidime, Ceftriaxone)	Rhinosinusitis, respiratory/ genitourinary tract infections, septicemia	Causes gut dysbiosis, disrupting bacterial balance.	(Li et al. 2014; Pauwels et al. 2021; Dahiya and Nigam 2023; Akhavan et al. 2025; Peechakara and Gupta 2025)
Metronidazole; Azithromycin	Sinusitis, pneumonia, respiratory/skin infections, urogenital and chlamydial infections	Decreases microbiome diversity; increases *Lactobacillus iners* in urinary and vaginal microbiota.	(Jakobsson and Forsum 2007; Rineh et al. 2014; Chee et al. 2020; Dahiya and Nigam 2023; Weir and Le 2025)
Beta-lactam-Macrolide; Beta-lactam-Nitrofuran; Beta-lactam-Nitroimidazole; Beta-lactam-Macrolide Nitroimidazole; Glycopeptide Nitroimidazole Quinolone	Tuberculosis, protozoal infections (trichomoniasis, amoebiasis, bacterial vaginosis, giardiasis, non-gonococcal urethritis), visceral leishmaniasis	Induces gut dysbiosis by disrupting bacterial composition.	(Li et al. 2014; Pauwels et al. 2021; Dahiya and Nigam 2023; Akhavan et al. 2025; Peechakara and Gupta 2025)

3.3. The Impact of Environmental Pollutants on the Gut Microbiota Composition and Cancer Risk

The rapid growth of microbiome research in the past ten years demonstrated how the external factors interact with the human microbiome in different ways, influencing health and disease. Recent findings suggest that environment-related chemicals have an impact on gut microbial communities and the gut microbiome may directly or indirectly alter xenobiotic metabolism, affecting human health (Gebrayel et al. 2022). The understanding of environmental exposure as a vital risk factor for cancer increases daily while this exposure type represents a major portion of worldwide cancer cases (Duvallet et al. 2017). Scientists have studied different types of environmental exposures that cause cancer while exploring occupational risks as well as air and water quality problems alongside life style choices between exercise and nutrition. Scientists demonstrated that lung cancer and multiple cancer types emerge from exposure to benzene together with nitrogen dioxide and particulate matter (PM2.5) in the air. Drinking water containing arsenic alongside industrial chemicals serves as a cause for various malignancies to affect the bladder, liver, and skin. Braking material exposure throughout particular professions substantially raises cancer risks because workers come in contact with asbestos, silica and particular pesticide types. Cancer development risks increase as individuals adopt lifestyle practices including alcohol use and cigarette smoking and unbalanced eating habits (Duvallet et al. 2017). The risk of environmental carcinogens exposure is typically higher among low-income communities as well as marginalized populations thus creating more significant health disparities that result in unequal cancer outcomes (Duvallet et al. 2017).

3.4. The Impact of Lifestyle on the Gut Microbiota Composition and Cancer Risk

Prior to cancer risk assessment one must consider both food consumption and physical activity as leading lifestyle components. The eating habits of people significantly influence cancer incidence because different nutrition patterns either raise or reduce the likelihood of tumor development. The consumption of processed and red meats in diets continues to increase the chance of developing colon cancer. Dietary agents that potentially cause cancer are nitrites and nitrates plus heterocyclic amines and polycyclic aromatic hydrocarbons found during meat preparation (Duvallet et al. 2017; Ajayi and Ogunjobi 2024). Dietary use of alcohol creates changes in cancer risk for individuals. The conversion of ethanol into the known carcinogen acetaldehyde then enables ROS to damage multiple cellular components as well as DNA. The hindering of essential nutrient absorption increases cancer risk since alcohol consumption can disrupt the body's nutrient utilization process (Duvallet et al. 2017; Diallo et al. 2018). The cancers primarily affected by obesity include colon, renal, pancreatic, endometrial, and breast malignancies. Several mechanisms related to sex hormone production and adipokine production as well as insulin resistance and chronic inflammation enable obesity to elevate cancer risk through enhanced cell growth and suppressed cellular death (Duvallet et al. 2017; Molina-Montes et al. 2021).

4. MECHANISMS OF GUT MICROBIOTA-MEDIATED CARCINOGENESIS

Gut microbiota can mediate carcinogenesis through various mechanisms, including the production of metabolites, effects on DNA repair and cellular pathways, the induction of chronic inflammation, and alterations in gene expression related to cancer progression (Andreeva et al. 2020). SCFAs like butyrate, propionate, and acetate, resulting from dietary fiber fermentation by microbiota, can suppress tumor development. SCFAs, such as butyrate, protect the intestinal barrier by upregulating claudin-1 and acting as the primary energy source for colonocytes. In tumor cells, butyrate accumulates and triggers apoptosis via histone deacetylase (HDAC) inhibition (Rivas-Domínguez et al. 2021). Bile acids, particularly secondary bile acids like deoxycholic and lithocholic, can cause reactive oxygen species (ROS) production and membrane damage in enterocytes, potentially leading to inflammation and inhibiting DNA repair systems. Secondary bile acids can also induce the degradation of p53 and activate survival pathways, promoting apoptosis-resistant clones.

Short-chain fatty acids, particularly butyrate, propionate, and acetate, generated by the fermentation of dietary fibers by gut microbiota, play a substantial role in modulating cancer development across various types. Their influence manifests through multiple biochemical pathways that impact cell growth, inflammation, and genomic stability. SCFAs have been shown to inhibit cancer stem cell proliferation, potentially delaying tumor progression and relapse by targeting specific genes and pathways associated with neoplastic growth. For example, butyrate functions as an HDAC inhibitor, which can lead to the differentiation of cancer cells, thereby promoting apoptosis in malignant tissues while preserving normal cells, a critical aspect that highlights the selective toxicity of SCFAs against cancer cells (Feitelson et al. 2023). In colorectal cancer (CRC), for instance, SCFAs attenuate inflammation by down-regulating pro-inflammatory cytokines and reducing oxidative stress, which has been primarily linked to tumorigenesis. The alteration of the gut microbiota composition, often characterized by reduced SCFA-producing bacteria during CRC, emphasizes the significance of these metabolites in maintaining homeostasis within the intestinal microenvironment and mitigating cancer risk. Furthermore, studies indicate that SCFAs can demethylate oncogenes, which helps to repress their expression and subsequently limits tumor growth (Feitelson et al. 2023). In hepatocellular carcinoma, SCFAs have shown potential to influence the activation of signaling pathways associated with cell proliferation and survival, thereby affecting tumor development. The multifaceted nature of SCFA action suggests they may alter tumor susceptibility depending on the specific genetic background and microenvironment of the cancer cells (Andreeva et al. 2020).

Additionally, SCFAs like butyrate, propionate, and acetate produced by beneficial gut bacteria exhibit anti-inflammatory properties and are vital for maintaining the health of intestinal epithelial cells. Butyrate, in particular, serves as a primary energy source for colonocytes and promotes the expression of tight junction proteins, including claudins and occludins, which are essential for the integrity of the gut barrier. The depletion of SCFAs in a leaky gut state can diminish the epithelial mucosal defense, making the intestinal lining susceptible to damage from pro-inflammatory cytokines and reactive oxygen species released during immune responses (Kalyanaraman et al. 2024). Moreover, the modulation of immune responses by SCFAs includes the promotion of regulatory T cells and inhibition of the NF-κB signaling pathway, which is activated by inflammatory stimuli and contributes to the persistent inflammatory state observed in leaky gut syndrome and associated carcinogenesis (Waldum and Fossmark 2023). The interplay between SCFAs and gut microbiota provides a promising avenue for therapeutic approaches targeting not only gut health but also inflammation-related diseases and cancer, suggesting that dietary interventions aimed at restoring or enhancing SCFA production may mitigate the detrimental effects of dysbiosis, leaky gut, and inflammation (Feitelson et al. 2023).

Dysbiosis can promote colorectal cancer (CRC) development, with certain bacteria directly secreting enzymes or molecules that influence NFkB activation, apoptosis pathways, or cytoskeleton reorganization. In dysbiosis, chemically modified nutrients from the diet can act as microbiota modulators, boosting ROS/RNS production, toxins, and the onset of CRC (Rivas-Domínguez et al. 2021). Some bacterial strains, such as *Helicobacter pylori*, can block the normal cell cycle by affecting oxidative environment-dependent DNA damage and disrupting the DNA mismatch-repair process (Sun et al. 2023). Specific bacteria, such as *E. coli* strains, produce toxins like colibactin that induce DNA double-strand breaks and chromosomal aberrations (Allen and Sears 2019).

The gut microbiota consists of diverse bacterial populations capable of producing various enzymes that contribute to homeostasis and influence the pathogenesis of cancer. One significant enzyme class involved in this process is the bile salt hydrolases produced by intestinal bacteria, which modulate bile acids' solubility and toxicity through deconjugation (Hsiao et al. 2020) . This enzymatic activity can alter bile acids' local concentration, promoting the formation of secondary bile acids known for their potential toxic effects on colonocytes. Furthermore, bacteria such as *E. coli* can synthesize the genotoxic compound colibactin, which induces double-strand breaks and chromosomal aberrations by altering DNA stability (Allen and Sears 2019).

Chronic inflammation is strongly linked to carcinogenesis in digestive organs such as the stomach, colon, and liver (Waldum and Fossmark 2023). The mechanisms by which chronic inflammation promotes malignancy include direct genotoxicity, release of genotoxic substances from inflammatory cells, increased cell proliferation due to inflammation-induced cell death, and hormonal disturbances affecting cellular proliferation. Pro-inflammatory molecules present during chronic inflammation can lead to mutations and genetic instability, promoting cell proliferation, survival, angiogenesis, and metastasis. The interactions between gut microbiota and the host can lead to the production of various genotoxic substances, significantly contributing to cancer development (Hsiao et al. 2020). One of the most well-documented examples is colibactin, a genotoxic compound produced by specific strains of *E. coli*. Colibactin is known to induce DNA double-strand breaks, chromosomal aberrations, and arrest the cell cycle, which can ultimately promote carcinogenesis (Allen and Sears 2019). The synthesis of colibactin involves intricate biochemical pathways, including the activity of non-ribosomal peptide synthases, which process a propeptide into its active form that can covalently link to DNA, disrupting replication and inducing mutational changes.

Another notable group of genotoxic agents comprises bile acids, particularly secondary bile acids such as deoxycholic acid and lithocholic acid, which are formed through microbial transformations. These compounds can cause oxidative damage to cellular membranes and DNA, inhibit essential DNA repair mechanisms, and induce genetic instability by promoting the formation of single-strand breaks and double-strand breaks (Režen et al. 2022). Their actions are significantly influenced by the microbiota composition, with dysbiosis often correlating with elevated levels of these harmful bile acids, leading to chronic inflammation and subsequent DNA damage. Gut microbes can transform cholesterol-derived bile acids into metabolites that block androgen signaling. This enhances the immune system's ability to combat cancer cells (Jin et al. 2025). Moreover, Enteropathogenic *E. coli* (EPEC) and the toxin Cdt (cytolethal distending toxin) exhibit similar genotoxic effects. EPEC can deplete components of the DNA mismatch repair system, increasing the mutation rate in host cells that may lead to neoplastic transformation. Similarly, toxins from organisms like *Fusobacterium nucleatum* and *Bacteroides fragilis* (such as *Bacteroides fragilis* toxin, BFT), significantly contribute to DNA damage through the promotion of inflammatory responses and direct interactions with DNA repair pathways (Režen et al. 2022). Through these mechanisms, microbial-produced toxins and metabolites can lead to significant alterations in the host's genome, promoting a state of genetic instability and enhancing the susceptibility to cancer development in individuals with dysbiosis or chronic inflammation. As shown in Table 2, trimethylamine N-oxide (TMAO) is associated with inflammation and fibrosis in liver cancer.

Table 2. Gut microbiome metabolites and their role in carcinogenesis across different cancer types

Cancer Type	Gut Microbiome Metabolites	Mechanism of Carcinogenesis	References
Colorectal Cancer (CRC)	Secondary bile acids (deoxycholate, lithocholate)	Induce DNA damage, inflammation, and apoptosis resistance.	(Liu et al. 2022)
	Hydrogen sulfide (H_2S)	Impairs DNA repair, promotes chronic inflammation.	(Szabo et al. 2013)
	SCFAs (butyrate, acetate, propionate)	Butyrate shows protective effects, but dysregulation can alter immune response.	(Mowat et al. 2023a)
	p-Cresol, phenol, indole	Increases epithelial permeability, DNA damage, and inflammation.	(Nowak and Libudzisz 2006)
Liver Cancer (HCC)	Trimethylamine N-oxide (TMAO)	Promotes inflammation, lipid accumulation, and fibrosis.	(Wu et al. 2022)
	Lipopolysaccharides (LPS)	Activates TLR4 signaling, leading to chronic inflammation and hepatocarcinogenesis.	(Wang et al. 2013)
	Secondary bile acids	Induce oxidative stress and DNA damage in hepatocytes.	(Ma et al. 2018)
Gastric Cancer	Nitrosamines	Produced by nitrate-reducing bacteria, leading to DNA alkylation and mutations.	(Xie et al. 2023)
	Ammonia	Causes DNA damage and promotes *Helicobacter pylori* colonization, increasing risk.	(Chen et al. 2022)
	Reactive oxygen species (ROS)	Induce oxidative DNA damage and epigenetic alterations.	(Srinivas et al. 2019)
Esophageal Cancer	Acetaldehyde	Produced by alcohol-metabolizing gut bacteria, causing DNA mutations and crosslinking.	(Nieminen and Salaspuro 2018)
	Lactic acid bacteria imbalance	Dysbiosis leads to chronic inflammation and increased carcinogen exposure.	(Zhang and Fu 2021)
Pancreatic Cancer	LPS	Chronic activation of NF-κB and cytokine production, promoting tumor growth.	(Jiang et al. 2022)
	Microbial dysbiosis	Alters immune response and promotes pro-tumorigenic environment.	(Jiang et al. 2022)
Breast Cancer	Estrogen metabolites (16α-hydroxyestrone)	Gut bacteria modify estrogen metabolism, increasing cancer risk.	(Parida and Sharma 2019)
	SCFAs imbalance	Alter immune response and systemic inflammation.	(Chapadgaonkar et al. 2023)

continued on following page

Table 2. Continued

Cancer Type	Gut Microbiome Metabolites	Mechanism of Carcinogenesis	References
Prostate Cancer	TMAO	Enhances oxidative stress and inflammatory pathways.	(Zhou et al. 2024)
	Dysregulated SCFAs	Affects hormonal regulation and immune modulation.	**(Li et al. 2025)**
Lung Cancer	Microbial dysbiosis	Alters systemic immunity, affecting lung inflammation and carcinogenesis.	(Li et al. 2024)
	LPS	Induces chronic inflammation and promotes tumor microenvironment.	(Liu et al. 2021)

5. SPECIFIC CANCERS AND GUT MICROBIOTA ALTERATIONS

Development of cancer may occur due to several factors among which an imbalance or dysbiosis in the gut microbiome can contribute to the onset and development of cancer. Certain bacteria like *Helicobacter pylori*, *Salmonella typhi*, *Helicobacter hepaticus* and viruses like hepatitis C virus (HCV) and hepatitis B virus (HBV) etc. support the process of tumorigenesis and cancer progression by disrupting various signalling pathways involved in cell cycle regulation and carcinogenesis. A detailed discussion of gut microbiota alterations and its related cancers is presented below (Sędzikowska and Szablewski 2021). As illustrated in Figure 3, specific gut microbiota secrete virulence factors and metabolites that trigger pro-inflammatory responses and DNA damage, promoting tumorigenesis.

5.1. Cancers of Digestive System

5.1.1. Colorectal Cancer (CRC)

Colorectal cancer is the third most prevalent cancer in males and second most in females which accounts for 9.4% of worldwide cancer deaths in 2020 (Pandey et al. 2023). Gut microbiota plays a crucial role in development and metastasis of CRC; especially gram-positive bacteria like – *Escherichia*, *Enterococcus*, *Klebsiella* and *Shigella* are present in increased levels in the stool sample of CRC patients (Wong et al. 2017). The gut microbiome of these patients are enriched with many opportunistic bacteria and pathogens like *Fusobacterium nucleatum*, *Escherichia coli*, *Streptococcus bovis*, *Enterococcus faecalis* and *Bacteroides fragilis*, whereas butyrate-producing bacteria like *Clostrium*, *Faecalibacterium*, *Roseburia* and *Bi-*

fidobacterium are found in lower levels (Sędzikowska and Szablewski 2021).Certain microbial species produce metabolites, such as short chain fatty acids (SCFAs), which help maintain intestinal integrity and modulate immune responses, but a decrease in SCFA-producing bacteria is associated with an increased risk of colorectal cancer. Diets rich in animal fats and proteins produce high amount of carcinogenic metabolites like bile salts that increase the risk of developing CRC (Sędzikowska and Szablewski 2021).

5.1.2. Gastric Cancer (GC)

Gastric cancer constitute 5.6% of all cancers and 7.7% of cancer-associated death worldwide and is mostly associated with the infection of *Helicobacter pylori,* which is about 90% (Sędzikowska and Szablewski 2021). Gastric microbiome has an acidic environment due to acidity of gastric juices, which in turns help the colonization of *Helicobacter pylori* and results in chronic inflammation. In antral-predominant gastritis, bacteria enhance secretion of gastrin that increases gastric acid production and also increases the risk of ulcer, whereas in corps-predominant gastritis, H. pylori reduced gastric acid production and favours growth of other nitrosating species of bacteria like *E. coli*, *Lactobacillus*, *Nitrospirae*, *Clostridium, Veillonella, Haemophilus*, and *Staphylococcus, Streptococcus, Prevotella*, and *Neisseria*. These bacteria increase nitride and N-nitrosamine levels that lowers the risk of GC. Patients with *H. pylori*-negative gastritis have increased levels of *Firmicutes*, *Fusobacteria, Bacteroidetes*, *Actinobacteria*, *Streptococcus* sp. and *Haemophilus influenzae*; whereas *H. pylori*-positive patients have *Treponema* sp. with low bacterial richness.

5.1.3 Pancreatic Ductal Adenocarcinoma (PDAC)

Pancreatic Ductal Adenocarcinoma (PDAC) is the most lethal type of pancreatic cancer which high malignancy rate. *H. pylori* plays an important role in prognosis of pancreatic carcinoma, it produce different pathogenic compounds such as LPS, ammonia, inflammatory cytokines which damages pancreatic tissues (Sędzikowska and Szablewski 2021). In 90% of the cases, *H. pylori* causes mutation of K-Ras by activating NF-κB and activator protein-1 (AP-1) (as shown in Figure 1). It also enhances activation of activator of transcription 3 (STAT3) and signal transducer, which results in overexpression of anti-apoptotic and pro-proliferative proteins like MCL-1, Bcl-xL, cyclin D1 and c-myc which promotes cancer progression (Lesina et al. 2011). Oral bacteria like *P. gingivalis, Fusobacterium, Neisseria elongata*, and *Streptococcus mitis* and *Aggregatibacter actinomycetemcomitans* increases the risk of developing PDAC by secreting peptidyl-arginine deiminase (PAD) enzymes that cause point mutations in p53 and K-Ras oncogene, whereas *Fusobacteria* and

Leptotrichia reduces the risk of PDAC (Magliano and Logsdon 2013). High levels of *Pseudoxanthoma*, *Saccharopolyspora*, *Bacillus clausii* and *Streptomyces* are associated with long-term survival in PDAC patients. Presence of *Gammaproteobacteria* has found to inhibit therapeutic effects of certain anticancer drugs in PDAC patients (Lesina et al. 2011).

5.1.4 Hepatocellular Carcinoma (HCC)

Hepatocellular Carcinoma (HCC) is the most prevalent type of liver cancer which accounts for 75-90% and has been found to associated with gut microbiota alterations (Sędzikowska and Szablewski 2021). HCC has shown higher levels of *Bacteroides*, *Ruminococcus*, *Escherichia coli*, *Gemmiger*, *Alistipes*, *Prevotella* and *Phascolarctobacterium* (LPS-producing bacteria) and lower levels of *Bifidobacterium*, *Klebsiella*, *Verrucomicrobia* and *Haemophilus* (butyrate-producing bacteria) (L'Hermitte et al. 2019). These LPS-producing bacteria stimulate hepatic Kupffer cells to produce inflammatory cytokines like IL-6 and TNF-α (as mentioned in Table 1), that induces precancerous hepatocellular proliferation (Jiang et al. 2019). Hepatic cancer is also associated with the production of secondary bile acids from primary bile acids by bacterial metabolism which in turns promote progression of liver cancer (Jia 2019). *Helicobacter pylori* is also responsible for development of liver cancer, but more precisely *H. pylori, H. bilis, H. hepaticus*, and *H. ganmani* are associated with cholangiocarcinoma (Jiang et al. 2019).

5.1.5 Esophageal Cancer (EC)

Esophageal Cancer (EC) is the eighth most common cancer and sixth most common cause of cancer-associated death worldwide. Esophagus houses different bacteria from 97 species which belongs to the phylum - Bacteroides, Firmicutes, Actinobacteria, Fusobacteria, Proteobacteria and TM7, in healthy condition. Esophageal cancer is divided into two types- Esophageal Squamous Cell Carcinoma (ESCC) and Esophageal Adenocarcinoma (EAC).

EAC is associated with high levels of *Streptococcus mitis*, *Treponema denticola*, *S. anginosus, Limosilactobacillus fermentum* and *Neisseria*, and decreased level of *Granulicatella* and *Veillonela*. However, chronic infection of *H. pylori* is inversely related to the risk of EAC. ESCC is related to the presence of *Porphyromonas gingivalis* and lower levels of *Bulleidia, Lautropia, Catonella, Moryella, Corynebacterium, Cardiobacterium* and *Peptococcus* (Sędzikowska and Szablewski 2021).

5.1.6 Oral Squamous Cell Carcinoma (OSCC)

Oral Squamous Cell Carcinoma (OSCC) constitute 90% of oral cavity cancer and is fourteenth most prevalent cancer worldwide. A healthy oral cavity includes 12 gram-positive genera, 15 gram-negative genera, 85 fungal genera and protozoa like *Trichomonas tenax* and *Entamoeba gingivalis* (Deo and Deshmukh 2019). OSCC is associated with biosynthesis of peptides and LPS from bacteria with a higher levels of *Peptostreptococcus, Filifactor, Fusobacterium, Peptococcus, Parvimonas* and *Catonella.* OSCC tissues were found to be enriched in six families- *Fusobacteriaceae, Prevotellaceae, Flavobacteriaceae, Peptostreptococcaceae, Lachnospiraceae, Campylobacteriaceae*, and 13 genera which includes *Fusobacterium, Porphyromonas* (Deo and Deshmukh 2019). Most of these bacteria causes chronic inflammation by stimulating production of inflammatory cytokines and matrix metalloproteinases (MMP). Oral cavity cancer is also caused by N-nitrosamine and acetaldehyde producing bacteria like *Candida sp.* and *Neisseria sp* (Healy and Moran 2019). The role of gut microbiota in carcinogenesis of digestive system are discussed below in Table 3 and the mechanisms are illustrated in Figure 2.

Table 3. List of microbes responsible for different types of cancers of digestive system and their mechanism of carcinogenesis.

Name of Cancer	Microbe Involved	Mechanism of Carcinogenesis	References
Colorectal Cancer	*Fusobacterium nucleatum*	Produce FadA, Fap2 that modulates E-cadherins/β-catenin pathway and blocks anti-tumor immune response	(Kostic et al. 2012; Wong et al. 2017; Pandey et al. 2023)
	E. coli	Produce B. fragilis toxin (BFT) that activates-catenin and STAT3 pathway, thereby increases expression of COX-2 and NF-kB	
	Enterotoxigenic Bacteroides fragilis	Produce colibactin, cyclolethal distending toxins (CDTs) that causes DNA double-stranded breaks	
	Enterococcus faecalis	Produce metalloprotease that damages DNA by producing reactive oxygen species (ROS) and extracellular superoxide	
	Streptococcus bovis/ gallolyticus	Produce Pil3 pilus which upregulates-catenin and promotes inflammation and cell proliferation	
	Helicobacter pylori	Produces CagA and VacA which activates-catenin/MAPK signalling pathway (as shown in Figure 1)	
	Peptostreptococcus anaerobius	Produce putative cell wall-binding repeat 2 (PCWBR2) protein that interacts with TLR-2 and TLR-4 on colon cells to induce ROS formation	
Gastric Cancer	*Helicobacter pylori*	Produces gastrin that causes chronic infection leads to inflammation, oxidative stress and DNA damage, thus promoting gastric carcinogenesis	(Schulz et al. 2019; Sędzikowska and Szablewski 2021; Fakharian et al. 2022)
	Escherichia coli	Produces colibactin, a genotoxin which causes DNA damage and promotes carcinogenesis	
	Streptococcus gastricus	Produces hydrogen peroxide that leads to oxidative stress and DNA damage	
	Bacteroides fragilis	Produces enterotoxin which leads to inflammation and promoting carcinogenesis	
	Fusobacterium nucleatum	Adheres to gastric epithelial cells, inducing inflammation and promoting carcinogenesis	

continued on following page

Table 3. Continued

Name of Cancer	Microbe Involved	Mechanism of Carcinogenesis	References
Pancreatic Ductal Adenocarcinoma	*Helicobacter pylori*	Causes mutation of K-Ras by activating NF-κB and activator protein-1 (AP-1) and also enhances activation of activator of transcription 3 (STAT3) and signal transducer	(Lesina et al. 2011; Magliano and Logsdon 2013; Thomas et al. 2018)
	Porphyromonas gingivalis	Produces gingipains that activate protease-activated receptors (PARs) and promote tumor growth, invasion, and metastasis (as shown in Figure 1)	
	Fusobacterium nucleatum	Promotes tumor progression through immune suppression, angiogenesis, and activation of pro-inflammatory signalling pathways	
	Neisseria elongata	Produces nitric oxide that promotes DNA damage	
Hepatocellular Carcinoma	*Prevotella intermedia*	Produces pro-inflammatory cytokines that causes chronic inflammation and promotes carcinogenesis.	(Jiang et al. 2019; Jia 2019; Sędzikowska and Szablewski 2021)
	Ruminococcus	Produces secondary bile acids that causes inflammation, oxidative stress and DNA damage	
	Gemmiger	Produces LPS that induces production of TNF-α and IL-6, promoting carcinogenesis	
Esophageal Cancer	*Treponema denticola*	Incudes production of pro-inflammatory cytokines like IL-1β and TNF-α	(May and Abrams 2018; Corning et al. 2018)
	Limosilactobacillus fermentum	Activate NF-kB signalling pathway by producing IL-6 & IL-8 and also produces reactive oxygen species (ROS)	
	Streptococcus mitis	Produces hydrogen peroxide that causes DNA damage	
Oral Squamous Cell Carcinoma	*Peptostreptococcus anaerobius*	Produces butyrate, which can induce DNA damage and promote carcinogenesis in high	(Deo and Deshmukh 2019; Al-Hebshi et al. 2019)
	Tannerella forsythia	Produces virulence factors, such as gingipains, which promote tumor growth, invasion, and metastasis.	
	Filifactor alocis	Produces LPS and activate NF-kB signalling pathway, thereby damaging oral cells	

Figure 2. Mechanism of carcinogenesis of different gut microbiota in causing different types of cancer and their related effects on Peyer's Patch (Figure created in Biorender.com)

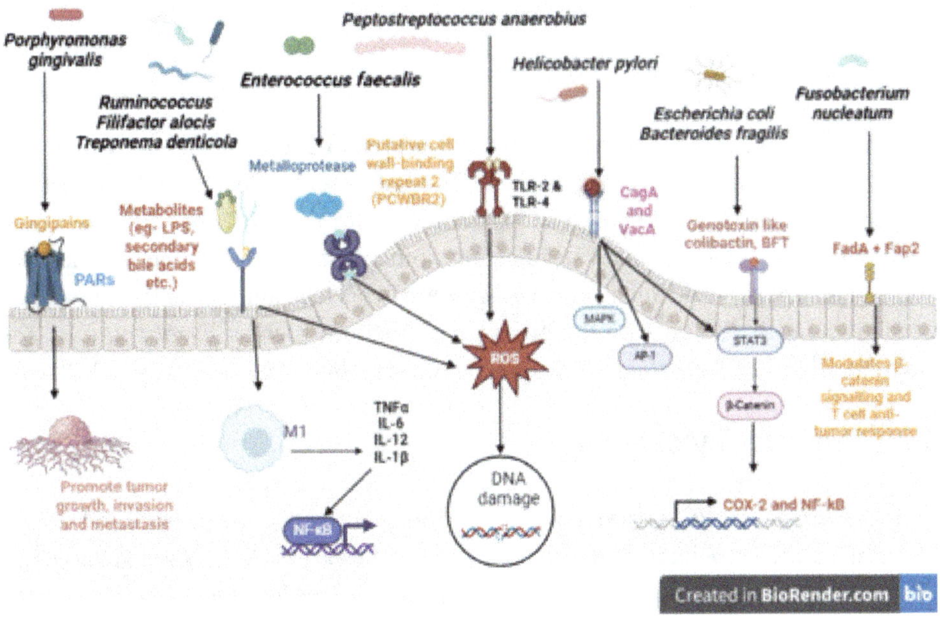

5.2. Cancers of Urogenital Tract

5.2.1 Bladder Cancer

Bladder cancer is the most common urinary system malignancy in men, which is associated with high levels of Actinomyces, A. europaeus and pro-tumorigenic pathogen, Fusobacterium. It results in lower levels of *Streptococcus*, *Veillonella* and *Corynebacterium.* Certain bacteria like *Lacticaseibacillus casei* present in bladder microbiota can prevent the occurrence of bladder cancer (Bi et al. 2019).

5.2.2 Ovarian Cancer (OC)

Ovarian Cancer (OC) is the second most common cancer of female reproductive system which accounts for 4.7% of cancer-associated death worldwide. Human microbiota has a crucial role in altering estrogen metabolism that might suppress or promote OC, among them *Mycoplasma genitalium* and *Chlamydia trachomatis* are of utmost importance (Baker et al. 2017). Other disease causing pathogens found in advanced stages of OC are – *Rikenellaceae* (estrogen responsive), *Akkermansia muciniphila* (anti-inflammatory properties), *Alphaproteobacteria* (vascular permeability), *Bacillus, Salmonella, Chryseobacterium, Prevotella* etc (Sędzikowska and Szablewski 2021).

5.2.3 Cervical Cancer (CC)

Cervical Cancer (CC) is the fourth most prevalent cancer in female which accounts for 6.5% of all cancer worldwide. The risk of CC is increased by infection of Human Papillomavirus (HPV) and an increased level of *Lactobacillus iners* and *Lactobacillus gasseri* is found in infected women (Sędzikowska and Szablewski 2021). HPV-positive women has high grade of cervical intraepithelial neoplasia which is also associated with the presence of bacteria such as *Fusobacterium sp, Lactobacillus iners, Sneathia, G. vaginalis* and *Atopobium vaginae* (Seo et al. 2016).

5.2.4 Prostate Cancer (PC)

Prostate Cancer (PC) is the most common cancer in men and is the second leading cause of cancer-associated death in men. Among the various factors responsible for PC, an elevated level of pro-inflammatory bacteria like *Streptococcus* and *Bacteroides*, responsible for carbohydrate metabolism are present in rectal microbiome. Patients with benign prostatic hyperplasia have lower levels of *Defluviicoccus* and *Eubacterium*, responsible for metabolism of riboflavin, biotin and folate (Yu et al. 2015).

5.3. Gut Microbiota and Lung Cancer

Lung Cancer (LC) is the leading cause of death worldwide, contributing 23.1% of all cancer deaths. Studies showed that gut microbiota can influence LC development through gut-lung axis that connects the gut and lung (Sędzikowska and Szablewski 2021). A significant shift in gut microbiota composition I observed in lung cancer patients across different stages and types - a higher level of *Klebsiella, Comamonas, Acidovorax* and *Polaromonas* are observed in small cell lung cancer (SCLC) (Greathouse et al. 2018). LC patient has lower counts of *Acinetobacter, Bifidobacterium* and *Acidovorax*, whereas fecal sample of LC patients has higher counts of *Proteobacteria* and *Verrucomicrobia* (Liu et al. 2019). Gut microbiota composition changes with LC metastasis – in adenocarcinoma patient without distant metastasis, has higher levels of genus *Streptococcus* and phylum Firmicutes; whereas SCLC patients with distant metastasis have higher counts of *Veillonella* and *Rothia* species. Thus composition of gut microbiota alters with LC progression and it also influences the effectiveness of therapy.

5.4. Gut Microbiota and Breast Cancer

Breast Cancer (BC) is the most common cancer in women which contribute 25% of all cancers in women and is the second most common cause of death worldwide. Studies showed a significant alteration in the gut microbiota of BC patients compared to healthy individuals. It is found that higher levels of *Staphylococcus*, *Bacillus*, *Comamonadaceae* are observed in BC patients; in fact the urinary tract microbiota differs in BC women than those without BC (Sampsell et al. 2020). There is a significant alteration in the gut microbiota with BC therapy. Chemotherapy often decreases the abundance of *Actinobacteria* and increases *Verrucomicrobia*; radiotherapy often increases levels of *Roseburia*, *Clostridium*, whereas hormonal therapies often alters the composition of estrogen responsive microbiome (Nandi et al. 2023).

6. STRATEGIES FOR CANCER PREVENTION BY MICROBIOME ALTERATION

Contrary to their role in mediating carcinogenesis, human microbiome has also been found to be involved in mediating the effects and outcomes of the host immune response to anticancer therapeutics. Microbiota modulates therapeutic efficacy of chemotherapy and immunotherapy (Kalmar et al. 2022). While some gut bacteria are required for chemotherapy to exert their therapeutic effect, others may induce chemoresistance. The mechanistic framework through which microbiota influences efficacy and toxicity of chemotherapy is collectively called 'TIMER, which is an acronym for translocation, immunomodulation, metabolism, enzymatic degradation, and reduced toxicity. Simplistically, when the intestinal barrier is damaged by chemotherapeutics, gastrointestinal bacteria translocate to various lymphoid organs modulating local and systemic immunity and boosting the activity of chemotherapeutics (Inamura 2021).

Promoting diets rich in fiber and marine omega-3 fatty acids can enhance beneficial microbial populations that produce short-chain fatty acids like butyrate, which have tumor-suppressive effects, support immune homeostasis, and lower intestinal pH to sustain the growth of beneficial microbes like *Bifidobacterium* and *Lactobacillus*. Aditionally, microbial species singly or in combination have been administered as probiotics to alter treatment outcomes in various gastrointestinal cancers. Utilization of probiotics, prebiotics, and synbiotics (a mix of prebiotics and probiotics) can help restore or maintain a favorable microbial balance to potentially reduce cancer risk.

For example, butyrate-producing bacteria or fiber supplementation has been linked to decreased colorectal tumorigenesis in animal models. Strategies such as fecal microbiota transplantation (FMT), administration of defined bacterial consortia, and bacterial isolates aim to modulate the gut microbiome to improve cancer prevention and treatment outcomes, including enhancing responses to immunotherapy. Circumventing the demerits associated with the use of antibiotics, bacteriophages are also being currently investigated for cancer treatment via alterations in the microbiome. Given interpersonal differences in microbiome composition and carcinogen metabolism, integrating microbiome profiling with genetic and environmental data may enable personalized prevention tailored to individual risk profiles. Together, these multidisciplinary strategies leverage the integral role of SCFAs in linking diet, microbiota, and host responses to effectively reduce colorectal cancer risk (Mowat et al. 2023b). Other strategies for cancer treatment by altering the microbiome include creation of genetically modified oncolytic bacteria capable of traveling and surviving in hypoxic tumor tissues and evoking immune response through TLR4 signaling (Zheng et al. 2017). Investigations pertaining to implementation of nanotechnology for cancer prevention via targeting of the microbiome are also underway. For instance, an engineered nanocarrier encapsulating antibiotic and presenting features of a gastric membrane lining have been deployed against *H. pylori* to tame gastric cancer (Angsantikul et al. 2018).

Metagenomics plays a crucial role in tracking antimicrobial resistance genes (ARGs) within microbial communities, which is vital for managing infection risks, especially in vulnerable populations like cancer patients. Metagenomic sequencing offers a culture-independent method that allows the direct analysis of microbial DNA from complex samples, circumventing the limitations of traditional culturing techniques, which misses out non-culturable bacteria. Advanced metagenomic workflows, such as HAM-ART, integrate Hi-C chromosome conformation capture with shotgun sequencing to link ARGs residing on mobile elements like plasmids with their bacterial hosts. This approach improves the resolution at which resistance genes can be attributed to specific bacteria in microbial communities (Kalmar et al. 2022). Metagenomics identifies both known and novel ARGs and elucidates resistance mechanisms, including enzymatic antibiotic degradation, target modification, efflux pump activation, and decreased permeability. These insights derived from sequence-based and functional metagenomic analyses, supported by bioinformatics tools and curated ARG databases such as ResFinder, CARD, MEGARes, and Resfams, which enable comprehensive annotation and interpretation of resistome data (de Abreu et al. 2021). Metagenomic next-generation sequencing (mNGS) facilitates rapid and precise identification of pathogens and resistance determinants in cancer patients, enabling stewardship programs to optimize antimicrobial use (Yan et al. 2024). Implementation of mNGS-guided protocols has been associated with lower antibiotic escalation rates and improved management of antiviral therapies in infections. Diagnostic stewardship partnerships between clinical microbiology and antimicrobial stewardship programs enhance test utilization, reducing unnecessary interventions, and tailoring antimicrobial prescriptions to patient-specific resistome profiles (Kalmar et al. 2022; Majeed and Rust 2025).

Understanding shifts in composition of microbiome through ML frameworks like MOFA+ (Multi-Omics Factor Analysis) or graph neural networks (GNNs) help reveal latent patterns and exposure-related pathways across omics layers towards the identification of individuals at risk (Kamel et al. 2024). Emerging studies are also examining the relationship between gut microbiota, the brain, and cancer. Understanding this axis may help in developing strategies that address psychological well-being in cancer patients alongside treatment (Lin et al. 2023).

7. CONCLUSION AND FUTURE DIRECTIONS

The gut microbiota significantly influences immunity and is implicated in various cancers through several mechanisms. Imbalances in the gut microbiota, or dysbiosis can modulate immune responses, alter metabolic pathways, and contribute to carcinogenesis. Specific bacterial species and their metabolites play critical roles in either promoting or inhibiting cancer development in different parts of the body. A diet high in meats and processed foods, and low in fresh vegetables, can harm gut flora and increase the risk of gastrointestinal cancers like colorectal cancer. New research suggests that imbalances in gut bacteria may play a significant role in the increasing rates of colorectal cancer in young adults. Dietary factors, antibiotics, and environmental pollutants are key modulators of gut microbiota composition, thereby influencing cancer risk. Dietary fiber, found in plant-based foods, promotes the growth of beneficial bacteria and the production of short-chain fatty acids, which have anti-inflammatory and immune-modulating effects. Conversely, diets high in animal fats and proteins can produce carcinogenic metabolites that increase cancer risk. Antibiotics can disrupt the natural microbiota, leading to dysbiosis and increasing the risk of pathogen colonization and various diseases, including cancer. Environmental factors, including exposure to pollutants and lifestyle choices, can also significantly alter the gut microbiota and influence cancer development. Exposure to environmental chemicals and pollutants can impact gut microbial communities, affecting xenobiotic metabolism and overall health. Lifestyle behaviors, such as diet, alcohol consumption, and physical activity, also play critical roles in modulating the gut microbiota and influencing cancer risk. Knowledge on the human microbiome and mechanisms of microbiome alteration-induced carcinogenesis would help to devise strategies for effective cancer treatment. These strategies may include targeted antibiotic therapy, administration of probiotics/ prebiotics, fecal microbiota transplantation, or for that matter simple dietary modifications. The mechanistic insights and causality intersection of environmental exposures, the microbiome, and cancer risk presents an array of challenges and opportunities for future research. However, most research has predominantly focused on bacterial components of the microbiome, leaving gaps in our understanding of other critical players like the mycobiome (fungi), virome, and archaea. Many current studies are limited by geographic and demographic homogeneity, which may obscure variations in microbiome responses to environmental exposures. Future research should involve diverse populations across different regions and socioeconomic backgrounds. Such studies will be essential for understanding global disparities in cancer risk, as well as for designing universally applicable public health strategies.

REFERENCES

Abdalkareem Jasim, S., Jade Catalan Opulencia, M., Alexis Ramírez-Coronel, A., Kamal Abdelbasset, W., Hasan Abed, M., Markov, A., Raheem Lateef Al-Awsi, G., Azamatovich Shamsiev, J., Thaeer Hammid, A., Nader Shalaby, M., Karampoor, S., & Mirzaei, R. (2022). The emerging role of microbiota-derived short-chain fatty acids in immunometabolism. *International Immunopharmacology, 110*, 108983. DOI: 10.1016/j.intimp.2022.108983 PMID: 35750016

Ajayi, R. O., & Ogunjobi, T. T. (2024). *Environmental Exposures and Cancer Risk: A Comprehensive Review*. Medinformatics. DOI: 10.47852/bonviewMEDIN42023598

Akhavan, B. J., Khanna, N. R., & Vijhani, P. (2025). Amoxicillin. In *StatPearls*. StatPearls Publishing.

Al-Hebshi, N. N., Borgnakke, W. S., & Johnson, N. W. (2019). The Microbiome of Oral Squamous Cell Carcinomas: A Functional Perspective. *Current Oral Health Reports*, *6*(2), 145–160. DOI: 10.1007/s40496-019-0215-5

Allen, J., & Sears, C. L. (2019). Impact of the gut microbiome on the genome and epigenome of colon epithelial cells: Contributions to colorectal cancer development. *Genome Medicine*, *11*(1), 11. DOI: 10.1186/s13073-019-0621-2 PMID: 30803449

Andreeva, N., Gabbasova, R., & Grivennikov, S. I. (2020). Microbiome in cancer progression and therapy. *Current Opinion in Microbiology*, *56*, 118–126. DOI: 10.1016/j.mib.2020.09.001 PMID: 33147555

Angsantikul, P., Thamphiwatana, S., Zhang, Q., Spiekermann, K., Zhuang, J., Fang, R. H., Gao, W., Obonyo, M., & Zhang, L. (2018). Coating nanoparticles with gastric epithelial cell membrane for targeted antibiotic delivery against Helicobacter pylori infection. *Advanced Therapeutics*, *1*(2), 1800016. DOI: 10.1002/adtp.201800016 PMID: 30320205

Baker, J. M., Al-Nakkash, L., & Herbst-Kralovetz, M. M. (2017). Estrogen–gut microbiome axis: Physiological and clinical implications. *Maturitas*, *103*, 45–53. DOI: 10.1016/j.maturitas.2017.06.025 PMID: 28778332

Bi, H., Tian, Y., Song, C., Li, J., Liu, T., Chen, Z., Chen, C., Huang, Y., & Zhang, Y. (2019). Urinary microbiota – a potential biomarker and therapeutic target for bladder cancer. *Journal of Medical Microbiology*, *68*(10), 1471–1478. DOI: 10.1099/jmm.0.001058 PMID: 31418671

Bosco, N., & Noti, M. (2021). The aging gut microbiome and its impact on host immunity. *Genes and Immunity*, *22*(5-6), 289–303. DOI: 10.1038/s41435-021-00126-8 PMID: 33875817

Bray, F., Laversanne, M., Sung, H., Ferlay, J., Siegel, R. L., Soerjomataram, I., & Jemal, A. (2024). Global cancer statistics 2022: GLOBOCAN estimates of incidence and mortality worldwide for 36 cancers in 185 countries. *CA: a Cancer Journal for Clinicians*, *74*(3), 229–263. DOI: 10.3322/caac.21834 PMID: 38572751

Bui, T., Patel, P., & Preuss, C. V. (2025). Cephalosporins. In *StatPearls*. StatPearls Publishing.

Burk, R. F. (2002). Selenium, an antioxidant nutrient. *Nutrition in Clinical Care*, *5*(2), 75–79. DOI: 10.1046/j.1523-5408.2002.00006.x PMID: 12134713

Chapadgaonkar, S. S., Bajpai, S. S., & Godbole, M. S. (2023). Gut microbiome influences incidence and outcomes of breast cancer by regulating levels and activity of steroid hormones in women. *Cancer Reports*, *6*(11), e1847. DOI: 10.1002/cnr2.1847 PMID: 37311575

Charmsaz, S., Collins, D. M., Perry, A. S., & Prencipe, M. (2019). Novel Strategies for Cancer Treatment: Highlights from the 55th IACR Annual Conference. *Cancers (Basel)*, *11*(8), 1125. DOI: 10.3390/cancers11081125 PMID: 31394729

Chee, W. J. Y., Chew, S. Y., & Than, L. T. L. (2020). Vaginal microbiota and the potential of Lactobacillus derivatives in maintaining vaginal health. *Microbial Cell Factories*, *19*(1), 203. DOI: 10.1186/s12934-020-01464-4 PMID: 33160356

Chen, L., Zhu, Y., Hou, X., Yang, L., & Chu, H. (2022). The Role of Gut Bacteria and Fungi in Alcohol-Associated Liver Disease. *Frontiers in Medicine*, *9*, 840752. DOI: 10.3389/fmed.2022.840752 PMID: 35308525

Corning, B., Copland, A. P., & Frye, J. W. (2018). The Esophageal Microbiome in Health and Disease. *Current Gastroenterology Reports*, *20*(8), 39. DOI: 10.1007/s11894-018-0642-9 PMID: 30069679

Crost, E. H., Coletto, E., Bell, A., & Juge, N. (2023). Ruminococcus gnavus: Friend or foe for human health. *FEMS Microbiology Reviews*, *47*(2), fuad014. Advance online publication. DOI: 10.1093/femsre/fuad014 PMID: 37015876

Dahiya, D., & Nigam, P. S. (2023). Antibiotic-Therapy-Induced Gut Dysbiosis Affecting Gut Microbiota-Brain Axis and Cognition: Restoration by Intake of Probiotics and Synbiotics. *International Journal of Molecular Sciences*, *24*(4), 3074. DOI: 10.3390/ijms24043074 PMID: 36834485 de Abreu, V. A. C., Perdigão, J., & Almeida, S. (2021). Metagenomic Approaches to Analyze Antimicrobial Resistance: An Overview. *Frontiers in Genetics, 11*, 575592. DOI: 10.3389/fgene.2020.575592 PMID: 33537056

den Besten, G., van Eunen, K., Groen, A. K., Venema, K., Reijngoud, D.-J., & Bakker, B. M. (2013). The role of short-chain fatty acids in the interplay between diet, gut microbiota, and host energy metabolism. *Journal of Lipid Research, 54*(9), 2325–2340. DOI: 10.1194/jlr.R036012 PMID: 23821742

Deo, P. N., & Deshmukh, R. (2019). Oral microbiome: Unveiling the fundamentals. *Journal of Oral and Maxillofacial Pathology : JOMFP, 23*(1), 122–128. DOI: 10.4103/jomfp.JOMFP_304_18 PMID: 31110428

di Magliano, M. P., & Logsdon, C. D. (2013). Roles for KRAS in Pancreatic Tumor Development and Progression. *Gastroenterology, 144*(6), 1220–1229. DOI: 10.1053/j.gastro.2013.01.071 PMID: 23622131

Diallo, A., Deschasaux, M., Latino-Martel, P., Hercberg, S., Galan, P., Fassier, P., Allès, B., Guéraud, F., Pierre, F. H., & Touvier, M. (2018). Red and processed meat intake and cancer risk: Results from the prospective NutriNet-Santé cohort study. *International Journal of Cancer, 142*(2), 230–237. DOI: 10.1002/ijc.31046 PMID: 28913916

Duarte-Mata, D. I., & Salinas-Carmona, M. C. (2023). Antimicrobial peptides´ immune modulation role in intracellular bacterial infection. *Frontiers in Immunology, 14*, 1119574. Advance online publication. DOI: 10.3389/fimmu.2023.1119574 PMID: 37056758

Duvallet, C., Gibbons, S. M., Gurry, T., Irizarry, R. A., & Alm, E. J. (2017). Meta-analysis of gut microbiome studies identifies disease-specific and shared responses. *Nature Communications, 8*(1), 1784. DOI: 10.1038/s41467-017-01973-8 PMID: 29209090

Fakharian, F., Asgari, B., Nabavi-Rad, A., Sadeghi, A., Soleimani, N., Yadegar, A., & Zali, M. R. (2022). The interplay between Helicobacter pylori and the gut microbiota: An emerging driver influencing the immune system homeostasis and gastric carcinogenesis. *Frontiers in Cellular and Infection Microbiology, 12*, 953718. DOI: 10.3389/fcimb.2022.953718 PMID: 36046747

Feitelson, M. A., Arzumanyan, A., Medhat, A., & Spector, I. (2023). Short-chain fatty acids in cancer pathogenesis. *Cancer and Metastasis Reviews, 42*(3), 677–698. DOI: 10.1007/s10555-023-10117-y PMID: 37432606

Fenech, M., Amaya, I., Valpuesta, V., & Botella, M. A. (2018). Vitamin C Content in Fruits: Biosynthesis and Regulation. *Frontiers in Plant Science*, *9*, 2006. DOI: 10.3389/fpls.2018.02006 PMID: 30733729

Fu, Y., Moscoso, D. I., Porter, J., Krishnareddy, S., Abrams, J. A., Seres, D., Chong, D. H., & Freedberg, D. E. (2020). Relationship Between Dietary Fiber Intake and Short-Chain Fatty Acid-Producing Bacteria During Critical Illness: A Prospective Cohort Study. *JPEN. Journal of Parenteral and Enteral Nutrition*, *44*(3), 463–471. DOI: 10.1002/jpen.1682 PMID: 31385326

Gebrayel, P., Nicco, C., Al Khodor, S., Bilinski, J., Caselli, E., Comelli, E. M., Egert, M., Giaroni, C., Karpinski, T. M., Loniewski, I., Mulak, A., Reygner, J., Samczuk, P., Serino, M., Sikora, M., Terranegra, A., Ufnal, M., Villeger, R., Pichon, C., & Edeas, M. (2022). Microbiota medicine: Towards clinical revolution. *Journal of Translational Medicine*, *20*(1), 111. DOI: 10.1186/s12967-022-03296-9 PMID: 35255932

Gill, P. A., Inniss, S., Kumagai, T., Rahman, F. Z., & Smith, A. M. (2022). The Role of Diet and Gut Microbiota in Regulating Gastrointestinal and Inflammatory Disease. *Frontiers in Immunology*, *13*, 866059. DOI: 10.3389/fimmu.2022.866059 PMID: 35450067

Greathouse, K. L., White, J. R., Vargas, A. J., Bliskovsky, V. V., Beck, J. A., von Muhlinen, N., Polley, E. C., Bowman, E. D., Khan, M. A., Robles, A. I., Cooks, T., Ryan, B. M., Padgett, N., Dzutsev, A. H., Trinchieri, G., Pineda, M. A., Bilke, S., Meltzer, P. S., Hokenstad, A. N., & Harris, C. C. (2018). Interaction between the microbiome and TP53 in human lung cancer. *Genome Biology*, *19*(1), 123. DOI: 10.1186/s13059-018-1501-6 PMID: 30143034

Hasan, N., & Yang, H. (2019). Factors affecting the composition of the gut microbiota, and its modulation. *PeerJ*, *7*, e7502. DOI: 10.7717/peerj.7502 PMID: 31440436

Healy, C. M., & Moran, G. P. (2019). The microbiome and oral cancer: More questions than answers. *Oral Oncology*, *89*, 30–33. DOI: 10.1016/j.oraloncology.2018.12.003 PMID: 30732955

Hickman, B., Salonen, A., Ponsero, A. J., Jokela, R., Kolho, K.-L., de Vos, W. M., & Korpela, K. (2024). Gut microbiota wellbeing index predicts overall health in a cohort of 1000 infants. *Nature Communications*, *15*(1), 8323. DOI: 10.1038/s41467-024-52561-6 PMID: 39333099

Hjorth, M. F., Blædel, T., Bendtsen, L. Q., Lorenzen, J. K., Holm, J. B., Kiilerich, P., Roager, H. M., Kristiansen, K., Larsen, L. H., & Astrup, A. (2019). Prevotella-to-Bacteroides ratio predicts body weight and fat loss success on 24-week diets varying in macronutrient composition and dietary fiber: Results from a post-hoc analysis. *International Journal of Obesity*, *43*(1), 149–157. DOI: 10.1038/s41366-018-0093-2 PMID: 29777234

Hsiao, Y.-C., Liu, C.-W., Chi, L., Yang, Y., & Lu, K. (2020). The Effects of Gut Microbiome on Carcinogenic DNA Damage. *Chemical Research in Toxicology*, *33*(8), 2130–2138. DOI: 10.1021/acs.chemrestox.0c00142 PMID: 32677427

Inamura, K. (2021). Gut microbiota contributes towards immunomodulation against cancer: New frontiers in precision cancer therapeutics. *Seminars in Cancer Biology*, *70*, 11–23. DOI: 10.1016/j.semcancer.2020.06.006 PMID: 32580023

Jakobsson, T., & Forsum, U. (2007). Lactobacillus iners: A marker of changes in the vaginal flora? *Journal of Clinical Microbiology*, *45*(9), 3145. DOI: 10.1128/JCM.00558-07 PMID: 17652481

Jia, B. (2019). Commentary: Gut microbiome–mediated bile acid metabolism regulates liver cancer via NKT cells. *Frontiers in Immunology*, *10*, 282. Advance online publication. DOI: 10.3389/fimmu.2019.00282 PMID: 30842777

Jiang, J.-W., Chen, X.-H., Ren, Z., & Zheng, S.-S. (2019). Gut microbial dysbiosis associates hepatocellular carcinoma via the gut-liver axis. *Hepatobiliary & Pancreatic Diseases International*, *18*(1), 19–27. DOI: 10.1016/j.hbpd.2018.11.002 PMID: 30527903

Jiang, Z., Wang, H., Mou, Y., Li, L., & Jin, W. (2022). Functions and clinical applications of exosomes in pancreatic cancer. *Molecular Biology Reports*, *49*(11), 11037–11048. DOI: 10.1007/s11033-022-07765-8 PMID: 36097109

Jin, W.-B., Xiao, L., Jeong, M., Han, S.-J., Zhang, W., Yano, H., Shi, H., Arifuzzaman, M., Lyu, M., Wang, D., Tang, Y. A., Qiao, S., Yang, X., Yang, H. S., Fu, J., Sonnenberg, G. F., Collins, N., Artis, D., & Guo, C.-J. (2025). Microbiota-derived bile acids antagonize the host androgen receptor and drive anti-tumor immunity. *Cell*, *188*(9), 2336–2353.e38. DOI: 10.1016/j.cell.2025.02.029 PMID: 40239649

Kalmar, L., Gupta, S., Kean, I. R. L., Ba, X., Hadjirin, N., Lay, E. M., de Vries, S. P. W., Bateman, M., Bartlet, H., Hernandez-Garcia, J., Tucker, A. W., Restif, O., Stevens, M. P., Wood, J. L. N., Maskell, D. J., Grant, A. J., & Holmes, M. A. (2022). HAM-ART: An optimised culture-free Hi-C metagenomics pipeline for tracking antimicrobial resistance genes in complex microbial communities. *PLOS Genetics*, *18*(3), e1009776. DOI: 10.1371/journal.pgen.1009776 PMID: 35286304

Kalyanaraman, B., Cheng, G., & Hardy, M. (2024). The role of short-chain fatty acids in cancer prevention and cancer treatment. *Archives of Biochemistry and Biophysics, 761*, 110172. DOI: 10.1016/j.abb.2024.110172 PMID: 39369836

Kamel, M., Aleya, S., Alsubih, M., & Aleya, L. (2024). Microbiome Dynamics: A Paradigm Shift in Combatting Infectious Diseases. *Journal of Personalized Medicine, 14*(2), 217. DOI: 10.3390/jpm14020217 PMID: 38392650

Kanoh, S., & Rubin, B. K. (2010). Mechanisms of action and clinical application of macrolides as immunomodulatory medications. *Clinical Microbiology Reviews, 23*(3), 590–615. DOI: 10.1128/CMR.00078-09 PMID: 20610825

Khelaifia, S., Caputo, A., Djossou, F., & Raoult, D. (2016). Draft genome sequence of a human-associated isolate of Haloferax alexandrinus strain Arc-hr, an extremely halophilic archaea. *New Microbes and New Infections, 15*, 44–45. DOI: 10.1016/j.nmni.2016.11.012 PMID: 28018603

Kostic, A. D., Gevers, D., Pedamallu, C. S., Michaud, M., Duke, F., Earl, A. M., Ojesina, A. I., Jung, J., Bass, A. J., Tabernero, J., Baselga, J., Liu, C., Shivdasani, R. A., Ogino, S., Birren, B. W., Huttenhower, C., Garrett, W. S., & Meyerson, M. (2012). Genomic analysis identifies association of Fusobacterium with colorectal carcinoma. *Genome Research, 22*(2), 292–298. DOI: 10.1101/gr.126573.111 PMID: 22009990

L'Hermitte, A., Pham, S., Cadoux, M., Couchy, G., Caruso, S., Anson, M., Crain-Denoyelle, A.-M., Celton-Morizur, S., Yamagoe, S., Zucman-Rossi, J., Desdouets, C., & Couty, J.-P. (2019). Lect2 Controls Inflammatory Monocytes to Constrain the Growth and Progression of Hepatocellular Carcinoma. *Hepatology (Baltimore, Md.), 69*(1), 160–178. DOI: 10.1002/hep.30140 PMID: 30070727

Lattimer, J. M., & Haub, M. D. (2010). Effects of dietary fiber and its components on metabolic health. *Nutrients, 2*(12), 1266–1289. DOI: 10.3390/nu2121266 PMID: 22254008

Lesina, M., Kurkowski, M. U., Ludes, K., Rose-John, S., Treiber, M., Klöppel, G., Yoshimura, A., Reindl, W., Sipos, B., Akira, S., Schmid, R. M., & Algül, H. (2011). Stat3/Socs3 Activation by IL-6 Transsignaling Promotes Progression of Pancreatic Intraepithelial Neoplasia and Development of Pancreatic Cancer. *Cancer Cell, 19*(4), 456–469. DOI: 10.1016/j.ccr.2011.03.009 PMID: 21481788

Li, B., Wang, D., Zhang, C., Wang, Y., Huang, Z., Yang, L., Yang, H., Liang, N., Li, S., & Liu, Z. (2024). Role of respiratory system microbiota in development of lung cancer and clinical application. *iMeta, 3*(5), e232. DOI: 10.1002/imt2.232 PMID: 39429871

Li, M., Wang, M., & Donovan, S. M. (2014). Early development of the gut microbiome and immune-mediated childhood disorders. *Seminars in Reproductive Medicine*, *32*(1), 74–86. DOI: 10.1055/s-0033-1361825 PMID: 24390924

Li, S., Duan, Y., Luo, S., Zhou, F., Wu, Q., & Lu, Z. (2025). Short-chain fatty acids and cancer. *Trends in Cancer*, *11*(2), 154–168. DOI: 10.1016/j.trecan.2024.11.003 PMID: 39638744

Lin, B., Ye, Z., Ye, Z., Wang, M., Cao, Z., Gao, R., & Zhang, Y. (2023). Gut microbiota in brain tumors: An emerging crucial player. *CNS Neuroscience & Therapeutics*, *29*(S1, Suppl 1), 84–97. DOI: 10.1111/cns.14081 PMID: 36627748

Liu, C.-H., Chen, Z., Chen, K., Liao, F.-T., Chung, C.-E., Liu, X., Lin, Y.-C., Keohavong, P., Leikauf, G. D., & Di, Y. P. (2021). Lipopolysaccharide-Mediated Chronic Inflammation Promotes Tobacco Carcinogen-Induced Lung Cancer and Determines the Efficacy of Immunotherapy. *Cancer Research*, *81*(1), 144–157. DOI: 10.1158/0008-5472.CAN-20-1994 PMID: 33122306

Liu, F., Li, J., Guan, Y., Lou, Y., Chen, H., Xu, M., Deng, D., Chen, J., Ni, B., Zhao, L., Li, H., Sang, H., & Cai, X. (2019). Dysbiosis of the Gut Microbiome is associated with Tumor Biomarkers in Lung Cancer. *International Journal of Biological Sciences*, *15*(11), 2381–2392. DOI: 10.7150/ijbs.35980 PMID: 31595156

Liu, Y., Zhang, S., Zhou, W., Hu, D., Xu, H., & Ji, G. (2022). Secondary Bile Acids and Tumorigenesis in Colorectal Cancer. *Frontiers in Oncology*, *12*, 813745. DOI: 10.3389/fonc.2022.813745 PMID: 35574393

Lobo, V., Patil, A., Phatak, A., & Chandra, N. (2010). Free radicals, antioxidants and functional foods: Impact on human health. *Pharmacognosy Reviews*, *4*(8), 118–126. DOI: 10.4103/0973-7847.70902 PMID: 22228951

Ma, C., Han, M., Heinrich, B., Fu, Q., Zhang, Q., Sandhu, M., Agdashian, D., Terabe, M., Berzofsky, J. A., Fako, V., Ritz, T., Longerich, T., Theriot, C. M., McCulloch, J. A., Roy, S., Yuan, W., Thovarai, V., Sen, S. K., Ruchirawat, M., & Greten, T. F. (2018). Gut microbiome-mediated bile acid metabolism regulates liver cancer via NKT cells. *Science*, *360*(6391), eaan5931. Advance online publication. DOI: 10.1126/science.aan5931 PMID: 29798856

Majeed, A., & Rust, T. (2025). Antimicrobial Stewardship in Patients With Cancer: Interventions and Future Directions to Combat the Rise of Antimicrobial Resistance. *JCO Oncology Practice*, *0*, OP-25–OP-00124. DOI: 10.1200/OP-25-00124 PMID: 40080740

Marant Micallef, C., Shield, K. D., Baldi, I., Charbotel, B., Fervers, B., Gilg Soit Ilg, A., Guénel, P., Olsson, A., Rushton, L., Hutchings, S. J., Straif, K., & Soerjomataram, I. (2018). Occupational exposures and cancer: A review of agents and relative risk estimates. *Occupational and Environmental Medicine*, *75*(8), 604–614. DOI: 10.1136/oemed-2017-104858 PMID: 29735747

Matza Porges, S., & Shamriz, O. (2022). Genetics of Immune Dysregulation and Cancer Predisposition: Two Sides of the Same Coin. *Clinical and Experimental Immunology*, *210*(2), 114–127. DOI: 10.1093/cei/uxac089 PMID: 36165533

May, M., & Abrams, J. A. (2018). Emerging Insights into the Esophageal Microbiome. *Current Treatment Options in Gastroenterology*, *16*(1), 72–85. DOI: 10.1007/s11938-018-0171-5 PMID: 29350339

Molina-Montes, E., Ubago-Guisado, E., Petrova, D., Amiano, P., Chirlaque, M.-D., Agudo, A., & Sánchez, M.-J. (2021). The Role of Diet, Alcohol, BMI, and Physical Activity in Cancer Mortality: Summary Findings of the EPIC Study. *Nutrients*, *13*(12), 4293. DOI: 10.3390/nu13124293 PMID: 34959845

Mowat, C., Dhatt, J., Bhatti, I., Hamie, A., & Baker, K. (2023a). Short chain fatty acids prime colorectal cancer cells to activate antitumor immunity. *Frontiers in Immunology*, *14*, 1190810. DOI: 10.3389/fimmu.2023.1190810 PMID: 37304266

Mowat, C., Dhatt, J., Bhatti, I., Hamie, A., & Baker, K. (2023b). Short chain fatty acids prime colorectal cancer cells to activate antitumor immunity. *Frontiers in Immunology*, *14*, 1190810. DOI: 10.3389/fimmu.2023.1190810 PMID: 37304266

Munteanu, C., & Schwartz, B. (2024). Interactions between Dietary Antioxidants, Dietary Fiber and the Gut Microbiome: Their Putative Role in Inflammation and Cancer. *International Journal of Molecular Sciences*, *25*(15), 8250. DOI: 10.3390/ijms25158250 PMID: 39125822

Nandi, D., Parida, S., & Sharma, D. (2023). The gut microbiota in breast cancer development and treatment: The good, the bad, and the useful! *Gut Microbes*, *15*(1), 2221452. DOI: 10.1080/19490976.2023.2221452 PMID: 37305949

Nieminen, M. T., & Salaspuro, M. (2018). Local Acetaldehyde-An Essential Role in Alcohol-Related Upper Gastrointestinal Tract Carcinogenesis. *Cancers (Basel)*, *10*(1), 11. DOI: 10.3390/cancers10010011 PMID: 29303995

Nowak, A., & Libudzisz, Z. (2006). Influence of phenol, p-cresol and indole on growth and survival of intestinal lactic acid bacteria. *Anaerobe*, *12*(2), 80–84. DOI: 10.1016/j.anaerobe.2005.10.003 PMID: 16701619

Pandey, H., Tang, D. W. T., Wong, S. H., & Lal, D. (2023). Gut Microbiota in Colorectal Cancer: Biological Role and Therapeutic Opportunities. *Cancers (Basel), 15*(3), 866. DOI: 10.3390/cancers15030866 PMID: 36765824

Parida, S., & Sharma, D. (2019). The Microbiome-Estrogen Connection and Breast Cancer Risk. *Cells, 8*(12), 1642. DOI: 10.3390/cells8121642 PMID: 31847455

Patangia, D. V., Anthony Ryan, C., Dempsey, E., Paul Ross, R., & Stanton, C. (2022). Impact of antibiotics on the human microbiome and consequences for host health. *MicrobiologyOpen, 11*(1), e1260. DOI: 10.1002/mbo3.1260 PMID: 35212478

Pauwels, I., Versporten, A., Drapier, N., Vlieghe, E., Goossens, H., Koraqi, A., Hoxha, I., Tafaj, S., Cornistein, W., Quiros, R., Hojman, M., Ghazaryan, L., Horne, K., Cairns, K., Doukas, F., Gottlieb, T., Sermijn, E., Verhamme, K., Brands, C., & Lindholm, D. A. (2021). Hospital antibiotic prescribing patterns in adult patients according to the WHO Access, Watch and Reserve classification (AWaRe): Results from a worldwide point prevalence survey in 69 countries. *The Journal of Antimicrobial Chemotherapy, 76*(6), 1614–1624. DOI: 10.1093/jac/dkab050 PMID: 33822971

Peechakara, B. V., & Gupta, M. (2025). Ampicillin/Sulbactam. In *StatPearls*. StatPearls Publishing.

Pisoschi, A. M., & Pop, A. (2015). The role of antioxidants in the chemistry of oxidative stress: A review. *European Journal of Medicinal Chemistry, 97*, 55–74. DOI: 10.1016/j.ejmech.2015.04.040 PMID: 25942353

Prasad, A. S. (2014). Zinc: an antioxidant and anti-inflammatory agent: role of zinc in degenerative disorders of aging. *Journal of Trace Elements in Medicine and Biology, 28*(4), 364–371. DOI: 10.1016/j.jtemb.2014.07.019 PMID: 25200490

Priyadarshini, M., Kotlo, K. U., Dudeja, P. K., & Layden, B. T. (2018). Role of Short Chain Fatty Acid Receptors in Intestinal Physiology and Pathophysiology. *Comprehensive Physiology, 8*(3), 1091–1115. DOI: 10.1002/j.2040-4603.2018.tb00038.x PMID: 29978895

Ren, Y., Wu, J., Wang, Y., Zhang, L., Ren, J., Zhang, Z., Chen, B., Zhang, K., Zhu, B., Liu, W., Li, S., & Li, X. (2023). Lifestyle patterns influence the composition of the gut microbiome in a healthy Chinese population. *Scientific Reports, 13*(1), 14425. DOI: 10.1038/s41598-023-41532-4 PMID: 37660184

Režen, T., Rozman, D., Kovács, T., Kovács, P., Sipos, A., Bai, P., & Mikó, E. (2022). The role of bile acids in carcinogenesis. *Cellular and Molecular Life Sciences : CMLS, 79*(5), 243. DOI: 10.1007/s00018-022-04278-2 PMID: 35429253

Rineh, A., Kelso, M. J., Vatansever, F., Tegos, G. P., & Hamblin, M. R. (2014). Clostridium difficile infection: Molecular pathogenesis and novel therapeutics. *Expert Review of Anti-Infective Therapy, 12*(1), 131–150. DOI: 10.1586/14787210.2014.866515 PMID: 24410618

Rivas-Domínguez, A., Pastor, N., Martínez-López, L., Colón-Pérez, J., Bermúdez, B., & Orta, M. L. (2021). The Role of DNA Damage Response in Dysbiosis-Induced Colorectal. *Cancer Cells (Cold Spring Harbor, N.Y.), 10*(8), 1934. DOI: 10.3390/cells10081934 PMID: 34440703

Ruiz, V. E., Battaglia, T., Kurtz, Z. D., Bijnens, L., Ou, A., Engstrand, I., Zheng, X., Iizumi, T., Mullins, B. J., Müller, C. L., Cadwell, K., Bonneau, R., Perez-Perez, G. I., & Blaser, M. J. (2017). A single early-in-life macrolide course has lasting effects on murine microbial network topology and immunity. *Nature Communications, 8*(1), 518. DOI: 10.1038/s41467-017-00531-6 PMID: 28894149

Sampsell, K., Hao, D., & Reimer, R. A. (2020). The Gut Microbiota: A Potential Gateway to Improved Health Outcomes in Breast Cancer Treatment and Survivorship. *International Journal of Molecular Sciences, 21*(23), 9239. DOI: 10.3390/ijms21239239 PMID: 33287442

Schirmer, M., Smeekens, S. P., Vlamakis, H., Jaeger, M., Oosting, M., Franzosa, E. A., ter Horst, R., Jansen, T., Jacobs, L., Bonder, M. J., Kurilshikov, A., Fu, J., Joosten, L. A. B., Zhernakova, A., Huttenhower, C., Wijmenga, C., Netea, M. G., & Xavier, R. J. (2016). Linking the Human Gut Microbiome to Inflammatory Cytokine Production Capacity. *Cell, 167*(4), 1125–1136.e8. DOI: 10.1016/j.cell.2016.10.020 PMID: 27814509

Schulz, C., Schütte, K., Mayerle, J., & Malfertheiner, P. (2019). The role of the gastric bacterial microbiome in gastric cancer: Helicobacter pylori and beyond. *Therapeutic Advances in Gastroenterology, 12*, 1756284819894062. DOI: 10.1177/1756284819894062 PMID: 31897087

Sędzikowska, A., & Szablewski, L. (2021). Human Gut Microbiota in Health and Selected Cancers. *International Journal of Molecular Sciences, 22*(24), 13440. DOI: 10.3390/ijms222413440 PMID: 34948234

Seekatz, A. M., Safdar, N., & Khanna, S. (2022). The role of the gut microbiome in colonization resistance and recurrent Clostridioides difficile infection. *Therapeutic Advances in Gastroenterology, 15*, 17562848221134396. DOI: 10.1177/17562848221134396 PMID: 36425405

Seo, S.-S., Oh, H. Y., Lee, J.-K., Kong, J.-S., Lee, D. O., & Kim, M. K. (2016). Combined effect of diet and cervical microbiome on the risk of cervical intraepithelial neoplasia. *Clinical Nutrition (Edinburgh, Lothian)*, *35*(6), 1434–1441. DOI: 10.1016/j.clnu.2016.03.019 PMID: 27075319

Srinivas, U. S., Tan, B. W. Q., Vellayappan, B. A., & Jeyasekharan, A. D. (2019). ROS and the DNA damage response in cancer. *Redox Biology*, *25*, 101084. DOI: 10.1016/j.redox.2018.101084 PMID: 30612957

Su, Q., & Liu, Q. (2021). Factors Affecting Gut Microbiome in Daily Diet. *Frontiers in Nutrition*, *8*, 644138. DOI: 10.3389/fnut.2021.644138 PMID: 34041257

Sun, J., Chen, F., & Wu, G. (2023). Potential effects of gut microbiota on host cancers: Focus on immunity, DNA damage, cellular pathways, and anticancer therapy. *The ISME Journal*, *17*(10), 1535–1551. DOI: 10.1038/s41396-023-01483-0 PMID: 37553473

Szabo, C., Coletta, C., Chao, C., Módis, K., Szczesny, B., Papapetropoulos, A., & Hellmich, M. R. (2013). Tumor-derived hydrogen sulfide, produced by cystathionine-β-synthase, stimulates bioenergetics, cell proliferation, and angiogenesis in colon cancer. *Proceedings of the National Academy of Sciences of the United States of America*, *110*(30), 12474–12479. DOI: 10.1073/pnas.1306241110 PMID: 23836652

Thomas, R. M., Gharaibeh, R. Z., Gauthier, J., Beveridge, M., Pope, J. L., Guijarro, M. V., Yu, Q., He, Z., Ohland, C., Newsome, R., Trevino, J., Hughes, S. J., Reinhard, M., Winglee, K., Fodor, A. A., Zajac-Kaye, M., & Jobin, C. (2018). Intestinal microbiota enhances pancreatic carcinogenesis in preclinical models. *Carcinogenesis*, *39*(8), 1068–1078. DOI: 10.1093/carcin/bgy073 PMID: 29846515

Turner, N. D., & Lupton, J. R. (2021). Dietary Fiber. *Advances in Nutrition*, *12*(6), 2553–2555. DOI: 10.1093/advances/nmab116 PMID: 34687531

Waldum, H., & Fossmark, R. (2023). Inflammation and Digestive Cancer. *International Journal of Molecular Sciences*, *24*(17), 13503. DOI: 10.3390/ijms241713503 PMID: 37686307

Wang, L., Zhu, R., Huang, Z., Li, H., & Zhu, H. (2013). Lipopolysaccharide-induced toll-like receptor 4 signaling in cancer cells promotes cell survival and proliferation in hepatocellular carcinoma. *Digestive Diseases and Sciences*, *58*(8), 2223–2236. DOI: 10.1007/s10620-013-2745-3 PMID: 23828139

Weir, C. B., & Le, J. K. (2025). Metronidazole. In *StatPearls*. StatPearls Publishing.

Wong, S. H., Zhao, L., Zhang, X., Nakatsu, G., Han, J., Xu, W., Xiao, X., Kwong, T. N. Y., Tsoi, H., Wu, W. K. K., Zeng, B., Chan, F. K. L., Sung, J. J. Y., Wei, H., & Yu, J. (2017). Gavage of Fecal Samples From Patients With Colorectal Cancer Promotes Intestinal Carcinogenesis in Germ-Free and Conventional Mice. *Gastroenterology, 153*(6), 1621–1633.e6. DOI: 10.1053/j.gastro.2017.08.022 PMID: 28823860

Wu, Y., Rong, X., Pan, M., Wang, T., Yang, H., Chen, X., Xiao, Z., & Zhao, C. (2022). Integrated Analysis Reveals the Gut Microbial Metabolite TMAO Promotes Inflammatory Hepatocellular Carcinoma by Upregulating POSTN. *Frontiers in Cell and Developmental Biology, 10,* 840171. DOI: 10.3389/fcell.2022.840171 PMID: 35676936

Xie, Y., Geng, Y., Yao, J., Ji, J., Chen, F., Xiao, J., Hu, X., & Ma, L. (2023). N-nitrosamines in processed meats: Exposure, formation and mitigation strategies. *Journal of Agriculture and Food Research, 13,* 100645. DOI: 10.1016/j.jafr.2023.100645

Xu, H., & Li, H. (2019). Acne, the Skin Microbiome, and Antibiotic Treatment. *American Journal of Clinical Dermatology, 20*(3), 335–344. DOI: 10.1007/s40257-018-00417-3 PMID: 30632097

Yan, M., Zou, X., Wang, Y., Wang, C., Wang, Y., Liu, Z., Shang, L., Cui, X., & Cao, B. (2024). Impact of Metagenomic Next-Generation Sequencing of Bronchoalveolar Lavage Fluid on Antimicrobial Stewardship in Patients With Lower Respiratory Tract Infections: A Retrospective Cohort Study. *The Journal of Infectious Diseases, 229*(1), 223–231. DOI: 10.1093/infdis/jiad296 PMID: 37506257

Yu, H., Meng, H., Zhou, F., Ni, X., Shen, S., & Das, U. N. (2015). Clinical research Urinary microbiota in patients with prostate cancer and benign prostatic hyperplasia. *Archives of Medical Science : AMS, 11,* 385–394. DOI: 10.5114/aoms.2015.50970 PMID: 25995756

Zafar H, Saier MH Gut Bacteroides species in health and disease. Gut Microbes 13:1848158. DOI: 10.1080/19490976.2020.1848158

Zhang, H., & Fu, L. (2021). The role of ALDH2 in tumorigenesis and tumor progression: Targeting ALDH2 as a potential cancer treatment. *Acta Pharmaceutica Sinica. B, 11*(6), 1400–1411. DOI: 10.1016/j.apsb.2021.02.008 PMID: 34221859

Zhang, P. (2022). Influence of Foods and Nutrition on the Gut Microbiome and Implications for Intestinal Health. *International Journal of Molecular Sciences, 23*(17), 9588. DOI: 10.3390/ijms23179588 PMID: 36076980

Zhao, L.-Y., Mei, J.-X., Yu, G., Lei, L., Zhang, W.-H., Liu, K., Chen, X.-L., Kołat, D., Yang, K., & Hu, J.-K. (2023a). Role of the gut microbiota in anticancer therapy: From molecular mechanisms to clinical applications. *Signal Transduction and Targeted Therapy*, *8*(1), 1–27. DOI: 10.1038/s41392-023-01406-7 PMID: 37179402

Zhao, M., Chu, J., Feng, S., Guo, C., Xue, B., He, K., & Li, L. (2023b). Immunological mechanisms of inflammatory diseases caused by gut microbiota dysbiosis: A review. *Biomedicine and Pharmacotherapy*, *164*, 114985. DOI: 10.1016/j.biopha.2023.114985 PMID: 37311282

Zheng, D., Liwinski, T., & Elinav, E. (2020). Interaction between microbiota and immunity in health and disease. *Cell Research*, *30*(6), 492–506. DOI: 10.1038/s41422-020-0332-7 PMID: 32433595

Zheng, J. H., Nguyen, V. H., Jiang, S.-N., Park, S.-H., Tan, W., Hong, S. H., Shin, M. G., Chung, I.-J., Hong, Y., Bom, H.-S., Choy, H. E., Lee, S. E., Rhee, J. H., & Min, J.-J. (2017). Two-step enhanced cancer immunotherapy with engineered Salmonella typhimurium secreting heterologous flagellin. *Science Translational Medicine*, *9*(376), eaak9537. Advance online publication. DOI: 10.1126/scitranslmed.aak9537 PMID: 28179508

Zhou, H., Yuan, Y., Wang, H., Xiang, W., Li, S., Zheng, H., Wen, Y., Ming, Y., Chen, L., & Zhou, J. (2021). Gut Microbiota: A Potential Target for Cancer Interventions. *Cancer Management and Research*, *13*, 8281–8296. DOI: 10.2147/CMAR.S328249 PMID: 34764691

Zhou, Y., Lv, J., Jin, S., Fu, C., Liu, B., Shen, Y., Li, M., Zhang, Y., & Feng, N. (2024). Gut microbiota derived metabolite trimethylamine N-oxide influences prostate cancer progression via the p38/HMOX1 pathway. *Frontiers in Pharmacology*, *15*, 1526051. DOI: 10.3389/fphar.2024.1526051 PMID: 39850572

Chapter 6
Cutting-Edge in Vitro Models and Multi-Omics Approaches for Carcinogen Exposome Studies

Fatima Ezzahra Elamrani
https://orcid.org/0009-0009-0248-1964
Cadi Ayyad University, Morocco

Souad Loqman
Faculty of Medicine and Pharmacy, Cadi Ayyad University, Morocco

Anass Belbachir
https://orcid.org/0009-0002-4828-0251
Faculty of Medicine and Pharmacy, Cadi Ayyad University, Morocco

ABSTRACT

The exposome concept has complemented the genome by opening new areas for cancer research. The in vitro models used in this context are fundamental for unraveling the molecular and cellular effects of carcinogenic agents in a controlled environment. Moreover, these models offer a new possibility for investigating the key mechanisms of tumor initiation and progression, bridging the gap between epidemiological data and mechanistic studies. In the same way, integrating recent technologies such as multiomics (genomics, transcriptomics, proteomics, metabolomics, etc.) expands the horizon for a deep understanding of cellular responses to carcinogenic exposures. This chapter reviews recent cutting-edge advances in using experimentation mod-

DOI: 10.4018/979-8-3373-2165-3.ch006

els to study the carcinogenic exposome. It emphasizes their role in understanding carcinogenesis pathways, focusing on the most up-to-date technologies.

INTRODUCTION

It is increasingly clear that cancer is a multifactorial disease, in which environmental factors play the crucial role in its appearance and progression. Daily exposure to harmful pollutant molecules induces stress that generates abnormal physiological responses with the potential to cause health anomalies, and above all increase serious disorders.

Cancer, on average, is heritable by approximately 10%, while non-genetic factors, such as environmental exposures, are not. The wide spectrum of harmful molecules to which humans are exposed on an everyday basis - food, environment, stress, life-style -is largely unknown and unmeasured. Yet gene-environment interactions may account for most of this missing heritability of cancer (Young et al., 2025) hence the interest in exposome research, which aims to explore exhaustively the non-genetic causes of diseases, including cancer.

Those harmful molecules influence cancer appearance and metastasis which are crucial components of carcinogenesis. They trigger epithelial-mesenchymal transition (EMT), a step essential for cancer cell migration and invasion, and may directly alter metastatic pathways. Additionally, xenobiotics can change the tumor microenvironmnt and may lead to an accelerate spread of cancer and cells capacity to escape the original tumor.

In this chapter, we give a summary of current state-of-the-art developments in the use of experimental models for the investigation of carcinogenic exposures. It highlights the importance of comprehending carcinogenesis pathways, finding novel biomarkers, and refining risk prediction techniques. It emphasizes their role for understanding carcinogenesis pathways, identifying new biomarkers and optimizing risk prediction strategies. Furthermore, a particular focus is devoted to the most up-to-date technologies, such as organ-on-chip, for improving interactions between the exposome and the tumor microenvironment. Finally, this chapter will discuss the strengths and limitations of current approaches, while proposing new perspectives for improving in vitro models and suggesting potential lines of research for a better understanding of the cumulative impact of exposures in the context of exposomic cancer.

I. KEY CONCEPTS IN CARCINOGENESIS: EXPOSOME, BIOACCUMULATION AND PERSISTENCE.

1.1. Exposome

Recent increases in cancer rates can be attributed to the improvements in diagnostic techniques, but also to the ever-increasing presence of carcinogens in the environment and the mutagenic mechanisms they cause. This exposition is dynamic and multifactorial in nature which makes its association to phenotypic outcomes challenging due to the complexity of the interaction involved.

The exposome concept, first introduced by Wild (2005), is a complement to the genome. It served to fill the gap in understanding the heritability of cancer as well as the degree of methodological development applied to the characterization of environmental exposures. This concept, although rarely investigated, has proved essential in human health, as it highlights the effect of exposure on the induction of complex diseases such as cancer.

Exposomics research explores the overall molecular or physiological effects, as well as the cumulative effects due to the physical, chemical, biological or psychosocial components of the internal or external environments of human beings (Figure 1). Susceptibility to xenobiotics depends on a variety of factors including genetic background (Exposition time, magnitude, duration, and interactions between chemical complexes), making it extremely variable between populations, with a long-term risk to health outcomes. This highlights the increased need to understand the effects of exposure on the population, individual and molecular levels (Wei et al., 2022).

The comprehensive approach of the exposome aims to improve the prevention, treatment and public health comprehension of illnesses, with better identification of the links between disease, and exposure. In addition, the exposome has greatly influenced research thanks to the models involved in its study; these models have enabled a reduction in reliance on animal testing, advances in personalized medicine, public health and regulatory policies, as well as the screening and classification of harmful chemicals.

1.1.1 Xenobiotics

The term xenobiotic in the exposome refers to any toxic product that may cause abnormalities due to exposure.

Table 1. Overview of Xenobiotics classifications.

Origin classification		Mode of action classification	Exposition sources	Potential health effect	Examples
Environmental pollutants	Atmospheric pollutants	Carcinogens Immunotoxic	o Industrial emissions o Exhaust gases o Cigarette smoke	■ Respiratory diseases. ■ Lung cancer. ■ Cardiovascular diseases.	- Polycyclic aromatic hydrocarbons (PAHs). - Nitrogen oxides (Nox). - Sulphur dioxide (SO_2)
	Water and soil pollutants	Neurotoxic Carcinogens Reprotoxic	o Industrial waste o Use of pesticide o Illegal landfill sites	■ kidney and liver toxicity ■ Neurological disorders ■ Various cancers	- Heavy metals (lead, mercury, cadmium, arsenic...) - Pesticides (glyphosate, atrazine…) - Persistent organic pollutants (PCBs, dioxins)
Industrial chemicals	Solvents and plasticizers	Endocrine perturbators Hepatotoxic	o Chemical industry. o Plastic packaging.	■ Endocrine disruptors. ■ Hepatic toxicity. ■ Cancerogenic effects.	- Benzene - Bisphenol A - Phthalates
	Flame retardants	Neurotoxic Immunotoxic	o Building materials o Electronics.	■ Neurological toxicity. ■ Immunotoxic effects	- PBDE. - TBBPA
Food contaminants	Additives and pesticide residues	Carcinogens Mutagens	o Industrial food. o Agricultural contaminants.	■ Metabolic disorders. ■ Gastrointestinal cancers.	- Nitrites. - Sulphites. - Acrylamide.
	Mycotoxins and heavy metals	Hepatotoxic Neurotoxic	o Food molds. o Water pollution.	■ Neurological disorders. ■ Hormonal disorders.	- Aflatoxin. - Arsenic.
Consumer products	Cosmetics and personal care	Endocrines perturbators Allergens	o Hygiene products. o Beauty products.	■ Skin irritations ■ Impaired fertility	- Parabens - Triclosan
	Household products and packaging	Endocrines perturbators Immunotoxic	o Detergents. o Food plastics.	■ Hormonal dysfunction ■ Allergic risks	- Alkylphenols. - BPA.
Drugs and medicine	Pharmaceutics and illicit substances	Hepatotoxic Neurotoxic	o Prescription medicine. o Recreational drugs.	■ Dependence. ■ Nervous system disorders.	- Antibiotics. - Opioids. - Amphetamines.
Emerging contaminants	Nanomaterials and pharmaceutical residues	Immunotoxic Unknown long-term effects	o Nanotechnologies industry. o Waste water pollution.	■ Chronic inflammation. ■ Ecotoxicological risks.	- Silver nanoparticles.

The toxic effects caused by xenobiotics are very variant, they may lead to:

- **Acute toxicity:** due to short-term exposure to high doses of xenobiotics.
- **Chronic toxicity:** resulting from long-term exposure to low levels of xenobiotics.
- **Carcinogenicity:** when they induce cancer.

- **Teratogenicity:** when they cause birth defects.
- **Endocrine disrupts** when they interfere with the endocrine system.
- **Immunotoxicity**: when they alter the immune system and increase infection and disease.

1.1.2 Exposome Types

Exposome studies are conducted at several levels, as illustrated in the figure below:

Figure 1. Overview of exposome types.

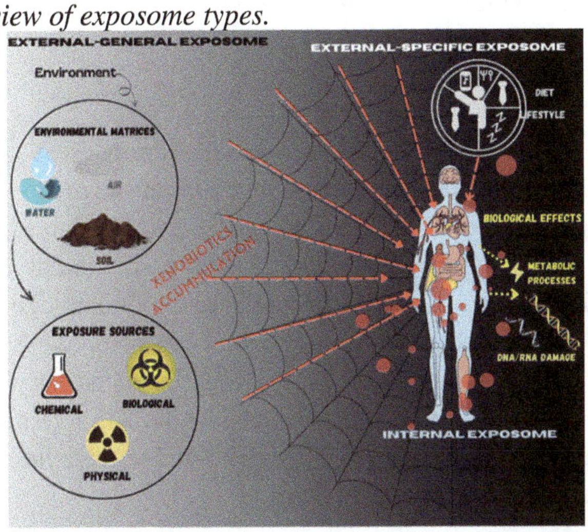

It covers all the environmental exposures we experience throughout our lives, from general environmental factors to specific ones. Their impact on health depends on their accumulation and interaction with physiological systems.

A. External-General Exposome

Populations are exposed to stress factors during the same period (Jiang et al., 2018). The primary source of human exposure to toxins is the environment, with a potential for exposure ranging from near-fields to far-fields (Gao et al., 2022). Sources of exposure are either direct biological, chemical or physical from environmental matrices (air, soil, water). This exposome concerns environmental exposures that influence the individual in a global and often involuntary way. Studying this exposome is both costly and very broad, since it is not associated with sufficient specific or lasting biomarkers and does not capture the doses that reach tissues in the body, which require measurement strategies, appropriate geospatial methods

(VoPham et al., 2024), remote sensing, sensors, personal external sampling devices, etc ...(Young et al., 2025).

B. External-Specific/Compartmental Exposome

The specific external exposome is complicated to uncode. The complexity stems from the fact that it involves personal and individual factors such as lifestyle, diet, substance use and occupation. Several studies have shown that exposome profiles are highly dynamic, with spatio-temporal differences between individuals living in the same geographical region (Gao et al., 2022).

C. Internal Exposome

Internal exposure covers biological and metabolic processes influenced by external exposure. It includes xenobiotics and their biotransformation products, DNA/RNA damage, bioactive molecules accumulated from exogenous sources (Gao et al., 2022), radiation, particles, drugs, food contaminants, pesticides, psychosocial factors (stress, household income, parental care, cultural traditions, education), lifestyle factors (sleep, work, diet, exercise, smoking, oral contraceptives), ecosystems and climate (green spaces, population density) and foods ingested early in life, including infant formula, breast milk and complementary foods. The internal exposome can be measured using multiomics techniques (metabolomics, methylomics, proteomics, transcriptomics etc.) (VoPham et al., 2024).

1.2. Exposition, Bioaccumulation, and Persistence Mechanisms

Figure 2. Carcinogens exposure pathways.

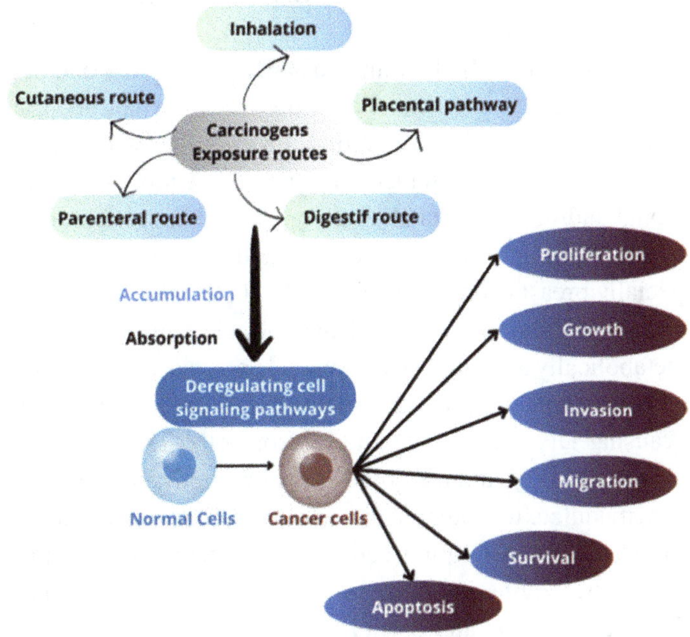

This figure illustrates the different ways of carcinogen exposition (Cutaneous, digestive, parenteral, placental) and their effects once accumulated and absorbed. These xenobiotics disrupt the cellular signaling pathways which may induce carcinogenesis.

1.2.1. Exposure Routes

Exposure to toxins occurs by various routes (Figure 2), contributing to their accumulation in the body:

- **Inhalation:** in the form of gases, vapors, aerosols or fine particles.
- **Dermal absorption:** through direct contact with the skin and mucous membranes.
- **Ingestion:** when the toxic agent is swallowed and absorbed by the digestive system.
- **Transplacental transfer:** when the toxic agent is transmitted from the mother to the fetus via the placenta.

- **Parenteral route**: when the toxic agent is introduced directly into the body through wounds, injections or insect bites.

1.2.2. Accumulation and Impact on Signaling Pathways

Xenobiotics, once in the body, binds to specific receptors and accumulate and deregulate cell signaling pathways. This influences normal and cancerous cells behavior, as well as their fate: proliferation, invasion, growth, survival, migration or apoptosis. Many of these substances are known as endocrine disruptors and can cause functional and/or structural changes or even disrupt hormonal homeostasis. Some have been reported to be carcinogenic and can lead to the development of tumors, especially breast cancer (Calafat et al., 2009).

Carcinogens have several characteristics. Some carcinogens are electrophilic, others are metabolically activated electrophiles, i.e. seek electrons that form adducts with cellular macromolecules, namely DNA, RNA, lipids and proteins. Others are genotoxic, causing DNA damage, mutations or both. Some alter DNA repair or cause genomic instability. Induce epigenetic alterations, oxidative stress, chronic inflammation, modulate receptor-mediated effects, immunosuppressive, cause immortalization, alter cell proliferation, cell death or nutrient supply (Smith et al., 2016).

Human exposure begins *in utero*, very early during the first phases of development. Chemical products and particles can accumulate in placental tissue and interfere with placental functions and the secretion of signaling mediators essential to the proper development of the gestation process and the health of the fetus. In addition to prenatal placental transfer, exposure can occur postnatally via the oral route (during the lactation phase), via baby food, drinking water, medicated products, parenteral route, inhalation route, cutaneous route or mucocutaneous route. Besides toxic metabolites that can be formed and secreted into the fetal circulation (Krausová et al., 2023).

1.2.3. Xenobiotics Sources

Toxins are omnipresent and consumed daily. Spices contained in every meal are one of the main human exposure routes to dangerous pollutants, especially heavy metals like cadmium (Cd), manganese (Mn), copper (Cu), iron (Fe), plomb (Pb) and zinc (Zn) (Ezez et al., 2024). Secondly, freshwater products are the other major source of exposure to polycyclic aromatic hydrocarbons (Qin et al., 2020). Even the air we breathe is in turn a source of carcinogens. Researchers suggest that relatively high levels of xenobiotics such as benzene may be associated with an increased risk of breast cancer (Madrigal et al., 2024).

One of the ubiquitous elements in the natural environment that humans find hard to avoid is plastics, which are classified as hazardous and carcinogenic substances that disrupt cellular homeostasis by numerous mechanisms (oxidative stress, biological membrane damage, activation of inflammatory factors, genotoxicity, apoptosis, genome instability causing the triggering of new mechanisms and signaling pathways responsible for malignant transformation). On another note, plastic additives (e.g. chlorinated paraffins, phthalates, phenols, bisphenols, etc.) are carcinogenic chemicals that are adsorbed by the environment and can be released when absorbed by the body. In addition, organic contaminants accumulated on the surface of plastics and toxic metals used in production also cause cancer (Dzierżyński et al., 2024).

Internal exposure to xenobiotics and their biotransformation products can be determined by biomonitoring. This process can be used to find correlations between exposure and disease outcomes and may therefore help to elucidate the mechanism of action. The most used biological biomatrices for this purpose are urine, breast milk and blood (serum or plasma), considering the population and the analyst being investigated when choosing the matrix to use (saliva, placenta, hair, nails, breath, umbilical cord blood, teeth, etc.) (Krausová et al., 2023).

Functional exposomics helps to improve the assessment of the root causes of indoor exposure. Zhang et al. (2021) proposed a functional exposomics approach that links measurements of external exposure to external environmental stressors with internal dose and biological response. In addition, functional exposomics can quantify internal biomarkers of responses to chemical and biological exposures to social determinants and investigate their interaction in cancer initiation (Young et al., 2025), even if cancers associated with exposure to harmful chemicals are very widespread (breast cancer (Go et al., 2023) (Parkinson et al., 2024) (Juarez et al., 2024), skin cancer (Gracia-Cazaña et al., 2020), colorectal cancer (N. Chen et al., 2022), prostate cancer (Wiese et al., 2024), oesophageal cancer (Lipenga et al., 2021), lung cancer (Sarlak, 2021), pancreatic cancer (Lauri et al., 2025), childhood cancers (Ghantous et al., 2015))...

1.3. Transport and Storage in Tissues

One of the major problems with exposure to toxins is their ability to gain access to cancer causing cells. Some polycyclic hydrocarbons, for example, can initiate carcinogenesis and reach the peripheral tissues after entering blood stream due the their lipophilic characteristic, enabling their accumulation in the body, especially in adipose tissue (Irigaray & Belpomme, 2010).

Lipid metabolism disorders play an important role in carcinogenesis as they are involved in causing abnormal genes, protein, expression, and dysregulation of cytokines and signaling pathways. Moreover, preclinical and clinical cancer studies have shown the crucial role of lipid metabolism in tumor growth and metastasis. This is due to the common pathway for lipid metabolism and cancer cell survival or proliferation involving many proteins as well as various cells, tissues and organelles (Long et al., 2018).

While physiological properties govern the uptake, intracellular distribution and binding of metal compounds, their interaction with proteins appears to be the more relevant process for the carcinogenicity of metals than binding to DNA.

A study has shown the role of metallic compounds and organic solvents in the development of breast cancer (Mulware, 2013). The physiology of the breast, particularly the parenchyma, is surrounded by a deposit of fat capable of storing lipophilic xenobiotics. The organic solvents are known as highly lipophilic and ae biotransformed mainly in the liver and kidney through successive oxidation and reduction reactions, some of which lead to bioactivation.

1.4. Excretion and Persistence

Excretion of carcinogens accumulated daily is a major difficulty. Their elimination from the body takes time (Z. Li et al., 2012) in some cases, or is impossible in other cases. For example, the carcinogenic polycyclic aromatic hydrocarbons (PAHs) are the most ubiquitous and the most concentrated. Certain exogenous and endogenous factors significantly modify their biological action.

Table 2. Endogenous and exogenous factors influencing carcinogen's biological actions (e.g. PAHs)

Exogenous factors	Endogenous factors
The simultaneous presence and action of anticarcinogenic agents in the environment.	The vehicle used by carcinogens affects persistence at the site of penetration and the rate of systemic distribution
Presence of anticarcinogenic in a physical state compatible with inhalation and deposition in the respiratory tract	The rate of metabolism in the hepatobiliary system
The presence of factors modifying the host response, particularly in relation to normal physiological defenses	The existence of anatomical or metabolic abnormalities modifying the tissue response

Excretion can be achieved through biotransformation reactions. Those biocatalytic conversions of toxic xenobiotics into hydrophilic forms facilitate their elimination from the body in the form of less toxic metabolites or conjugates. Those reactions are catalyzed by enzymes, which mainly exist in the sites of biotransformation, i.e. the liver, skin, kidneys, lungs, intestines, placenta, gonads, aorta, lymphocytes, blood platelets, adrenal cortex and spinal cord, but not in the nervous system. The mechanism involves two reactions:

- First-phase reactions, which introduce a polar functional group onto the xenobiotic, and are referred to as non-synthetic reactions (oxidation, reduction and hydrolysis).
- Second-phase reactions, which are synthetic, increase the solubility of xenobiotics by binding endogenous molecules. They involve glucoronidation, sulphoconjugation, acetylation, methylation and glutathione conjugation (Bhaskar Mahanayak, 2024)..

Despite these reactions, several molecules are persistent and escape excretion. This is due to the limits of their biodegradation and to the fact that there is no technology available to clean up the environment, given the wide dispersion of persistent substances (Langenbach, 2013).

II. CARCINOGENESIS

2.1. Carcinogens Classification

Figure 3. IARC classification of carcinogens and their distribution by group.

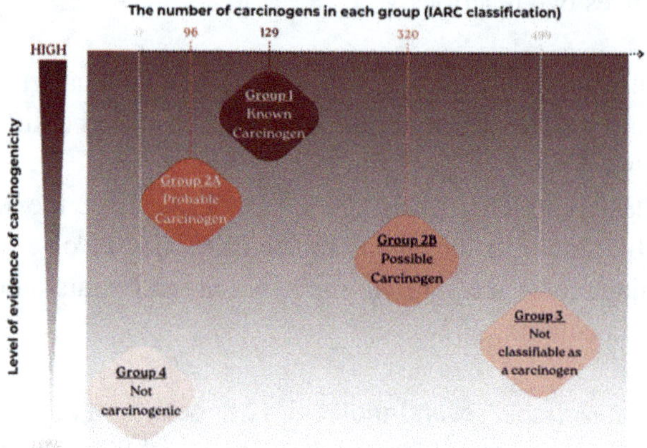

Carcinogens are classified by the International Agency for Research on Cancer (IARC) into five groups (Figure 3):

- **Group 1:** covers agents that have been shown to be carcinogenic in humans.
- **Group 2A:** covers agents with limited evidence of carcinogenicity in humans but with sufficient evidence in laboratory animals.
- **Group 2B:** concerns agents with limited evidence of carcinogenicity in humans and insufficient evidence of carcinogenicity in animals.
- **Group 3:** contains agents with insufficient evidence of carcinogenicity in both humans and animals.
- **Group 4:** concerns agents for which there is evidence suggesting a lack of carcinogenicity in humans and animals (WHO, 2025).

2.2. Signalization Pathways Involved in Carcinogenesis

The carcinogenic process complexity may be due often to non-carcinogenic factors, involved in the pathogenesis of neoplastic diseases. Toxins, which accumulate and persist in the body, can disrupt cellular homeostasis and contribute to carcinogenesis via various pathways.

Figure 4. Insights into xenobiotic metabolism pathways (XMPs).

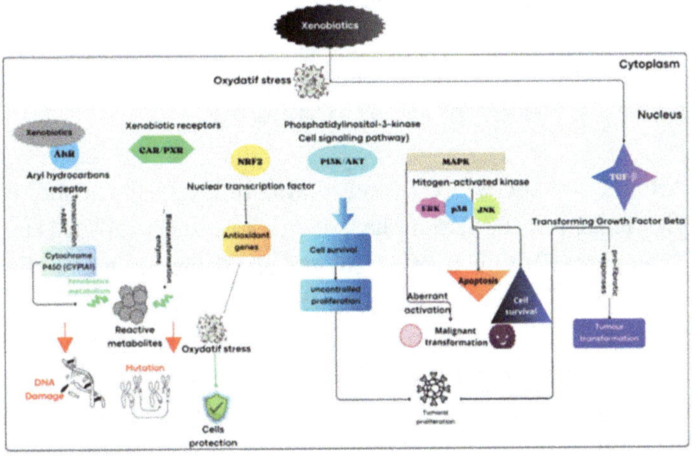

This figure illustrates the principles signalization pathways activated by xenobiotics and their role in stress oxidative, cell survival and tumoral transformation.

2.2.1. Xenobiotics Initial Response Pathway via Aryl Hydrocarbon Receptor Pathway (AhR)

Xenobiotics initial response takes place thanks to specific receptors such as Aryl hydrocarbons receptor (Ahr) which stimulate genes transcription encoding biotransformation enzymes including cytochrome P450 (CYP1A1) (Figure 4). This receptor is a cytoplasmic transcription factor which is activated once bind to xenobiotics. It undergoes a translocation to the nucleus and forms a complex with ARNT (AhR Nuclear Translocator). This activation led to the formation of reactive metabolite that may cause DNA damage which can initiate carcinogenesis and influences cellular proliferation (D. Lim, 2015).

This activation promotes xenobiotic metabolism and enhances reactive metabolites production and biotransformation. These reactive metabolites may induce DNA damage and mutations, which, if left unrepaired, promote malignant transformation.

Ahr was found constitutively active in many cancers, including aggressive breast cancers. Researchers used organoid models to study Endocrine disrupting chemicals (EDCs) effects on breast cancer. Organoids in culture were treated with EDV mixture at estimated in human exposure. They demonstrated that even the low PAH concentration may increase AhR expression and CYP activity in estrogen receptor positive cancer cells. Upregulated AhR signaling match the increased cell proliferation and expression of antiapoptotic and antioxidant proteins and it was validated by a mathematical model (Gearhart-Serna et al., 2020).

2.2.2. Constitutive Androstane Receptor (CAR) and Pregnanes X Receptor (PXR) Pathway

PXR, CAR and Ahr are related xenoreceptors linked to the xenobiotic's metabolism(Tomkiewicz et al., 2024) and play a major role in homeostasis maintenance. Pregnane X receptor (PXR) is a key regulator of xenobiotic metabolism which is highly expressed in the liver (Vázquez-Gómez et al., 2023).

These nuclear receptors are activated once they detect toxins presence and modulate biotransformation enzyme expression (Figure 4). They contribute to detoxification, but, if excessively activated, they could disrupt cellular homeostasis and contribute to carcinogenesis (Corcos et al., 2002).

2.2.3. Oxidative Stress Defense Pathway via Nuclear Factor Linked to Factor 2 (NRF2) Pathway

NFE2L2 or NRF2 is a transcription factor located in human chromosome 2. This transcription factor regulates antioxidant response. Xenobiotics cause oxidative stress, and NRF2 dissociates from its inhibitor, translocate to the nucleus and activates the expression of protective genes. However, this activation can protect cancer cells from oxidative damage (Nault, 2015).

The transcription factor NRF2 is the main factor that resolve inflammation by reducing oxidative stress and inhibiting pro-inflammatory signalization. This factor, once activated, may promote antioxidants genes expression and promotes cells protection against oxidative stress.

2.2.4. Tumoral Progression Pathway via Transforming Growth Factor Beta (TGF-β)

Transforming growth factor beta TGF-β, a growth factor protein implicated in a multitude of functions such as regulating cells proliferation and differentiation. It prevents the production of autoantibody by controlling cellular differentiation. It is produced by tumoral cells and tumoral microenvironment cells and plays the role of brake to the immune system anti-tumoral action, contributes to a pro-fibrotic response and participates in tumoral transformation. It facilitates the evolution towards more aggressive cancer Xenobiotics can influence this pathway and may lead to pro-fibrotic responses and promoting tumoral progression(Sandy Fellah, 2024).

2.2.5. Malignant Transformation Due to Mitogen-Activated Kinase (MAPK) Activation Pathways

Xenobiotics can activate these pathways, including ERK, JNK and p38 (Figure 4) which are involved in cell proliferation regulation, differentiation and apoptosis. The malignant transformation is caused when these pathways are aberrantly activated (IARC, 2006).

The family of Mitogen activated kinase, inoculant ERK, p38 and JNK play a double role; if activated normally it triggers apoptosis and eliminates damaged cells. But in aberrant activation cases, they may promote cell survival and malignant transformation, which lead to tumoral proliferation.

2.2.6. Cells Survival and Proliferation via Phosphatidylinositol-3-Kinase PI3K/AKT Pathways

Xenobiotics may influence this pathway and enhance the uncontrolled cell proliferation and apoptosis resistance. The PI3K/AKT pathway, a signalization cascade activated in response to oxidative stress which promotes cell survival. The excessive activation of this pathway may lead to uncontrolled proliferation, which is a major factor of malignant transformation.

A series of studies have shown the link between exposure to xenobiotics and the risk of both cancer and other diseases. This underlines the need for further research focusing on the mechanisms behind, and the long-term effects of, the toxic agents to which we are exposed. Among other properties, these xenobiotics are carcinogens with several characteristics: genotoxicity, altered gene expression, metabolic activation, cell proliferation, altered energy and disruption of receptor proteins and signaling, each of which has interactions, crosstalk and feedback through multiomics that have the capacity to elucidate both genotoxic and non-genotoxic mechanisms of environmental carcinogens. Non-carcinogenic chemical agents, although not the cause behind cancer, can act with low dose effects on signaling pathways linked to carcinogenesis as their cumulative effects with other non-genotoxic chemical agents which can act adversely and contribute to carcinogenesis (Young et al., 2025).

The equilibria between oxidative stress responses, apoptosis and cell survival determines if the cell undergoes reparable damage, apoptosis or may evaluate towards tumoral state. The dysregulation of those pathways, caused essentially by the prolonged xenobiotics expositions may lead to cancer development and progression.

2.3. Carcinogenesis Mechanism

The process that transforms a normal cell into a cancerous one is called 'carcinogenesis'. It is a multi-steps process, which can last from a few months to several years, depending on the tumor's aggressivity and the influence of daily exposure to xenobiotics (*Figure 5*).

Several models of carcinogenesis have been proposed; the first is mainly mutation-based and focuses on the chemical environment, radiation and viruses. The second is mainly linked to genome instability and focuses on familiarity, while the third is based on non-genotoxic mechanisms, clonal expansion and epigenetics. The fourth model encompasses the three previous models and is based on the concept of cellular selection. The fifth model is based on tissue organization. It can be grouped into two broad models; the first where physiological changes in the epithelium alone lead to malignancy, and the second where changes in the stroma/extracellular matrix are important, in addition to changes in the epithelium for malignancy (Vineis et al., 2010).

Figure 5. Carcinogenic stages induced by toxin exposure.

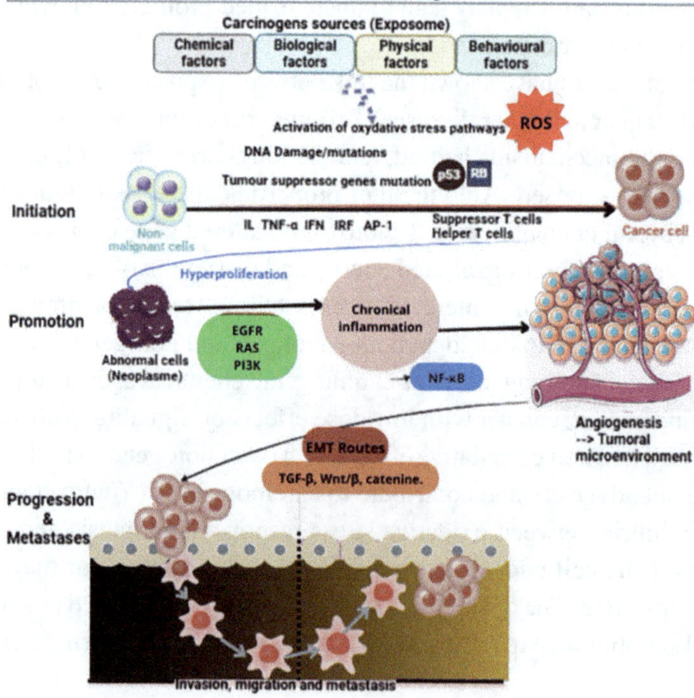

EGFR: Epithelial growth factor receptor, produce a surface cell receptor, and induce cell multiplication once activated.

RAS: Rasmark pathway, is a chain of proteins implicated in cell signaling from surface receptor the cell's DNA.

PI3K: a signal transduction pathway that promotes survival and growth in response to extracellular signals.

NF-κB1: Nuclear factor kappa-light-chain-enhancer of activated B cells, a group of transcription factors implicated in signal transduction pathways.

p53: a tumor suppressor gene, implicated in cell cycle control and apoptosis.

RB: affects tumor cell responses to genotoxic drugs.

TGF-β: Transforming growth factor, produced by cancer cells and microenvironmental tumor cells.

Wnt/β-catenin: a signaling pathway, regulate cell proliferation and polarity, cell determination and tissue homeostasis.

Carcinogenesis consists of four phases; The initiation involves irreversible genetic damage in a normal cell, which is either spontaneous or influenced by xenobiotics, leading to its conversion into an initiated cell via interleukins: IL-1, IL-6, IL-8, tumor necrosis factor α (TNF-α), interferons (IFN), suppressor T cells, helper T cells, interferon regulatory factors (IRF), activator protein 1 (AP-1).

The second phase is promotion, during which the initiated cells undergo mass growth of abnormal cells. This development results from the long uncontrolled proliferation of initiated cells which may take place due to drugs administration that affect the neoplastic cells divisions.

In the third phase, the pre-neoplastic cells transform into neoplastic cells acquiring additional genetic mutations that promote the ability of neoplastic cells to become malignant, invade other tissues and spread to other parts of the body (metastasis).

Tumoral progression, metastasis and chemoresistance are influenced by cancer stemness in cellular stress case (Kim et al., 2024).

2.4. Xenobiotics Roles in Metastasis

Carcinogens may cause or accentuate metastasis via their action on cell receptors and disrupted signaling pathways which lead to an impaired cellular function. At this stage angiogenesis is promoted by the vascular endothelial growth factor (VEGF) and supplies tumors with oxygen and nutrients.

In addition, TGF-β alters tight junctions and promotes EMT essential for preserving epithelial integrity. This causes the loss of cell adhesion and polarity and develops invasiveness and migration traits like mesenchymal cells, as it facilitates the separation of cells from the initial tumor, and infiltrates close to tissues, and reaches the extracellular matrix. This transition is crucial in metastasis, and these changes increase the invasion and motility of cancer cells, which accelerates the development of the disease (Pal & Firdous, 2024).

On the other hand, carcinogens affect prostate carcinogenesis at every stage via influencing cytochrome P450, which metabolizes a wide range of endogenous and foreign xenobiotic chemicals (Maksymchuk & Kashuba, 2019).

III. EPIGENETIC MODIFICATIONS

In studying the exposome, it is particularly interesting to conduct epigenetic profiling (Colwell et al., 2023), since several chemicals associated with carcinogenesis are involved in epigenetic alterations in cells. These alterations are used to identify epigenetics marks changes because carcinogens exert their effects via genotoxic and non-genotoxic mechanisms, which makes the assessment of potential epigenetic effects and the underlying mechanisms of action the main element in assessing the safety of chemicals omnipresent in the environment.

Furthermore, pollutants to which we are exposed are actors in inducing oxidative stress that generate reactive oxygen species (ROS), which in turn cause direct DNA damage, or interfere with the functioning of methyltransferases (DNMTS), leading to DNA methylation alteration.

In addition, environmental factors may cause post-translational modifications of histones (phosphorylation, methylation or ubiquitination) that create binding sites for other regulating proteins responsible for chromatin structure regulation and transcription. Those modifications can disrupt the functioning of multi-protein complexes involved in histone modifications and cause gene expression deregulation.

3.1. Methylation

Methylation, a chemical modification that consists on adding a methyl group to CpG sites of the DNA where cytosine C is followed by guanine G. Once carried out, this modification can tighten the DNA, making it difficult to activate genes, or loosen it, causing an easy activation of genes (Danieli et al., 2024).

Environmental stimuli may alter chromatin structure and gene expression. It can trigger signaling pathways that recruit histone acetyl transferase (HATs) responsible for adding an acetyl group to histone proteins, or histone deacetylases (HDACs) responsible for removing an acetyl group from histone proteins for specific regions of the gene.

3.2. The Non-Coding RNAs

microRNAs (miRs) and long-non-coding RNAs (lncRNAs) are involved in a major regulatory mechanism in biological an pathological processes. They modulate gene expressions without altering the underlying DNA sequence by binding to mRNA promoting inhibition by a translation or a degradation. Their deregulation is implicated in several diseases, making them a potential target for personalized therapeutic intervention(Isachesku et al., 2023).

Environmental toxins cause epigenetic alterations. For example, respiratory exposure to ozone may cause airway damages and increase inflammation markers and extracellular vesicle-sized particles number in bronchovascular lavage fluid. This was highlighted by high-throughput smal RNA sequencing that shows the expression of several mRNAs in pulmonary extracellular vesicles (Li et al., 2019).

Water toxins have epigenetic effects. Glyphosate, for example, has been detected in blood and urine and was associated with DNA methylation alteration in various tissues. It has been associated with non-Hodgkin's lymphoma, acute leukemia and several deregulatory endocrine activities (Woźniak et al., 2020) (Olmedo-Suárez et al., 2022).

Moreover, orthotoluidine, another example of carcinogens in the epigenetic context, known as a human carcinogen. It is absorbed by inhalation, ingestion and/or via skin contact (Nakano et al., 2025). And similarly asbestos, they must therefore be properly eliminated to prevent asbestos-related diseases such as mesothelioma and lung cancer (TAKATA et al., 2024).

The evaluation of epigenetic alterations induced by chemical compounds has yet to be developed. This highlights the need to identify specific genes to broaden the scope and usefulness of these epigenetic tests for assessing and monitoring the risks of environmental exposure (Yamada et al., 2025).

IV. *IN VITRO* MODELS AND EXPERIMENTAL APPROACHES FOR STUDYING CARCINOGENIC EXPOSURES

4.1. Toxicity and Bioassays

Numerous toxicity tests have been carried out using different techniques; non-targeted high-resolution mass spectrometry is one of the essential advances in exposome methodologies. It enables the systematic measurement, on an omic scale, of both the chemical exposome and the metabolome in biological samples in a single analysis cycle (Young et al., 2025). This technique can detect over 100,000 signals in biological samples, including exogenous environmental chemicals, endogenous metabolites, microbiome-related compounds and pharmaceuticals.

In the other hand, liquid chromatography and gas chromatography are used for exogenous chemicals optimal detection and do not require a priori selection of chemical analytes and can therefore produce new hypotheses and discoveries beyond what we can anticipate. Although these methods are non-targeted, they are accurate, cheaper, higher throughput, feasible for smaller sample volumes and more streamlined through data pipelines (Young et al., 2025).

More than just measuring the original chemicals, the internal exposome reveals their biotransformation products, which reflect an individual's unique physiology and are often responsible for inducing toxic effects. Non-targeted chemical profiling using exposomic methods is a powerful tool for assessing exposures to complex mixtures of tens of thousands of environmental chemicals (Manz et al., 2023).

4.2. Experimental Models

In the exposome, the investigation of carcinogen exposure is based on the development of *in vitro* models that enable in-depth holistic analysis of the molecular and cellular mechanisms involved in carcinogenesis. These models offer an environment that mimics physiological conditions in a controlled, reproducible and ethical manner to examine the effects of xenobiotics on the human organism.

Cell lines, primary cultures, organoids and spheroids have proved to be essential models for research in general, and for studying and understanding the underlying mechanisms due to exposure to environmental pollutants more specifically. These models are also essential tools for understanding the impact of genetic and environmental factors in the development of cancer (Silva et al., 2025). They have proved to be an effective alternative to animal models. Although the latter faithfully reproduce *in vivo* physiology, they present ethical concerns, high costs and long lead times. They are also unsuitable for several advanced applications such as drug screening and studies of exposure to toxins, due to the fundamental differences between animals and humans in terms of metabolism and genetic make-up (Kim et al., 2024).

Advances in tissue engineering, such as micro-fluidic systems and organ-on-chip, have made it possible to better simulate pathophysiological conditions, thereby refining the analysis of interactions between cells and their microenvironments. They better mimic the structure, function, development and homeostasis of natural organs (Wan et al., 2024).

4.2.1. Simple Culture (2D) Model

Two-dimensional (2D) cell culture is the classic model for a wide range of studies, including the exposome. It allows the impact of xenobiotics to be analyzed in a simple and reproducible way, with direct access to the cells. This model has the advantage of rapid development in confluent and polarized monolayers, that can be used in coculture, or in studies of drug and xenobiotic transport. However, this model is limited by the absence of cell-matrix interactions, and by the fact that it is not representative of the original structure of the tissue microenvironment, which means that the resulting physiological response remains incomplete.

In addition, its ability to represent *in situ* phenotypes, genetic drift and culture conditions make it difficult to rapidly and reliably generate new cell lines from patient samples. This may be because cell lines and primary cells are only relatively simplified models compared with the complex tumor microenvironment of the human body. They do not interact with other cell types, extracellular matrix components or physiological conditions present in living tissue. In addition, mechanical and/or enzymatic disruption disrupts normal tissue architecture and cell-cell connections. When cell lines are established from primary cultures of tissue removed during surgical procedures, mechanical fragmentation is necessary to allow the separation of tissue cells into a homogenous suspension. This facilitates their subsequent culture and study in the laboratory. Consequently, the results of cell culture experiments need to be validated using more accurate models (Silva et al., 2025).

This model is therefore far from recapitulating the cellular functions of human tissues and physiology. In addition, genetic drift and culture conditions make it difficult to rapidly and reliably generate new cell lines from patient samples. The growth and maintenance of cell lines begins with the choice of suitable culture medium, supplements and culture flasks.

4.2.2. Tridimensional (3D) Culture Models

Tissue engineering has helped to overcome the disadvantages of the 2D culture system by developing cellular models that mimic physiological conditions better than animal models, enabling us to study the impact of exposure on the body.

Figure 6. Comparative overview of 3D cell culture models: organoids, spheroids, and organ-on-chip.

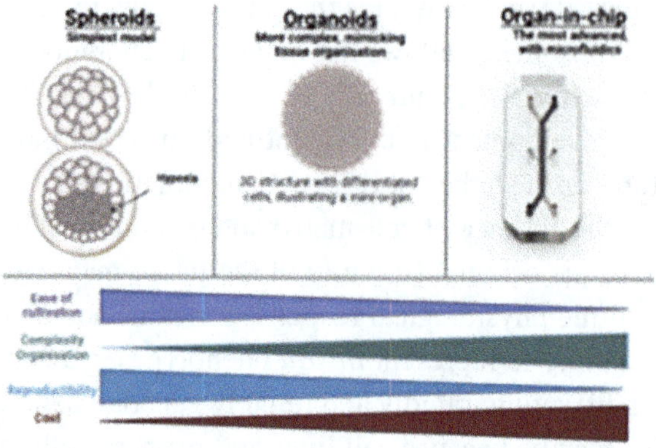

The three *in vitro* models differ as illustrated from the ease of cultivation, complexity, organization, reproducibility, and cost. The model choice is crucial while considering the present advantages/ disadvantages of each model, the aim of the study and the type of results to obtain.

A. Spheroids

Spheroids are three-dimensional cell culture models of grown cell aggregates in suspension, with or without extracellular matrix, which bridge the gap between conventional two-dimensional cell culture and the complexity of tumors *in vivo*. They better reproduce the architecture and metabolism of their tissue of origin, considering the complexity of the tumor microenvironment in the body as well as intracellular signaling, extracellular matrix arrangement and internal transport properties (Costa et al., 2016) (Kim et al., 2024). The initial aim of their development is to gain a better understanding of carcinogenesis and develop new therapeutic approaches, thanks to their cost-effectiveness compared with other *ex vivo* models and their suitability for a wide range of studies, including the exposome (Silva et al., 2025).

Figure 7. Formation, culture, and analysis of cellular spheroids.

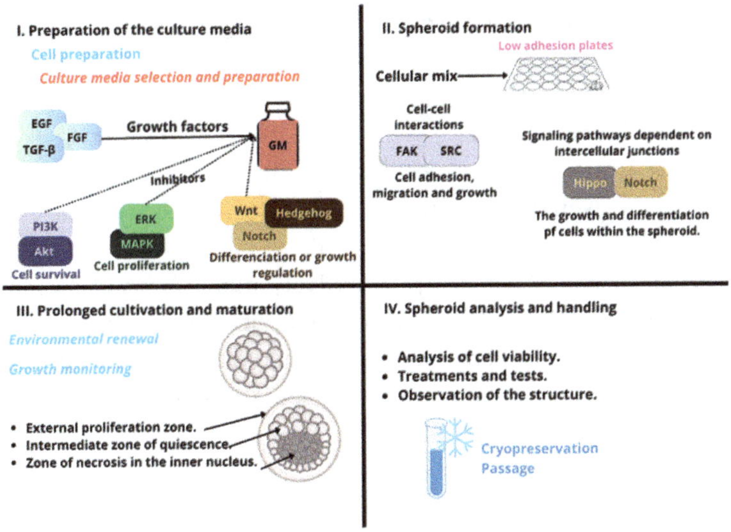

PI3K- AKT: Phosphoinositide 3-kinase and Protein kinase B, a signal transduction pathway that promotes survival and growth in response to extracellular signals.

MAPK-ERK: Microtubule-associated protein kinases and Extracellular signal-regulated kinases, a proteins chain in the cells that communicates a signal from a receptor on the cell surface to the DNA in the cell nucleus.

WNT-Notch-Hedgehog: a major signaling pathway for the dynamic transformation of single celled-zygote into a highly complex multicellular organism (Kumar et al., 2021)

FAK-Src: Focal adhesion kinase and steroid receptor coactivator, intracellular nonreceptor tyrosine kinase, playing a major role in cellular responses (tumoral angiogenesis, epithelial mesenchymal stem cells promotion, cancer resistance…) (Bolós et al., 2010).

Hippo-Notch: Hippo signaling is an evolutionarily conserved pathway, it regulates cell proliferation, apoptosis, and stem cells renewal. Notch mediates cellular signaling and it may be considered as the intermediary of hippo pathway.

This figure describes the principles spheroids formation steps, from the media preparation to their analyses and manipulation. The first phase highlights the media selection, with multiple agents that regulate cells survival, proliferation and differentiation via affectiong cellular pathways.

Next, cells are cultured on low-adhesion microplates to promote their aggregation and spheroid formation. Maturation involves media renewal and growth monitoring with a caracteristic interne organization. In carcinogenesis study case the tumor spheres are composed of three layers:

- External proliferation zone.
- Intermediate zone of quiescence.
- Zone of necrosis in the inner nucleus.

The zone of necrosis becomes progressively more apparent as the spheroid increases in size. And its viability is linked to its size, the smaller it is, there is no difference between the inside and outside and there is no significant distinction in terms of oxygen and nutrients between the inside and outside of the spheroid with most proliferating cells (Huang et al., 2025).

B. Organoids

This model has similarities with spheroids, yet they are two different models.

Table 3. Comparison between spheroids and organoids.

Characteristics	Spheroids (Figure *7*)	Organoids (Figure *8*)
Historically	Used since the 70's for tumor culture.	Recently developed with the advances in stem cells and bioengineering.
Origin	Cell lines. Primary cells. Tumor cells.	Pluripotent stem cells (Induced pluripotent stem cells) Adult stems cells.
Complexity	Low to moderate because of simple cellular aggregation with no specific architecture.	Very high complexity due to the organization in tissular structures close to the organ.
Architecture	Homogenous or heterogenous cell masse, without any tissue organization.	Like real tissue (compartmentation, cellular polarization, different cell types).
Cellular differentiation	Not possible, cells keep their initial phenotype.	Possible, allow structural and functional specification.
Physiological functions reproduction	Not possible, or limited	Possible
Cellular polarization	Not possible, cells are randomly disposed.	Possible, cells are oriented / Organized.

continued on following page

Table 3. Continued

Characteristics	Spheroids (Figure 7)	Organoids (Figure 8)
Formation	Spontaneous cells aggregation in adapted conditions (low attachment plates, ultra-low adherence)	Auto-organization is influenced by the extracellular matrix and growth factors.
Development time	Short (few hours to few days)	Long (several days to weeks)
Typical size	Small size (50-500μm)	Variable, (100-1000 μm)
Reproducibility	High, because cell lines derived from spheroids are homogenous.	Moderated to high, depends on the protocol and cell source.
Research use	Cancerology studies. Toxicology. Drugs studies. Tumoral responses studies...	Organ modelisation. Exposome studies. Diseases studies. Regenerative medicine. Drugs screening. Cells interactions studies ....
Therapeutic applications	Used more for preclinical tests and oncology research.	High potential for regenerative medicine, organ transplantation.

Despite their similarity, spheroids and organoids are two quite distinct models. The first is the simpler to design, using different cell types (even primary adult cells), while the second is more complex and expensive to develop, even if it offers better options than spheroids, such as vascularization, which avoids the hypoxia found in spheroids (Figure 7).

The first pioneering work in this field was carried out in 1907 by Henry Van Peters Wilson. He reported the self-assembly of dissociated sponge cells into a whole organism, but the actual evolution has only taken place over the last two decades. The term organoid was first used in 1946 in an unusual way, and its meaning has evolved to refer to structures that resemble organs and has been progressively used *in vitro*.

The organoid is more valid than animal models and patient-derived xenograft models in terms of accuracy, specificity, efficacy, and disease modelling(Inamura et al., 2022). It can use cell types specific to an organ and show structural, functional and molecular similarities with the tissue of origin to obtain mechanistic information on the absorption and penetration of xenobiotics.

Figure 8. Key steps and functional characteristics of organoid in vitro culture.

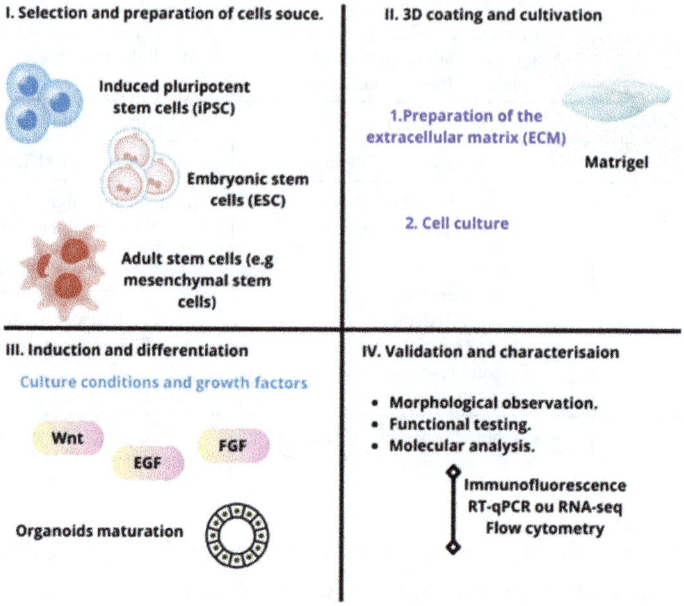

The culture of organoids as a three-dimensional self-organizing model is interesting. Their growth and differentiation are supported by a cocktail of media that provides the essential signaling molecules required for the process. The media choice may depend on the cells involved for the organoid elaboration. They can be either embryonic stem cells, induced pluripotent stem cells, adult stem cells or even cells from well-established cancer cell lines commonly used as single cell cancer models.

Tumoroids or tumor organoids are a well-tested genetic representation of tumors with personalized characteristics. They provide a platform to help bridge the gap between molecular characteristics and patient outcomes. For example, they can be used in organ transplantation in patients with organ failure. Although they are less mature than natural organs, due to a heterotypic cell population or functional immaturity, their use can still be significant as an alternative strategy to real organ transplantation (Ahammed & Kalangi, 2024). In this context, zero-pass organoids have proved to be a rapid and scalable means of studying the properties of cancer in order to test the mechanisms of action of drugs in different clinical cohorts (Przanowska et al., 2024)..

Drug exposome interactions are the future approach for precision medicine (Pristner & Warth, 2020).

In addition, this model has shown significant utility for the study and screening of toxicity and is moving towards the development of treatments for cancer caused by exposure to xenobiotics (Wan et al., 2024). It implements high-throughput drug screening, combining information on drug sensitivity with detailed genomic information to stratify patients.

Studies have targeted the detection of acute toxicity for environmental toxins. They have demonstrated the ability of organoids to investigate the physiological effects of these toxins in a shorter timeframe, using less time-consuming and less complicated methods. These results help to create a picture of toxicity that demonstrates the value of multiple tests to investigate the progression of toxicity in organoids, compare levels found in blood plasma and show that the system effectively mimics human toxicity (Forsythe et al., 2018).

Organoids are promoting in renal carcinoma studies as a model of glomerular and tubular disease. Kidney organoids include kidney organoids derived from pluripotent stem cell, tubuloids derived from renal epithelial cells, collecting duct organoids, uteric bud progenitor cells, duct organoids (Tong, 2022).

The use of a matrix that facilitates organoid development influences the reproducibility of results, which is one of the critical factors in research. Organoids cultured over a long period undergo apoptosis and necrosis due to anoxia. Research has been carried out in this area where organoids have been reincorporated into their base matrix with endothelial cells to vascularize them (Ahammed & Kalangi, 2024).

Although these models are expensive, time-consuming and require monolayer culture, they still do not fully capture the complex physiological structure, function and dynamics of human tissues. They are useful for pre-selecting compounds for transfer because of their reproducibility, standardization, and accessibility (Silva et al., 2025).

C. Organ-on-chip (OOC):

Organ-on-chip (OOC) engineering is the emerging technology of the last few years. First mentioned by Huh et al. (2010), it is based on biophysical principles of microfluidics to simulate real organs in a controlled culture-on-a-chip system. It has been able to stimulate *in vivo* research thanks to the small volume of liquid it uses, which gives it a low Reynold's number (indicating laminar flow) whereas a high Reynold's number means turbulent flow.

The organ-on-chip elaboration can be delicate, and complex due to the adjustable parameters. Device design is crucial for the whole process of human organism simulation, the channels choice, their deposition and the cells used for the study are highly inter-dependent. Once conceived, this model may be useful for a large spectrum of applications.

Dynamic organ-on-chip culture has not only revolutionized *in vitro* culture but also offered innovative solutions for characterizing chemicals and their specific modes of action (Nitsche et al., 2022). This biomimetic micro-dispositive model mimics the physiological functions of organs in culture. It reproduces the micro-environment of cells (Table 1) under physiological conditions more faithfully than the three-dimensional models cited above.

The three-dimensional (3D) chip is bio-printed in a shorter time, incorporate multiple biomaterials, living cells, controlled porosity, record accuracy, and integrate channels and connections. Its advanced microfluidic platform gives it the ability to reproduce the complex interactions between different cell types, the extracellular matrix, and the flow of fluids such as blood or lymph (Farhang Doost & Srivastava, 2024).

a) Chip material

There are several properties that need to be considered when choosing a chip material; surface roughness and wettability are the most important, as they affect cell adhesion and migration. Rigidity is equally significant, as it influences the later stages of cell growth (Galateanu et al., 2022).

b) Porous-compartment-separation membranes

Several polymers may be suitable for the manufacture of the porous membrane used to separate the compartments.

- Natural polymers are highly compatible (collagen, gelatin or polysaccharides) and allow the reproduction of native tissues with channel interactions, allowing the perfusion of oxygen and nutrients to mimic the natural behavior of cell differentiation, spreading and adhesion (Galateanu et al., 2022).
- Synthetic polymers (e.g., polydimethylsiloxane PDMS, polycarbonate PC, polyethylene terephthalate PET, aliphatic polyesters, and polyurethanes) can easily adjust porosity, surface roughness and mechanical properties.

c) Surface treatment

To improve cell adherence and biocompatibility, the chip in contact with cells must be treated.

- With Pluronic acid (in 3D spheroid or organoid culture) to passivate the chip surface and avoid the unwanted breakups through possible cell attachment.

- With protein and extracellular matrix (fibrin, collagen, Matrigel) to increase cell adhesion to the ship substrate (Leung et al., 2022).

d) Cell microenvironment control

Studies mentioned the employment of the original culture media used for the cell type which show positive results (Leung et al., 2022). This can be solved by dividing cell compartments across permeable membranes without the need for a common coculture medium, while allowing paracrine interactions between compartments.

Thanks to this ability to create a realistic model of human organs, this model is remarkably interesting for the study of toxicology (Cho & Yoon, 2017). This model has been used to study the effect on cancer cells and to assess potential side effects on healthy tissues (Silva et al., 2025).

Organ-on-a-chip systems can recapitulate an environment like the *in vivo* environment.

Liver OOC, for example, developed from induced pluripotent stem cells iPSCs have shown advantages and have demonstrated the possibility of developing OOC from the same donor (Messelmani et al., 2022). One study, using a multi-organ-on-chip approach, involved topical exposure of the buccal mucosa to metals to study systemic toxicity and the effect on health (Koning et al., 2021).

The organ-on-chip can be useful to study environmental exposure impacts on human physiology. This model has demonstrated its potential for improving drugs and chemical compounds toxicity prediction, offering more accurate and ethical alternatives to traditional models.

Table 4. Main organs-on-a-chip developed so far.

Organ-on-chip	Principle	References
Hair-on-chip	Evaluating hair follicle biology	(Ataç et al., 2013)
Skin-on-chip	To create more realistic models of the various layers of skin.	(Jones et al., 2022)
Muscle-on-chip	Mimics the morphological and structural intricacies of muscle.	(Agrawal et al., 2017)
Bone-on-chip	Researching cell-cell contact at physiologically significant distances and understanding the cells interaction to cause bone illness such as osteoporosis or metastasis.	(Riquelme et al., 2020)
Spleen-on-chip	Replicate the spleen's filtration function on a chip	(Rigat-Brugarolas et al., 2014)
Eye-on-chip	Facilitates the recapitulation on choroidal neovascularization (CNV) or for drug discovery.	(Chung et al., 2018) (Peng et al., 2020)
Brain-on-chip	To reduce the cost and time used to evaluate drugs that correlate to central nervous system diseases.	(Maoz, 2021)

continued on following page

Table 4. Continued

Organ-on-chip	Principle	References
Blood brain barrier-on-chip	Mimics the protective barrier of the brain to assess drug penetration and neurotoxicity	(Griep et al., 2013)
Nerve-on-chip	Enables the study of neuronal interactions and the neurotoxicity of chemical substances.	(A. D. Sharma et al., 2019)
Bone Marrow-on-chip	Sustain the type of stem cells and preserves the spatial structure within *in vitro* developed 3D bone marrow niche.	(Sieber et al., 2018)
Lung-on-chip	Reproduces the alveolar-capillary barrier to study gas exchange and responses to pathogens.	(Guenat & Berthiaume, 2018)
Heart-on-chip	Stimulates the heartbeat to analyze the effects of drugs on cardiac contractility and electrophysiology.	(Marsano et al., 2016)
Artery-on-chip	To explore underlying mechanisms of high blood pressure.	(Günther et al., 2010)
Stomach-on-chip	Mimicking human gastrointestinal disorders.	(K. K. Lee et al., 2018)
Gut-on-chip	Stimulate the intestinal environment to analyze nutrient absorption and interaction with microbiota.	(Kasendra et al., 2018)
Kidney-on-chip	Models glomerular filtration and tubular reabsorption to test the nephrotoxicity of compounds.	(Musah et al., 2018)
Liver-on-chip	Reproduces hepatic metabolic functions to study drug metabolism and liver toxicity	(Y. B. A. Kang et al., 2015)
Pancreas-on-chip	To evaluate the pancreas islet cell function in specific pancreas dysfunction.	(Shik Mun et al., 2019)
Uterus-on-chip	Integrates models of the ovary, fallopian tube, uterus, and liver to study the menstrual cycle and reproduction	(W. X. Li et al., 2013)
Cervix-on-chip	Studying the physiology of the cervix in real time.	(Tantengco et al., 2022)
Placenta-on-chip	To solve the primary drawback of existing placenta model systems and provide research platform for reproductive biology and medicine.	(J. S. Lee et al., 2016)
Testis-on-chip	Investigates new avenues for the analysis and implementation of *in vitro* testicular function.	(Abumadighem et al., 2022)
Bladder-on-chip	Detecting early uropathogenic Escherichia coli infection.	(K. Sharma et al., 2021)
Lymph nodes-on-chip	Examining the immune system related to pathologies like cancer and inflammation diseases.	(Shanti et al., 2021)
Vagina-on-chip	To improve the understanding of the interaction between the host and microbiome.	(Stone, 2023)

This broad spectrum of studies carried out in the development of on-chip organs clearly illustrates the model's potential to mimic the most complex physiological conditions. It is increasingly important to develop organ-on-chips to satisfy the need for better test systems for diseases studies to overcome the poor knowledge of diseases mechanisms in human model systems and to accelerate drugs development. This development is crucial, it may speed up the time it takes for therapeutic compounds to enter clinical trials. In which, due to the lack of a good human model system, nine out of ten drug candidates failed at late stages of development. It may be applied also for toxicity testing, personalized medicine, and research on disease mechanisms.

D. In silico models

Mathematics and complex equations can be used to study an area as complex as the exposome. Powerful computer tools have the capacity to simulate and analyze biological mechanisms. Based on data collected from *in vitro* or *in vivo* studies. They offer modelling, predicting effects or consequences so that we can avoid them before they materialize.

In silico models are attracting attention because of their ability to integrate and evaluate large quantities of biological and clinical data. They provide a computational framework for understanding the subtleties of disease, generating predictions, guiding experimental design and promoting personalized medicine approaches.

Bioinformatics tools to identify genes associated with tumor progression for validation of their potential as prognostic indicators or new therapeutic targets in the study of cancers.

E. Multiomics

Human biomonitoring is facilitated by advanced methods such as omics, biomonitoring and microphysiological systems (Sillé et al., 2024). It is based on the measurement of chemical substances and their metabolites in biological tissues and fluids (blood, urine, etc.) to assess exposure levels. However, biomonitoring is not limited to biological fluids. As part of the exposome, it also extends to the environment by measuring contaminants in environmental media such as air, water, and soil, providing a context for holistic assessment of human exposure (Sillé et al., 2024).

In this sense, molecular biology techniques are being used in the context of exposome to better integrate equity, diversity, and inclusion into exposure research. Multiomics technologies (genomics, transcriptomics, proteomics, macrobiotics and metabolomics) offer a new field for studying the complex interactions of the exposome across biological layers. These technologies enable detailed analysis of genes, RNA, proteins, metabolites, and biological mechanisms underlining human phenotypes through the integration of multiomics. Gao et al. carried out a study aimed at annotating biological and chemical expressions in the external exposome and human blood. They then integrated it with internal multi-omics to investigate the effect of the exposome on phenotypes and molecular pathways and to show the correlation of environmental components through clinical measurements to associate them with health effects in the external exposome. This has been achieved by integrating DATA from thousands of biological and chemical compounds measured longitudinally with physical factors to see how different stressors influence the proteome, metabolome, and the gut microbiome, as well as cytokines and blood markers. This encourages the use and development of large biobanks, which are essential to guarantee the necessary resources for research in this area. They have had long latency periods, and the continued collection of data from biobanks and pre-existing repositories represents an important priority in the epidemiology of the exposome.

Integrating the exposome and metabolome involves identifying exposures significantly associated with disease, determining metabolic pathways significantly associated with disease, and networking the intersection between exposures associated with disease, and networking the intersection between exposures associated with disease and metabolic pathways, thereby identifying the metabolic mechanisms that intersect between exposure and outcome.

Recent technological and statistical advances in the field of high-resolution metabolomics (HRM) have enabled omic-scale biomonitoring of chemicals derived from the environment, endogenous metabolism and chemicals from food, the gut microbiome, food supplements, pharmaceuticals, and personal use products. As metabolome is a functional indicator of interactions between a person's genes and exposures, HRM of biological samples is one of the most accessible ways of linking environmental exposures to biological status to anticipate breast cancer. Many exposure factors interact with each other against a genetic background to produce a specific biological response (Molina-García et al., 2022).

A study showed that these methods can be used with network and pathway analysis to identify suspect environmental chemicals and functional communities linked to breast cancer outcomes. Such network approaches can be widely applied to discover how lifelong exposures influence personal cancer risk. In the case of breast cancer, we believe that this approach will enable the development of much-needed protocols to enhance protection or mitigate risks associated with pregnancy (Go et al., 2023).

A study has shown the first evidence of assessing the carcinogenic potential of particles generated during 3D printing based on carcinogenic mechanisms (C. H. Lim & Seo, 2024)

V. CHALLENGES AND PROSPECTS:

Table 5. A look at exposome challenges and opportunities.

Challenges			Opportunities
Technical and logistic challenges	Exposure diversity and complexity	The multitude and variability of exposures sources.	Recent progress in high-throughput, real time survey technologies, portable sensors enhance the capacity of measuring with precision diverse expositions.
	Scale and scope pf data collection.	The immense data volume required for exposome (biological samples, environmental measures, personal exposition…).	Infrastructure exploitation of big data and informatics in louds facilitate the storage, management and data analysis.
Normalizing data collection protocol	Resources and infrastructure need.	Setting up and maintaining exposome infrastructure (laboratories, informatic resources).	Strategic partnerships between businesses and governmental agencies.
Data integration and interpretations.	Data sources heterogeneity.	Exposome data sources are diverse (omics technologies, biomonitoring, environmental captors, personal dispositive.	Bioinformatics tools and IA algorithms development to improve data integration.
	Complex data analysis.	Analyzing complex and multidimensional data to identify significant patterns and correlations.	Machine learning use and learning-by-doing techniques to improve the accuracy and efficiency of data analysis.
	Interpretation of causality relations.	Difficulty in establishing causality relation between expositions and effects due to their multifactorial nature and the interaction on diverse expositions.	The use of advanced modeling technics (systems biology, network analysis may help elucidate causality pathways.

A great deal of research has been conducted to elucidate the mechanisms of carcinogenesis of a single metal. But less is known about the synergistic effect of multiple metal pollutants on the development of cancer in humans. Certain carcinogenic metals may influence similar pathways when promoting tumorigenesis, which could lead to a combined mechanism of action. However, given the scale of our daily exposure to a conglomeration of carcinogens, it is important that future research examines the risks of the combined action of several metals and carcinogens, as well as their potential mechanisms for health (Q. Y. Chen et al., 2019).

Environmental exposures complexity and variability poses significant challenges for data collection, analysis and interpretation. Critics argue that the exposome concept may be too broad and ambitious, leading to difficulties in drawing meaningful conclusions from the enormous amount of data generated. There is also a risk of over-interpreting correlations as cause-and-effect relationships, given the multifactorial nature of many diseases. The Human Exposome project needs to consider the variations of the exposome in different populations and environments around the world to truly realize its potential (Sillé et al., 2024).

On the other hand, despite the constant evolution of technology to study exposure, there is a lack of synthesized information on how it has been applied to the study of cancer. The various data sources identified present several obstacles. These include the integration of social exposures and their related challenges, the interpretation, cohesion, and understanding of multiomics datasets both within and between studies, statistical power, exposome cohorts with omics data that are generally small scale <1000 individuals, which calls into question the ability to identify statistically significant trends at the biomolecular level between exposure and effect.

Moreover, the definition of generational impacts and the difficulties in distinguishing between genetic and non-genetic inheritance make it necessary to have intergenerational cohorts. Among the challenges encountered in exposome studies is the short half-life of certain endocrine disruptors in humans, and exposure to chemicals, which confound the results(J. H. Kang et al., 2006). The need to manipulate exposure at the individual level by integrating internal multi-omic profiles. Potential benefits for policy development by dealing holistically with cumulative exposures over the life course. It is therefore necessary and appropriate to provide further evidence of associations of environmental and molecular effects through defined, hypothesis-driven research in closed systems.

The research directions demonstrate the crucial role that xenobiotics play at different stages of cancer development. Degradation enzymes such as cytochrome P450 that degrade xenobiotics (XMEs) play a role in the transformation of procarcinogens into carcinogens, including colorectal cancer, and studies have shown that these enzymes influence drug elimination and treatment resistance. This highlights the importance of further research into the mechanisms by which xenobiotics affect carcinogenesis to develop more effective preventive and therapeutic approaches.

The use of a range of cell types and culture techniques, such as 2D monolayers, 3D spheroids and organoids, significantly improves cancer prevention strategies by providing more realistic models of the tumor microenvironment. While 2D monolayers lack the complexity of in vivo tissues, they provide a simple platform for studying cancer cell behavior and screening for potential chemo preventive drugs. In contrast, 3D spheroids mimic the structure of tumors, providing researchers with a more realistic setting in which to study the efficacy of treatments and the interactions between cancer cells and stromal cells. The most sophisticated model is offered by organoids, which are made from cancer cells or stem cells and faithfully reproduce human tumors while preserving the complexity of the tissues. To fully assess tumor growth and relapse, these models make it easy to study the interplay between cancer cells and the extracellular matrix as well as immune cells and stromal components. Using these tumor models, scientists can identify substances that interfere with cancer cell proliferation as well as with the tumor's beneficial microenvironment, providing more valuable cancer prevention approaches. In another respect, patient-derived organoids can lead to tailor-made methods, which adapt preventive measures to specific genetic contexts, leading to more targeted and successful results. All in all, sophisticated culture methods make it possible to create reliable, patient-specific cancer prevention techniques that are more likely to work in the clinical setting.

VI. CONCLUSION AND PERSPECTIVES:

The human exposome still needs to be deciphered, and existing studies in this context, ranging from basic research to epigenetic studies and environmental toxicology, could provide a new avenue for solidifying the determination of the causal link. There is an urgent need to create a global cancer exposome atlas on the same scale as the Cancer Genome Atlas Program (TCGA) to provide studies with sufficient sample sizes to study the full complexity of the exposome (with tens of thousands of biomarkers) and of cancer (with more than 200 types in addition to subtypes). The cancer exposome will require going beyond looking at one exposure at a time or one cancer at a time and pooling studies into a cumulative resource across populations and diseases. While there are limitations to pooling data from heterogeneous cohorts, harmonizing laboratory methods for analyzing biological samples will improve the comparability of exposome measurements across pooled cohorts. Such an exposome atlas enables a streamlined and agnostic approach to the discovery of new environmental risk factors and biological pathways in disease, which can then inform targeted research by further investigating specific hypotheses-(Young et al., 2025).

On the other hand, longitudinal sampling in the context of the exposome could improve the detection of associations between exposure and cancer, given that the exposome is highly dynamic, not fixed in time and sometimes short-lived in the body. Toxins can affect cancer at various stages during its long latency, including the initiation, promotion or evaluation phases. Repeated sampling would also make it possible to study the intermediate biological response pathways between the exposome and the outcome without relying on cross-sectional data. Finally, multi-analysis per individual considerably increases the statistical power of omics studies by reducing intra-individual variability and the technical variability of metabolites (Young et al., 2025).

REFERENCES

Abumadighem, A., Shuchat, S., Lunenfeld, E., Yossifon, G., & Huleihel, M. (2022). Testis on a chip - A microfluidic three-dimensional culture system for the development of spermatogenesis in-vitro. *Biofabrication*, *14*(3), 035004. Advance online publication. DOI: 10.1088/1758-5090/ac6126 PMID: 35334473

Agrawal, G., Aung, A., & Varghese, S. (2017). Skeletal muscle-on-a-chip: An in vitro model to evaluate tissue formation and injury. *Lab on a Chip*, *17*(20), 3447–3461. DOI: 10.1039/C7LC00512A PMID: 28871305

Ahammed, B., & Kalangi, S. K. (2024). A Decade of Organoid Research: Progress and Challenges in the Field of Organoid Technology. *ACS Omega*, *9*(28), 30087–30096. DOI: 10.1021/acsomega.4c03683 PMID: 39035960

Ataç, B., Wagner, I., Horland, R., Lauster, R., Marx, U., Tonevitsky, A. G., Azar, R. P., & Lindner, G. (2013). Skin and hair on-a-chip: In vitro skin models versus ex vivo tissue maintenance with dynamic perfusion. *Lab on a Chip*, *13*(18), 3555–3561. DOI: 10.1039/c3lc50227a PMID: 23674126

Bolós, V., Gasent, J. M., López-Tarruella, S., & Grande, E. (2010). The dual kinase complex FAK-src as a promising therapeutic target in cancer. In *OncoTargets and Therapy* (Vol. 3, pp. 83–97). Dove Medical Press Ltd. DOI: 10.2147/OTT.S6909

Calafat, A. M., Weuve, J., Ye, X., Jia, L. T., Hu, H., Ringer, S., Huttner, K., & Hauser, R. (2009). Exposure to bisphenol A and other phenols in neonatal intensive care unit premature infants. *Environmental Health Perspectives*, *117*(4), 639–644. DOI: 10.1289/ehp.0800265 PMID: 19440505

Chen, N., Liang, H., Huang, T., & Huang, N. (2022). Exposome approach for identifying modifiable factors for the prevention of colorectal cancer. *Scientific Reports*, *12*(1), 21615. Advance online publication. DOI: 10.1038/s41598-022-25832-9 PMID: 36517625

Chen, Q. Y., DesMarais, T., & Costa, M. (2019). Metals and mechanisms of carcinogenesis. In *Annual Review of Pharmacology and Toxicology* (Vol. 59, pp. 537–554). Annual Reviews Inc. DOI: 10.1146/annurev-pharmtox-010818-021031

Chung, M., Lee, S., Lee, B. J., Son, K., Jeon, N. L., & Kim, J. H. (2018). Wet-AMD on a Chip: Modeling Outer Blood-Retinal Barrier In Vitro. *Advanced Healthcare Materials*, *7*(2), 1700028. Advance online publication. DOI: 10.1002/adhm.201700028 PMID: 28557377

Colwell, M. L., Townsel, C., Petroff, R. L., Goodrich, J. M., & Dolinoy, D. C. (2023). Epigenetics and the exposome: DNA methylation as a proxy for health impacts of prenatal environmental exposures. *Exposome, 3*(1), osad001. Advance online publication. DOI: 10.1093/exposome/osad001 PMID: 37333730

Corcos, C., Brey, J., & Corcos, L. (2002). The nuclear receptors CAR and PXR control induction of cytochromes P450 by phenobarbital. In *Medecine/Sciences* (Vol. 18, pp. 429–437). Elsevier Masson SAS. DOI: 10.1051/medsci/2002184429

Costa, E. C., Moreira, A. F., de Melo-Diogo, D., Gaspar, V. M., Carvalho, M. P., & Correia, I. J. (2016). 3D tumor spheroids: an overview on the tools and techniques used for their analysis. In *Biotechnology Advances* (Vol. 34, pp. 1427–1441). Elsevier Inc. DOI: 10.1016/j.biotechadv.2016.11.002

Danieli, M. G., Casciaro, M., Paladini, A., Bartolucci, M., Sordoni, M., Shoenfeld, Y., & Gangemi, S. (2024). Exposome: Epigenetics and autoimmune diseases. In *Autoimmunity Reviews* (Vol. 23). Elsevier B.V. DOI: 10.1016/j.autrev.2024.103584

Dzierżyński, E., Gawlik, P. J., Puźniak, D., Flieger, W., Jóźwik, K., Teresiński, G., Forma, A., Wdowiak, P., Baj, J., & Flieger, J. (2024). Microplastics in the Human Body: Exposure, Detection, and Risk of Carcinogenesis: A State-of-the-Art Review. *Cancers (Basel), 16*(21), 3703. Advance online publication. DOI: 10.3390/cancers16213703 PMID: 39518141

Ezez, D., Birhanu, H., Shamena, S., & Engidaw, S. (2024). Bioaccumulation of heavy metals, assessment of carcinogenic and non-carcinogenic health risk in various spices. *Journal of Hazardous Materials Advances, 15*, 100441. Advance online publication. DOI: 10.1016/j.hazadv.2024.100441

Farhang Doost, N., & Srivastava, S. K. (2024). A Comprehensive Review of Organ-on-a-Chip Technology and Its Applications. In *Biosensors* (Vol. 14). Multidisciplinary Digital Publishing Institute (MDPI). DOI: 10.3390/bios14050225

Fellah, S. (2024). *Stratégies thérapeutiques permettant de limiter l'agression chimique des xénobiotiques : ciblage du long ARN non codant DNM3OS et du récepteur à l'adénosine A2A.* https://doi.org/HALId:tel-04642293https://theses.hal.science/tel-04642293v1

Forsythe, S. D., Devarasetty, M., Shupe, T., Bishop, C., Atala, A., Soker, S., & Skardal, A. (2018). Environmental toxin screening using human-derived 3D bioengineered liver and cardiac organoids. *Frontiers in Public Health, 6*, 103. Advance online publication. DOI: 10.3389/fpubh.2018.00103 PMID: 29755963

Galateanu, B., Hudita, A., Biru, E. I., Iovu, H., Zaharia, C., Simsensohn, E., Costache, M., Petca, R. C., & Jinga, V. (2022). Applications of Polymers for Organ-on-Chip Technology in Urology. In *Polymers* (Vol. 14). MDPI., DOI: 10.3390/polym14091668

Gao, B., Shu, Z., Ren, S., & Gao, D. (2022). Biobanking: A foundation of life-science research and advancement. *Biosafety and Health, 4*(5), 285–289. DOI: 10.1016/j.bsheal.2022.09.003

Gearhart-Serna, L. M., Davis, J. B., Jolly, M. K., Jayasundara, N., Sauer, S. J., Di Giulio, R. T., & Devi, G. R. (2020). A polycyclic aromatic hydrocarbon-enriched environmental chemical mixture enhances AhR, antiapoptotic signaling and a proliferative phenotype in breast cancer cells. *Carcinogenesis, 41*(12), 1648–1659. DOI: 10.1093/carcin/bgaa047 PMID: 32747956

Ghantous, A., Hernandez-Vargas, H., Byrnes, G., Dwyer, T., & Herceg, Z. (2015). Characterising the epigenome as a key component of the fetal exposome in evaluating in utero exposures and childhood cancer risk. In *Mutagenesis* (Vol. 30, pp. 733–742). Oxford University Press. DOI: 10.1093/mutage/gev010

Go, Y. M., Weinberg, J., Teeny, S., Cirillo, P. M., Krigbaum, N. Y., Singer, G., Tran, V. L., Cohn, B. A., & Jones, D. P. (2023a). Exposome epidemiology for suspect environmental chemical exposures during pregnancy linked to subsequent breast cancer diagnosis. *Environment International, 178*, 108112. Advance online publication. DOI: 10.1016/j.envint.2023.108112 PMID: 37517180

Go, Y. M., Weinberg, J., Teeny, S., Cirillo, P. M., Krigbaum, N. Y., Singer, G., Tran, V. L., Cohn, B. A., & Jones, D. P. (2023b). Exposome epidemiology for suspect environmental chemical exposures during pregnancy linked to subsequent breast cancer diagnosis. *Environment International, 178*, 108112. Advance online publication. DOI: 10.1016/j.envint.2023.108112 PMID: 37517180

Gracia-Cazaña, T., González, S., Parrado, C., Juarranz, Á., & Gilaberte, Y. (2020). Influence of the Exposome on Skin Cancer. [English Edition]. *Actas Dermo-Sifiliográficas, 111*(6), 460–470. DOI: 10.1016/j.adengl.2020.04.011 PMID: 32507282

Griep, L. M., Wolbers, F., De Wagenaar, B., Ter Braak, P. M., Weksler, B. B., Romero, I. A., Couraud, P. O., Vermes, I., Van Der Meer, A. D., & Van Den Berg, A. (2013). BBB on CHIP: Microfluidic platform to mechanically and biochemically modulate blood-brain barrier function. *Biomedical Microdevices, 15*(1), 145–150. DOI: 10.1007/s10544-012-9699-7 PMID: 22955726

Guenat, O. T., & Berthiaume, F. (2018). Incorporating mechanical strain in organs-on-a-chip: Lung and skin. *Biomicrofluidics*, *12*(4), 042207. DOI: 10.1063/1.5024895 PMID: 29861818

Günther, A., Yasotharan, S., Vagaon, A., Lochovsky, C., Pinto, S., Yang, J., Lau, C., Voigtlaender-Bolz, J., & Bolz, S. S. (2010). A microfluidic platform for probing small artery structure and function. *Lab on a Chip*, *10*(18), 2341–2349. DOI: 10.1039/c004675b PMID: 20603685

Huang, C. Y., Xie, R. H., Li, P. H., Chen, C. Y., You, B. H., Sun, Y. C., Chou, C. K., Chang, Y. H., Lin, W. C., & Chen, G. Y. (2025). Environmental Exposure to Bisphenol A Enhances Invasiveness in Papillary Thyroid Cancer. *International Journal of Molecular Sciences*, *26*(2), 814. Advance online publication. DOI: 10.3390/ijms26020814 PMID: 39859529

Huh, D., Matthews, B. D., Mammoto, A., Montoya-Zavala, M., Yuan Hsin, H., & Ingber, D. E. (2010). Reconstituting organ-level lung functions on a chip. *Science*, *328*(5986), 1662–1668. DOI: 10.1126/science.1188302 PMID: 20576885

IARC. (2006). *Mécanismes du développement tumoral.*

Inamura, K., Hamada, T., Bullman, S., Ugai, T., Yachida, S., & Ogino, S. (2022). Cancer as microenvironmental, systemic and environmental diseases: opportunity for transdisciplinary microbiomics science. In *Gut* (Vol. 71, pp. 2107–2122). BMJ Publishing Group., DOI: 10.1136/gutjnl-2022-327209

Irigaray, P., & Belpomme, D. (2010). Basic properties and molecular mechanisms of exogenous chemical carcinogens. In *Carcinogenesis* (Vol. 31, pp. 135–148). DOI: 10.1093/carcin/bgp252

Isachesku, E., Braicu, C., Pirlog, R., Kocijancic, A., Busuioc, C., Pruteanu, L. L., Pandey, D. P., & Berindan-Neagoe, I. (2023). The Role of Non-Coding RNAs in Epigenetic Dysregulation in Glioblastoma Development. In *International Journal of Molecular Sciences* (Vol. 24). Multidisciplinary Digital Publishing Institute (MDPI). DOI: 10.3390/ijms242216320

Jiang, C., Wang, X., Li, X., Inlora, J., Wang, T., Liu, Q., & Snyder, M. (2018). Dynamic Human Environmental Exposome Revealed by Longitudinal Personal Monitoring. *Cell*, *175*(1), 277–291.e31. DOI: 10.1016/j.cell.2018.08.060 PMID: 30241608

Jones, C. F. E., Di Cio, S., Connelly, J. T., & Gautrot, J. E. (2022). Design of an Integrated Microvascularized Human Skin-on-a-Chip Tissue Equivalent Model. *Frontiers in Bioengineering and Biotechnology, 10*, 915702. DOI: 10.3389/fbioe.2022.915702 PMID: 35928950

Juarez, M. N., McDermott, A., Wade, M. G., & Plante, I. (2024). Exposure to brominated flame retardants in utero and through lactation delays the development of DMBA-induced mammary cancer: Potential effects on subtypes? *Frontiers in Endocrinology, 15*, 1429142. DOI: 10.3389/fendo.2024.1429142 PMID: 39610845

Kang, J. H., Kondo, F., & Katayama, Y. (2006). Human exposure to bisphenol A. In *Toxicology* (Vol. 226, pp. 79–89). DOI: 10.1016/j.tox.2006.06.009

Kang, Y. B. A., Sodunke, T. R., Lamontagne, J., Cirillo, J., Rajiv, C., Bouchard, M. J., & Noh, M. (2015). Liver sinusoid on a chip: Long-term layered co-culture of primary rat hepatocytes and endothelial cells in microfluidic platforms. *Biotechnology and Bioengineering, 112*(12), 2571–2582. DOI: 10.1002/bit.25659 PMID: 25994312

Kasendra, M., Tovaglieri, A., Sontheimer-Phelps, A., Jalili-Firoozinezhad, S., Bein, A., Chalkiadaki, A., Scholl, W., Zhang, C., Rickner, H., Richmond, C. A., Li, H., Breault, D. T., & Ingber, D. E. (2018). Development of a primary human Small Intestine-on-a-Chip using biopsy-derived organoids. *Scientific Reports, 8*(1), 2871. Advance online publication. DOI: 10.1038/s41598-018-21201-7 PMID: 29440725

Kim, K. H., Lee, S. J., Kim, J., & Moon, Y. (2024). Leveraging Xenobiotic-Responsive Cancer Stemness in Cell Line-Based Tumoroids for Evaluating Chemoresistance: A Proof-of-Concept Study on Environmental Susceptibility. *International Journal of Molecular Sciences, 25*(21), 11383. Advance online publication. DOI: 10.3390/ijms252111383 PMID: 39518936

Koning, J. J., Rodrigues Neves, C. T., Schimek, K., Thon, M., Spiekstra, S. W., Waaijman, T., de Gruijl, T. D., & Gibbs, S. (2021). A Multi-Organ-on-Chip Approach to Investigate How Oral Exposure to Metals Can Cause Systemic Toxicity Leading to Langerhans Cell Activation in Skin. *Frontiers in Toxicology, 3*, 824825. Advance online publication. DOI: 10.3389/ftox.2021.824825 PMID: 35295125

Krausová, M., Braun, D., Buerki-Thurnherr, T., Gundacker, C., Schernhammer, E., Wisgrill, L., & Warth, B. (2023). Understanding the Chemical Exposome During Fetal Development and Early Childhood: A Review. In *Annual Review of Pharmacology and Toxicology* (Vol. 63, pp. 517–540). Annual Reviews Inc. DOI: 10.1146/annurev-pharmtox-051922-113350

Kumar, V., Vashishta, M., Kong, L., Wu, X., Lu, J. J., Guha, C., & Dwarakanath, B. S. (2021). The Role of Notch, Hedgehog, and Wnt Signaling Pathways in the Resistance of Tumors to Anticancer Therapies. In *Frontiers in Cell and Developmental Biology* (Vol. 9). Frontiers Media S.A. DOI: 10.3389/fcell.2021.650772

Langenbach, T. (2013). Persistence and Bioaccumulation of Persistent Organic Pollutants (POPs). In *Applied Bioremediation - Active and Passive Approaches.* InTech. DOI: 10.5772/56418

Lauri, G., Mills, K., Majumder, S., & Capurso, G. (2025). The exposome as a target for primary prevention and a tool for early detection of pancreatic cancer. In *Best Practice and Research: Clinical Gastroenterology*. Bailliere Tindall Ltd. DOI: 10.1016/j.bpg.2025.101991

Lee, J. S., Romero, R., Han, Y. M., Kim, H. C., Kim, C. J., Hong, J. S., & Huh, D. (2016). Placenta-on-A-chip: A novel platform to study the biology of the human placenta. *The Journal of Maternal-Fetal & Neonatal Medicine, 29*(7), 1046–1054. DOI: 10.3109/14767058.2015.1038518 PMID: 26075842

Lee, K. K., McCauley, H. A., Broda, T. R., Kofron, M. J., Wells, J. M., & Hong, C. I. (2018). Human stomach-on-a-chip with luminal flow and peristaltic-like motility. *Lab on a Chip, 18*(20), 3079–3085. DOI: 10.1039/C8LC00910D PMID: 30238091

Leung, C. M., de Haan, P., Ronaldson-Bouchard, K., Kim, G. A., Ko, J., Rho, H. S., Chen, Z., Habibovic, P., Jeon, N. L., Takayama, S., Shuler, M. L., Vunjak-Novakovic, G., Frey, O., Verpoorte, E., & Toh, Y. C. (2022). A guide to the organ-on-a-chip. In *Nature Reviews Methods Primers* (Vol. 2). Springer Nature., DOI: 10.1038/s43586-022-00118-6

Li, W. X., Liang, G. T., Yan, W., Zhang, Q., Wang, W., Zhou, X. M., & Liu, D. Y. (2013). Artificial uterus on a microfluidic chip. *Fenxi Huaxue. Chinese Journal of Analytical Chemistry, 41*(4), 467–472. DOI: 10.1016/S1872-2040(13)60639-8

Li, Z., Ma, J., Li, X., Chan, M. T. V., Wu, W. K. K., Wu, Z., & Shen, J. (2019). Aberrantly expressed long non-coding RNAs in air pollution-induced congenital defects. *Journal of Cellular and Molecular Medicine, 23*(11), 7717–7725. DOI: 10.1111/jcmm.14645 PMID: 31557384

Li, Z., Romanoff, L., Bartell, S., Pittman, E. N., Trinidad, D. A., McClean, M., Webster, T. F., & Sjödin, A. (2012). Excretion Profiles and half-lives of ten urinary polycyclic aromatic hydrocarbon metabolites after dietary exposure. *Chemical Research in Toxicology, 25*(7), 1452–1461. DOI: 10.1021/tx300108e PMID: 22663094

Lim, C. H., & Seo, D. S. (2024). Assessment of the carcinogenic potential of particulate matter generated from 3D printing devices in Balb/c 3T3-1-1 cells. *Scientific Reports, 14*(1), 23981. DOI: 10.1038/s41598-024-75491-1 PMID: 39402095

Lim, D. (2015). *Rôle du récepteur des hydrocarbures aromatiques chez les cellules T auxiliaires dans le contrôle de la réponse immunitaire*. Https://Www.Semanticscholar.Org/Paper/R%C3%B4le-Du-R%C3%A9cepteur-Des-Hydrocarbures-Aromatiques-Les-Lim/2acbff8244f316a8a47469d7625c0a4817cc5376

Lipenga, T., Matumba, L., Vidal, A., Herceg, Z., McCormack, V., De Saeger, S., & De Boevre, M. (2021). A concise review towards defining the exposome of oesophageal cancer in sub-Saharan Africa. In *Environment International* (Vol. 157). Elsevier Ltd. DOI: 10.1016/j.envint.2021.106880

Long, J., Zhang, C.-J., Zhu, N., Du, K., Yin, Y.-F., Tan, X., Liao, D.-F., & Qin, L. (2018). Lipid metabolism and carcinogenesis, cancer development. In *Am J Cancer Res* (Vol. 8, Issue 5). www.ajcr.us/ISSN:2156-6976/ajcr0076971

Madrigal, J. M., Pruitt, C. N., Fisher, J. A., Liao, L. M., Graubard, B. I., Gierach, G. L., Silverman, D. T., Ward, M. H., & Jones, R. R. (2024). Carcinogenic industrial air pollution and postmenopausal breast cancer risk in the National Institutes of Health AARP Diet and Health Study. *Environment International, 191*, 108985. DOI: 10.1016/j.envint.2024.108985 PMID: 39226766

Mahanayak, B. (2024). Biotransformation reactions of xenobiotics: Mechanisms and implications for environmental and human health. *World Journal of Biology Pharmacy and Health Sciences, 19*(1), 158–164. DOI: 10.30574/wjbphs.2024.19.1.0406

Maksymchuk, O., & Kashuba, V. (2019). Dietary lipids and environmental xenobiotics as risk factors for prostate cancer: The role of cytochrome P450. *Pharmacological Reports, 71*(5), 826–832. DOI: 10.1016/j.pharep.2019.04.011 PMID: 31382168

Manz, K. E., Feerick, A., Braun, J. M., Feng, Y. L., Hall, A., Koelmel, J., Manzano, C., Newton, S. R., Pennell, K. D., Place, B. J., Godri Pollitt, K. J., Prasse, C., & Young, J. A. (2023). Non-targeted analysis (NTA) and suspect screening analysis (SSA): a review of examining the chemical exposome. In *Journal of Exposure Science and Environmental Epidemiology* (Vol. 33, pp. 524–536). Springer Nature. DOI: 10.1038/s41370-023-00574-6

Maoz, B. M. (2021). Brain-on-a-Chip: Characterizing the next generation of advanced in vitro platforms for modeling the central nervous system. *APL Bioengineering, 5*(3), 030902. DOI: 10.1063/5.0055812 PMID: 34368601

Marsano, A., Conficconi, C., Lemme, M., Occhetta, P., Gaudiello, E., Votta, E., Cerino, G., Redaelli, A., & Rasponi, M. (2016). Beating heart on a chip: A novel microfluidic platform to generate functional 3D cardiac microtissues. *Lab on a Chip*, *16*(3), 599–610. DOI: 10.1039/C5LC01356A PMID: 26758922

Messelmani, T., Morisseau, L., Sakai, Y., Legallais, C., Le Goff, A., Leclerc, E., & Jellali, R. (2022). Liver organ-on-chip models for toxicity studies and risk assessment. In *Lab on a Chip* (Vol. 22, pp. 2423–2450). Royal Society of Chemistry. DOI: 10.1039/D2LC00307D

Molina-García, M., Malvehy, J., Granger, C., Garre, A., Trullàs, C., & Puig, S. (2022). Exposome and Skin. Part 2. The Influential Role of the Exposome, Beyond UVR, in Actinic Keratosis, Bowen's Disease and Squamous Cell Carcinoma: A Proposal. In *Dermatology and Therapy* (Vol. 12, Issue 2, pp. 361–380). Adis. DOI: 10.1007/s13555-021-00644-3

Mulware, S. J. (2013). The Mammary Gland Carcinogens: The Role of Metal Compounds and Organic Solvents. *International Journal of Breast Cancer*, *2013*, 1–10. DOI: 10.1155/2013/640851 PMID: 23762568

Musah, S., Dimitrakakis, N., Camacho, D. M., Church, G. M., & Ingber, D. E. (2018). Directed differentiation of human induced pluripotent stem cells into mature kidney podocytes and establishment of a Glomerulus Chip. *Nature Protocols*, *13*(7), 1662–1685. DOI: 10.1038/s41596-018-0007-8 PMID: 29995874

Nakano, M., Gi, M., Toyooka, T., Suzuki, S., Wanibuchi, H., & Takebayashi, T. (2025). Occupational health topics series on the effects of chemicals: Epidemiological and toxicological risk assessments of ortho-toluidine for bladder cancer. *Journal of Occupational Health*, *67*(1), uiaf005. Advance online publication. DOI: 10.1093/joccuh/uiaf005 PMID: 39930727

Nault, J.-C. (2015). *Spécialité : Bases Fondamentales de l'Oncogenèse Présentée par Identification de nouveaux mécanismes de carcinogenèse et facteurs pronostiques des tumeurs hépatocellulaires.*

Nitsche, K. S., Müller, I., Malcomber, S., Carmichael, P. L., & Bouwmeester, H. (2022). Implementing organ-on-chip in a next-generation risk assessment of chemicals: a review. In *Archives of Toxicology* (Vol. 96, Issue 3, pp. 711–741). Springer Science and Business Media Deutschland GmbH. DOI: 10.1007/s00204-022-03234-0

Olmedo-Suárez, M. Á., Ramírez-Díaz, I., Pérez-González, A., Molina-Herrera, A., Coral-García, M. Á., Lobato, S., Sarvari, P., Barreto, G., & Rubio, K. (2022). Epigenetic Regulation in Exposome-Induced Tumorigenesis: Emerging Roles of ncRNAs. *Biomolecules, 12*(4), 513. Advance online publication. DOI: 10.3390/biom12040513 PMID: 35454102

Pal, S., & Firdous, S. M. (2024). Unraveling the role of heavy metals xenobiotics in cancer: a critical review. In *Discover Oncology* (Vol. 15). Springer Science and Business Media B.V. DOI: 10.1007/s12672-024-01417-y

Parkinson, L. V., Geueke, B., & Muncke, J. (2024). Potential mammary carcinogens used in food contact articles: Implications for policy, enforcement, and prevention. *Frontiers in Toxicology, 6*, 1440331. DOI: 10.3389/ftox.2024.1440331 PMID: 39381597

Pristner, M., & Warth, B. (2020). Drug–Exposome Interactions: The Next Frontier in Precision Medicine. In *Trends in Pharmacological Sciences* (Vol. 41, pp. 994–1005). Elsevier Ltd. DOI: 10.1016/j.tips.2020.09.012

Przanowska, R. K., Labban, N., Przanowski, P., Hawes, R. B., Atkins, K. A., Showalter, S. L., & Janes, K. A. (2024). Patient-derived response estimates from zero-passage organoids of luminal breast cancer. BioRxiv *: The Preprint Server for Biology.*

Qin, N., He, W., Liu, W., Kong, X., Xu, F., & Giesy, J. P. (2020). Tissue distribution, bioaccumulation, and carcinogenic risk of polycyclic aromatic hydrocarbons in aquatic organisms from Lake Chaohu, China. *The Science of the Total Environment, 749*, 141577. Advance online publication. DOI: 10.1016/j.scitotenv.2020.141577 PMID: 32829278

Rigat-Brugarolas, L. G., Elizalde-Torrent, A., Bernabeu, M., De Niz, M., Martin-Jaular, L., Fernandez-Becerra, C., Homs-Corbera, A., Samitier, J., & Del Portillo, H. A. (2014). A functional microengineered model of the human splenon-on-a-chip. *Lab on a Chip, 14*(10), 1715–1724. DOI: 10.1039/C3LC51449H PMID: 24663955

Riquelme, M. A., Cardenas, E. R., & Jiang, J. X. (2020). Osteocytes and Bone Metastasis. *Frontiers in Endocrinology, 11*, 567844. DOI: 10.3389/fendo.2020.567844 PMID: 33162934

Sarlak, S. (2021). *Exposome du cancer : reprogrammation métabolique du cancer du poumon par les nitrosamines spécifiques de la fumée de tabac.* Https://Hal.Science/Tel-04138441/

Shanti, A., Hallfors, N., Petroianu, G. A., Planelles, L., & Stefanini, C. (2021). Lymph Nodes-On-Chip: Promising Immune Platforms for Pharmacological and Toxicological Applications. *Frontiers in Pharmacology, 12*, 711307. DOI: 10.3389/fphar.2021.711307 PMID: 34483920

Sharma, A. D., McCoy, L., Jacobs, E., Willey, H., Behn, J. Q., Nguyen, H., Bolon, B., Curley, J. L., & Moore, M. J. (2019). Engineering a 3D functional human peripheral nerve in vitro using the Nerve-on-a-Chip platform. *Scientific Reports, 9*(1), 8921. Advance online publication. DOI: 10.1038/s41598-019-45407-5 PMID: 31222141

Sharma, K., Dhar, N., Thacker, V. V., Simonet, T. M., Signorino-Gelo, F., Knott, G., & McKinney, J. D. (2021). Dynamic persistence of intracellular bacterial communities of uropathogenic escherichia coli in a human bladder-chip model of urinary tract infections. *eLife, 10*. Advance online publication. DOI: 10.7554/eLife.66481 PMID: 34219648

Shik Mun, K., Arora, K., Huang, Y., Yang, F., Yarlagadda, S., Ramananda, Y., Abu-El-Haija, M., Palermo, J. J., Appakalai, B. N., Nathan, J. D., & Naren, A. P. (2019). Patient-derived pancreas-on-a-chip to model cystic fibrosis-related disorders. *Nature Communications, 10*(1), 3124. Advance online publication. DOI: 10.1038/s41467-019-11178-w PMID: 31311920

Sieber, S., Wirth, L., Cavak, N., Koenigsmark, M., Marx, U., Lauster, R., & Rosowski, M. (2018). Bone marrow-on-a-chip: Long-term culture of human haematopoietic stem cells in a three-dimensional microfluidic environment. *Journal of Tissue Engineering and Regenerative Medicine, 12*(2), 479–489. DOI: 10.1002/term.2507 PMID: 28658717

Sillé, F. C. M., Busquet, F., Fitzpatrick, S., Herrmann, K., Leenhouts-Martin, L., Luechtefeld, T., Maertens, A., Miller, G. W., Smirnova, L., Tsaioun, K., & Hartung, T. (2024). The Implementation Moonshot Project for Alternative Chemical Testing (IMPACT) toward a Human Exposome Project. *ALTEX, 41*(3), 344–362. DOI: 10.14573/altex.2407081 PMID: 39016082

Silva, J., Oliveira, P. A., Duarte, J. A., & Faustino-Rocha, A. I. (2025). Mammary Cancer Models: An Overview from the Past to the Future. *In Vivo (Athens, Greece), 39*(1), 1–16. DOI: 10.21873/invivo.13800 PMID: 39740866

Smith, M. T., Guyton, K. Z., Gibbons, C. F., Fritz, J. M., Portier, C. J., Rusyn, I., DeMarini, D. M., Caldwell, J. C., Kavlock, R. J., Lambert, P. F., Hecht, S. S., Bucher, J. R., Stewart, B. W., Baan, R. A., Cogliano, V. J., & Straif, K. (2016). Key characteristics of carcinogens as a basis for organizing data on mechanisms of carcinogenesis. In *Environmental Health Perspectives* (Vol. 124, pp. 713–721). Public Health Services, US Dept of Health and Human Services. DOI: 10.1289/ehp.1509912

Stone, L. (2023). A vagina on a chip to model microbiome–host interactions. In *Nature Reviews Urology* (Vol. 20, p. 64). Nature Research., DOI: 10.1038/s41585-022-00717-8

Takata, A., Yamauchi, H., Yamashita, K., Aminaka, M., Hitomi, T., Toya, T., & Kohyama, N. (2025). Mesothelioma carcinogenesis of chrysotile and forsterite compared and validated by intraperitoneal injection in rat. *Industrial Health*, *63*(1), 14–28. Advance online publication. DOI: 10.2486/indhealth.2024-0025

Tantengco, O. A. G., Richardson, L., Radnaa, E., Kammala, A. K., Kechichian, T., Ganguly, E., Kim, S., Han, A., Medina, P. M., & Menon, R. (2022). Cervix-on-a-chip for investigating ascending Ureaplasma parvum infection in pregnancy. *American Journal of Obstetrics and Gynecology*, *226*(1), S12–S13. DOI: 10.1016/j.ajog.2021.11.068

Tomkiewicz, C., Coumoul, X., Nioche, P., Barouki, R., & Blanc, E. B. (2024). Costs of molecular adaptation to the chemical exposome: A focus on xenobiotic metabolism pathways. *Philosophical Transactions of the Royal Society of London. Series B, Biological Sciences*, *379*(1898), 20220510. Advance online publication. DOI: 10.1098/rstb.2022.0510 PMID: 38310928

Vázquez-Gómez, G., Petráš, J., Dvořák, Z., & Vondráček, J. (2023). Aryl hydrocarbon receptor (AhR) and pregnane X receptor (PXR) play both distinct and common roles in the regulation of colon homeostasis and intestinal carcinogenesis. In *Biochemical Pharmacology* (Vol. 216). Elsevier Inc. DOI: 10.1016/j.bcp.2023.115797

Vineis, P., Schatzkin, A., & Potter, J. D. (2010). Models of carcinogenesis: An overview. In *Carcinogenesis* (Vol. 31, pp. 1703–1709). Oxford University Press. DOI: 10.1093/carcin/bgq087

VoPham, T., White, A. J., & Jones, R. R. (2024). Geospatial Science for the Environmental Epidemiology of Cancer in the Exposome Era. *Cancer Epidemiology, Biomarkers & Prevention*, *33*(4), 451–460. DOI: 10.1158/1055-9965.EPI-23-1237 PMID: 38566558

Wan, Y., Ding, J., Jia, Z., Hong, Y., Tian, G., Zheng, S., Pan, P., Wang, J., & Liang, H. (2024). Current trends and research topics regarding organoids: A bibliometric analysis of global research from 2000 to 2023. *Heliyon, 10*(12), e32965. DOI: 10.1016/j.heliyon.2024.e32965 PMID: 39022082

Wei, X., Huang, Z., Jiang, L., Li, Y., Zhang, X., Leng, Y., & Jiang, C. (2022). Charting the landscape of the environmental exposome. In *iMeta* (Vol. 1). John Wiley and Sons Inc. DOI: 10.1002/imt2.50

Wiese, D., DuBois, T. D., Sorice, K. A., Fang, C. Y., Ragin, C., Daly, M., Reese, A. C., Henry, K. A., & Lynch, S. M. (2024). An exploratory analysis of the impact of area-level exposome on geographic disparities in aggressive prostate cancer. *Scientific Reports, 14*(1), 16900. Advance online publication. DOI: 10.1038/s41598-024-63726-0 PMID: 39075110

Wild, C. P. (2005). Complementing the genome with an "exposome": The outstanding challenge of environmental exposure measurement in molecular epidemiology. In *Cancer Epidemiology Biomarkers and Prevention* (Vol. 14, pp. 1847–1850). DOI: 10.1158/1055-9965.EPI-05-0456

Yamada, H., Odagiri, M., Yamakita, K., Chiba, A., Ukai, A., Yasui, M., Honma, M., Sugiyama, K.-I., Ura, K., & Sassa, A. (2025). Dual-directional epi-genotoxicity assay for assessing chemically induced epigenetic effects utilizing the housekeeping TK gene. *Scientific Reports, 15*(1), 7780. DOI: 10.1038/s41598-025-92121-6 PMID: 40044744

Young, A. S., Mullins, C. E., Sehgal, N., Vermeulen, R. C. H., Kolijn, P. M., Vlaanderen, J., Rahman, M. L., Birmann, B. M., Barupal, D., Lan, Q., Rothman, N., & Walker, D. I. (2025). The need for a cancer exposome atlas: a scoping review. In *JNCI Cancer Spectrum* (Vol. 9). Oxford University Press. DOI: 10.1093/jncics/pkae122

Zhang, P., Carlsten, C., Chaleckis, R., Hanhineva, K., Huang, M., Isobe, T., Koistinen, V. M., Meister, I., Papazian, S., Sdougkou, K., Xie, H., Martin, J. W., Rappaport, S. M., Tsugawa, H., Walker, D. I., Woodruff, T. J., Wright, R. O., & Wheelock, C. E. (2021). Defining the Scope of Exposome Studies and Research Needs from a Multidisciplinary Perspective. In *Environmental Science and Technology Letters* (Vol. 8, Issue 10, pp. 839–852). American Chemical Society. DOI: 10.1021/acs.estlett.1c00648

Chapter 7
Environmental DNA and RNA Metabarcoding:
Advancing Insights in Cancer Research

Odangowei Inetiminebi Ogidi
https://orcid.org/0000-0002-9961-893X
Bayelsa Medical University, Yenagoa, Nigeria

Ejeomo Christopher
Michael and Cecilia Ibru University, Ughelli, Nigeria

Happiness Adaekwu Orlu
https://orcid.org/0000-0001-7142-487X
River State University, Port-Harcourt, Nigeria

ABSTRACT

Environmental DNA (eDNA) and RNA (eRNA) technologies, when integrated with metabarcoding, have emerged as significant instruments in cancer research particularly in exposomics and environmental carcinogenesis. These approaches facilitate the identification and monitoring of genetic material from many environmental sources, yielding insights into the biological and chemical factors that influence cancer risk. Environmental samples can be examined to identify pollutants, microbiota, and other molecular markers that contribute to carcinogenesis through the use of eDNA and eRNA. Metabarcoding enhances this technique by employing high-throughput sequencing to facilitate the comprehensive characterisation of complex ecosystems, the detection of potential carcinogenic exposures, and the elucidation of their interactions with human health. This methodology possesses significant potential for enhancing our comprehension of the environmental factors associated

DOI: 10.4018/979-8-3373-2165-3.ch007

with early detection, prevention, and treatments. This chapter explores the concept of the human exposome as evidenced by eDNA and eRNA.

INTRODUCTION

Environmental DNA (eDNA) and RNA (eRNA) metabarcoding have revolutionised molecular ecology by facilitating the identification of genetic material excreted by organisms into their surroundings. These approaches, first designed for ecological study and biodiversity evaluation, are currently being investigated for biological applications, including cancer research. Blood, urine, and saliva contain extracellular nucleic acids, holding potential new gateways in precision medicine, monitoring disease, and cancer diagnosis using non-invasive techniques. Biomarkers for cancer are determined and dynamics of and progression of cancer are revealed using bioinformatics and high-throughput sequencing (Wan et al., 2020; Ogidi et al., 2024a).

Early cancer diagnosis is one of the biggest problems in oncology because conventional methods of diagnosis are not very sensitive and specific. Conventional tumour sample approaches are invasive, costly, and cannot capture all tumour heterogeneity. According to Heitzer et al. (2019), liquid biopsy approaches offer a non-invasive solution to identifying genetic mutations, epigenetic changes, and other molecular alterations in cancer. These techniques measure cell-free DNA (cfDNA) and cell-free RNA (cfRNA) in body fluids. Improved genetic stratification by eDNA and eRNA metabarcoding technologies drives early diagnosis, risk assessment, and patient stratification for therapeutic targeting (Heitzer et al., 2019).

The tumour microenvironment plays an important role in cancer development, such as tumour growth, immune evasion, and metastasis, beyond the early detection phase. Extracellular nucleic acids serve as significant markers of malignant processes derived from cell death of cancer cells, necrosis, and active secretion (Mohan et al., 2022). Metabarcoding analysis of extracellular nucleic acids allows researchers to follow the development of cancer in real-time, the treatment response, and new drug resistance in real-time. It is a useful tool for personalization of therapy in precision oncology, where tumour genomes are dynamically changing. Environmental oncology and cancer epidemiology were established utilizing eDNA metabarcoding and eRNA cancer research. The research has discovered that carcinogens and environmental pollutants can alter the structure and nucleic acid content of extracellular nucleic acids, thereby opening the door to cancer formation (Cheng et al., 2021). Analysis of how environmental determinants affect cancer occurrence and development can be supported by analysis of environmental eDNA and eRNA and hence improve public health interventions and prevention.

While there is huge potential for eDNA and eRNA metabarcoding in cancer research, there are problems to be solved. Some of the most significant challenges to overcome are contamination, degradation of nucleic acids, and difficulties in interpreting sequencing data (Cheng et al., 2021). To enable clinical reproducibility and utility, strategies need to be standardized, biomarkers need to be validated, and efficient bioinformatics pipelines need to be developed (Ogidi & Emaikwu, 2024). Metabarcoding in clinical oncology will become more achievable and a part of standard procedure over the coming years with the advancement in sequencing technologies and computational power. The chapter examines environmental DNA and RNA metabarcoding's prospects to advance cancer research, diagnostics, disease monitoring, precision medicine, and epidemiology. These methods offer new solutions through the integration of molecular ecology and oncology, improving cancer diagnosis, tracking disease progression, and personalising treatment for patients. Continued refinement and evolution of these methods could significantly enhance our ability to fight cancer and enable us to come up with more effective and personalised treatments.

Objectives of the Chapter

The aims of this chapter are as follows:

(1) To review the fundamentals of environmental DNA and RNA metabarcoding.
(2) To evaluate the applications in cancer research.
(3) To determine the methodologies and technological advances.
(4) To assess the challenges and limitations.
(5) To X ray the future directions and clinical implications of environmental DNA and RNA metabarcoding in cancer research.

Organization of the Chapter

The rest of this chapter is organized as follows: Section 2 explores fundamentals of environmental DNA and RNA metabarcoding Section 3 evaluate the applications in cancer research Section 4 determine the methodologies and technological advances.. Section 5 assess the challenges and limitations. Section 6 X rayed the future directions and clinical implications of environmental DNA and RNA metabarcoding in cancer research. Finally, a concluding section summarizes the key takeaways of the chapter.

FUNDAMENTALS OF ENVIRONMENTAL DNA AND RNA METABARCODING

Definition and Mechanisms of eDNA and eRNA Metabarcoding

Environmental DNA (eDNA) and environmental RNA (eRNA) metabarcoding are scientific methods applied to analyze genetic material that is released by organisms into their environment. These methods have transformed disease monitoring and biodiversity inventory by enabling non-invasive detection of species and biological processes. eDNA contains extracellular remnants of DNA formed from biological activities like secretion, excretion, or decomposition (Ogidi 2024b). In contrast, eRNA consists of just-transcribed RNA molecules and captures information regarding the pattern of gene expression and, therefore, bears testimony to continuous biological processes (Cristescu & Hebert, 2018).

The general metabarcoding method includes amplification and sequencing of specific genetic markers that are common to most taxonomic groups. The method allows researchers to recognize species composition within an environmental sample without direct observation or conventional culture techniques (Deiner et al., 2017). For example, in aquatic ecosystems, eDNA extracted from water samples can identify fish, amphibians, and microbial communities, while eRNA from soil samples can examine microbial activity and plant-microbe relationships. These are now being utilized in cancer research to measure tumor-derived nucleic acids in liquid biopsies, offering a minimally invasive approach to disease detection and tracking progression (Barnes & Turner, 2016; Ogidi, 2024).

Differences Between eDNA and eRNA in Biological Research

The fundamental difference between eDNA and eRNA lies in how stable they are and their purpose. Environmental DNA (eDNA) is extremely stable and can remain within ecosystems for extended durations, thereby making it an effective tool for retroactive biodiversity and species distribution analyses (Stewart et al., 2021). This stability enables researchers to reconstruct past environmental shifts and identify rare or cryptic species. The persistence of eDNA can blur the distinction between contemporary and historical biological activity, causing false positives during monitoring of existing populations (Lafferty et al., 2021).

In contrast, eRNA is extremely unstable because it is prone to enzymatic degradation. This instability, once thought to be a limitation, renders eRNA a perfect marker for real-time biological activity (Best et al., 2019). Detection of RNA in an environmental sample signals active gene transcription and the presence of living organisms because RNA degrades quickly after cell death. This feature is especially helpful in cancer research as eRNA analysis can detect actively transcribed oncogenes and tumor-suppressor genes, giving vital information on disease progression (Stewart et al., 2021). Secondly, eRNA profiling can be employed in monitoring the response to treatment in cancer patients as transcript abundance changes can reflect therapeutic response (Best et al., 2019; Ogidi & Tawariowei, 2023).

One of the main distinctions between eDNA and eRNA lies in their use. Environmental DNA (eDNA) is routinely used in ecological and evolutionary research to study species diversity and community dynamics, while environmental RNA (eRNA) is primarily utilized in functional genomics and biomedical research. In oncology, the identification of circulating tumour RNA (ctRNA) in blood samples is an attractive approach to liquid biopsies as it offers a dynamic snapshot of tumour activity with the potential to disclose cancer-specific mutations in near real-time (Heitzer et al., 2019). Table 1 presents the distinction between eDNA and eRNA in biological research.

Table 1. Differences between eDNA and eRNA in biological research

Feature	Environmental DNA (eDNA)	Environmental RNA (eRNA)
Definition	DNA fragments released from cells into the environment, including bodily fluids, soil, and water.	RNA molecules actively transcribed from DNA, found in circulating fluids and extracellular vesicles.
Source	Released from dead cells, lysed cells, or shed by living organisms.	Comes from actively transcribing cells and extracellular vesicles.
Stability	Highly stable due to its double-stranded structure; persists in the environment for extended periods.	Highly unstable due to rapid degradation by ribonucleases (RNases) and environmental factors.
Primary Function	Provides genetic information for species identification, population genetics, and evolutionary studies.	Reflects real-time gene expression and dynamic cellular activities.
Applications in Cancer Research	Used for detecting genetic mutations, tumor DNA profiling, and microbial diversity in tumor microenvironments.	Used for identifying cancer-specific gene expression patterns, tracking treatment response, and biomarker discovery.
Detection Methods	PCR, qPCR, next-generation sequencing (NGS), and whole-genome sequencing (WGS).	RNA-seq, quantitative PCR (qPCR), microarrays, and single-cell RNA sequencing (scRNA-seq).
Clinical Utility	Useful for identifying hereditary cancer risks, detecting tumor DNA in blood (liquid biopsy), and studying microbiome-cancer interactions.	Helps in precision oncology by analyzing gene expression, immune responses, and therapy resistance mechanisms.
Role in Metabarcoding	Used for species identification and microbial diversity studies in cancer-associated microbiomes.	Used for transcriptomic profiling, tracking tumor evolution, and distinguishing active tumor cells.

continued on following page

Table 1. Continued

Feature	Environmental DNA (eDNA)	Environmental RNA (eRNA)
Persistence in Samples	Can persist for weeks to months in environmental and clinical samples.	Degrades within minutes to hours unless preserved under optimal conditions.
Challenges	Risk of contamination from environmental sources; difficulty in distinguishing between historical and recent DNA signals.	Requires immediate stabilization and careful handling to prevent RNA degradation.

Techniques and Methodologies Used for Metabarcoding

The first step in metabarcoding is sampling of environmental materials, i.e., water, soil, air, or body fluids. The samples should be preserved to prevent the breakdown of nucleic acids through various methods depending on the eDNA or eRNA analysis. In eDNA studies, samples are usually filtered and stored at low temperatures to preserve DNA integrity, whereas eRNA samples need to be immediately stabilized using RNA preservatives like RNAlater to avoid degradation (Callahan et al., 2016). Nucleic acids are subsequently purified after extraction to remove impurities that will interfere with downstream applications. DNA and RNA extraction kits for environmental samples are often used to maximize recovery efficiency. eRNA analysis involves a second step of reverse transcription, in which RNA is transcribed into complementary DNA (cDNA) using reverse transcriptase enzymes. The step specifically analyzes actively transcribed genetic material, giving feedback on functional gene expression (Callahan et al., 2016). Polymerase chain reaction (PCR) amplification of the specific genetic markers is the next step.

Marker genes are chosen based on the species of interest and research purpose. Mitochondrial cytochrome c oxidase I (COI) is widely utilized for the identification of animal species, whereas bacterial and eukaryotic taxon prefer 16S and 18S ribosomal RNA genes, respectively. According to Stewart et al. (2021), ITS region is the most commonly used genetic marker in fungal research. Cordier et al. (2019) found that RNA biomarkers, including miRNAs and long non-coding RNAs (lncRNAs), sequencing allowed scientists to establish tumour-specific patterns of gene expression. Next-generation sequencing technologies like PacBio, Illumina, and Oxford Nanopore facilitate the rapid generation of millions of reads from DNA or RNA sequences. The methods are optimally suited for various research applications due to their distinctive sequencing depths, read lengths, and error rates. Heitzer et al. (2019) say that Illumina sequencing is suitable for metabarcoding analysis because, in addition to its high precision and short-read benefit, Oxford Nanopore offers long-read sequencing, which is useful in the construction of complicated genomes. Bioinformatics pipelines enhance raw sequencing data by re-assembling reads, eliminating sequencing errors, and assigning taxonomy against reference databases such as GenBank, SILVA, or UNITE. Metabarcoding pipelines are also employing machine learning techniques to enhance accuracy and data interpretation. Open-source software packages such as QIIME2 and DADA2 provide taxonomy classification (Callahan et al., 2016; Cordier et al., 2019). It is the contention of Heitzer et al. (2019) that bioinformatics techniques are utilized in cancer research with a view to predicting patient outcomes based on eRNA signatures, determining gene expression profiles, and detecting cancer-associated mutations. Metabarcoding is susceptible to a number of limitations despite its usefulness.

Some taxa can be over-represented due to the bias in PCR amplification used, thus affecting the accuracy of species identification. The possibility of poor-quality or incorrect reference databases also discourages sequence classification (Ogidi et al., 2024c). Contamination is also a major issue, where small amounts of exogenous DNA or RNA may affect results. Researchers always endeavor to create bioinformatics software, employ more rigorous sampling and analysis protocols, and refine primer design to overcome those issues. Ecological and biological sciences increasingly view the promise of the use of metabarcoding technology innovation. Best et al. (2019) propose that the application of eRNA metabarcoding in conjunction with artificial intelligence and big data analysis has tremendous possibilities to enhance early detection, precision therapy, and treatment monitoring of cancer research. High-throughput sequencing and computer processing enable pioneering advancements in pathogenic and environmental processes, immensely contributing to medicinal and research growth (Ogidi et al., 2024d).

APPLICATIONS OF ENVIRONMENTAL DNA AND RNA METABARCODING IN CANCER RESEARCH

Environmental DNA (eDNA) and RNA (eRNA) metabarcoding have transformed cancer research by facilitating non-invasive biomarker identification, tumour surveillance, and tailored therapeutic approaches. These kinds of methodologies are utilized in early cancer detection through the identification of oncogenic mutations and aberrant gene expression within circulating nucleic acids in biofluids including blood, urine, and saliva (Best et al., 2019). Liquid biopsy uses eDNA and eRNA in applications for tracking tumour progression, therapeutic resistance, and minimal residual disease following treatment, and hence improves real-time tracking of cancer development (Heitzer et al., 2019). Moreover, tumour microenvironment analyses by eDNA metabarcoding enable the characterisation of cancer-associated microbiomes, which reveal microbial impacts on carcinogenesis (Flemer et al., 2017;

Ogidi & Felagha, 2024). Single-cell RNA sequencing enhances characterisation of tumour heterogeneity by revealing treatment-refractory subpopulations in tumours (Stewart et al., 2021). Combining machine learning and AI with metabarcoding further improves biomarker discovery, cancer subclassification, prediction of response to immunotherapy, and personalization of clinical interventions (Min et al., 2017; Ogidi & Ajoko, 2024). Better sequencing technologies are likely to revolutionize oncology by offering very accurate, less-invasive diagnoses and treatments. Figure 1 and Table 2 illustrate the applicability of environmental DNA and RNA metabarcoding in oncological research.

Figure 1. Some applications of environmental DNA and RNA metabarcoding in cancer research

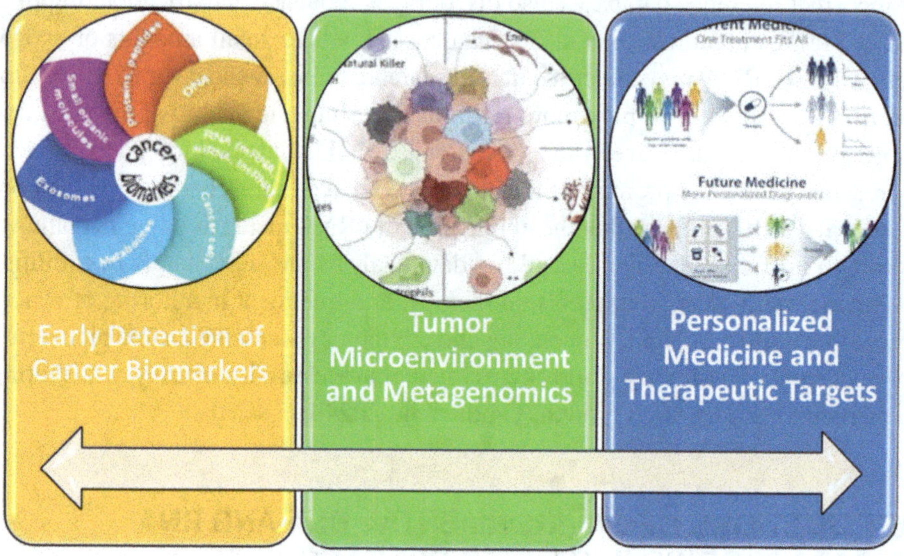

Early Detection of Cancer Biomarkers

Role of eRNA in Identifying Oncogenes and Tumor Suppressor Genes

An important aspect of cancer research lies in the identification of genes governing cell growth, apoptosis, and genome integrity; oncogenes and tumour suppressors, in turn. Metabarcoding of eRNA is an efficient method to analyze the gene expression levels so that genetic aberrations linked to malignancies may be identified without delay. Carcinogenesis may be facilitated through mutations or overexpression of the oncogenes KRAS, BRAF, and MYC. Researchers are able to sequence patient sample eRNA to identify oncogenes with high transcript levels and thereby offer important diagnostic and prognostic data (Best et al., 2019). TP53, RB1, and PTEN are tumor suppressor genes that restrict cell growth without regulation. Cancer can be more easily formed if the tumor-suppressing activities of these genes are lost due to mutations or epigenetic suppression. Stewart et al. (2021) indicated that metabarcoding eRNA can discriminate between benign and cancerous conditions through the determination of low levels of expression for these essential genes. eRNA profiling identifies changes in genes and measures carcinogenesis pathway activation with a general outline of cancer biology and enabling precision oncology therapy construction (Cristescu & Hebert, 2018).

Detection of Circulating Tumor DNA (ctDNA) and RNA for Prognosis

It is crucial that major biomarkers for non-invasive cancer tracking, circulating tumour DNA (ctDNA) and RNA (ctRNA), offer real-time tumour evolution. The genomic content of the original tumour is reflected in ctDNA, which consists of DNA fragments released into the bloodstream by cancer cells (Heitzer et al., 2019). Therapeutic methods and results could be guided by the identification of certain ctDNA abnormalities, for example, PIK3CA mutations in breast cancer and EGFR mutations in non-small cell lung cancer. Likewise, ctRNA, like mRNA, miRNA, and lncRNA, is also important in determining the prognosis of cancer. Since tumour cells are translating ctRNA in real time, having ctRNA in the blood or other body fluids reflects real-time tumour activity. The prognosis for certain cancers is poor owing to increased oncogenic microRNA miR-21 expression (Best et al., 2019). Stewart et al. (2021) found that clinicians are able to track alterations in gene expression, tumour burden evaluation, and minimum residual disease identification using a combination of eRNA metabarcoding and liquid biopsy approaches.

Tumor Microenvironment and Metagenomics

Influence of Microbial Diversity on Cancer Progression

The tumour microenvironment (TME) is composed of cancer cells, immune cells, stromal cells, and microbiome that interact with one another to affect tumour growth and response to treatment. Emerging evidence demonstrates that microbial diversity within the tumour microenvironment has a significant effect on carcinogenesis, whereby certain bacteria can promote or suppress tumour formation (Deiner et al., 2017). Fusobacterium nucleatum is associated with colorectal cancer through promoting inflammation and suppressing anti-tumour immunity, whereas

Lactobacillus species have protective functions through modifying host immunity (Deiner et al., 2017). eRNA metabarcoding enables researchers to describe tumour-associated microbial communities, revealing information about their functional contribution to cancer progression. RNA transcript sequencing of microorganisms enables separation between tumour-associated, metabolically active bacteria and pathogenic commensal microorganisms (Cristescu & Hebert, 2018). The exposure of such microbial interactions may provide insight into new targets for therapy, such as microbiome-modulating compounds that manipulate the tumor-associated microbial milieu for the facilitation of treatment effect (Stewart et al., 2021).

Metabarcoding for Profiling Microbiomes Linked to Carcinogenesis

Metabarcoding and metagenomic techniques have transformed carcinogenic microbiome studies, enabling high-resolution tumour bacterial, viral, and fungal community characterization. Researchers can define carcinogenesis-involving species, e.g., Helicobacter pylori in gastric cancer and Epstein-Barr virus (EBV) in nasopharyngeal carcinoma, through sequencing microbial RNA and DNA extracted from tumour tissues (Deiner et al., 2017). In addition to bacterial and viral elements, fungal populations are increasingly being seen as key contributors to cancer progression. Research indicates that Candida species can enhance the inflammatory milieu in gastrointestinal cancers, whereas Malassezia has been associated with pancreatic ductal adenocarcinoma (Stewart et al., 2021). eRNA metabarcoding provides greater insight into these interactions by identifying transcriptionally active microbial populations, rather than using DNA-based presence/absence data (Cordier et al., 2019). This strategy provides a more accurate definition of microbiome function that enhances the identification of cancer-associated microbial signatures and candidate biomarkers for early diagnosis.

Personalized Medicine and Therapeutic Targets

Role of eRNA in Gene Expression Profiling for Targeted Therapy

Precision medicine aims to tailor therapy based on an individual's molecular and genetic tumor profile. metabarcoding eRNA has proven helpful in this regard as it allows for reliable gene expression profiling for matching to appropriate targeted therapy (Best et al., 2019). In contrast to DNA-based methods that examine fixed genetic mutations, RNA-based profiling identifies dynamic alterations in gene expression due to environmental stress, treatment, and evolution of the tumor. For example, subtypes of breast cancer such as luminal A, luminal B, HER2-enriched, and triple-negative breast cancer all have distinct patterns of gene expression that inform treatment. Endocrine therapy is sensitive in hormone receptor-positive cancers, while those with HER2 overexpression are treated with HER2 inhibitors such as trastuzumab (Stewart et al., 2021). Using eRNA expression, oncologists can personalize treatment and improve therapeutic response. Additionally, eRNA profiling has allowed the discovery of novel drug targets, including non-coding RNAs that regulate oncogenic processes (Heitzer et al., 2019).

Identifying Tumor-Specific Mutations and Epigenetic Changes

Apart from gene expression profiling, eRNA metabarcoding also facilitates the detection of tumor-specific mutations and epigenetic alterations affecting cancer development. The majority of cancers harbor mutations in key regulatory genes, e.g., IDH1 in glioma and BRAF V600E in melanoma. Detection of such mutations through eRNA analysis allows for precise molecular classification and targeted therapy selection (Stewart et al., 2021). There exist a number of epigenetic alterations, including DNA, histone, and RNA-mediated gene silencing, involved in cancer development and progression. Post-transcriptional regulation has provided important regulatory components, including microRNAs and long non-coding RNAs, through eRNA-based epigenomic analysis (Cristescu & Hebert, 2018). Epithelial-to-mesenchymal transition (EMT), implicated in the miR-200 family, is a process of metastasis. By characterizing these epigenetic regulators, researchers can engineer epigenetic therapy to reestablish normal patterns of gene expression and identify candidate biomarkers for early cancer diagnosis.

Table 2. Applications of environmental DNA and RNA metabarcoding in cancer research

Application	Description	Key Benefits	Example Cancer Types	Reference
Early Detection of Cancer Biomarkers	eRNA metabarcoding helps identify oncogenes and tumor suppressor genes from circulating nucleic acids in biofluids.	Enables non-invasive, early detection of cancer before symptoms arise.	Lung cancer, Breast cancer, Colorectal cancer	Best et al. (2019)
Liquid Biopsy for Cancer Monitoring	eDNA and eRNA sequencing of blood-derived ctDNA/ctRNA provides real-time insights into tumor evolution.	Tracks treatment response and minimal residual disease (MRD) with high sensitivity.	Breast cancer, Prostate cancer, Pancreatic cancer	Heitzer et al. (2019)
Microbiome Profiling and Tumor Microenvironment Analysis	eDNA metabarcoding identifies microbial communities influencing cancer progression.	Uncovers microbial signatures associated with tumorigenesis and potential therapeutic targets.	Colorectal cancer, Gastric cancer, Liver cancer	Flemer et al. (2017)
Gene Expression Profiling for Precision Medicine	eRNA sequencing reveals tumor-specific gene expression patterns for targeted therapy selection.	Enhances personalized treatment strategies by identifying actionable mutations.	Leukemia, Lung cancer, Melanoma	Stewart et al. (2021)
AI and Machine Learning for Biomarker Discovery	AI-driven analysis of metabarcoding data improves cancer classification and prognosis.	Automates biomarker identification, increasing diagnostic accuracy.	Pancreatic cancer, Brain cancer, Breast cancer	Min et al. (2017)
Epigenetic Modifications and Cancer Progression	eRNA metabarcoding detects methylation changes and histone modifications linked to tumor biology.	Helps in understanding cancer progression and identifying new drug targets.	Gastric cancer, Ovarian cancer, Colorectal cancer	Sun et al. (2021)
Single-Cell RNA Sequencing for Tumor Heterogeneity Analysis	eRNA sequencing at the single-cell level helps characterize tumor subpopulations.	Reveals tumor heterogeneity and identifies treatment-resistant clones.	Small-cell lung cancer, Glioblastoma, Ovarian cancer	Stewart et al. (2021); Ogidi et al., 2024b
Metabarcoding for Identifying Fusion Genes in Leukemia	Long-read sequencing of eRNA detects oncogenic fusion transcripts in hematologic malignancies.	Improves leukemia classification and aids in targeted therapy selection.	Acute myeloid leukemia (AML), Chronic myeloid leukemia (CML)	Smith et al. (2020)

continued on following page

Table 2. Continued

Application	Description	Key Benefits	Example Cancer Types	Reference
Metabarcoding-Based Immunotherapy Response Prediction	eRNA profiling identifies immune-related gene signatures predictive of immunotherapy success.	Helps stratify patients for immune checkpoint inhibitors and CAR-T cell therapies.	Melanoma, Non-small cell lung cancer (NSCLC), Bladder cancer	Chen et al. (2021)
Tracking Metastatic Evolution with Metabarcoding	eRNA sequencing reveals transcriptomic changes associated with metastasis.	Enables real-time monitoring of tumor progression and metastasis risk.	Breast cancer, Prostate cancer, Pancreatic cancer	Heitzer et al. (2019)
Detecting Minimal Residual Disease (MRD) After Cancer Treatment	eRNA metabarcoding identifies trace amounts of residual tumor-derived RNA after therapy.	Helps detect recurrence at earlier stages than imaging-based techniques.	Leukemia, Colorectal cancer, Lung cancer	Best et al. (2019)

THE POTENTIAL OF ENVIRONMENTAL DNA AND RNA METABARCODING IN ADVANCING CANCER RESEARCH

Environmental DNA (eDNA) and RNA (eRNA) metabarcoding provides a paradigm in cancer diagnosis by enabling the detection of cancer-related genetic markers through non-invasive liquid biopsies. Traditional cancer diagnosis through tissue biopsies is possibly invasive, costly, and laborious to repeat while tracking the disease (Heitzer et al., 2019). In contrast, eDNA and eRNA metabarcoding allow the identification of circulating tumor DNA (ctDNA) and RNA in bodily fluids such as blood, urine, and saliva, a minimally invasive but highly sensitive approach to cancer detection (Wan et al., 2020). This approach enhances presymptomatic cancer diagnosis through the detection of mutations, epigenetic changes, and oncogene expression profiles before advanced tumors develop, improving patient survival through earlier intervention (Ogidi et al., 2025a,b).

Other than diagnostics, disease monitoring is also one very important application of eDNA and eRNA metabarcoding in cancer. Monitoring of cancer development and therapy response can be done in real time using circulating nucleic acids from apoptotic and necrotic cancer cells (Mohan et al., 2022). Such extracellular nucleic acids contain informative data regarding tumor dynamics, and clinicians can monitor the response to treatment as well as residual disease or relapse prior to its visibility through standard imaging procedures (Siravegna et al., 2017). Continuous monitoring of eDNA and eRNA allows for individualized treatment adjustment, reducing the risk of overtreatment or useless therapies while improving patient outcomes.

In precision medicine, metabarcoding of eDNA and eRNA is critically significant in identifying patient-specific genetic mutations which can guide targeted therapy. Cancer illness is highly heterogeneous and requires the therapy to be customized according to the tumor profile in order to deliver the best therapeutic responses (Cheng et al., 2021). Next-generation sequencing technologies can detect new genetic mutations and resistance patterns, which can help oncologists prescribe drugs best suited for the individual patient (Heitzer et al., 2019). For example, the identification of specific mutations in ctDNA can determine whether or not a patient is eligible for immunotherapy or targeted therapy programs, markedly improving treatment with reduced side effects.

Furthermore, metabarcoding of eRNA and eDNA is used in cancer epidemiology in the sense that it allows for the facilitation of extensive population studies of genetic risk factors and environmental effects on cancer development. Researchers can ascertain how carcinogen exposure, pollutants, and lifestyle factors impact the development of cancer through extracellular nucleic acid analysis of environmental and biological matrices (Cheng et al., 2021). This approach can detect new biomarkers of susceptibility to cancer, leading to improved public health policy and prevention. Longitudinal eDNA and eRNA study can also track cancer occurrence in different populations, providing improved early detection schemes and resource planning in healthcare systems (Ogidi, 2025).

While promising, eDNA and eRNA metabarcoding clinically combined for cancer studies faces challenges. Sample degradation, contamination, and bioinformatics analysis complexity are some of the challenges that require attention for robustness and reproducibility (Mohan et al., 2022). It further requires standardized protocols and regulatory clearances to be used widely clinically. However, with ongoing improvement in sequencing technology and data interpretation, eDNA and eRNA metabarcoding will most probably be a treasured resource in cancer diagnosis, disease surveillance, precision medicine, and epidemiology, and ultimately translate into improved patient care and survival.

MICROBIAL eDNA/eRNA AS A POWERFUL TOOL IN CANCER PREVENTION

Recent advances in metagenomic next-generation sequencing (mNGS) technology have been successful in revolutionizing the detection and characterization of microbial DNA (eDNA) and RNA (eRNA) in clinical samples, yielding unprecedented insights into infectious agents' involvement in cancerogenesis. Different from the pathogen-specific diagnostic methodology, mNGS provides room for profiling comprehensive microbial genetic material in a sample, thereby determining known and even unknown microorganisms involved in cancer causation (Simner et al., 2017). This unbiased tool has helped elucidate relationships between a diverse array of microbes including parasites, viruses, fungi, and bacteria with carcinomas, also informing on microbe roles in the development of cancer.

Application of eDNA and eRNA metabarcoding techniques has shown the complex interplay between the human microbiome and cancer. For instance, studies have established the existence of some bacterial species, such as Fusobacterium nucleatum, in colorectal cancer tissues, suggesting a potential tumor-initiating and growth-promoting role (Kostic et al., 2013). In a similar vein, viral pathogens such as human papillomavirus (HPV) have been found to cause cervical and other anogenital cancers, underlining the relevance of viral eDNA detection in cancer prevention strategies (Walboomers et al., 1999). These findings emphasize the necessity of rigorous microbial profiling in the detection of oncogenic pathogens and in describing their mechanism of action.

Apart from pathogen detection, mNGS can give functional characterization of microbial communities such as metabolic and immunologic pathways through which microbes can influence carcinogenesis. Metabolite detection from microbes and their engagement with host signaling networks, for example, can reveal mechanisms by which the microbiome controls inflammation, immune response, and cell proliferation—all critical determinants in cancer development (Garrett, 2015). Furthermore, the integration of microbial genomic data with host transcriptomic and epigenomic signatures enables a holistic interpretation of the tumor microenvironment and its modulation by microbial effects.

In order to maximize optimally the therapeutic potential of microbial eDNA and eRNA profiling for cancer prevention, there is an imperative need to standardize and validate mNGS technologies. The existence of standardized protocols for sample collection, nucleic acid extraction, sequencing, and bioinformatics analysis will ensure comparability and consistency of results between studies, with eventual translation of the findings to clinical use (Chiu & Miller, 2019). In addition, the development of robust bioinformatics pipelines with the capacity to accurately detect pathogenic signals against background noise is essential for unambiguous interpretation of advanced metagenomic data. With these hurdles overcome, the integration of microbial genomics into oncology stands to develop new diagnostic, prognostic, and therapeutic modalities to reduce the global cancer burden.

METHODOLOGIES AND TECHNOLOGICAL ADVANCES IN EDNA/ERNA METABARCODING FOR CANCER RESEARCH

Metabarcoding of eDNA and eRNA has transformed cancer studies with the provision for non-invasive, high-throughput analysis of tumour genomics and transcriptomics with eDNA and eRNA metabarcoding. Shendure et al. (2017) and Amarasinghe et al. (2020) showed that mutations, fusion genes, and alternative splicing events associated with tumours are optimally revealed by NGS and long-read sequencing technologies like PacBio and Oxford Nanopore. Whole-genome sequencing (WGS) and whole-exome sequencing (WES) are enhancing genomic profiling by enabling the identification of novel oncogenic mutations and tumour suppressor gene mutations (Shendure et al., 2017). Machine learning algorithms enhance biomarker discovery through the identification of intricate gene expression signatures linked to tumour development, whereas bioinformatics software such as STAR, HISAT2, and QIIME2 enable sequencing data processing and analysis (Callahan et al., 2016; Min et al., 2017). Liquid biopsy technology has advanced in recent years to enable real-time monitoring of tumours without the need for surgery.

This enables the assessment and determination of treatment response at an early stage (Heitzer et al., 2019). MeDIP-seq, WGBS (Methylation Sequencing), ChIP-seq, and ATAC-seq are epigenetic and transcriptomic technologies that disclose cancer progression and resistance to treatment mechanisms by gene regulation and chromatin accessibility (Sun et al., 2021). Furthermore, single-cell RNA sequencing (scRNA-seq) enables quantification of gene expression at the single-cell level and offers valuable insights into tumour heterogeneity and treatment-resistant subpopulations (Stewart et al., 2021). The intersection of AI-driven analytics and multi-omics will likewise transform cancer biomarker discovery and precision medicine applications as these technologies evolve further (Ogidi & Tobia, 2024). Recent advancements in sequencing technology, bioinformatics, and machine learning herald a new era of precision, individualisation, and efficacy in cancer diagnosis and therapy. Table 3 presents methods and technical advancements in eDNA/eRNA metabarcoding for cancer research.

Figure 2. Methodologies and technological advances in eDNA/eRNA metabarcoding for cancer research

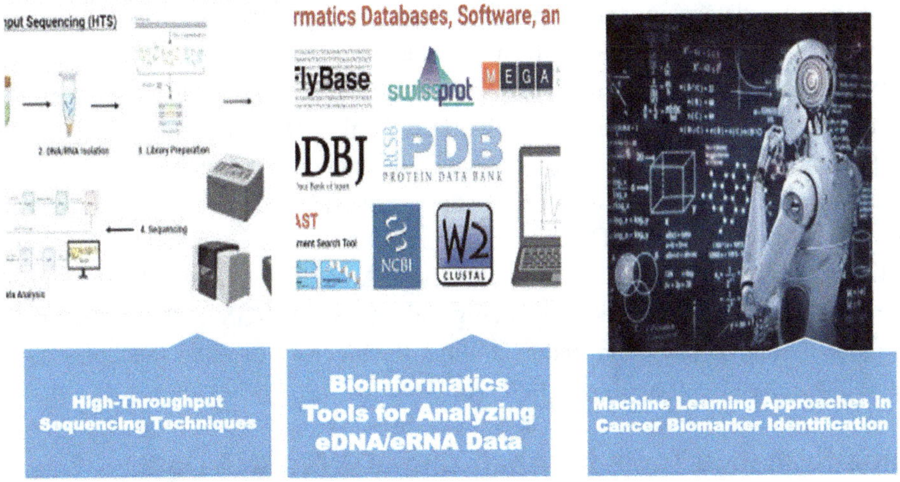

High-Throughput Sequencing Techniques

Next-Generation Sequencing (NGS) in eDNA/eRNA Analysis

Next-Generation Sequencing (NGS) has facilitated the rapid and efficient sequencing of eDNA and eRNA molecules, which has revolutionized cancer genetics. Next-generation sequencing (NGS) technologies are suitable for large-scale biomarker discovery since they can sequence millions of DNA or RNA fragments simultaneously, in contrast to the conventional Sanger sequencing (Shendure et al., 2017). This technology enables cancer to be diagnosed and monitored non-surgically through liquid biopsies through the detection of circulating tumour DNA (ctDNA) and RNA (ctRNA) (Heitzer et al., 2019). NGS is of utmost application with eRNA metabarcoding because of its ability to enable transcriptome-scale analysis of gene expression within cancer cells. RNA transcript sequencing can ascertain the active transcription of genes, therefore defining tumor-specific signatures and the related carcinogenic mechanisms (Best et al., 2019). RNA sequencing, one of the standard uses of next-generation sequencing (NGS), has facilitated the identification of new biomarkers that are associated with resistance to therapy and tumour heterogeneity characterization (Cristescu & Hebert, 2018).

Single-Molecule Sequencing Technologies

While it has the potential for high-throughput sequencing, NGS is not flawless and does not detect epigenetic modifications or large structural rearrangements. PacBio and ONT are single-molecule sequencing technologies that bypass these limitations by generating long-read sequences, thereby providing more genomic context (Amarasinghe et al., 2020). Stewart et al. (2021) confirm that long-read sequencing is especially efficient in identifying cancer-associated fusion genes and alternative splicing mechanisms. One of the strongest aspects of cancer epigenetics is base modifications, and ONT sequencing enables real-time analysis and the identification of alterations such as DNA methylation (Amarasinghe et al., 2020). Through the combination of long-read sequencing and traditional NGS methods, researchers are able to develop a clearer understanding of cancer's molecular mechanisms and establish more effective diagnostic tools.

Bioinformatics Tools for Analyzing eDNA/eRNA Data

Preprocessing and Quality Control of Sequencing Data

Comprehensive bioinformatics analysis is essential to extract valuable insights from the substantial volumes of sequencing data generated by next-generation sequencing (NGS) and single-molecule sequencing. Quality control and preprocessing constitute the preliminary phases of bioinformatics analysis. They consist of adaptor sequence trimming, sequencing error, and low-quality reads (Bolger et al., 2014). Sequencing quality is typically verified and error data filtered out by software such as FastQC and Trimmomatic (Andrews, 2010). rRNA sequence removal, typically a high percentage of total RNA, is also a pre-processing requirement for eRNA analysis. Kopylova et al. (2012) stated that SortMeRNA and ribo-zero depletion kits are both methods that improve the specificity of RNA sequencing through the detection of protein-coding transcripts. Minimizing biases in gene expression quantitation, correct preprocessing ensures reproducible and accurate downstream outcomes.

Alignment, Assembly, and Quantification of eDNA/eRNA Reads

Preprocessing of sequencing data, and then read alignment onto a reference genome or de novo transcript assembly is performed. The alignment tools such as STAR and HISAT2 are generally applied to ensure the correct mapping of RNA-seq sequences to reference genomes. For organisms lacking a good-annotated reference genome, transcript sequences can be reconstructed from short reads through de novo transcriptome assembly programs such as Trinity (Grabherr et al., 2011). Quantitative gene expression level estimation is enabled through the use of programs such as Salmon and featureCounts that quantify transcript abundance in terms of read depth (Patro et al., 2017). Researchers can identify principal causes of cancer and potential treatment targets using differential patterns of gene expression to investigate. Pawlowski et al. (2018) found that eRNA expression quantification in biomarker studies can reveal molecular markers associated with the development of a disease and how a disease develops.

Taxonomic and Functional Annotation in eDNA/eRNA Metabarcoding

Taxonomic classification of eDNA and eRNA sequences and functional annotation are required before cancer and environmental microbiome studies. For the identification of microbial species in tumor-associated microbiomes, SILVA, Greengenes, and UNITE databases offer curated reference sequences (Quast et al., 2013). In order to allow for identification of microbial communities that participate in cancer, packages such as QIIME2 (Bolyen et al., 2019) and DADA2 (Callahan et al., 2016) cluster and classify microbial reads. Functional annotation tools such as KEGG and EggNOG and taxonomic profiling are used to assist in the prediction of tumour microbiome microbial community metabolic functions (Kanehisa & Goto, 2000; Huerta-Cepas et al., 2019). The impact of microbial diversity on tumour development and responsiveness to treatment can be better comprehended by combining taxonomic and functional analysis.

Machine Learning Approaches in Cancer Biomarker Identification

Supervised Learning for Cancer Classification

Machine learning has revolutionized cancer biomarker discovery by allowing the prediction of tumour types from genomic and transcriptome data. Supervised learning techniques like random forests and support vector machines (SVMs) are widely employed to differentiate between carcinogenic and non-cancerous tissues according to gene expression profiles (Libbrecht & Noble, 2015). These models are able to enhance diagnostic performance and stratify patients based on the detection of eRNA biomarkers that distinguish between various subtypes of cancer. In order to find patterns that are associated with certain kinds of cancer, for instance, transcriptome data has been passed through CNNs (Leung & Pang, 2020). Models can be trained on very large datasets and create highly accurate classifiers for early cancer diagnosis; this would reduce the workload for patients and doctors performing invasive biopsy tests.

Unsupervised Learning for Biomarker Discovery

There are not well-characterized cancer subtypes, therefore, researchers can apply unsupervised learning techniques such as hierarchical clustering and principal component analysis (PCA) to identify new biomarkers. These techniques can identify novel molecular cancer subgroups that are not seen in gene expression data (Zhao & Simon 2020). Best et al. (2019) applied the k-means and t-distributed stochastic neighbour embedding (t-SNE) clustering algorithms to explore eRNA data from liquid biopsies. The outcomes were that there existed distinct profiles of transcriptomes which were treatment resistance-correlated. Precision oncology biomarkers may be detected sooner using a mixture of high-throughput sequencing and unsupervised learning.

Deep Learning for Multi-Omics Data Integration

Deep learning techniques have also been put forward to integrate information from genomes, transcriptomics, proteomics, and epigenomics, all of which are becoming increasingly relevant to cancer studies. Min et al. (2017) suggest that DNNs can be employed to investigate complex interactions across numerous molecular levels and obtain a better understanding of cancer biology. A case in point is employing variational autoencoders (VAEs) to describe new regulatory processes governing cancer development in multi-omics data (Rampášek et al., 2019). Molecular profile analysis with deep learning allows researchers to identify new drug targets and design individualized therapy protocols.

Table 3. Methodologies and technological advances in eDNA/eRNA metabarcoding for cancer research

Category	Methodology/Technology	Description	Key Benefits	Reference
High-Throughput Sequencing	Next-Generation Sequencing (NGS)	Short-read sequencing of eDNA/eRNA from biofluids and tumor samples	High sensitivity, cost-effective for large-scale cancer biomarker discovery	Shendure et al. (2017)
	Single-Molecule Sequencing (PacBio, Oxford Nanopore)	Long-read sequencing for detecting fusion genes, isoforms, and structural variants	Resolves complex mutations, useful for leukemia and solid tumor profiling	Amarasinghe et al. (2020)
	Whole-Exome Sequencing (WES)	Focuses on protein-coding regions of the genome to identify cancer-related mutations	Cost-effective for detecting mutations in known oncogenes and tumor suppressors	Shendure et al. (2017)
	Whole-Genome Sequencing (WGS)	Captures all genetic variants across the entire genome	Provides comprehensive mutation profiles for tumor evolution studies	Kim et al. (2019)
Bioinformatics Tools for eDNA/eRNA Analysis	QIIME2, DADA2	Computational pipelines for analyzing microbiome composition in tumor microenvironments	Enables identification of cancer-associated microbial species	Callahan et al. (2016)
	HISAT2, STAR, Trinity	Tools for aligning and assembling RNA sequencing data to study gene expression	Identifies cancer-specific transcripts, alternative splicing, and fusion genes	Kim et al. (2019)
	Salmon, Kallisto	Algorithms for quantifying RNA abundance in transcriptomic studies	High-speed, accurate gene expression quantification for biomarker analysis	Patro et al. (2017)
	GATK (Genome Analysis Toolkit)	Variant calling tool for identifying somatic mutations in tumor DNA/RNA	Detects point mutations, insertions/deletions, and structural variants	McKenna et al. (2010)
Machine Learning and AI in Biomarker Discovery	Deep Learning for eRNA Classification	AI-driven pattern recognition for cancer subtype classification	Improves accuracy in predicting tumor types and progression	Min et al. (2017)

continued on following page

Table 3. Continued

Category	Methodology/Technology	Description	Key Benefits	Reference
	Unsupervised Learning for Biomarker Identification	Clustering techniques (PCA, t-SNE) for detecting unknown cancer biomarkers	Identifies novel RNA signatures linked to therapy resistance	Zhao & Simon, (2020)
	Neural Networks for Mutation Prediction	AI models trained on sequencing data predict functional impact of mutations	Helps prioritize target genes for precision oncology	Libbrecht & Noble (2015)
Liquid Biopsy Technologies	Circulating Tumor DNA (ctDNA) & RNA (ctRNA) Analysis	Metabarcoding of eDNA/eRNA from blood for real-time cancer monitoring	Detects minimal residual disease (MRD) and therapy response	Heitzer et al. (2019)
	Extracellular Vesicle RNA Profiling	Isolation and sequencing of tumor-derived exosomal RNA	Enhances non-invasive detection of brain, breast, and prostate cancer	Akers et al. (2017)
	Cell-Free DNA (cfDNA) Sequencing	Analyzes DNA fragments released from tumor cells into the bloodstream	Detects tumor-specific mutations and epigenetic changes	Wan et al. (2020)
Epigenetic and Transcriptomic Analysis	Methylation Sequencing (MeDIP-seq, WGBS)	Identification of epigenetic modifications in tumor eDNA/eRNA	Helps in understanding cancer progression and drug resistance	Sun et al. (2021)
	Single-Cell RNA Sequencing (scRNA-seq)	High-resolution transcriptomic analysis of individual cancer cells	Reveals tumor heterogeneity and identifies treatment-resistant clones	Stewart et al. (2021)
	Chromatin Immunoprecipitation Sequencing (ChIP-seq)	Identifies genome-wide protein-DNA interactions and histone modifications	Helps in mapping epigenetic regulation of oncogenes	Akers et al. (2017)
	ATAC-seq (Assay for Transposase-Accessible Chromatin sequencing)	Maps chromatin accessibility and regulatory regions in cancer cells	Reveals epigenetic changes driving tumor progression	Buenrostro et al. (2013)

CASE STUDIES ON ENVIRONMENTAL DNA AND RNA METABARCODING IN CANCER RESEARCH

Metabarcoding of environmental DNA (eDNA) and environmental RNA (eRNA) has been increasingly employed in cancer research to enhance the identification of biomarkers, the development of personalised medications, and the early detection of cancer. Numerous case studies have demonstrated the efficacy of these methods in cancer diagnosis without invasion, tumour microenvironmental analysis, and therapy monitoring (Table 4). Through the help of bioinformatics and high-throughput sequencing, researchers have unraveled microbial interactions that are responsible for tumour formation and tumour growth and cancer-specific gene signatures. For instance, Best et al. (2019) employed eRNA metabarcoding in testing for RNA circulating in the blood sample for the purpose of detecting lung cancer. The determination of the levels of oncogene overexpression EGFR and KRAS by the study allowed early, very sensitive, and specific detection of NSCLC. Flemer et al. (2017), on their part, employed eDNA metabarcoding to analyze the gastrointestinal microbiota of participants diagnosed with CRC. They identified a higher prevalence of Fusobacterium nucleatum, a carcinogenesis-related bacterium. This research provided insight into the relationship between microbial dysbiosis and cancer development, as well as potential interventions that target the microbiome directly.

Metabarcoding is also heavily engaged with breast cancer liquid biopsy result follow-up. Heitzer et al. (2019), for instance, demonstrated that PI3K/AKT signalling pathway was employed to interpret tumour development and activity of therapeutic resistance pathways by following up eRNA and circulating tumour DNA (ctDNA) in breast cancer patients. In addition, Stewart et al. (2021) employed AI with eRNA metabarcoding to predict pancreatic cancer prognosis. By identifying the major RNA biomarkers (GATA6 and SMAD4), their AI-driven algorithm outperformed conventional clinical markers in predicting disease progression. These examples demonstrate the potential of eDNA and eRNA metabarcoding to revolutionize cancer treatment. These approaches will offer the non-invasive real-time genomic profiling of tumours and their microenvironments, improving cancer diagnosis, precision medicine, and patient management as technologies in sequencing continue to develop. New studies involving integration of metabarcoding with AI and multi-omics technology are envisioned to enable enhanced early cancer detection and therapeutic responses.

Table 4. Experimental data/case studies on eDNA and eRNA metabarcoding in cancer research

Case Study	Cancer Type	Methodology	Key Findings	Reference
eRNA Metabarcoding for Early Lung Cancer Detection	Lung Cancer (NSCLC)	Next-Generation Sequencing (NGS) of circulating RNA in blood samples	Identified upregulated oncogenes (*EGFR*, *KRAS*) for early lung cancer detection with high sensitivity and specificity. eRNA metabarcoding enables non-invasive early cancer screening.	Best et al. (2019)
eDNA and the Role of the Microbiome in Colorectal Cancer	Colorectal Cancer (CRC)	16S rRNA sequencing of fecal samples to analyze gut microbiome composition	Enrichment of *Fusobacterium nucleatum* and *Bacteroides fragilis* in CRC patients; depletion of *Bifidobacterium* in CRC-associated microbiomes. Microbial profiling aids in cancer diagnostics and potential microbiome-targeted therapies.	Flemer et al. (2017)
Liquid Biopsy and Metabarcoding for Tracking Breast Cancer Progression	Breast Cancer	eRNA and circulating tumor DNA (ctDNA) sequencing from serial blood samples	Tracked dynamic gene expression and mutation profiles. Identified *PI3K/AKT* pathway activation as a resistance mechanism to therapy. Enabled real-time treatment monitoring.	Heitzer et al. (2019)
AI-Driven eRNA Metabarcoding for Predicting Pancreatic Cancer Outcomes	Pancreatic Cancer	eRNA metabarcoding combined with machine learning	AI models identified RNA biomarkers (*GATA6*, *SMAD4*) predictive of poor prognosis. Outperformed traditional clinical markers in forecasting disease progression.	Stewart et al. (2021)
Circulating Tumor RNA (ctRNA) Metabarcoding for Prostate Cancer Screening	Prostate Cancer	RNA-seq analysis of blood-derived exosomal RNA	Identified prostate-specific RNA biomarkers, including *KLK3* (PSA) and *PCA3*, improving early detection accuracy. eRNA-based screening provided a non-invasive alternative to PSA blood tests.	Saini et al. (2018)
Metabarcoding for Identifying Tumor-Derived Exosomal RNA in Glioblastoma	Glioblastoma	Small RNA sequencing of exosomes isolated from cerebrospinal fluid (CSF)	Detected tumor-specific microRNAs (*miR-21*, *miR-221*) in CSF samples, enabling non-invasive brain cancer diagnostics. eRNA profiling helped distinguish glioblastomas from other brain tumors.	Akers et al. (2017)

continued on following page

Table 4. Continued

Case Study	Cancer Type	Methodology	Key Findings	Reference
Long-Read Sequencing for Metabarcoding-Based Leukemia Classification	Leukemia (AML, CML)	Oxford Nanopore sequencing of fusion transcripts in leukemia patients	Successfully identified oncogenic fusion genes (*BCR-ABL, RUNX1-RUNX1T1*) in leukemia subtypes. Long-read sequencing improved detection of complex structural variants.	Smith et al. (2020)
Microbiome-Epigenome Interactions in Gastric Cancer	Gastric Cancer	eDNA sequencing of stomach microbiota and methylation profiling of host DNA	Identified *Helicobacter pylori* in tumor-associated microbiomes. Found significant methylation changes in tumor suppressor genes (*CDH1, MLH1*) linked to gastric carcinogenesis.	Sun et al. (2021)

CHALLENGES AND LIMITATIONS IN ENVIRONMENTAL DNA AND RNA METABARCODING FOR CANCER RESEARCH

Technical Limitations in Data Extraction and Sequencing

Complexity of eDNA/eRNA Extraction From Clinical and Environmental Samples

One of the significant eDNA and eRNA metabarcoding issues is the complexity of nucleic acid recovery from wide-ranging environmental and biological samples. Unlike DNA extracted from fresh tissue, eDNA can be degraded and trace in nature, and it is problematic to recover enough material for sequencing (Cristescu & Hebert, 2018). eRNA is even worse since it is not stable in nature, as it degrades immediately when exposed to environmental conditions such as heat, UV light, and enzymatic activity (Stewart et al., 2021). Isolation of good-quality eRNA from physiological fluids such as blood, urine, and saliva in cancer research requires special preservation methods such as RNA stabilizing buffers and immediate freezing of samples (Best et al., 2019).

In addition, various materials have varying extraction efficiency of nucleic acids. The concentration of extracellular RNA in normal cells is high and can inhibit detection of circulating RNA derived from tumor in blood (Pawlowski et al., 2018). Also, obstacles to the process of extraction can be triggered by environmental conditions like soil chemistry or microbial contamination; this hinders sequencing efficiency and increases data loss (Deiner et al., 2017).

Limitations in Sequencing Technologies

Current methods remain limited in their capacity to get and interpret eDNA and eRNA accurately, even with the development of sequencing technology. Though Illumina and other short-read sequencing technologies have massive throughput, they are not able to address the complex genomic rearrangements and large-scale structural variations prevalent in cancer genomes (Shendure et al., 2017). While long-read sequencing technologies such as PacBio and ONT have higher genome coverage, they are also prone to more errors that may lead to misinterpretation of sequencing data (Amarasinghe et al., 2020). Moreover, sequencing depth and coverage are required for identifying rare mutations and low-abundance transcripts in cancer studies. Too low sequencing depth may lead to the exclusion of informative genetic variants, whereas too high sequencing can lead to unnecessary costs and computational demands (Amarasinghe et al., 2020). Sequencing of highly degraded or low-input samples generally produces data representation biases, for which enhanced library preparation techniques as well as bioinformatics pipelines are needed to address these limitations (Amarasinghe et al., 2020).

False Positives and Contamination Issues in Environmental Sampling

Risk of Cross-Contamination in Sample Handling and Processing

Contamination is a pertinent concern in eDNA and eRNA metabarcoding because even trace amounts of extraneous nucleic acids are capable of grossly biasing sequencing outcomes. Nichols et al. (2018) disclose several instances of potential contamination in clinical and ecological research. Sample locations include sites, DNA/RNA extraction, polymerase chain reaction amplification, and sequencing. The adventitious addition of non-tumor origin nucleic acids may cause false positives for cancer biomarker detection and, thus, cause misleading clinical diagnosis and treatment (Best et al., 2019). Sterilization, negative controls, and strict quality control procedures are essential in order to reduce contamination. To reduce contamination, it is essential to use single-use reagents and have separate rooms for pre- and post-PCR activities (Deiner et al., 2017). A few labs have further implemented automated liquid-handling instruments in order to improve sequencing data quality and mitigate human-mediated contamination (Callahan et al., 2016).

Challenges in Differentiating True Positives From Background Noise

False positives in eDNA and eRNA analyses occur when sequencing picks up non-target DNA or RNA, which misleads conclusions of species presence or gene expression level. False positives in cancer biology may be due to sequencing mistakes, PCR bias in amplification, or genomics sequence misannotation (Cristescu & Hebert, 2018). Sequencing errors as a result of polymerase slippage or misincorporation during PCR can produce spurious mutations that are not representative of the true genomic landscape of tumours (Heitzer et al., 2019). Furthermore, environmental influences can introduce unwanted genetic material that complicates results. In microbiome analysis of the tumour microenvironment, it is an important challenge to separate cancer-specific microbial species from transient contaminants introduced during handling samples. Scientists use bioinformatics filtering algorithms and statistical modeling to identify true signals from sequencing artefacts, enhancing data validity and reliability (Pawlowski et al., 2018).

Ethical Concerns in Genetic Data Usage for Cancer Research

Privacy and Data Security Challenges

The ethical significance of guarding against genetic information regarding patients has expanded over the past few decades with increasing applications of genomic and transcriptomic information in studies of cancer (Ogidi et al., 2025c). Genetic information can be abused and illicitly obtained while it is accrued, stored, and transferred, particularly if it gains a connection to identifiable individuals (Kaye et al., 2018). Maintaining patient confidentiality while enabling collaborative research has been an important issue in the backdrop of vast genomic databases (Knoppers & Chadwick, 2021). Genetic data is safeguarded by de-identification technology, controlled-access databases, and encryption. According to Lunshof et al. (2017), the European General Data Protection Regulation (GDPR) and the United States Health Insurance Portability and Accountability Act (HIPAA) regulatory regimes provide frameworks for ethical genomic data management in research. Ethical rules should, however, be repeatedly updated to align the challenge of data accessibility towards scientific development with consideration for patients' rights.

Consent and Ethical Considerations in Genetic Research

Even though informed consent is a basic research ethical principle, substantive consent for genetic testing is hindered by a wide range of barriers despite being released. The long-term impact of releasing genetic data is the potential re-identification or accidental findings that could influence medical care decisions, a situation that even few patients may not fully appreciate (Kaye et al., 2018). Issues of ownership and management of data are raised by environmental eDNA and eRNA metabarcoding studies based on uncertainty of genetic material sampled from public or shared spaces (Knoppers & Chadwick, 2021). Further, ethical problems might arise due to unforeseen consequences from genetic research, for instance, vulnerabilities to hereditary disorders. Researchers are faced with the challenging task of releasing findings to participants in the context of delayed clinical interventions (Lunshof et al., 2017). Open communication among researchers, patients, and policymakers is central to the development of public trust in genomic medicine and the implementation of ethical research practices.

FUTURE DIRECTIONS AND CLINICAL IMPLICATIONS OF EDNA/ERNA METABARCODING IN CANCER RESEARCH

Integration of eDNA/eRNA Metabarcoding in Clinical Oncology

Advancing Cancer Diagnostics With Metabarcoding Approaches

Environmental RNA (eRNA) and environmental DNA (eDNA) metabarcoding in clinical oncology offers a very sensitive, non-invasive method for the detection of cancer biomarkers, and can potentially revolutionize cancer diagnosis. Terminal cancer patients cannot tolerate the painful and invasive tissue biopsies employed in conventional cancer diagnosis (Heitzer et al., 2019). Metabarcoding techniques provide easy identification of cancer-associated genetic material through the analysis of circulating nucleic acids in different biofluids (Cristescu & Hebert, 2018). Clinical oncology application of metabarcoding enables thorough molecular profiling of tumours, which is a significant benefit. Clinicians can enable precise subtyping and personalized selection of treatment by examining eRNA transcripts to identify patterns of gene expression associated with specific cancer subtypes (Best et al., 2019). Therapists can also gain useful information about tumour development by monitoring temporal patterns of eRNA expression. This allows dynamic adjustment of treatment protocols to maximize patient recovery (Stewart et al., 2021).

Enhancing Early Cancer Detection and Prognostic Accuracy

Early diagnosis of cancer is an overarching challenge in oncology because the majority of cancers are not symptomatic while they are first developing and appear to get noticed only when cancer has progressed, and by then treatments have few options. eRNA metabarcoding is promising for the early detection of cancers by the identification of unusual transcriptional activity prior to the appearance of morphological abnormalities, according to Pawlowski et al. (2018). Best et al. (2019) stated that the majority of cancers can be detected at the initial stage if circulating RNA samples show high levels of expression for carcinogenic transcripts such as KRAS, TP53, and MYC. Minimum residual disease (MRD) can be defined as the extremely low proportion of residual cancer cells present in the body after treatment that can lead to relapse. Metabarcoding is utilized in enabling real-time monitoring of the disease (Heitzer et al., 2019). Ongoing surveillance of eRNA signals allows practitioners to evaluate therapy response and identify potential recurrences at an earlier stage than with traditional imaging techniques. This role can lead to significant improvements in long-term cancer patient survival and relief of recurrent cancer burden.

Potential for Liquid Biopsy Advancements Using Environmental RNA

Non-Invasive Cancer Monitoring Through Liquid Biopsies

Liquid biopsies represent a notable improvement in oncology, facilitating the diagnosis and monitoring of cancer by the analysis of circulating biomarkers in biological fluids. Rather of employing conventional tissue biopsies, physicians can regularly utilise liquid biopsies to track disease progression (Cristescu & Hebert, 2018). Metabarcoding of extended RNA (eRNA) improves the viability of liquid biopsies by identifying a broader array of biomarkers, including messenger RNA (mRNA), microRNA (miRNA), and long non-coding RNA (lncRNA), which collectively elucidate cancer biology (Best et al., 2019). A notable benefit of employing eRNA in liquid biopsies is its capacity to indicate dynamic fluctuations in tumour activity. The ongoing transcription and degradation of RNA in circulation offer an immediate perspective on the cellular activity taking place in malignant tissues (Pawlowski et al., 2018). This real-time monitoring capability allows oncologists to adjust treatment plans based on patient responses, thereby enhancing the effectiveness of targeted drugs and immunotherapies.

Detecting Rare and Heterogeneous Tumor Populations

Tumour heterogeneity, defined by unique genetic and molecular characteristics among individual tumour cells within a single patient, is a significant obstacle in cancer therapy. Heitzer et al. (2019) note that traditional biopsy techniques may fail to recognise this heterogeneity, thus resulting in insufficient therapeutic approaches.

To tackle this issue, eRNA metabarcoding analyses RNA signatures from various extracellular vesicles and tumor-derived exosomes found in circulation, offering a more thorough comprehension of cancer biology (Stewart et al., 2021). Furthermore, liquid biopsies employing eRNA have demonstrated potential in identifying rare cancer cell types, including CTCs and CSCs, which are essential in disease progression and metastasis (Best et al., 2019). The capacity to non-invasively define these uncommon cells improves the precision of prognostic and therapeutic determinations. Due to advancements in sequencing technologies, eRNA metabarcoding-based liquid biopsy applications are poised to become essential in precision oncology.

Role of AI and Big Data in Refining Cancer Biomarker Discovery

Machine Learning for Pattern Recognition in Metabarcoding Data

The domain of cancer research is undergoing a transformation due to the implementation of artificial intelligence (AI) and big data analytics. These tools facilitate the fast study of intricate transcriptomic and genomic datasets. A growing array of machine learning techniques is being utilised to discern tendencies in eRNA sequencing data that may indicate malignancy (Libbrecht & Noble, 2015). These algorithms include support vector machines (SVMs) and deep learning techniques. Training AI models on comprehensive datasets of eRNA signatures, encompassing both malignant and benign signatures, enhances the accuracy of cancer classification and biomarker discovery (Leung & Pang, 2020). To further diminish the likelihood of diagnostic false positives, AI-powered classification models can differentiate between benign and malignant lesions by analysing gene expression patterns (Cristescu & Hebert, 2018). This trait is essential for the early diagnosis of malignancy. The ability to identify even slight fluctuations in RNA expression levels can dictate the promptness of diagnosis or the loss of an intervention opportunity.

Integrating Multi-Omics Data for Personalized Medicine

The amalgamation of data from many omics platforms—genomics, transcriptomics, proteomics, and epigenomics—constitutes a substantial use of artificial intelligence in cancer research. AI-driven models may integrate various data sets to generate detailed molecular profiles of certain tumours, so enabling personalised therapy recommendations according to each patient's distinct genetic composition (Min et al., 2017). Artificial intelligence algorithms have been employed to connect eRNA expression patterns with treatment response data, thus identifying predictive biomarkers for targeted therapy (Rampášek et al., 2019). This technique reduces trial-and-error prescribing and the likelihood of unpleasant side effects, allowing oncologists to choose the most effective therapy alternatives for each patient. Precision medicine endeavours will progress markedly through the incorporation of artificial intelligence and eRNA metabarcoding. This will facilitate the personalisation of cancer therapy based on the molecular attributes of each tumour.

Enhancing Predictive Modeling for Cancer Progression and Recurrence

AI and big data analytics are as essential as biomarker discovery for predicting cancer progression and recurrence. Machine learning algorithms can analyse longitudinal eRNA sequencing data from cancer patients to detect early indicators of disease relapse, according to Pawlowski et al. (2018). This enables timely intervention. Predictive modelling approaches, like Bayesian networks and recurrent neural networks (RNNs), have proven capable of properly forecasting disease trajectories (Min et al., 2017). The advancement of AI-driven clinical decision support systems is allowing oncologists to interpret complex sequencing data and propose individualised treatment strategies (Heitzer et al., 2019). Ultimately, these systems improve patient outcomes and optimise healthcare budget allocation by providing evidence-based recommendations generated from comprehensive cancer research data repositories. eDNA/eRNA metabarcoding possesses substantial clinical relevance for cancer research, as demonstrated in Table 5.

Table 5. Clinical implications of eDNA/eRNA metabarcoding in cancer research

Clinical Application	Description	Key Benefits	Example Cancer Types	Reference
Early Cancer Detection	eRNA metabarcoding identifies circulating tumor RNA (ctRNA) and oncogenic transcripts in biofluids.	Non-invasive, high-sensitivity detection of early-stage cancer before symptoms appear.	Lung cancer, Breast cancer, Colorectal cancer	Best et al. (2019)
Liquid Biopsy for Cancer Monitoring	Sequencing of ctDNA/ctRNA from blood and other biofluids for real-time tumor surveillance.	Enables dynamic tracking of tumor evolution, treatment response, and minimal residual disease (MRD).	Breast cancer, Prostate cancer, Pancreatic cancer	Heitzer et al. (2019)
Microbiome-Cancer Interaction Analysis	eDNA sequencing of tumor-associated microbiota to assess microbial influence on cancer.	Identifies microbial risk factors, improves diagnostics, and opens new therapeutic avenues (e.g., microbiome-targeted therapies).	Colorectal cancer, Gastric cancer, Liver cancer	Flemer et al. (2017)
Personalized Medicine and Targeted Therapy Selection	eRNA profiling reveals patient-specific gene expression patterns and druggable mutations.	Enhances precision medicine by tailoring therapies based on molecular tumor profiles.	Leukemia, Lung cancer, Melanoma	Stewart et al. (2021)
AI and Big Data for Biomarker Discovery	Machine learning applied to metabarcoding data for cancer classification and prognosis prediction.	Improves diagnostic accuracy and aids in early identification of therapy-resistant tumors.	Pancreatic cancer, Brain cancer, Breast cancer	Min et al. (2017)
Epigenetic and Transcriptomic Profiling	eRNA metabarcoding detects DNA methylation, histone modifications, and chromatin accessibility changes in tumors.	Provides insights into tumor progression, immune evasion, and potential epigenetic drug targets.	Gastric cancer, Ovarian cancer, Colorectal cancer	Sun et al. (2021)
Single-Cell RNA Sequencing for Tumor Heterogeneity Analysis	scRNA-seq analyzes transcriptomic variations in individual cancer cells within a tumor.	Identifies treatment-resistant subclones and predicts therapy failure risk.	Small-cell lung cancer, Glioblastoma, Ovarian cancer	Stewart et al. (2021)
Metabarcoding for Immunotherapy Response Prediction	eRNA sequencing of immune-related genes to assess response to checkpoint inhibitors.	Helps in patient stratification for immunotherapies such as PD-1/PD-L1 and CAR-T cell therapy.	Melanoma, NSCLC, Bladder cancer	Chen et al. (2021)

continued on following page

Table 5. Continued

Clinical Application	Description	Key Benefits	Example Cancer Types	Reference
Metastasis and Tumor Evolution Tracking	Longitudinal sequencing of eRNA to monitor transcriptomic changes associated with metastasis.	Enables early intervention in metastatic disease and personalized treatment modifications.	Breast cancer, Prostate cancer, Pancreatic cancer	Heitzer et al. (2019)
Detection of Minimal Residual Disease (MRD) Post-Treatment	eRNA metabarcoding detects low levels of tumor-derived RNA after surgery or chemotherapy.	Allows for earlier detection of relapse compared to traditional imaging methods.	Leukemia, Colorectal cancer, Lung cancer	Best et al. (2019)
Tumor Microenvironment Characterization	eDNA/eRNA sequencing maps interactions between cancer cells, immune cells, and stromal cells.	Improves understanding of tumor-immune evasion mechanisms and therapy resistance.	Ovarian cancer, Triple-negative breast cancer	Binnewies et al. (2018)
Non-Invasive Monitoring of Pediatric Cancers	eRNA metabarcoding from blood or urine samples for pediatric oncology applications.	Reduces the need for invasive biopsies and facilitates treatment adjustments.	Neuroblastoma, Wilms tumor, Pediatric leukemia	Klega et al. (2018)
Detection of Cancer Predisposition and Hereditary Risk	eRNA profiling identifies germline mutations and epigenetic risk markers.	Assists in genetic counseling and early intervention for at-risk individuals.	BRCA1/BRCA2-associated breast cancer, Lynch syndrome	Lu et al. (2020)
Radiotherapy and Chemotherapy Sensitivity Prediction	eRNA metabarcoding identifies gene expression patterns predicting radiation and chemotherapy response.	Helps in optimizing treatment plans to minimize side effects and improve efficacy.	Cervical cancer, Head and neck cancer	Buqué et al. (2021)
Monitoring of Post-Surgical Complications	eRNA sequencing detects inflammatory and immune response signatures in post-operative cancer patients.	Allows early intervention in cases of recurrence or complications like infections.	Pancreatic cancer, Colorectal cancer	Cata et al. (2020)

CONCLUSION

Recent breakthroughs in cancer research have brought environmental DNA (eDNA) and environmental RNA (eRNA) metabarcoding as revolutionary approaches. These technologies provide innovative strategies for early cancer detection, biomarker discovery, and the use of precision oncology. The non-invasive examination of circulating nucleic acids provides essential insights into cancer biology, gene expression patterns, and interactions within the tumour microenvironment. Metabarcoding enables precise identification of oncogenic mutations, tracking of cancer progression, and assessment of therapy responses. This substantially impacts the increasing prevalence of cancer diagnosis, the decrease in invasive biopsy requirements, and the improvement of patient outcomes via real-time molecular profiling. Significant ethical and technological obstacles persist in realising the complete promise of electronic DNA and RNA metabarcoding. The dependability of data may be undermined by sequencing mistakes, contamination, and limitations in nucleic acid extraction; hence, there remains a continual need for improvements in bioinformatics tools and sequencing technology. To guarantee a responsible and ethical implementation in clinical settings, it is imperative to tackle concerns regarding genetic data privacy, informed consent, and equitable access to precision medicine. To resolve these challenges and enhance the application of metabarcoding in cancer, it is imperative to continue refining techniques, expanding genetic reference libraries, and integrating machine learning models.

Metabarcoding, along with liquid biopsy technology and artificial intelligence, is anticipated to significantly transform cancer research. AI-driven analytics can enhance the development of personalised treatment plans by synthesising multi-omics data, hence refining predictive models for cancer progression and biomarker identification. Improvements in long-read sequencing and real-time transcriptome analysis will augment the sensitivity and specificity of cancer diagnostics, enabling the development of more personalised therapeutics. Integrating advancements in these technologies into standard clinical practice could revolutionise early cancer detection, therapeutic resistance, and patient care. Metabarcoding of environmental DNA and RNA is a significant advancement in cancer research, with the potential to revolutionise cancer diagnosis, treatment, and disease surveillance. High-throughput sequencing, bioinformatics, and artificial intelligence collectively empower scientists and clinicians to deepen their comprehension of tumour biology and formulate more efficacious cancer therapies. Translating metabarcoding findings into actionable therapeutic interventions can improve cancer treatment and elevate patient survival rates. Despite challenges, continuous progress and interdisciplinary collaboration are vital.

Underlying fundamentals must be tackled head-on because cancer research is increasingly making use of environmental DNA and RNA metabarcoding. Standardization of methods, utilization of sound validation approaches, and establishment of clearly defined and functional bioinformatics pipelines are at the core. Without these underlying pillars, use of exposomics and its integration into clinical oncology will be hampered. This is a transformative moment. Research centers, regulatory authorities, and the clinic can be presented with a harmonized reproducibility, validity, and pragmatic information package by bringing them together. Exposomics, a convergence of innovation and practical application, presents a new instrument in probing the influence of the environment and shaping preventive oncology therapy with unrivaled specificity. Uncoordinate growth cannot be allowed to shape the future. Promoting combined initiatives of data science and molecular biology, worldwide standards support, and investments in sophisticated informatics technology is pivotal. These steps, while necessary, trigger the process of cancer preventive transformation.

ABBREVIATIONS

AI Artificial intelligence
AML Acute myeloid leukemia
cDNA complementary DNA
cfDNA cell-free DNA
cfRNA cell-free RNA
ChIP-seq Chromatin Immunoprecipitation Sequencing
CML Chronic myeloid leukemia
CNNs convolutional neural networks
CRC colorectal cancer
CSF cerebrospinal fluid
ctDNA circulating tumour DNA
ctRNA circulating tumour RNA
DNA Deoxyribonucleic Acid
DNNs Domain name systems
EBV Epstein-Barr virus
eDNA Environmental DNA
eRNA Environmental RNA
GDPR General Data Protection Regulation
HIPAA Health Insurance Portability and Accountability Act
lncRNA long non-coding RNA
lncRNAs long non-coding RNAs
miRNA microRNA

MRD minimal residual disease
mRNA messenger RNA
NGS next-generation sequencing
NSCLC Melanoma, Non-small cell lung cancer
PCA principal component analysis
PCR Polymerase Chain reaction
qPCR quantitative PCR
RNA Ribonucleic Acid
RNases ribonucleases
RNNs recurrent neural networks
scRNA-seq single-cell RNA sequencing
SVMs support vector machines
TME tumor microenvironment
VAEs variational autoencoders
WES whole-exome sequencing
WGS whole-genome sequencing

REFERENCES

Akers, J. C., Ramakrishnan, V., Kim, R., Skog, J., Nakano, I., & Hochberg, F. H. (2017). MiR-21 in the extracellular vesicles (EVs) of cerebrospinal fluid: A novel biomarker for glioblastoma. *Journal of Neuro-Oncology, 134*(1), 1–10. DOI: 10.1007/s11060-013-1084-8 PMID: 28555425

Amarasinghe, S. L., Su, S., Dong, X., Zappia, L., Ritchie, M. E., & Gouil, Q. (2020). Opportunities and challenges in long-read sequencing data analysis. *Genome Biology, 21*(1), 30. DOI: 10.1186/s13059-020-1935-5 PMID: 32033565

Andrews, S. (2010). *FastQC: A quality control tool for high throughput sequence data.* https://www.bioinformatics.babraham.ac.uk/projects/fastqc/

Barnes, M. A., & Turner, C. R. (2016). The ecology of environmental DNA and implications for conservation genetics. *Conservation Genetics, 17*(1), 1–17. DOI: 10.1007/s10592-015-0775-4

Best, M. G., Sol, N., Kooi, I., Tannous, J., Westerman, B. A., & Wurdinger, T. (2019). RNA sequencing of tumor-educated platelets enables blood-based pan-cancer, multiclass, and molecular pathway cancer diagnostics. *Cancer Cell, 36*(6), 881–895. DOI: 10.1016/j.ccell.2019.11.005

Binnewies, M., Roberts, E. W., Kersten, K., Chan, V., Fearon, D. F., Merad, M., & Krummel, M. F. (2018). Understanding the tumor immune microenvironment (TIME) for effective therapy. *Nature Medicine, 24*(5), 541–550. DOI: 10.1038/s41591-018-0014-x PMID: 29686425

Bolger, A. M., Lohse, M., & Usadel, B. (2014). Trimmomatic: A flexible trimmer for Illumina sequence data. *Bioinformatics (Oxford, England), 30*(15), 2114–2120. DOI: 10.1093/bioinformatics/btu170 PMID: 24695404

Bolyen, E., Rideout, J. R., Dillon, M. R., Bokulich, N. A., Abnet, C. C., Al-Ghalith, G. A., Alexander, H., Alm, E. J., Arumugam, M., Asnicar, F., Bai, Y., Bisanz, J. E., Bittinger, K., Brejnrod, A., Brislawn, C. J., Brown, C. T., Callahan, B. J., Caraballo-Rodríguez, A. M., Chase, J., & Caporaso, J. G. (2019). Reproducible, interactive, scalable and extensible microbiome data science using QIIME 2. *Nature Biotechnology, 37*(8), 852–857. DOI: 10.1038/s41587-019-0209-9 PMID: 31341288

Buenrostro, J. D., Giresi, P. G., Zaba, L. C., Chang, H. Y., & Greenleaf, W. J. (2013). Transposition of native chromatin for fast and sensitive epigenomic profiling of open chromatin, DNA-binding proteins, and nucleosome position. *Nature Methods, 10*(12), 1213–1218. DOI: 10.1038/nmeth.2688 PMID: 24097267

Buqué, A., Galluzzi, L., & Zitvogel, L. (2021). Immunological determinants of radiotherapy response. *Radiotherapy and Oncology : Journal of the European Society for Therapeutic Radiology and Oncology, 160*, 61–69. DOI: 10.1016/j.radonc.2021.04.001

Callahan, B. J., McMurdie, P. J., Rosen, M. J., Han, A. W., Johnson, A. J. A., & Holmes, S. P. (2016). DADA2: High-resolution sample inference from Illumina amplicon data. *Nature Methods, 13*(7), 581–583. DOI: 10.1038/nmeth.3869 PMID: 27214047

Callahan, B. J., McMurdie, P. J., Rosen, M. J., Han, A. W., Johnson, A. J. A., & Holmes, S. P. (2016). DADA2: High-resolution sample inference from Illumina amplicon data. *Nature Methods, 13*(7), 581–583. DOI: 10.1038/nmeth.3869 PMID: 27214047

Cata, J. P., Bachmann, D., & Pedraza, R. (2020). Perioperative inflammatory response and cancer recurrence risk. *Anesthesia and Analgesia, 130*(6), 1686–1695. DOI: 10.1213/ANE.0000000000004711 PMID: 32384350

Chen, R., Caserto, J. S., & Chiu, D. (2021). RNA-based immune signatures for predicting response to immunotherapy in cancer patients. *Nature Communications, 12*(1), 1878. DOI: 10.1038/s41467-021-22129-x PMID: 33767163

Cheng, Y., Wang, T., Li, T., & Yan, Y. (2021). Challenges and opportunities of circulating tumor DNA detection using next-generation sequencing. *Frontiers in Medicine, 8*, 674474. DOI: 10.3389/fmed.2021.674474

Chiu, C. Y., & Miller, S. A. (2019). Clinical metagenomics. *Nature Reviews. Genetics, 20*(6), 341–355. DOI: 10.1038/s41576-019-0113-7 PMID: 30918369

Cordier, T., Alonso-Sáez, L., Apothéloz-Perret-Gentil, L., Aylagas, E., Bohan, D. A., Bouchez, A., & Pawlowski, J. (2019). Ecosystems monitoring powered by environmental genomics: A review of current strategies with an implementation roadmap. *Molecular Ecology, 28*(14), 2937–2954. DOI: 10.1111/mec.15176 PMID: 32416615

Cristescu, M. E., & Hebert, P. D. N. (2018). Uses and misuses of environmental DNA in biodiversity science and conservation. *Annual Review of Ecology, Evolution, and Systematics, 49*(1), 209–230. DOI: 10.1146/annurev-ecolsys-110617-062306

Deiner, K., Bik, H. M., Mächler, E., Seymour, M., Lacoursière-Roussel, A., Altermatt, F., & Bernatchez, L. (2017). Environmental DNA metabarcoding: Transforming how we survey animal and plant communities. *Molecular Ecology, 26*(21), 5872–5895. DOI: 10.1111/mec.14350 PMID: 28921802

Flemer, B., Warren, R. D., Barrett, M. P., Cisek, K., Das, A., Jeffery, I. B., & O'Toole, P. W. (2017). The oral microbiota in colorectal cancer is distinctive and predictive. *Gut, 67*(4), 1454–1463. DOI: 10.1136/gutjnl-2016-313173 PMID: 28988196

Garrett, W. S. (2015). Cancer and the microbiota. *Science, 348*(6230), 80–86. DOI: 10.1126/science.aaa4972 PMID: 25838377

Grabherr, M. G., Haas, B. J., Yassour, M., Levin, J. Z., Thompson, D. A., Amit, I., Adiconis, X., Fan, L., Raychowdhury, R., Zeng, Q., Chen, Z., Mauceli, E., Hacohen, N., Gnirke, A., Rhind, N., di Palma, F., Birren, B. W., Nusbaum, C., Lindblad-Toh, K., & Regev, A. (2011). Full-length transcriptome assembly from RNA-Seq data without a reference genome. *Nature Biotechnology, 29*(7), 644–652. DOI: 10.1038/nbt.1883 PMID: 21572440

Heitzer, E., Haque, I. S., Roberts, C. E. S., & Speicher, M. R. (2019). Current and future perspectives of liquid biopsies in genomics-driven oncology. *Nature Reviews. Genetics, 20*(2), 71–88. DOI: 10.1038/s41576-018-0071-5 PMID: 30410101

Huerta-Cepas, J., Szklarczyk, D., Heller, D., Hernández-Plaza, A., Forslund, S. K., Cook, H., Mende, D. R., Letunic, I., Rattei, T., Jensen, L. J., von Mering, C., & Bork, P. (2019). eggNOG 5.0: A hierarchical, functionally and phylogenetically annotated orthology resource based on 5090 organisms and 2502 viruses. *Nucleic Acids Research, 47*(D1), D309–D314. DOI: 10.1093/nar/gky1085 PMID: 30418610

Kanehisa, M., & Goto, S. (2000). KEGG: Kyoto Encyclopedia of Genes and Genomes. *Nucleic Acids Research, 28*(1), 27–30. DOI: 10.1093/nar/28.1.27 PMID: 10592173

Kaye, J., Whitley, E. A., Lund, D., Morrison, M., Teare, H., & Melham, K. (2018). Data sharing in genomics—Re-shaping scientific practice. *Nature Reviews. Genetics, 19*(2), 111. PMID: 19308065

Kim, D., Paggi, J. M., Park, C., Bennett, C., & Salzberg, S. L. (2019). Graph-based genome alignment and genotyping with HISAT2 and HISAT-genotype. *Nature Biotechnology, 37*(8), 907–915. DOI: 10.1038/s41587-019-0201-4 PMID: 31375807

Klega, K., Imamovic-Tuco, L., & An, E. (2018). Clinical applications of cell-free RNA sequencing in pediatric oncology. *Pediatric Blood & Cancer, 65*(5), e26936. DOI: 10.1002/pbc.26936 PMID: 29286573

Knoppers, B. M., & Chadwick, R. (2021). Human genetics and genomics: A new paradigm. *Annual Review of Genomics and Human Genetics, 22*, 1–24.

Kopylova, E., Noé, L., & Touzet, H. (2012). SortMeRNA: Fast and accurate filtering of ribosomal RNAs in metatranscriptomic data. *Bioinformatics (Oxford, England), 28*(24), 3211–3217. DOI: 10.1093/bioinformatics/bts611 PMID: 23071270

Kostic, A. D., Gevers, D., Pedamallu, C. S., Michaud, M., Duke, F., Earl, A. M., Ojesina, A. I., Jung, J., Bass, A. J., Tabernero, J., Baselga, J., Liu, C., Shivdasani, R. A., Ogino, S., Birren, B. W., Huttenhower, C., Garrett, W. S., & Meyerson, M. (2013). Genomic analysis identifies association of Fusobacterium with colorectal carcinoma. *Genome Research*, *22*(2), 292–298. DOI: 10.1101/gr.126573.111 PMID: 22009990

Leung, A., & Pang, K. M. (2020). Utilizing deep learning to predict cancer diagnoses from gene expression profiles. *Scientific Reports*, *10*(1), 1–11. DOI: 10.1038/s41598-020-67447-6 PMID: 31913322

Libbrecht, M. W., & Noble, W. S. (2015). Machine learning applications in genetics and genomics. *Nature Reviews. Genetics*, *16*(6), 321–332. DOI: 10.1038/nrg3920 PMID: 25948244

Lu, C., Thompson, J. R., & Schwartz, A. G. (2020). Hereditary cancer risk assessment in clinical oncology. *The Lancet. Oncology*, *21*(2), 189–200. DOI: 10.1016/S1470-2045(19)30735-5 PMID: 31838012

Lunshof, J. E., Church, G. M., & Prainsack, B. (2017). From genetic privacy to open consent. *Nature Reviews. Genetics*, *18*(8), 512. PMID: 18379574

McKenna, A., Hanna, M., Banks, E., Sivachenko, A., Cibulskis, K., Kernytsky, A., Garimella, K., Altshuler, D., Gabriel, S., Daly, M., & DePristo, M. A. (2010). The genome analysis toolkit: A MapReduce framework for analyzing next-generation DNA sequencing data. *Genome Research*, *20*(9), 1297–1303. DOI: 10.1101/gr.107524.110 PMID: 20644199

Min, S., Lee, B., & Yoon, S. (2017). Deep learning in bioinformatics. *Briefings in Bioinformatics*, *18*(5), 851–869. DOI: 10.1093/bib/bbw068 PMID: 27473064

Mohan, S., Heitzer, E., Ulz, P., Lafer, I., Lax, S., Auer, M., & Speicher, M. R. (2022). Beyond the blood: Circulating tumor DNA in the liquid biopsies of other body fluids. *Nature Reviews. Clinical Oncology*, *19*(9), 600–618. DOI: 10.1038/s41571-022-00660-y PMID: 35915225

Nichols, T. A., Einarsson, A., & Willerslev, E. (2018). Contamination and DNA degradation in ancient DNA. *Science and Technology of Archaeological Research*, *4*(1), 63–73.

Ogidi, O. I. (2024). Recent advances in anticancer activity and Bioinformatics Approach from Potential Plants. In: Computational Approaches in Biomaterials, Bioinformatics and Biomedical Engineering Applications. *CRC Press, Taylor and Francis Group, Florida, USA*. DOI: 10.1201/9781003354437-3

Ogidi, O. I. (2025). Natural Products Modulating Mitophagy: Implications for Cancer Therapy. In Pandurangan, A. (Ed.), *Roles of Mitophagy in Cancer Regulation* (pp. 325–358). IGI Global Scientific Publishing, DOI: 10.4018/979-8-3693-3836-0.ch012

Ogidi, O. I., & Ajoko, I. (2024). Neuroprotective Potentials of Phytochemicals. In: M.S. Rajput, T. Sarachana, P.D. Sarkar, M. Raval (eds) NeuroPhytomedicine. *CRC Press, Routledge Taylor and Francis Group.*

Ogidi, O. I., Ajoko, I. T., & Tawariowei, A. M. (2024c). Sustainable Application of Genetic Ecotoxicological Techniques. In *Biomonitoring For Environmental Sustainability. In: Biomonitoring of Pollutants in the Global South.* Springer Nature Singapore Pte Ltd. DOI: 10.1007/978-981-97-1658-6_19

Ogidi, O. I., Barwant, M. M., & Okara, E. (2024a). Biomarker Discovery: Protein Phosphorylation State. In *Spatially Variable Genes in Cancer: Development, Progression, and Treatment Response.* IGI Global. DOI: 10.4018/979-8-3693-7728-4.ch005

Ogidi, O. I., Chukwunonso, O. A., Afakwu-Adimoha, H. C., & Barwant, M. M. (2025c). Ethical Considerations in Generative Artificial Intelligence in Healthcare. In: Generative Artificial Intelligence in Healthcare: Current Practice and Future Development. *CRC Press, Taylor and Francis Group, Florida, USA.* DOI: 10.1201/9781003488255-5

Ogidi, O. I., & Emaikwu, N. G. (2024). Plant Phenolic compound isolation and its Bioinformatics Approaches of Molecular Mechanisms in Antimicrobial activities and Resistance. In: Computational Approaches in Biomaterials, Bioinformatics and Biomedical Engineering Applications. *CRC Press, Taylor and Francis Group, Florida, USA.* DOI: 10.1201/9781003354437-8

Ogidi, O. I., Erho, S. A., & Omu, O. (2025a). Reactive Oxygen Species in Cancer. In Prabhakar, P. (Ed.), *The Role of Reactive Oxygen Species in Human Health and Disease* (pp. 339–376). IGI Global Scientific Publishing. DOI: 10.4018/979-8-3693-7919-6.ch010

Ogidi, O. I., & Felagha, I. (2024). Gut Microbiome and Diet Interaction. In *Nutrition Controversies and Advances in Autoimmune Disease.* IGI Global. DOI: 10.4018/979-8-3693-5528-2.ch012

Ogidi, O. I., Ijere, N. D., & Sogoi, P. B. (2025b). Neural and Endocrine Regulation of Immunity. In Reddy, K. (Ed.), *Research Methodologies and Practical Applications in Psychoneuroimmunology* (pp. 17–42). IGI Global Scientific Publishing. DOI: 10.4018/979-8-3693-7432-0.ch002

Ogidi, O. I., Ogoun, T. R., Alex, E. I., Edward, R. B., Joshua, M. T., & Bunu, E. M. (2024b). Radiogenomics and Genetic Diversity of Glioblastoma Characterization. In: Radiomics and Radiogenomics in Neuro-Oncology: An Artificial Intelligence Paradigm- volume 2: Genetics and clinical applications. *Elsevier*. DOI: 10.1016/B978-0-443-18509-0.00002-5

Ogidi, O. I., Onwuagba, C. G., & Richard-Nwachukwu, N. (2024d). Biomonitoring Tools, Techniques and Approaches For Environmental Assessments. In *Biomonitoring of Pollutants in the Global South*. Springer Nature Singapore Pte Ltd. DOI: 10.1007/978-981-97-1658-6_7

Ogidi, O. I., & Tawariowei, A. M. (2023). Endocrine Disrupting Chemicals and their Role in Cancer-A review. *Molecular Sciences And Applications.*, *3*, 5–14. DOI: 10.37394/232023.2023.3.2

Ogidi, O. I., & Tobia, P. S. (2024). Harnessing Artificial Intelligence (AI) Techniques for the prevention of Microbial Disease in Humans. In *Artificial Intelligence in Microbiology: scopes and Challenges*. Elsevier.

Patro, R., Duggal, G., Love, M. I., Irizarry, R. A., & Kingsford, C. (2017). Salmon provides fast and bias-aware quantification of transcript expression. *Nature Methods*, *14*(4), 417–419. DOI: 10.1038/nmeth.4197 PMID: 28263959

Pawlowski, J., Audic, S., Adl, S., Bass, D., Belbahri, L., Berney, C., & de Vargas, C. (2018). CBOL protist working group: Barcoding eukaryotic richness beyond the animal, plant, and fungal kingdoms. *PLoS Biology*, *16*(10), e2005849. DOI: 10.1371/journal.pbio.2005849 PMID: 23139639

Quast, C., Pruesse, E., Yilmaz, P., Gerken, J., Schweer, T., Yarza, P., Peplies, J., & Glöckner, F. O. (2013). The SILVA ribosomal RNA gene database project: Improved data processing and web-based tools. *Nucleic Acids Research*, *41*(D1), D590–D596. DOI: 10.1093/nar/gks1219 PMID: 23193283

Rampášek, L., Hidru, D., Smirnov, P., Haibe-Kains, B., & Goldenberg, A. (2019). Dr.VAE: Drug Response Variational Autoencoder. *bioRxiv*. DOI: 10.1101/602607

Saini, S., PSA, K. L. K., & PCA3. (2018). Non-coding RNA in prostate cancer: Molecular functions and clinical implications. *The Prostate*, *78*(14), 1057–1074. DOI: 10.1002/pros.23673

Shendure, J., Balasubramanian, S., Church, G. M., Gilbert, W., Rogers, J., Schloss, J. A., & Waterston, R. H. (2017). DNA sequencing at 40: Past, present, and future. *Nature*, *550*(7676), 345–353. DOI: 10.1038/nature24286 PMID: 29019985

Simner, P. J., Miller, S., & Carroll, K. C. (2017). Understanding the promises and hurdles of metagenomic next-generation sequencing as a diagnostic tool for infectious diseases. *Clinical Infectious Diseases*, *66*(5), 778–788. DOI: 10.1093/cid/cix881 PMID: 29040428

Siravegna, G., Marsoni, S., Siena, S., & Bardelli, A. (2017). Integrating liquid biopsies into the management of cancer. *Nature Reviews. Clinical Oncology*, *14*(9), 531–548. DOI: 10.1038/nrclinonc.2017.14 PMID: 28252003

Smith, C. C., Selitsky, S. R., Chai, S., Liu, W., Busman-Sahay, K., & Parker, J. S. (2020). Long-read sequencing for improved detection of oncogenic fusions in acute leukemia. *Leukemia*, *34*(3), 799–810. DOI: 10.1038/s41375-019-0677-9 PMID: 31628430

Stewart, C. A., Gay, C. M., Xi, Y., Sivajothi, S., Sivakumar, S., Fujimoto, J., & Wistuba, I. I. (2021). Single-cell analyses reveal increased intratumoral heterogeneity after the onset of therapy resistance in small-cell lung cancer. *Nature Cancer*, *2*(4), 404–421. DOI: 10.1038/s43018-021-00184-1 PMID: 33521652

Sun, Y., Zhang, Y., Qi, X., Zhou, Y., & Yu, J. (2021). Helicobacter pylori-induced DNA methylation alterations in gastric carcinogenesis: A pathway-based analysis of whole-genome methylation sequencing data. *Frontiers in Oncology*, *11*, 654230. DOI: 10.3389/fonc.2021.654230

Walboomers, J. M., Jacobs, M. V., Manos, M. M., Bosch, F. X., Kummer, J. A., Shah, K. V., & Meijer, C. J. (1999). Human papillomavirus is a necessary cause of invasive cervical cancer worldwide. *The Journal of Pathology*, *189*(1), 12–19. DOI: 10.1002/(SICI)1096-9896(199909)189:1<12::AID-PATH431>3.0.CO;2-F PMID: 10451482

Wan, J. C. M., Massie, C., Garcia-Corbacho, J., Mouliere, F., Brenton, J. D., Caldas, C., & Rosenfeld, N. (2020). Liquid biopsies come of age: Towards implementation of circulating tumor DNA. *Nature Reviews. Cancer*, *17*(4), 223–238. DOI: 10.1038/nrc.2017.7 PMID: 28233803

Zhao, M., & Simon, R. (2020). Identification of cancer subtypes using unsupervised clustering and cancer gene expression data. *Cancers (Basel)*, *12*(10), 2767. DOI: 10.3390/cancers12102767 PMID: 32992445

ADDITIONAL READING

Adamo, M., Voyron, S., Chialva, M., Marmeisse, R., & Girlanda, M. (2020). Metabarcoding on both environmental DNA and RNA highlights differences between fungal communities sampled in different habitats. *PLoS One*, *15*(12), e0244682. DOI: 10.1371/journal.pone.0244682 PMID: 33378355

Farrell, J. A., Whitmore, L., & Duffy, D. J. (2021). The Promise and Pitfalls of Environmental DNA and RNA Approaches for the Monitoring of Human and Animal Pathogens from Aquatic Sources. *Bioscience*, *71*(6), biab027. Advance online publication. DOI: 10.1093/biosci/biab027

Macher, T. H., Arle, J., Beermann, A. J., Frank, L., Hupało, K., Koschorreck, J., Schütz, R., & Leese, F. (2024). Is it worth the extra mile? Comparing environmental DNA and RNA metabarcoding for vertebrate and invertebrate biodiversity surveys in a lowland stream. *PeerJ*, *12*, e18016. DOI: 10.7717/peerj.18016 PMID: 39465159

Thakur, I. S., & Roy, D. (2020). Environmental DNA and RNA as Records of Human Exposome, Including Biotic/Abiotic Exposures and Its Implications in the Assessment of the Role of Environment in Chronic Diseases. *International Journal of Molecular Sciences*, *21*(14), 4879. DOI: 10.3390/ijms21144879 PMID: 32664313

Ye, P., Cheng, J., Lo, L. S. H., Liu, J., Li, C., So, K. J. Y., Xia, F., Yan, M., Wang, J., U, C., Qiu, J.-W., Cai, W., & Leung, K. M. Y. (2025). Environmental DNA/RNA metabarcoding for noninvasive and comprehensive monitoring and assessment of marine fishes. *Marine Pollution Bulletin*, *211*, 117422. DOI: 10.1016/j.marpolbul.2024.117422 PMID: 39689660

Chapter 8
Digital Exposome:
A Digital Age Approach to Environmental Exposure and Cancer Risk Assessment

Kholis Ernawati
https://orcid.org/0000-0002-3582-5294
Universitas YARSI, Jakarta Pusat, Indonesia

Hamzah Hasyim
Universitas Sriwijaya, Indonesia

Ahmad Rusdan Handoyo Utomo
https://orcid.org/0000-0003-3092-3714
Universitas YARSI, Jakarta Pusat, Indonesia

Dicky Budiman
Universitas YARSI, Jakarta Pusat, Indonesia

Dian Widiyanti
Universitas YARSI, Jakarta Pusat, Indonesia

ABSTRACT

The digital exposome integrates digital technologies, multi-omics analysis, and artificial intelligence to holistically assess environmental exposures across human life, particularly their contribution to cancer risk. Chemical, physical, biological, social, and behavioral factors are critically examined, emphasizing prenatal vulnerability. Wearable sensors, geographic information systems (GIS), and spatial mapping technologies enable real-time biomonitoring and precise visualization of exposures. Multi-omics and epigenetic modeling further clarify biological mecha-

DOI: 10.4018/979-8-3373-2165-3.ch008

nisms linking exposure to cancer, while machine learning supports big data-driven risk classification and identification of vulnerable populations. This approach enhances early detection and targeted prevention strategies and supports inclusive, evidence-based public health policies.

INTRODUCTION

Cancer is the second leading cause of death worldwide, accounting for more than 19.3 million new cases and 10 million deaths in 2020 (IARC, 2020). The World Health Organization projects that the number of new cancer cases will rise to 28.4 million by 2040, primarily driven by factors such as population aging, urbanization, and changes in lifestyle patterns (Lewandowska et al., 2019) Recent studies have highlighted that the majority of cancer risks are linked to modifiable factors, including environmental exposures, smoking habits, and social inequalities (Bryere et al., 2019; IARC, 2020) It is estimated that more than half of cancer cases could be prevented through effective risk management strategies. Notably, environmental carcinogens such as delicate particulate matter (PM2.5), volatile organic compounds (VOCs) like benzene and formaldehyde, and endocrine-disrupting chemicals (EDCs) such as phthalates and bisphenol A (BPA) have been associated with an elevated risk of cancer development (Ahn & Jeung, 2023; Tseng et al., 2019).

Social determinants—such as poverty, pollution, and limited access to healthcare—exacerbate this burden, particularly in developing nations (Bhattacharjee et al., 2022). To address this complexity, the exposome framework—introduced by Wild in 2005—captures lifelong environmental exposures and their biological effects. It highlights mechanisms like inflammation, oxidative stress, and epigenetic changes linked to carcinogenesis (Go et al., 2023). With digital innovation, the digital exposome enhances this framework by integrating wearable sensors, GIS, multi-omics, and machine learning for real-time exposure mapping and personalized analysis (Vermeulen et al., 2020). These tools help identify exposure hotspots and decode molecular responses. The digital exposome significantly advances cancer research by enabling real-time mapping of external exposures—such as pollutants, diet, and social environment—and internal biological responses like metabolism and stress regulation. It facilitates precise exposure tracking through sensors, mobile devices, GPS, air quality monitors, and citizen science data. It facilitates cancer patients to further connect exposure events with biological changes, enhancing early detection, risk stratification, and understanding of metastasis mechanisms.

Particularly critical is the prenatal period, where exposures to pollutants such as PAHs and EDCs may cause long-term epigenetic changes and cancer risk (Sun et al., 2019). In vitro models and organoids now facilitate studying exposure-induced carcinogenesis at the tissue level. The digital exposome represents a research tool and a public health strategy. By embedding exposure data into health systems, countries like Finland and the Netherlands enhance precision prevention for high-risk populations (Combarnous & Nguyen, 2019).

This paper aims to explore the digital exposome's role in cancer risk assessment, discuss its technological foundations, highlight its application in policy, and advocate for its use in reducing health disparities.

METHODS

This article was prepared using the narrative literature review method to integrate current scientific knowledge on digital exposomes and their relevance in cancer risk assessment. References included indexed scientific journals, reports from global health agencies (such as WHO, IARC, and NIH), and recent academic books in epidemiology, toxicology, data science, and environmental health.

The literature search process was conducted through several major databases, including PubMed, Scopus, ScienceDirect, and Google Scholar, using keywords such as: "digital exposome," 'cancer risk assessment,' 'machine learning in environmental health,' 'prenatal exposure and cancer,' and 'multi-omics and carcinogenesis.' The literature selected was prioritized from the last ten years (2019-2025) to maintain relevance with the latest technological developments and research.

Inclusion criteria included:

- Peer-reviewed articles that focus on the relationship between environmental exposures and cancer.
- Studies that apply digital approaches, such as wearable technology, machine learning, GIS, and multi-omics.
- Studies that highlighted prenatal aspects, vulnerable populations, and health inequalities.

The analysis was done thematically by grouping the findings based on the dimensions of the technology used, the type of environmental exposure studied, the biomarkers identified, the policy approach, and its public health implications. The final results are organized into a comprehensive discussion framework, providing a comprehensive understanding of digital exposomes as a modern approach to environmental exposure-based cancer risk mitigation.

RESULTS AND DISCUSSION

The following results and discussion section elaborates on the classification of different types of cancer-causing environmental exposures, the biological mechanisms behind them, and the contribution of digital exposome technologies, wearables, multi-omics, machine learning, and GIS in detecting, mapping, and mitigating cancer risk in a more targeted and data-driven manner.

1. CLASSIFICATION OF TYPES OF CANCER-CAUSING ENVIRONMENTAL EXPOSURES

The classification of cancer-causing environmental exposures covers various chemical, physical, biological, social, and behavioral agents. Each category comprises different substances or conditions contributing to the complex mechanisms behind cancer occurrence, as evidenced by numerous scientific studies.

a. Chemical agents

Chemical agents are significant contributors to cancer risk. Examples include persistent organic pollutants (POPs), heavy metals such as arsenic and mercury, volatile organic compounds (VOCs), and polycyclic aromatic hydrocarbons (PAHs). These substances can cause genetic mutations through DNA damage, which alters cellular processes and leads to the growth of cancer cells. Long-term exposure to these chemicals is associated with cumulative and synergistic effects, especially in developing lung and skin cancers (Lewandowska et al., 2019). Some substances, such as diethylnitrosamine (DENA), which is commonly found in food products, can form DNA adducts that trigger cellular abnormalities, including chromosomal abnormalities, as a precursor to tumors (Arnaud et al., 2021). Toxicological evaluations have also shown that many chemical agents are carcinogenic due to their genotoxic profile. Findings from the National Toxicology Program (NTP) confirm that chemicals can have long-term carcinogenic effects that are only apparent through intensive testing and classification systems such as the Oncologic database. In addition, recent studies highlight the importance of understanding food contaminants' genotoxic and non-genomic mechanisms, particularly in colorectal cell carcinogenesis (Arnaud et al., 2021).

b. Physical agents

Physical agents also play an important role in cancer causation, especially about radiation exposure. Ultraviolet (UV) radiation is known to be a potent carcinogen due to its ability to damage DNA through the formation of pyrimidine dimers, which are directly linked to skin cancer. Ionizing radiation, such as radon, has also been linked to lung cancer through genetic damage (Lewandowska et al., 2019). Exposure to electromagnetic fields (EMF), especially from electronic devices, is still controversial in carcinogenic risk assessment. Despite being a common concern, there is no conclusive scientific evidence regarding the carcinogenic mechanism of EMFs (Chapman et al., 2021). Research suggests that structural signals in chemical molecules may help classify potential carcinogens more accurately, providing insight into mechanisms of action and helping to identify risk factors from physical exposures.

c. Biological agents

Biological agents, particularly viruses, play a crucial role in cancer development. High-risk types of human papillomavirus (HPV), Epstein-Barr virus (EBV), and hepatitis B and C viruses are classified as oncogenic pathogens. These viruses can disrupt standard cellular mechanisms by inactivating tumor suppressor genes, promoting chronic inflammation, and inducing genomic instability, ultimately facilitating uncontrolled cell proliferation and tumorigenesis (Lewandowska et al., 2019).

Recent advancements in oncology have explored the therapeutic potential of viruses through the development of oncolytic virotherapy. This strategy involves genetically engineered or naturally occurring viruses that selectively infect and destroy cancer cells while sparing normal tissues. Oncolytic viruses cause direct tumor cell lysis and stimulate systemic anti-tumor immune responses, offering a dual therapeutic benefit. Despite promising clinical outcomes, challenges such as immune clearance, delivery efficiency, and tumor microenvironment barriers remain active research areas (Chen et al., 2023).

d. Social and Behavioral Factors

Social and behavioral factors are increasingly recognized as contributors to cancer risk. Unhealthy lifestyles such as poor diet, physical inactivity, and stress have been associated with increased cancer risk. Psychosocial factors also have a significant influence on patient outcomes, where social support and emotional-mental interventions can affect the prognosis of cancer patients. Research suggests that a comprehensive cancer risk assessment should include biological and chemical exposures and social determinants of health that influence lifestyle and mental state. Developing interventions that promote healthy behaviors and address socio-cultural barriers to healthcare access is critical to reducing cancer morbidity and mortality (Tamer & Yuksel, 2020).

2. PRENATAL EXPOSURE AND EPIGENETIC MECHANISMS IN CARCINOGENESIS

Prenatal exposure represents a critical and highly sensitive window in human development, during which environmental factors can exert profound and lasting influences on health trajectories through various epigenetic mechanisms, including DNA methylation, histone modifications, and the regulation of gene expression by non-coding RNAs. These molecular alterations are increasingly recognized as central to the pathogenesis of several diseases, particularly in the context of carcinogenesis. Evidence suggests that early-life exposure to environmental toxicants, such as industrial chemicals, pollutants, and dietary factors, can significantly modify the epigenome, thereby predisposing individuals to an elevated risk of malignancies such as leukemia and neuroblastoma later in life (Go et al., 2023; Pramana et al., 2020).

DNA methylation has emerged as a critical regulatory mechanism governing gene expression and genomic stability among the various epigenetic processes. Aberrant DNA methylation patterns have been extensively studied in cancer biology, demonstrating their key role in tumor initiation and progression. Environmental exposures, particularly to polycyclic aromatic hydrocarbons (PAHs) and heavy metals like arsenic and cadmium, have been shown to disrupt normal methylation homeostasis. Hypomethylation of oncogene promoters can lead to their aberrant activation, while hypermethylation of tumor suppressor gene promoters often results in their transcriptional silencing, collectively contributing to tumorigenesis.

Recent advances in molecular epidemiology have further demonstrated that DNA methylation alterations are not only involved in the late stages of carcinogenesis but may also serve as early molecular events detectable prior to the appearance of clinical symptoms. This has positioned DNA methylation signatures as promising non-invasive biomarkers for various cancers' early detection, prognosis, and risk stratification (Chen et al., 2021; Shao et al., 2021). Furthermore, studies have indicated that these methylation changes can sometimes be reversed or modulated, opening avenues for preventive interventions and targeted therapies to restore normal epigenetic regulation (Lee et al., 2020; Park et al., 2020).

Understanding the impact of prenatal environmental exposures on epigenetic programming thus holds critical implications for elucidating the mechanisms underlying cancer susceptibility and developing early diagnostic tools and preventive strategies. Continued research into exposure-epigenome interactions during early development remains essential for advancing precision medicine approaches and reducing the long-term burden of environmentally-induced cancers.

Histone modification is also an important epigenetic mechanism that affects chromatin structure and, in turn, gene transcription. Histones can be modified in various ways, including methylation, acetylation, and phosphorylation, all of which can alter the accessibility of DNA for transcription machinery. Research shows that modified histones allow for significant changes in gene regulation that are important for cancer development, such as cell cycle control and response to DNA damage (Mollah & Subramaniam, 2020). For example, SETDB1, as a histone methyltransferase, has been shown to play a role in the silencing of tumor suppressor genes, and its increased expression has been linked to the development of several forms of cancer, such as colon cancer and breast cancer (Kim et al., 2020).

In addition to DNA and histone modifications, the regulation of non-coding RNAs also has important implications for carcinogenesis. MicroRNAs (miRNAs), for example, can regulate the stability of mRNAs and their translation. Prenatal exposure to harmful compounds can modify miRNA expression, potentially altering signaling pathways involved in cell growth and development. These distorted miRNAs can have long-term impacts on biological systems, including increasing the risk of developing neoplasms (Perri et al., 2019). Recent studies have shown that exposure to environmental chemicals such as plasticizers and pesticides can alter the expression of microRNAs (miRNAs), which play a role in genetic regulation and carcinogenesis. These changes in miRNA expression may increase the incidence of cancer, particularly in early-age populations that are more susceptible to environmental toxicants (Ferrante et al., 2021).

Consistent longitudinal data show a significant association between prenatal environmental exposures and cancer development in children. In-depth research is needed to understand more about the timing and duration of carcinogen exposure, as well as how epigenetic patterns may serve as markers for later cancer risk. Moreover, utilizing new technologies in epigenetic biology has the potential to identify early biomarkers that can guide more targeted treatment and prevention (Chen et al., 2021; Xue et al., 2019). Emphasis on early intervention and screening monitoring may increase the likelihood of success in addressing cancers associated with prenatal exposure.

With the advancement of epigenetic research, new therapeutic avenues have emerged, focusing on correcting aberrant histone modifications. Recent studies have identified prognostic models based on histone modification-related genes, suggesting potential targets for innovative cancer therapies (Chen et al., 2021). A theoretical and practical understanding of the underpinnings of these mechanisms provides an important foundation for further exploration into the utilization of epigenetics as a diagnostic and therapeutic tool in the context of carcinogenesis.

Prenatal exposure to various environmental factors and epigenetic mechanisms such as DNA methylation, histone modification, and non-coding RNA regulation play an important role in increased cancer risk. Through a better understanding of these mechanisms, health sciences can begin to target more effective preventive interventions, building new hope for cancer disease management in future generations. Further research should focus on the potential of epigenetic biomarkers for early detection and developing more effective therapies based on a deep understanding of epigenetic changes associated with carcinogenesis.

3. THE ROLE OF MULTI-OMICS IN EARLY DETECTION AND CANCER RISK PROFILING

The integration of multi-omics approaches—encompassing genomics, epigenomics, transcriptomics, proteomics, and metabolomics—has revolutionized the landscape of early cancer detection by providing a comprehensive framework to capture the intricate interplay between genetic predispositions, molecular dynamics, and environmental exposures. By leveraging multiple layers of biological information, multi-omics identifies subtle, early biological changes that often remain undetectable through single-omics analyses, thereby enhancing the sensitivity and specificity of cancer diagnostics (Heo et al., 2021).

Recent advancements in exposome research, particularly through mechanistic molecular biology and metabolomic profiling, have expanded the capacity to elucidate environmental contributions to carcinogenesis. The development of sensitive analytical platforms has facilitated the identification of biomarkers associated with specific toxicants, such as benzene and formaldehyde, offering critical insights into the molecular mechanisms driving environmental carcinogenesis (Foreman et al., 2024). In parallel, proteomic analyses have emerged as vital tools in detecting changes in tissue protein expression profiles, assisting in early tumor characterization and distinguishing between distinct tumor subtypes.

To address tumors' inherent complexity and heterogeneity, sophisticated computational algorithms have been developed to optimize multi-omics data integration. Methods such as MONET (Multi-Omic clustering by Non-Exhaustive search Technique) and NEMO (Network Module Clustering for Multi-Omics) cluster patients based on integrated molecular signatures, thereby revealing novel tumor phenotypes that transcend traditional histopathological classifications (Rappoport et al., 2020). Such stratification is particularly valuable for understanding intra-tumor variability, a significant obstacle to effective cancer management, and paves the way for more refined patient risk profiling and tailored therapeutic strategies (Heo et al., 2021; Sharifi-Noghabi et al., 2019).

The advent of liquid biopsy technologies, which integrate circulating tumor DNA (ctDNA) analysis with proteomic and metabolomic biomarkers, represents another significant advancement, offering a minimally invasive method for early cancer detection and dynamic disease monitoring. Liquid biopsy approaches hold particular promise in capturing tumor heterogeneity and evolutionary changes over time, further underscoring the importance of integrative multi-omics frameworks.

Moreover, exposome-based metabolomic studies have illuminated the critical role of gene-environment interactions in cancer development, emphasizing that carcinogenesis is rarely driven by genetic mutations alone but often by complex and cumulative environmental influences modulating biological pathways (Foreman et al., 2024). This perspective reinforces the necessity of adopting holistic approaches that consider intrinsic and extrinsic factors in cancer risk assessment and prevention.

The burgeoning field of artificial intelligence (AI) further amplifies the potential of multi-omics research. AI-based analytical models, such as autoencoders, support vector machines, and logistic regression frameworks, have demonstrated remarkable capabilities in mining large-scale, high-dimensional omics datasets to uncover novel biomarkers and predict individualized therapeutic responses (Milner & Lennerz, 2024; Xiaoyi et al., 2023). Through integrating AI with multi-omics data, researchers can now construct more robust predictive models that enhance early detection accuracy and inform precision oncology initiatives.

In summary, integrating multi-omics technologies, empowered by exosome advances, proteomics, and AI-driven analytics, fundamentally transforms the understanding of cancer biology. By offering unprecedented insights into the complex molecular and environmental determinants of cancer, multi-omics approaches are poised to drive the next generation of individualized cancer prevention, early detection, and therapeutic strategies, ultimately improving patient outcomes and advancing the paradigm of personalized medicine.

4. MACHINE LEARNING FOR EXPOSOME BIG DATA ANALYTICS

Machine learning (ML) has emerged as a pivotal tool in analyzing digital exposomes, which generate vast, complex, and multidimensional datasets encompassing environmental and lifestyle factors such as air pollution, chemical exposures, dietary patterns, and occupational hazards. The application of ML allows for the systematic processing and extraction of meaningful patterns from these extensive datasets, facilitating a more nuanced understanding of the relationships between environmental exposures and health outcomes. Advanced ML algorithms, including random forest, support vector machine (SVM), and increasingly, deep learning models, are instrumental in detecting subtle, non-linear associations that traditional statistical methods often fail to capture (Ernawati et al., 2022; Peng et al., 2020). ML enables more precise, data-driven health interventions through such sophisticated approaches, transforming the landscape of exposure assessment and disease prevention.

One concrete application of ML lies in developing individualized cancer risk stratification models. These models integrate diverse data streams, encompassing genetic, environmental, and behavioral variables, to predict an individual's risk of developing cancer more accurately. In addition to classical algorithms such as random forest and SVM, deep learning techniques, particularly convolutional neural networks (CNNs), have demonstrated substantial efficacy in enhancing risk prediction by accommodating complex feature hierarchies and high-dimensional interactions. For instance, Go et al. (2023) employed random forest models to identify subgroups of women with prenatal exposure to hazardous chemicals who exhibited a higher propensity for developing breast cancer later in life. Similarly, Gong et al. (2023) demonstrated how deep learning-based analysis of satellite imagery and environmental monitoring data could spatially map areas of elevated air pollution, correlating them with increased lung cancer incidence. These advances enable geographically informed public health interventions while incorporating individual-level behavioral and genetic susceptibilities.

Beyond risk prediction, ML is a powerful tool for population stratification based on risk profiles derived from demographic characteristics, medical history, and environmental exposure trajectories. By identifying high-risk subpopulations, ML-driven analytics enhances the precision of public health strategies, allowing for targeted resource allocation and tailored preventive measures. Predictive analytics supported by ML strengthens public health surveillance and early warning systems and informs the design of intervention programs responsive to the dynamic nature of environmental exposures and societal changes (Dixit et al., 2024; Ernawati et al., 2024). These developments signify a transition from traditional, population-based prevention models to more personalized, data-driven cancer prevention and control approaches.

Nevertheless, the integration of ML into exposome analysis is accompanied by significant challenges. Critical concerns surrounding data privacy, security, ethical use, and the fragmentation of data sources pose barriers to seamless implementation. The diversity of data types — including genomics, environmental monitoring, wearable device outputs, and electronic health records — requires standardized data harmonization and interoperability frameworks. To address these issues, continuous efforts in policy integration are imperative, aiming to strike an optimal balance between protecting individual privacy and fostering innovation. Regulatory frameworks must evolve with technological advancements to ensure that ML applications remain ethically sound and socially acceptable.

Moreover, ML-based exposome analysis holds immense potential for elucidating the complex interplay between environmental, genetic, and behavioral determinants of health across the life course. By capturing dynamic exposures and biological responses in real-time, these approaches deepen our understanding of disease etiology and offer opportunities for earlier and more effective intervention (Di et al., 2022). The convergence of ML with exosomes thus represents a paradigm shift in precision public health, moving towards interventions that are not only reactive but anticipatory.

The success of such integrative efforts depends heavily on cross-disciplinary collaboration, bringing together expertise from computer science, biostatistics, environmental health, epidemiology, and bioethics (Chen et al., 2021). Building theoretical and methodological foundations that are robust, transparent, and generalizable across populations is essential to advance the field. Additionally, a commitment to embedding ethical principles — including transparency, fairness, accountability, and inclusivity — into the design and deployment of ML models is crucial to ensure that data-driven innovations enhance, rather than exacerbate, health equity.

Machine learning offers unprecedented opportunities to revolutionize exposure assessment, risk prediction, and disease prevention. However, realizing its full potential requires careful navigation of technical, ethical, and societal challenges. By fostering interdisciplinary partnerships and prioritizing ethical governance, ML can contribute to a future where public health strategies are more responsive, personalized, and equitable, thereby addressing individual and population-level health risks in an increasingly complex and dynamic environment.

5. ENHANCING DATA FUSION AND SPATIAL MODELING IN EXPOSOME ANALYTICS

In the realm of exposome-based cancer risk assessments, the integration of diverse datasets is pivotal for accurate spatial modeling. Data fusion techniques such as early, Integrating heterogeneous data for exposome-based cancer risk mapping necessitates selecting appropriate data fusion strategies and AI algorithms. Early fusion merges raw demographic, geographic, and environmental data before feature extraction, yet it may suffer from format incompatibilities (Feng et al., 2021). Alternatively, intermediate fusion, which extracts features separately before integration, enhances flexibility and interpretability, as suggested by studies focusing on integrating high-resolution demographic and environmental variables (Wijaya et al., 2022).

Late fusion, which combines predictions from independent models, supports modular design and has practical utility in urban health risk assessments. Random Forests are frequently employed in spatial modeling for their robustness and interpretability; however, deep learning methods such as Convolutional Neural Networks have demonstrated superior capabilities in capturing complex spatial patterns from satellite imagery (Morandeira et al., 2019). Thus, selecting a fusion and modeling technique is contingent upon data quality, spatial resolution, and specific research objectives, underscoring the need for tailored AI strategies in risk assessment.

6. WEARABLE AND SENSOR TECHNOLOGY IN REAL-TIME BIOMONITORING

Recent advancements in wearable and sensor technologies have revolutionized real-time environmental biomonitoring. Smart devices, such as air quality trackers and UV exposure monitors, enable continuous assessment of pollutants like PM2.5, CO, NO2, and UV radiation, thereby empowering communities to understand better and mitigate environmental health risks (Marfo & Obeng-Gyasi, 2024). One key feature of wearables is GPS integration, allowing location-based exposure tracking. For instance, urban studies in cities like New York and Tokyo used portable air sensors to assess participants' exposure throughout the day, integrating variables like indoor/outdoor time and sleep patterns to enhance exposure modeling (Fu et al., 2022).

Smartphone connectivity is another essential component. Apps linked to wearables enable self-reporting and deliver alerts about harmful exposure levels. UV sensors, for example, can prompt users to reapply sunscreen, reducing skin cancer risk. Research shows wearables increase environmental health awareness, particularly empowering marginalized communities to monitor their exposure and health risks (Marfo & Obeng-Gyasi, 2024; Tundjungsari et al., 2020). This promotes collaboration between citizens and policymakers to improve air quality monitoring and public health efforts.

Miniaturized sensors provide vital data for understanding pollutant exposure and health impacts, as Fu et al. (2022). highlighted. Integrating physiological and environmental sensor data in pediatric asthma research offers more profound insights, enhancing care outcomes for vulnerable children. Wearables also support environmental justice by democratizing access to exposure data in underserved communities and fostering active participation in environmental decision-making (Marfo & Obeng-Gyasi, 2024).

In addition, advances in wearable sensor technologies allow real-time monitoring of environmental exposures such as air pollutants and heat, aiming to reduce health incidents related to extreme weather conditions. Recent innovations, such as wearable carbon monoxide sensors using hybrid PANI/SWCNT/Ferrocene-based layers, demonstrate high sensitivity and portability for personal environmental monitoring (Savin et al., 2021). In modeling environmental threats, wearables help link environmental data to individual health, strengthening community resilience (Savin et al., 2021). Integrating digital exposome tools, including remote sensing technologies, Surface Acoustic Wave (SAW) sensors, and self-heating nanomaterial-based sensors, enables more precise, continuous, and scalable environmental exposure monitoring. This advancement overcomes traditional exposome limitations by providing real-time, personalized data on diet, occupational exposures, lifestyle factors, and environmental pollutants.

Table 1. Comparison of Digital Exposome Monitoring Tools

Tool	Function	Advantages	Challenges
Wearable Sensor (UV, PM2.5)	Individual exposure monitoring	Real-time, portable	Battery life, privacy issues
GPS Smartphone	Geospatial exposure tracking	Easy access, accurate	Data privacy concerns
GIS	Spatial analysis of exposure patterns	Visualizing risk clusters	Data quality limitations
Crowdsourced Mobile Apps	Community-reported pollution data	Broad community participation	Reporting bias
Remote Sensing (Satellite)	Regional pollutant detection	Large scale, frequent updates	Low spatial resolution

Table 1 shows the main tools in digital exposure monitoring, including wearable sensors, smartphone GPS, GIS, crowdsourcing applications, and remote sensing. Each tool has advantages in enriching environmental exposure data spatially and temporally but also faces challenges such as technical limitations and privacy issues. The integration of these technologies strengthens digital exposome analysis to support early detection and evidence-based cancer prevention.

By understanding the advantages and limitations of these digital exposure monitoring tools, further spatial analysis through GIS-based mapping is the next strategic step in identifying the geographic distribution of cancer risk.

7. CANCER RISK MAPPING BASED ON GIS AND SPATIAL DATA

Geographic Information Systems (GIS) is an important tool in cancer risk mapping, enabling spatial analysis of the distribution of carcinogen exposure and cancer incidence in different regions. Researchers can identify correlations between environmental exposure levels and cancer incidence using spatial data, such as air and water pollution levels, land use maps, access to health facilities, and socioeconomic factors. For example, a study in South Korea by Jang et al. (2021) showed a significant relationship between hepatitis infection, poverty level, and liver cancer incidence, confirming the importance of geospatial approaches in understanding cancer epidemiology. GIS-based mapping improves the ability to visualize data distribution and supports public decision-making in cancer prevention efforts. This spatial visualization clarifies high-risk areas that require more targeted public health interventions.

One important aspect of cancer risk analysis is the impact of air and water pollution as significant risk factors. Research by Mungi et al. (2019) found that industrial benzene emissions were not significantly correlated with cancer incidence at the district level. However, exposure to delicate particulate matter (PM2.5) was positively associated with cancer incidence. These findings underscore the importance of spatial data accuracy in evaluating the health impacts of environmental pollutants, where GIS plays a vital role in collecting, mapping, and analyzing environmental exposure data.

Using GIS in cancer risk mapping also highlights the importance of access to health facilities. Studies in Japan found an association between income levels and cancer incidence, with areas of lower economic status tending to have poorer health outcomes. This is in line with findings in France, which showed that poverty contributes to an increased risk of cancer-related to alcohol and tobacco consumption (Bryere et al., 2019). With GIS, areas that need health interventions can be identified more precisely, formulating more focused and effective public health policies.

Geospatial analysis focused on identifying cancer clusters within a limited area provides important insights into existing risk factors. The study by Jang et al. (2021) illustrates how spatial analysis was used to determine liver cancer incidence and its influencing factors, focusing on the link between hepatitis infection and poverty. These findings show that GIS is a data collection tool and an analytic platform for understanding the complex relationship between risk factors and cancer incidence.

Advances in GIS technology have significantly increased the capacity of researchers to map and analyze cancer risk by integrating multiple complex factors, including environmental exposures, demographic characteristics, and social determinants of health. Through sophisticated spatial modeling and geostatistical approaches, studies have revealed significant geographic disparities in cancer incidence and mortality, highlighting the important role of socioeconomic inequalities and local environmental conditions in shaping health outcomes (Jang et al., 2021).

The application of GIS in cancer epidemiology improves precision in risk assessment. It enables policymakers to identify high-risk areas, allocate health resources more efficiently, and design targeted intervention strategies. Thus, using GIS contributes to creating more equitable public health outcomes in different regions. Independence in data analysis is an important aspect of using GIS. Studies show that applying more complex modeling, considering indices such as the Townsend Index, which reflects socioeconomic status, can improve the validity of spatial analysis results (Bryere et al., 2019). This approach is needed to ensure that the resulting cancer risk maps are accurate and helpful in planning preventive measures and health promotion.

Further research on data management in cancer-prone areas can deepen the understanding of the contribution of environmental exposures to cancer epidemiology. This is important for developing more effective monitoring and intervention strategies, focusing on the most affected areas. GIS provides a robust framework for integrating exposure and social and health data, revealing the deep interconnections between the environment and human health.

8. TOXICOGENOMICS AND VULNERABLE POPULATIONS

Toxicogenomics, the integration of toxicology and genomics, provides important insights into the interaction between environmental toxicants and genetic predisposition, especially in vulnerable groups such as children and pregnant women. The still-developing physiological conditions in these groups increase susceptibility to toxic exposures, where gene-environment interactions are crucial in determining health risks (Go et al., 2023).

Genetic variations, such as gene polymorphisms, can modify xenobiotic metabolic pathways, increasing the risk of disease, including cancer, through mechanisms involving DNA damage and immune system dysfunction (Foreman et al., 2024). Recent epidemiological studies have also shown that children and pregnant women living in agricultural zones are exposed to higher contaminants, such as nitrate levels, due to heightened biological sensitivity (Feng et al., 2021).

Socioeconomic status exacerbates this vulnerability. Low-income communities often face higher environmental exposure levels and have limited access to preventive health information and services (Bryere et al., 2019). Furthermore, genetic variation between ethnic groups also influences susceptibility to environmental toxins, underscoring the importance of public health approaches that consider genetic diversity (Juarez et al., 2023).

In this context, public health strategies tailored to individual genetic characteristics are crucial to reducing health disparities from environmental exposures (Matus et al., 2024). Digital exposome-based approaches have offered new opportunities to map the impact of pollutants on gene expression, deepening our understanding of gene-environment interactions and their impact on public health (Foreman et al., 2024).

Integrating toxicogenomics data into evidence-based health policies is critical to protect high-risk populations. This requires close collaboration between researchers, policymakers, and local communities. Public education on environmental and genetic risks and implementing better environmental management practices are key to empowering communities to play an active role in disease prevention efforts (Carter et al., 2019).

Furthermore, the development of interdisciplinary research that combines epidemiology, genomics, and data science accelerates the development of effective policies to reduce toxic exposures. Improved research infrastructure and utilization of advanced analytics support more individualized public health responses (Foreman et al., 2024). Increased public awareness of the links between genetic factors and environmental exposures is fundamental to building more inclusive community-based health strategies. A deeper understanding of toxicogenomic linkages and environmental exposures plays a key role in reducing health inequalities and achieving more equitable health outcomes.

Several developed countries have seen tangible implementations of using the digital exposome in public health policy. In Finland, for example, environmental monitoring systems have been integrated with national electronic health data, enabling early detection of cancer risk based on exposure levels to air pollutants such as PM2.5 and ozone (Matus et al., 2024). Meanwhile, in the Netherlands, exposome data has been used to map high-exposure areas and design community-based interventions, especially for vulnerable groups such as pregnant women and children in industrial areas (Foreman et al., 2024). This approach emphasizes how applying the digital exposome strengthens the public health system in evidence-based preventive efforts.

9. INTEGRATION OF DIGITAL EXPOSURE IN PUBLIC POLICY

Integrating the digital exposome into public policy is crucial to promoting improved public health and reducing the impact of various environmental risks. The exposome, which covers an individual's entire exposure to environmental factors throughout their lifetime, is a scientific analysis tool and a foundation for more effective and evidence-based policy decision-making.

As described by Andrianou et al., exposome-based tools can be applied in environmental exposure-oriented public health interventions, particularly in addressing urban infectious diseases (Andrianou et al., 2021). Policy developers can design more targeted and effective interventions by deriving information from exposome studies. One of the key recommendations is the implementation of exposure risk-based industrial zoning. This aligns with the concept proposed by Matus et al., who emphasized the importance of utilizing Big Data and the exposome approach in national health monitoring (Matus et al., 2024).

Combining exposome data with spatio-temporal analysis offers opportunities to identify biomarkers indicating potential health risks in specific populations. This enables earlier and more appropriate interventions, potentially reducing the prevalence of chronic diseases and cancers, especially those linked to environmental exposures. Air and water quality standards should also be developed based on newly discovered scientific evidence. Juárez et al. highlights the need for novel biomarkers to monitor exposure and its impacts on health (Juarez et al., 2023).

Appropriate air quality measurements should include continuous exposure monitoring linked to long-term health outcomes. Concurrently, research has shed light on how air pollution affects immune responses, findings that can be corroborated with exposome data (Orešič et al., 2020). Thus, developing quality standards should integrate considerations of exposures throughout the human life cycle that influence health outcomes.

Prenatal exposure-based cancer prevention policies are another important aspect of digital exposome integration. Studies have shown that exposure before birth can significantly affect a child's long-term health, as Foreman et al. highlighted the importance of mechanistic understanding in exposome research to elucidate the pathways between exposure and disease development (Foreman et al., 2024). Consequently, prevention programs should be designed to address risk factors experienced by pregnant women, particularly those living in heavily industrialized or heavily polluted environments.

Furthermore, a national digital environmental monitoring program must be established to integrate exposome data with public health systems. This supports the argument by Adeyinka and Adewumi regarding the need for agile governance systems to adapt to the digital era (Adeyinka & Adewumi, 2023). Such a program would incorporate digital technologies for real-time environmental exposure data collection, enabling authorities to rapidly adjust public health investment strategies, implement evidence-based interventions, and foster more effective cross-sector collaboration.

The practical application of the digital exposome in public policy has been demonstrated in Finland, the Netherlands, and Canada. In Finland, real-time air quality data is utilized to prioritize region-specific health interventions, thereby enhancing the responsiveness of public health actions (Matus et al., 2024). In the Netherlands, exposome data is integrated into the national e-health system to identify communities at high risk of industrial pollutant exposure, illustrating how the digital exposome can strengthen evidence-based health policies. Meanwhile, initiatives incorporating digital environmental exposure data into urban planning in Canada have shown promising outcomes in reducing community health risks.

Countries like Finland and the Netherlands illustrate how integrating exposome data into e-health systems can support environmentally-based early cancer detection. Finland, for instance, has implemented an air quality monitoring network that assesses real-time pollution levels and analyzes historical data to understand long-term health trends (Matus et al., 2024b). Other countries could adopt this model to promote public health policies that integrate exposome insights as a foundational consideration.

In this context, the digital exposome is no longer viewed merely as an academic concept but as a transformational tool capable of reshaping public health and safety policies. To effectively implement evidence-based policies, stakeholders must foster partnerships with academics and researchers to ensure that policy practices reflect the latest findings in exposome research. Such collaborations will encourage a broader application of scientific knowledge to real-world settings, translating research into tangible public health benefits.

Nonetheless, a significant challenge in implementing exposome-based policies lies in the multidisciplinary complexity involved, encompassing epidemiology, toxicology, public health, and environmental science (Bültmann et al., 2024). Therefore, policy development processes must incorporate interdisciplinary reviews to identify challenges and opportunities in applying exposome-based approaches. Ultimately, leveraging the exposome in public health decision-making will enhance our understanding of health risks and shape more proactive and preventive public health policies against emerging threats.

CONCLUSION

Integrating the digital exposome framework into cancer risk assessment marks a transformative advancement in environmental health research and public health strategy. By leveraging cutting-edge technologies such as wearable sensors, spatial analysis through GIS, multi-omics platforms, and machine learning algorithms, the digital exposome offers a holistic, real-time, and individualized approach to mapping environmental exposures and their biological impacts. This paradigm facilitates the early detection of cancer risk factors, enables personalized prevention strategies, and supports more precise public health interventions.

Environmental exposures—chemical, physical, biological, social, and behavioral—play a significant role in the multifactorial processes of carcinogenesis, with prenatal exposures presenting particularly critical windows of vulnerability through epigenetic modifications such as DNA methylation, histone alterations, and non-coding RNA regulation. Multi-omics technologies have further refined the ability to capture these molecular signatures. At the same time, machine learning enables integrating and interpreting high-dimensional exposome data to identify hidden patterns and generate predictive risk models with unprecedented accuracy.

Moreover, wearable technology and real-time spatial data have strengthened exposure mapping at individual and population levels, enabling geographically targeted health interventions and improving resource allocation in public health systems. Significantly, the digital exposome enriches scientific understanding and has direct applicability in evidence-based policymaking, particularly in designing equitable health interventions for vulnerable populations disproportionately affected by environmental risks.

However, the successful implementation of digital exposome approaches demands addressing critical challenges related to data privacy, ethical governance, interdisciplinary collaboration, and the harmonization of complex data systems. Strengthening cross-sectoral partnerships between health, environment, data science, and policy sectors will translate digital exposome innovations into sustainable and equitable health outcomes.

In conclusion, the digital exposome represents not merely an academic advancement but a powerful, transformative tool for precision public health, capable of reshaping cancer prevention, promoting environmental justice, and advancing toward a more responsive, preventive, and personalized healthcare future.

SUGGESTIONS

To optimize the application of digital exposomes in cancer prevention, several strategic recommendations need to be considered:

a. **Integration in the national health system:** The government must adopt the digital exposome approach into the public health surveillance system and data-driven policymaking.
b. **Strengthening technological and human resource capacity:** Training for health workers, researchers, and policymakers in wearable technology, omic analysis, and spatial data is needed.
c. **Multidisciplinary and cross-sector collaboration:** Addressing environmental exposures and cancer risk requires synergy between the health, environment, information technology, and education sectors.
d. **Focus on vulnerable populations:** Exposure data collection and analysis efforts should actively reach high-risk groups such as children, pregnant women, and low-income communities.

e. **Funding and sustainable research:** Financial and policy support for digital exposome research should be strengthened to accelerate innovation in cancer risk mitigation.

Through these steps, the digital exposome is a sophisticated diagnostic and predictive tool and the foundation for transforming the health system towards a more preventive, personalized, and equitable era.

REFERENCES

Adeyinka, F. M., & Adewumi, A. P. (2023). Enhancing Public Service Delivery in Nigeria Through Agile Practice. *Jurnal Administrasi Publik Public Administration Journal, 13*(2), 192–206. DOI: 10.31289/jap.v13i2.10647

Ahn, C., & Jeung, E.-B. (2023). Endocrine-Disrupting Chemicals and Disease End-points. *International Journal of Molecular Sciences, 24*(6), 5342. DOI: 10.3390/ijms24065342 PMID: 36982431

Andrianou, X. D., Pronk, A., Galea, K. S., Stierum, R., Loh, M., Riccardo, F., Pezzotti, P., & Makris, K. C. (2021). Exposome-based public health interventions for infectious diseases in urban settings. *Environment International, 146*, 106246. DOI: 10.1016/j.envint.2020.106246 PMID: 33181410

Arnaud, L. C., Gauthier, T., Le Naour, A., Hashim, S., Naud, N., Shay, J. W., Pierre, F. H., Boutet-Robinet, E., & Huc, L. (2021). Short-Term and Long-Term Carcinogenic Effects of Food Contaminants (4-Hydroxynonenal and Pesticides) on Colorectal Human Cells: Involvement of Genotoxic and Non-Genomic Mechanisms. *Cancers (Basel), 13*(17), 4337. DOI: 10.3390/cancers13174337 PMID: 34503147

Bhattacharjee, N., Sarkar, S., & Giri, B. (2022). Impact of endocrine disrupting chemicals (EDCs) on the predisposition of cancer and polycystic ovary syndrome (PCOS): A Note. *Journal of Drug Delivery and Therapeutics, 12*(5), 3–7. DOI: 10.22270/jddt.v12i5.5582

Bryere, J., Tron, L., Menvielle, G., & Launoy, G. (2019). The respective parts of incidence and lethality in socioeconomic differences in cancer mortality. An analysis of the French network Cancer registries (FRANCIM) data. *International Journal for Equity in Health, 18*(1), 189. DOI: 10.1186/s12939-019-1087-y PMID: 31796079

Bültmann, U., Broberg, K., & Selander, J. (2024). Integrating a life course perspective in work environment and health research: Empirical challenges and interdisciplinary opportunities. *Scandinavian Journal of Work, Environment & Health, 50*(5), 311–316. DOI: 10.5271/sjweh.4174 PMID: 38934300

Carter, S. E., Ong, M. L., Simons, R. L., Gibbons, F. X., Lei, M. K., & Beach, S. R. H. (2019). The effect of early discrimination on accelerated aging among African Americans. *Health Psychology, 38*(11), 1010–1013. DOI: 10.1037/hea0000788 PMID: 31343220

Chapman, K. E., Wilde, E. C., Chapman, F. M., Verma, J. R., Shah, U.-K., Stannard, L. M., Seager, A. L., Tonkin, J. A., Brown, M. R., Doherty, A. T., Johnson, G. E., Doak, S. H., & Jenkins, G. J. S. (2021). Multiple-endpoint in vitro carcinogenicity test in human cell line TK6 distinguishes carcinogens from non-carcinogens and highlights mechanisms of action. *Archives of Toxicology*, *95*(1), 321–336. DOI: 10.1007/s00204-020-02902-3 PMID: 32910239

Chen, C. X., Park, H. S., Price, H., & Wax, A. (2021). Automated Classification of Breast Cancer Cells Using High-Throughput Holographic Cytometry. *Frontiers in Physics (Lausanne)*, *9*, 759142. Advance online publication. DOI: 10.3389/fphy.2021.759142

Chen, K., Zhang, F., Ding, J., Liang, Y., Zhan, Z., Zhan, Y., Chen, L., & Ding, Y. (2017). Histone Methyltransferase SETDB1 Promotes the Progression of Colorectal Cancer by Inhibiting the Expression of TP53. *Journal of Cancer*, *8*(16), 3318–3330. DOI: 10.7150/jca.20482 PMID: 29158805

Chen, L., Zuo, M., Zhou, Q., & Wang, Y. (2023). Oncolytic virotherapy in cancer treatment: Challenges and optimization prospects. *Frontiers in Immunology*, *14*, 1308890. Advance online publication. DOI: 10.3389/fimmu.2023.1308890 PMID: 38169820

Chen, Y., Xu, R., Ruze, R., Yang, J., Wang, H., Song, J., You, L., Wang, C., & Zhao, Y. (2021). Construction of a prognostic model with histone modification-related genes and identification of potential drugs in pancreatic cancer. *Cancer Cell International*, *21*(1), 291. DOI: 10.1186/s12935-021-01928-6 PMID: 34090418

Combarnous, Y., & Nguyen, T. M. D. (2019). Comparative Overview of the Mechanisms of Action of Hormones and Endocrine Disruptor Compounds. *Toxics*, *7*(1), 5. DOI: 10.3390/toxics7010005 PMID: 30682876

Di, S., Petch, J., Gerstein, H. C., Zhu, R., & Sherifali, D. (2022). Optimizing Health Coaching for Patients With Type 2 Diabetes Using Machine Learning: Model Development and Validation Study. *JMIR Formative Research*, *6*(9), e37838. DOI: 10.2196/37838 PMID: 36099006

Dixit, A., Gupta, A. K., Chaplot, N., & Bharti, V. (2024). Emoji Support Predictive Mental Health Assessment Using Machine Learning: Unveiling Personalized Intervention Avenues. *International Journal of Experimental Research and Review*, *42*, 228–240. DOI: 10.52756/ijerr.2024.v42.020

Ernawati, K., Burhan, A., Albar, A. S., Al Khaliel, A. T., & Al Fatich, A. S. F. (2024). *Professional Development of Environmental Health Workers*. DOI: 10.4018/979-8-3693-4334-0.ch010

Ernawati, K., Nugroho, B. S., Suryana, C., Riyanto, A., & Fatmawati, E. (2022). advantages of digital applications in public health services on automation era. *International Journal of Health Sciences*, *6*(1), 174–186. DOI: 10.53730/ijhs.v6n1.3684

Feng, C., Li, R., Shamim, A. A., Ullah, M. B., Li, M., Dev, R., Wang, Y., Zhao, T., Liao, J., Du, Z., Ling, Y., Lai, Y., & Hao, Y. (2021). High-resolution mapping of reproductive tract infections among women of childbearing age in Bangladesh: A spatial-temporal analysis of the demographic and health survey. *BMC Public Health*, *21*(1), 342. DOI: 10.1186/s12889-021-10360-4 PMID: 33579253

Ferrante, M., Cristaldi, A., & Oliveri Conti, G. (2021). Oncogenic Role of miRNA in Environmental Exposure to Plasticizers: A Systematic Review. *Journal of Personalized Medicine*, *11*(6), 500. DOI: 10.3390/jpm11060500 PMID: 34199666

Foreman, A. L., Warth, B., Hessel, E. V. S., Price, E. J., Schymanski, E. L., Cantelli, G., Parkinson, H., Hecht, H., Klánová, J., Vlaanderen, J., Hilscherova, K., Vrijheid, M., Vineis, P., Araujo, R., Barouki, R., Vermeulen, R., Lanone, S., Brunak, S., Sebert, S., & Karjalainen, T. (2024). Adopting Mechanistic Molecular Biology Approaches in Exposome Research for Causal Understanding. *Environmental Science & Technology*, *58*(17), 7256–7269. DOI: 10.1021/acs.est.3c07961 PMID: 38641325

Fu, X., Cai, Q., Yang, Y., Xu, Y., Zhao, F., Yang, J., Qiao, L., Yao, L., & Li, W. (2022). Application of Mobile Monitoring to Study Characteristics of Air Pollution in Typical Areas of the Yangtze River Delta Eco-Green Integration Demonstration Zone, China. *Sustainability (Basel)*, *15*(1), 205. DOI: 10.3390/su15010205

Go, Y.-M., Weinberg, J., Teeny, S., Cirillo, P. M., Krigbaum, N. Y., Singer, G., Tran, V., Cohn, B. A., & Jones, D. P. (2023). Exposome epidemiology for suspect environmental chemical exposures during pregnancy linked to subsequent breast cancer diagnosis. *Environment International*, *178*, 108112. DOI: 10.1016/j.envint.2023.108112 PMID: 37517180

Heo, Y. J., Hwa, C., Lee, G.-H., Park, J.-M., & An, J.-Y. (2021). Integrative Multi-Omics Approaches in Cancer Research: From Biological Networks to Clinical Subtypes. *Molecules and Cells*, *44*(7), 433–443. DOI: 10.14348/molcells.2021.0042 PMID: 34238766

International Agency for Research on Cancer (IARC). (2020). *Global Cancer Observatory: Cancer Today.* The Global Cancer Observatory (GCO) World Health Organization. https://gco.iarc.fr/today(https://gco.iarc.fr/today

Jang, J., Yoo, D.-S., & Chun, B. C. (2021). Spatial epidemiologic analysis of the liver cancer and gallbladder cancer incidence and its determinants in South Korea. *BMC Public Health*, *21*(1), 2090. DOI: 10.1186/s12889-021-12184-8 PMID: 34774036

Juarez, P. D., Hood, D. B., Song, M., & Ramesh, A. (2023). Applying an Exposome-wide Association Study (ExWAS) Approach to Latino Cancer Disparities. In *Advancing the Science of Cancer in Latinos* (pp. 17–32). Springer International Publishing. DOI: 10.1007/978-3-031-14436-3_2

Kim, H. G., Sung, J.-Y., Na, K., & Kim, S.-W. (2020). Low H3K9me3 Expression Is Associated With Poor Prognosis in Patients With Distal Common Bile Duct Cancer. *In Vivo (Athens, Greece)*, *34*(6), 3619–3626. DOI: 10.21873/invivo.12207 PMID: 33144476

Lee, H.-J., Lee, Y., & Yun, J. (2020). Factors Associated with Physical Activity in Older Adults by Region: Based on the 2017 Community Health Survey. *Journal of Korean Academy of Community Health Nursing*, *31*(Suppl), 563. DOI: 10.12799/jkachn.2020.31.S.563

Lewandowska, A., Rudzki, M., Rudzki, S., Lewandowski, T., & Laskowska, B. (2019a). Environmental risk factors for cancer – review paper. *Annals of Agricultural and Environmental Medicine*, *26*(1), 1–7. DOI: 10.26444/aaem/94299 PMID: 30922021

Lewandowska, A., Rudzki, M., Rudzki, S., Lewandowski, T., & Laskowska, B. (2019b). Environmental risk factors for cancer – review paper. *Annals of Agricultural and Environmental Medicine*, *26*(1), 1–7. DOI: 10.26444/aaem/94299 PMID: 30922021

Marfo, A., & Obeng-Gyasi, E. (2024). *Empowering communities: The role of wearable devices in environmental justice*. DOI: 10.22541/au.170965072.20316399/v1

Matus, P., Urquidi, C., Cárcamo, M., & Vidal, V. (2024). Integrating the exposome and one health approach to national health surveillance: An opportunity for Latin American countries in health preventive management. *Frontiers in Public Health*, *12*, 1376609. Advance online publication. DOI: 10.3389/fpubh.2024.1376609 PMID: 39211902

Milner, D. A.Jr, & Lennerz, J. K. (2024). Technology and Future of Multi-Cancer Early Detection. *Life (Chicago, Ill.)*, *14*(7), 833. DOI: 10.3390/life14070833 PMID: 39063587

Mollah, S. A., & Subramaniam, S. (2020). Histone Signatures Predict Therapeutic Efficacy in Breast Cancer. *IEEE Open Journal of Engineering in Medicine and Biology*, *1*, 74–82. DOI: 10.1109/OJEMB.2020.2967105 PMID: 32412527

Morandeira, N. S., Castesana, P. S., Cardo, M. V., Salomone, V. N., Vadell, M. V., & Rubio, A. (2019). An interdisciplinary approach to assess human health risk in an urban environment: A case study in temperate Argentina. *Heliyon*, *5*(10), e02555. DOI: 10.1016/j.heliyon.2019.e02555 PMID: 31687482

Mungi, C., Lai, D., & Du, X. L. (2019). Spatial Analysis of Industrial Benzene Emissions and Cancer Incidence Rates in Texas. *International Journal of Environmental Research and Public Health*, *16*(15), 2627. DOI: 10.3390/ijerph16152627 PMID: 31344779

Orešič, M., McGlinchey, A., Wheelock, C. E., & Hyötyläinen, T. (2020). Metabolic Signatures of the Exposome—Quantifying the Impact of Exposure to Environmental Chemicals on Human Health. *Metabolites*, *10*(11), 454. DOI: 10.3390/metabo10110454 PMID: 33182712

Park, H.-M., Kim, H., Lee, K.-H., & Cho, J.-Y. (2020). Analysis of opposing histone modifications H3K4me3 and H3K27me3 reveals candidate diagnostic biomarkers for TNBC and gene set prediction combination. *BMB Reports*, *53*(5), 266–271. DOI: 10.5483/BMBRep.2020.53.5.045 PMID: 32317088

Peng, C., He, M., Cutrona, S. L., Kiefe, C. I., Liu, F., & Wang, Z. (2020). Theme Trends and Knowledge Structure on Mobile Health Apps: Bibliometric Analysis. *JMIR mHealth and uHealth*, *8*(7), e18212. DOI: 10.2196/18212 PMID: 32716312

Perri, A. M., Agosti, V., Olivo, E., Concolino, A., De Angelis, M., Tammè, L., Fiumara, C. V., Cuda, G., & Scumaci, D. (2019). Histone proteomics reveals novel post-translational modifications in breast cancer. *Aging (Albany NY)*, *11*(23), 11722–11755. DOI: 10.18632/aging.102577 PMID: 31816600

Pramana, C., Peranawengrum, K. B., & Juliani, V. (2020). Maternal characteristics and perinatal outcomes in women with severe preeclampsia. *Systematic Reviews in Pharmacy*, *11*, 549–553.

Rappoport, N., Safra, R., & Shamir, R. (2020). MONET: Multi-omic module discovery by omic selection. *PLoS Computational Biology*, *16*(9), e1008182. DOI: 10.1371/journal.pcbi.1008182 PMID: 32931516

Savin, M., Mihailescu, C.-M., Avramescu, V., Dinulescu, S., Firtat, B., Craciun, G., Brasoveanu, C., Pachiu, C., Romanitan, C., Serban, A.-B., Ion, A. C., & Moldovan, C. (2021). A New Hybrid Sensitive PANI/SWCNT/Ferrocene-Based Layer for a Wearable CO Sensor. *Sensors (Basel)*, *21*(5), 1801. DOI: 10.3390/s21051801 PMID: 33807640

Shao, K., Pu, W., Zhang, J., Guo, S., Qian, F., Glurich, I., Jin, Q., Ma, Y., Ju, S., Zhang, Z., & Ding, W. (2021). DNA hypermethylation contributes to colorectal cancer metastasis by regulating the binding of CEBPB and TFCP2 to the CPEB1 promoter. *Clinical Epigenetics*, *13*(1), 89. DOI: 10.1186/s13148-021-01071-z PMID: 33892791

Sharifi-Noghabi, H., Zolotareva, O., Collins, C. C., & Ester, M. (2019). MOLI: Multi-omics late integration with deep neural networks for drug response prediction. *Bioinformatics (Oxford, England)*, *35*(14), i501–i509. DOI: 10.1093/bioinformatics/btz318 PMID: 31510700

Sun, L., Yang, H., Cai, Y., Li, W., Liu, G., & Tang, Y. (2019). *In Silico* Prediction of Endocrine Disrupting Chemicals Using Single-Label and Multilabel Models. *Journal of Chemical Information and Modeling*, *59*(3), 973–982. DOI: 10.1021/acs.jcim.8b00551 PMID: 30807141

Tamer, F., & Yuksel, M. E. (2020). Colonoscopy in patients with psoriasis before the initiation of treatment with biological agents. *Dermatologic Therapy*, *33*(4). Advance online publication. DOI: 10.1111/dth.13720 PMID: 32506694

Tseng, C.-H., Tsuang, B.-J., Chiang, C.-J., Ku, K.-C., Tseng, J.-S., Yang, T.-Y., Hsu, K.-H., Chen, K.-C., Yu, S.-L., Lee, W.-C., Liu, T.-W., Chan, C.-C., & Chang, G.-C. (2019). The Relationship Between Air Pollution and Lung Cancer in Non-smokers in Taiwan. *Journal of Thoracic Oncology*, *14*(5), 784–792. DOI: 10.1016/j.jtho.2018.12.033 PMID: 30664991

Tundjungsari, V., Ernawati, K., & Mutia, N. (2020). *Public Health Surveillance to Promote Clean and Healthy Life Behaviours Using Big Data Approach (An Indonesian Case Study)* (pp. 761–775). DOI: 10.1007/978-3-030-23162-0_69

Vermeulen, R., Schymanski, E. L., Barabási, A.-L., & Miller, G. W. (2020). The exposome and health: Where chemistry meets biology. *Science*, *367*(6476), 392–396. DOI: 10.1126/science.aay3164 PMID: 31974245

Wijaya, A. P., Nugraha, A. L., Sukmono, A., & Firdaus, H. S. (2022). Study on the analysis of demographic data based on spatial information systems. *IOP Conference Series. Earth and Environmental Science*, *1098*(1), 012029. DOI: 10.1088/1755-1315/1098/1/012029

Xiaoyi, Z., Yang, H., Kumar, N., Bhutto, M. H., Kun, W., & Hu, T. (2023). Assessing Chinese Textile and Apparel Industry Business Sustainability: The Role of Organization Green Culture, Green Dynamic Capabilities, and Green Innovation in Relation to Environmental Orientation and Business Sustainability. *Sustainability (Basel)*, *15*(11), 8588. Advance online publication. DOI: 10.3390/su15118588

Xue, B., Zhao, J., Feng, P., Xing, J., Wu, H., & Li, Y. (2019). Epigenetic mechanism and target therapy of UHRF1 protein complex in malignancies. *OncoTargets and Therapy*, *12*, 549–559. DOI: 10.2147/OTT.S192234 PMID: 30666134

Compilation of References

Aakula, M., Kedare, M. M., Satyam, S., Patra, S., & Singha, S. (2024). Unraveling Microbial Dynamics in Hydrocarbon Contaminated Sites: A Comparative Metagenomic Perspective. *Available at SSRN* 5035502. DOI: 10.2139/ssrn.5035502

Abdalkareem Jasim, S., Jade Catalan Opulencia, M., Alexis Ramírez-Coronel, A., Kamal Abdelbasset, W., Hasan Abed, M., Markov, A., Raheem Lateef Al-Awsi, G., Azamatovich Shamsiev, J., Thaeer Hammid, A., Nader Shalaby, M., Karampoor, S., & Mirzaei, R. (2022). The emerging role of microbiota-derived short-chain fatty acids in immunometabolism. *International Immunopharmacology*, *110*, 108983. DOI: 10.1016/j.intimp.2022.108983 PMID: 35750016

Abdelmonem, B. H., Abdelaal, N. M., Anwer, E. K., Rashwan, A. A., Hussein, M. A., Ahmed, Y. F., Khashana, R., Hanna, M. M., & Abdelnaser, A. (2024). Decoding the role of CYP450 enzymes in metabolism and disease: A comprehensive review. *Biomedicines*, *12*(7), 1467. DOI: 10.3390/biomedicines12071467 PMID: 39062040

Abudahab, S., Kronfol, M. M., Dozmorov, M. G., Campbell, T., Jahr, F. M., Nguyen, J., AlAzzeh, O., Al Saeedy, D. Y., Victor, A., Lee, S., Malay, S., Lapato, D. M., Halquist, M. S., McRae, M. P., Deshpande, L. S., Slattum, P. W., Price, E. T., & McClay, J. L. (2024). Genome-wide analysis of hepatic DNA methylation reveals impact of epigenetic aging on xenobiotic metabolism and transport genes in an aged mouse model. *GeroScience*, *46*(6), 1–14. DOI: 10.1007/s11357-024-01137-9 PMID: 38558216

Abumadighem, A., Shuchat, S., Lunenfeld, E., Yossifon, G., & Huleihel, M. (2022). Testis on a chip - A microfluidic three-dimensional culture system for the development of spermatogenesis in-vitro. *Biofabrication*, *14*(3), 035004. Advance online publication. DOI: 10.1088/1758-5090/ac6126 PMID: 35334473

Abusara, O. H., Agha, A. S. A. A., & Bardaweel, S. K. (2025). Advancements and innovations in liquid biopsy through microfluidic technology for cancer diagnosis. *Analyst, 150*(9), 1711–1725. Advance online publication. DOI: 10.1039/D5AN00105F PMID: 40181713

Acharya, D., & Mukhopadhyay, A. (2024). A comprehensive review of machine learning techniques for multi-omics data integration: Challenges and applications in precision oncology. *Briefings in Functional Genomics, 23*(5), elae013. Advance online publication. DOI: 10.1093/bfgp/elae013 PMID: 38600757

Achkar, M. E., Atieh, O., Ghadban, C., Awad, T., Ghadban, E., Grandjean, V., Yarkiner, Z., Raad, G., & Khalife, M.-C. F. (2024). Preconceptional paternal obesity may increase the risk of congenital urogenital anomalies in offspring: A case–control study. *Andrology*. DOI: 10.1111/andr.13673

Adeyinka, F. M., & Adewumi, A. P. (2023). Enhancing Public Service Delivery in Nigeria Through Agile Practice. *Jurnal Administrasi Publik Public Administration Journal, 13*(2), 192–206. DOI: 10.31289/jap.v13i2.10647

Agrawal, G., Aung, A., & Varghese, S. (2017). Skeletal muscle-on-a-chip: An in vitro model to evaluate tissue formation and injury. *Lab on a Chip, 17*(20), 3447–3461. DOI: 10.1039/C7LC00512A PMID: 28871305

Aguilar, D.Jr, & Colacino, J. A. (2024). Single cell approaches to understand environmental impacts on aggressive breast cancers. *Current Opinion in Toxicology, 37*, 100459. DOI: 10.1016/j.cotox.2024.100459

Ahammed, B., & Kalangi, S. K. (2024). A Decade of Organoid Research: Progress and Challenges in the Field of Organoid Technology. *ACS Omega, 9*(28), 30087–30096. DOI: 10.1021/acsomega.4c03683 PMID: 39035960

Ahn, C., & Jeung, E.-B. (2023). Endocrine-Disrupting Chemicals and Disease Endpoints. *International Journal of Molecular Sciences, 24*(6), 5342. DOI: 10.3390/ijms24065342 PMID: 36982431

Ajayi, R. O., & Ogunjobi, T. T. (2024). *Environmental Exposures and Cancer Risk: A Comprehensive Review*. Medinformatics. DOI: 10.47852/bonviewMEDIN42023598

Akers, J. C., Ramakrishnan, V., Kim, R., Skog, J., Nakano, I., & Hochberg, F. H. (2017). MiR-21 in the extracellular vesicles (EVs) of cerebrospinal fluid: A novel biomarker for glioblastoma. *Journal of Neuro-Oncology, 134*(1), 1–10. DOI: 10.1007/s11060-013-1084-8 PMID: 28555425

Akhatova, A., Jones, C., Coward, K., & Yeste, M. (2025). How do lifestyle and environmental factors influence the sperm epigenome? Effects on sperm fertilising ability, embryo development, and offspring health. *Clinical Epigenetics, 17*(1), 1. Advance online publication. DOI: 10.1186/s13148-025-01815-1 PMID: 39819375

Akhavan, B. J., Khanna, N. R., & Vijhani, P. (2025). Amoxicillin. In *StatPearls*. StatPearls Publishing.

Albuquerque, C., Manguinhas, R., Costa, J. G., Gil, N., Codony-Servat, J., Castro, M., Miranda, J. P., Fernandes, A. S., Rosell, R., & Oliveira, N. G. (2021). A narrative review of the migration and invasion features of non-small cell lung cancer cells upon xenobiotic exposure: Insights from in vitro studies. *Translational Lung Cancer Research, 10*(6), 2698–2714. DOI: 10.21037/tlcr-21-121 PMID: 34295671

Alemu, R., Sharew, N. T., Arsano, Y. Y., Ahmed, M., Tekola-Ayele, F., Mersha, T. B., & Amare, A. T. (2025). Multi-omics approaches for understanding gene-environment interactions in noncommunicable diseases: Techniques, translation, and equity issues. *Human Genomics, 19*(1), 1. Advance online publication. DOI: 10.1186/s40246-025-00718-9 PMID: 39891174

Al-Hebshi, N. N., Borgnakke, W. S., & Johnson, N. W. (2019). The Microbiome of Oral Squamous Cell Carcinomas: A Functional Perspective. *Current Oral Health Reports, 6*(2), 145–160. DOI: 10.1007/s40496-019-0215-5

Alipour, M., Moghanibashi, M., Naeimi, S., & Mohamadynejad, P. (2024). Integrative bioinformatics analysis reveals ECM and nicotine-related genes in both LUAD and LUSC, but different lung fibrosis-related genes are involved in LUAD and LUSC. *Nucleosides, Nucleotides & Nucleic Acids, 43*(9), 1–20. DOI: 10.1080/15257770.2023.2300982 PMID: 38198447

Allen, J., & Sears, C. L. (2019). Impact of the gut microbiome on the genome and epigenome of colon epithelial cells: Contributions to colorectal cancer development. *Genome Medicine, 11*(1), 11. DOI: 10.1186/s13073-019-0621-2 PMID: 30803449

Ally, A., Balasundaram, M., Carlsen, R., Chuah, E., Clarke, A., Dhalla, N., Holt, R. A., Jones, S. J. M., Lee, D., Ma, Y., Marra, M. A., Mayo, M., Moore, R. A., Mungall, A. J., Schein, J. E., Sipahimalani, P., Tam, A., Thiessen, N., Cheung, D., & Laird, P. W. (2017). Comprehensive and Integrative Genomic Characterization of Hepatocellular Carcinoma. *Cell, 169*(7), 1327–1341.e23. DOI: 10.1016/j.cell.2017.05.046 PMID: 28622513

Altamirano, G. A., Ramos, J. G., Gomez, A. L., Luque, E. H., Muñoz-de-Toro, M., & Kass, L. (2017). Perinatal exposure to bisphenol A modifies the transcriptional regulation of the β-Casein gene during secretory activation of the rat mammary gland. *Molecular and Cellular Endocrinology*, *439*, 407–418. DOI: 10.1016/j.mce.2016.09.032 PMID: 27697584

Amarasinghe, S. L., Su, S., Dong, X., Zappia, L., Ritchie, M. E., & Gouil, Q. (2020). Opportunities and challenges in long-read sequencing data analysis. *Genome Biology*, *21*(1), 30. DOI: 10.1186/s13059-020-1935-5 PMID: 32033565

Ananthakumar, B., Nanjundeshwara, N., Lakshmaiah, A., & Raghavan, R. (2024). Synthetic Gene Circuits as a Promising Approach in Cancer Immunotherapy. *Critical Developments in Cancer Immunotherapy*, 391–418. DOI: 10.4018/979-8-3693-3976-3.ch011

Anderson, L. M., Chhabra, S. K., Nerurkar, P. V., Souliotis, V. L., & Kyrtopoulos, S. A. (1995). Alcohol-related cancer risk: A toxico kinetic hypothesis. *Alcohol (Fayetteville, N.Y.)*, *12*(2), 97–104. DOI: 10.1016/0741-8329(94)00089-1 PMID: 7772272

Andreeva, N., Gabbasova, R., & Grivennikov, S. I. (2020). Microbiome in cancer progression and therapy. *Current Opinion in Microbiology*, *56*, 118–126. DOI: 10.1016/j.mib.2020.09.001 PMID: 33147555

Andrews, S. (2010). *FastQC: A quality control tool for high throughput sequence data*. https://www.bioinformatics.babraham.ac.uk/projects/fastqc/

Andrianou, X. D., Pronk, A., Galea, K. S., Stierum, R., Loh, M., Riccardo, F., Pezzotti, P., & Makris, K. C. (2021). Exposome-based public health interventions for infectious diseases in urban settings. *Environment International*, *146*, 106246. DOI: 10.1016/j.envint.2020.106246 PMID: 33181410

Angsantikul, P., Thamphiwatana, S., Zhang, Q., Spiekermann, K., Zhuang, J., Fang, R. H., Gao, W., Obonyo, M., & Zhang, L. (2018). Coating nanoparticles with gastric epithelial cell membrane for targeted antibiotic delivery against Helicobacter pylori infection. *Advanced Therapeutics*, *1*(2), 1800016. DOI: 10.1002/adtp.201800016 PMID: 30320205

Annalora, A. J., Coburn, J. L., Jozic, A., Iversen, P. L., & Marcus, C. B. (2024). Global transcriptome modulation by xenobiotics: The role of alternative splicing in adaptive responses to chemical exposures. *Human Genomics*, *18*(1), 127. DOI: 10.1186/s40246-024-00694-6 PMID: 39558396

Aoyama, Y., Naiki-Ito, A., Xiaochen, K., Komura, M., Kato, H., Nagayasu, Y., Inaguma, S., Tsuda, H., Tomita, M., Matsuo, Y., Takiguchi, S., & Takahashi, S. (2021). Lactoferrin Prevents Hepatic Injury and Fibrosis via the Inhibition of NF-κB Signaling in a Rat Non-Alcoholic Steatohepatitis Model. *Nutrients*, *14*(1), 42. DOI: 10.3390/nu14010042 PMID: 35010924

Argentieri, M. A., Amin, N., Nevado-Holgado, A. J., Sproviero, W., Collister, J. A., Keestra, S. M., Kuilman, M. M., Ginos, B. N. R., Ghanbari, M., Doherty, A., Hunter, D. J., Alvergne, A., & van Duijn, C. M. (2025). Integrating the environmental and genetic architectures of aging and mortality. *Nature Medicine*, *31*(3), 1–10. DOI: 10.1038/s41591-024-03483-9 PMID: 39972219

Arnaud, L. C., Gauthier, T., Le Naour, A., Hashim, S., Naud, N., Shay, J. W., Pierre, F. H., Boutet-Robinet, E., & Huc, L. (2021). Short-Term and Long-Term Carcinogenic Effects of Food Contaminants (4-Hydroxynonenal and Pesticides) on Colorectal Human Cells: Involvement of Genotoxic and Non-Genomic Mechanisms. *Cancers (Basel)*, *13*(17), 4337. DOI: 10.3390/cancers13174337 PMID: 34503147

Ataç, B., Wagner, I., Horland, R., Lauster, R., Marx, U., Tonevitsky, A. G., Azar, R. P., & Lindner, G. (2013). Skin and hair on-a-chip: In vitro skin models versus ex vivo tissue maintenance with dynamic perfusion. *Lab on a Chip*, *13*(18), 3555–3561. DOI: 10.1039/c3lc50227a PMID: 23674126

Athreya, A., Iyer, R., Neavin, D., Wang, L., Weinshilboum, R., Kaddurah-Daouk, R., Rush, J., Frye, M., & Bobo, W. (2018). Augmentation of Physician Assessments with Multi-Omics Enhances Predictability of Drug Response: A Case Study of Major Depressive Disorder. *IEEE Computational Intelligence Magazine*, *13*(3), 20–31. DOI: 10.1109/MCI.2018.2840660 PMID: 30467458

Baccarelli, A., & Bollati, V. (2009). Epigenetics and environmental chemicals. *Current Opinion in Pediatrics*, *21*(2), 243–251. DOI: 10.1097/MOP.0b013e32832925cc PMID: 19663042

Baeker Bispo, J., Lee, H., Jemal, A., & Islami, F. (2025). Associations of social support, living arrangements, and residential stability with cancer screening in the United States. *Cancer Causes & Control*, *36*(2), 157–169. DOI: 10.1007/s10552-024-01913-0 PMID: 39422870

Baker, B. H., Zhang, S., Simon, J. M., McLarnan, S. M., Chung, W. K., & Pearson, B. L. (2023). Environmental carcinogens disproportionally mutate genes implicated in neurodevelopmental disorders. *Frontiers in Neuroscience*, *17*, 1106573. Advance online publication. DOI: 10.3389/fnins.2023.1106573 PMID: 37599994

Baker, J. M., Al-Nakkash, L., & Herbst-Kralovetz, M. M. (2017). Estrogen–gut microbiome axis: Physiological and clinical implications. *Maturitas*, *103*, 45–53. DOI: 10.1016/j.maturitas.2017.06.025 PMID: 28778332

Balcells, C., Xu, Y., Gil-Solsona, R., Maitre, L., Gago-Ferrero, P., & Keun, H. C. (2024). Blurred lines: Crossing the boundaries between the chemical exposome and the metabolome. *Current Opinion in Chemical Biology*, *78*, 102407. DOI: 10.1016/j.cbpa.2023.102407 PMID: 38086287

Bannister, A. J., & Kouzarides, T. (2011). Regulation of chromatin by histone modifications. *Cell Research*, *21*(3), 381–395. DOI: 10.1038/cr.2011.22 PMID: 21321607

Barnes, M. A., & Turner, C. R. (2016). The ecology of environmental DNA and implications for conservation genetics. *Conservation Genetics*, *17*(1), 1–17. DOI: 10.1007/s10592-015-0775-4

Beigh, S. (2024). A Phytochemicals Approach towards the Role of Dioxins in Disease Progression Targeting Various Pathways: Insights. *Ind. J. Pharm. Edu. Res*, *58*(3s), s732–s756. DOI: 10.5530/ijper.58.3s.76

Benak, D., Alanova, P., Holzerova, K., Chalupova, M., Opletalova, B., Kolar, F., Pavlinkova, G., & Hlavackova, M. (2025). Epitranscriptomic regulation of HIF-1: Bidirectional regulatory pathways. *Molecular Medicine (Cambridge, Mass.)*, *31*(1), 1. Advance online publication. DOI: 10.1186/s10020-025-01149-x PMID: 40102715

Benavent, N., Cañete, A., Moreno, L., Gros, L., Verdú-Amorós, J., Salinas, J. A., Navarro, S., Álvaro, T., Carbonell-Asins, J. A., & Noguera, R. (2025). Risk of developing neuroblastoma influenced by maternal stressful life events during pregnancy and congenital pathologies. *Pediatric Blood & Cancer*, *72*(2), e31402. DOI: 10.1002/pbc.31402 PMID: 39618320

Benítez, L., Castro-Barquero, S., Crispi, F., Youssef, L., Crovetto, F., Fischer, U., Kameri, E., Bueno, C., Camos, M., Menéndez, P., Heinäniemi, M., Borkhardt, A., & Gratacós, E. (2024). Maternal Lifestyle and Prenatal Risk Factors for Childhood Leukemia: A Review of the Existing Evidence. *Fetal Diagnosis and Therapy*, *51*(4), 395–410. DOI: 10.1159/000539141 PMID: 38710162

Bernardo, J., & Valentão, P. (2024). Herb-drug interactions: A short review on central and peripheral nervous system drugs. *Phytotherapy Research*, *38*(4), 1903–1931. DOI: 10.1002/ptr.8120 PMID: 38358734

Berrandou, T., Mulot, C., Cordina-Duverger, E., Arveux, P., Laurent-Puig, P., Truong, T., & Guénel, P. (2019). Association of breast cancer risk with polymorphisms in genes involved in the metabolism of xenobiotics and interaction with tobacco smoking: A gene-set analysis. *International Journal of Cancer, 144*(8), 1896–1908. DOI: 10.1002/ijc.31917 PMID: 30303517

Bersanelli, M., Mosca, E., Remondini, D., Giampieri, E., Sala, C., Castellani, G., & Milanesi, L. (2016). Methods for the integration of multi-omics data: Mathematical aspects. *BMC Bioinformatics, 17*(S2), S15. DOI: 10.1186/s12859-015-0857-9 PMID: 26821531

Best, M. G., Sol, N., Kooi, I., Tannous, J., Westerman, B. A., & Wurdinger, T. (2019). RNA sequencing of tumor-educated platelets enables blood-based pan-cancer, multiclass, and molecular pathway cancer diagnostics. *Cancer Cell, 36*(6), 881–895. DOI: 10.1016/j.ccell.2019.11.005

Betts, A. C., Roth, M. E., Albritton, K., Pruitt, S. L., Lupo, P. J., Wang, J. S., Shay, L. A., Allicock, M. A., & Murphy, C. C. (2024). Racialized inequities in live birth after cancer: A population-based study of 63,000 female adolescents and young adults with cancer. *Cancer, 130*(17), 2928–2937. DOI: 10.1002/cncr.35341 PMID: 38696087

Bhagyaraj, E., Ahuja, N., Kumar, S., Tiwari, D., Gupta, S., Nanduri, R., & Gupta, P. (2019). TGF-β induced chemoresistance in liver cancer is modulated by xenobiotic nuclear receptor PXR. *Cell Cycle (Georgetown, Tex.), 18*(24), 3589–3602. DOI: 10.1080/15384101.2019.1693120 PMID: 31739702

Bhan, A., Hussain, I., Ansari, K. I., Bobzean, S. A. M., Perrotti, L. I., & Mandal, S. S. (2014). Histone Methyltransferase EZH2 Is Transcriptionally Induced by Estradiol as Well as Estrogenic Endocrine Disruptors Bisphenol-A and Diethylstilbestrol. *Journal of Molecular Biology, 426*(20), 3426–3441. DOI: 10.1016/j.jmb.2014.07.025 PMID: 25088689

Bhardwaj, A., Sharma, R. K., & Singh, G. B. (2021). Contagious Progression and Distribution of Arsenic in India: A Key Towards Bioremediation. *Nature Environment & Pollution Technology, 20*(2). Advance online publication. DOI: 10.46488/NEPT.2021.v20i02.037

Bhattacharjee, N., Sarkar, S., & Giri, B. (2022). Impact of endocrine disrupting chemicals (EDCs) on the predisposition of cancer and polycystic ovary syndrome (PCOS): A Note. *Journal of Drug Delivery and Therapeutics, 12*(5), 3–7. DOI: 10.22270/jddt.v12i5.5582

Bhattacharyya, A., Chattopadhyay, R., Mitra, S., & Crowe, S. E. (2014). Oxidative Stress: An Essential Factor in the Pathogenesis of Gastrointestinal Mucosal Diseases. *Physiological Reviews*, *94*(2), 329–354. DOI: 10.1152/physrev.00040.2012 PMID: 24692350

Biedermann, L., Zeitz, J., Mwinyi, J., Sutter-Minder, E., Rehman, A., Ott, S. J., Steurer-Stey, C., Frei, A., Frei, P., Scharl, M., Loessner, M. J., Vavricka, S. R., Fried, M., Schreiber, S., Schuppler, M., & Rogler, G. (2013). Smoking Cessation Induces Profound Changes in the Composition of the Intestinal Microbiota in Humans. *PLoS One*, *8*(3), e59260. DOI: 10.1371/journal.pone.0059260 PMID: 23516617

Bi, H., Tian, Y., Song, C., Li, J., Liu, T., Chen, Z., Chen, C., Huang, Y., & Zhang, Y. (2019). Urinary microbiota – a potential biomarker and therapeutic target for bladder cancer. *Journal of Medical Microbiology*, *68*(10), 1471–1478. DOI: 10.1099/jmm.0.001058 PMID: 31418671

Binnewies, M., Roberts, E. W., Kersten, K., Chan, V., Fearon, D. F., Merad, M., & Krummel, M. F. (2018). Understanding the tumor immune microenvironment (TIME) for effective therapy. *Nature Medicine*, *24*(5), 541–550. DOI: 10.1038/s41591-018-0014-x PMID: 29686425

Biradar, S., Korrapati, C., Krishna, R. J., & Nanjundeshwara, N. (2025). Spatial Omics and Gene Circuits: The Future in Cancer Biology. *Spatially Variable Genes in Cancer: Development, Progression, and Treatment Response*, 383–408. DOI: 10.4018/979-8-3693-7728-4.ch014

Biradar, S., Suresh, C., Nanjundeshwara, N., & Raghavan, R. (2025). Spatially Variable Genes. *Spatially Variable Genes in Cancer*, 1–28. DOI: 10.4018/979-8-3693-7728-4.ch001

Birben, E., Sahiner, U. M., Sackesen, C., Erzurum, S., & Kalayci, O. (2012). Oxidative Stress and Antioxidant Defense. *The World Allergy Organization Journal*, *5*(1), 9–19. DOI: 10.1097/WOX.0b013e3182439613 PMID: 23268465

Bisen, A. C., Sanap, S. N., Agrawal, S., Biswas, A., & Bhatta, R. S. (2023). Chemical metabolite synthesis and profiling: Mimicking in vivo biotransformation reaction. *Bioorganic Chemistry*, *106722*, 106722. Advance online publication. DOI: 10.1016/j.bioorg.2023.106722

Blériot, C., Dunsmore, G., Alonso-Curbelo, D., & Ginhoux, F. (2024). A temporal perspective for tumor-associated macrophage identities and functions. *Cancer Cell*, *42*(5), 747–758. DOI: 10.1016/j.ccell.2024.04.002 PMID: 38670090

Boffetta, P., & Hashibe, M. (2006). Alcohol and cancer. *The Lancet. Oncology*, *7*(2), 149–156. DOI: 10.1016/S1470-2045(06)70577-0 PMID: 16455479

Bojić, M., Debeljak, Ž., & Guengerich, F. P. (2024). Principles of Xenobiotic Metabolism (Biotransformation). In *Pharmacogenomics in Clinical Practice* (pp. 13–33). Springer International Publishing. DOI: 10.1007/978-3-031-45903-0_2

Bolger, A. M., Lohse, M., & Usadel, B. (2014). Trimmomatic: A flexible trimmer for Illumina sequence data. *Bioinformatics (Oxford, England)*, *30*(15), 2114–2120. DOI: 10.1093/bioinformatics/btu170 PMID: 24695404

Bolós, V., Gasent, J. M., López-Tarruella, S., & Grande, E. (2010). The dual kinase complex FAK-src as a promising therapeutic target in cancer. In *OncoTargets and Therapy* (Vol. 3, pp. 83–97). Dove Medical Press Ltd. DOI: 10.2147/OTT.S6909

Bolyen, E., Rideout, J. R., Dillon, M. R., Bokulich, N. A., Abnet, C. C., Al-Ghalith, G. A., Alexander, H., Alm, E. J., Arumugam, M., Asnicar, F., Bai, Y., Bisanz, J. E., Bittinger, K., Brejnrod, A., Brislawn, C. J., Brown, C. T., Callahan, B. J., Caraballo-Rodríguez, A. M., Chase, J., & Caporaso, J. G. (2019). Reproducible, interactive, scalable and extensible microbiome data science using QIIME 2. *Nature Biotechnology*, *37*(8), 852–857. DOI: 10.1038/s41587-019-0209-9 PMID: 31341288

Borankova, K., Krchniakova, M., Leck, L. Y. W., Kubistova, A., Neradil, J., Jansson, P. J., Hogarty, M. D., & Skoda, J. (2023). Mitoribosomal synthetic lethality overcomes multidrug resistance in MYC-driven neuroblastoma. *Cell Death & Disease*, *14*(11), 1–17. DOI: 10.1038/s41419-023-06278-x PMID: 37973789

Bosco, N., & Noti, M. (2021). The aging gut microbiome and its impact on host immunity. *Genes and Immunity*, *22*(5-6), 289–303. DOI: 10.1038/s41435-021-00126-8 PMID: 33875817

Boyce, M., Favela, K. A., Bonzo, J. A., Chao, A., Lizarraga, L. E., Moody, L. R., Owens, E. O., Patlewicz, G., Shah, I., Sobus, J. R., Thomas, R. S., Williams, A. J., Yau, A., & Wambaugh, J. F. (2023). Identifying xenobiotic metabolites with *in-silico* prediction tools and LCMS suspect screening analysis. *Frontiers in Toxicology*, *5*, 1051483. DOI: 10.3389/ftox.2023.1051483 PMID: 36742129

Boysen, G., Alexandrov, L. B., Rahbari, R., Nookaew, I., Ussery, D., Chao, M.-R., Hu, C.-W., & Cooke, M. S. (2025). Investigating the origins of the mutational signatures in cancer. *Nucleic Acids Research*, *53*(1), gkae1303. Advance online publication. DOI: 10.1093/nar/gkae1303 PMID: 39778866

Bray, F., Laversanne, M., Sung, H., Ferlay, J., Siegel, R. L., Soerjomataram, I., & Jemal, A. (2024). Global cancer statistics 2022: GLOBOCAN estimates of incidence and mortality worldwide for 36 cancers in 185 countries. *CA: a Cancer Journal for Clinicians, 74*(3), 229–263. DOI: 10.3322/caac.21834 PMID: 38572751

Brouwer, K. L., Evers, R., Hayden, E., Hu, S., Li, C. Y., Meyer zu Schwabedissen, H. E., Neuhoff, S., Oswald, S., Piquette-Miller, M., Saran, C., Sjöstedt, N., Sprowl, J. A., Stahl, S. H., & Yue, W. (2022). Regulation of drug transport proteins—From mechanisms to clinical impact: A white paper on behalf of the international transporter consortium. *Clinical Pharmacology and Therapeutics, 112*(3), 461–484. DOI: 10.1002/cpt.2605 PMID: 35390174

Bryere, J., Tron, L., Menvielle, G., & Launoy, G. (2019). The respective parts of incidence and lethality in socioeconomic differences in cancer mortality. An analysis of the French network Cancer registries (FRANCIM) data. *International Journal for Equity in Health, 18*(1), 189. DOI: 10.1186/s12939-019-1087-y PMID: 31796079

Bucher, M. L., Anderson, F. L., Lai, Y., Dicent, J., Miller, G. W., & Zota, A. R. (2023). Exposomics as a tool to investigate differences in health and disease by sex and gender. *Exposome, 3*(1), osad003. Advance online publication. DOI: 10.1093/exposome/osad003 PMID: 37122372

Bučko, M., Kaniaková, K., Hronská, H., Gemeiner, P., & Rosenberg, M. (2023). Epoxide hydrolases: Multipotential biocatalysts. *International Journal of Molecular Sciences, 24*(8), 7334. DOI: 10.3390/ijms24087334 PMID: 37108499

Buenrostro, J. D., Giresi, P. G., Zaba, L. C., Chang, H. Y., & Greenleaf, W. J. (2013). Transposition of native chromatin for fast and sensitive epigenomic profiling of open chromatin, DNA-binding proteins, and nucleosome position. *Nature Methods, 10*(12), 1213–1218. DOI: 10.1038/nmeth.2688 PMID: 24097267

Bültmann, U., Broberg, K., & Selander, J. (2024). Integrating a life course perspective in work environment and health research: Empirical challenges and interdisciplinary opportunities. *Scandinavian Journal of Work, Environment & Health, 50*(5), 311–316. DOI: 10.5271/sjweh.4174 PMID: 38934300

Buqué, A., Galluzzi, L., & Zitvogel, L. (2021). Immunological determinants of radiotherapy response. *Radiotherapy and Oncology : Journal of the European Society for Therapeutic Radiology and Oncology, 160*, 61–69. DOI: 10.1016/j.radonc.2021.04.001

Burk, R. F. (2002). Selenium, an antioxidant nutrient. *Nutrition in Clinical Care, 5*(2), 75–79. DOI: 10.1046/j.1523-5408.2002.00006.x PMID: 12134713

Cadet, J., Davies, K. J. A., Medeiros, M. H., Di Mascio, P., & Wagner, J. R. (2017). Formation and repair of oxidatively generated damage in cellular DNA. *Free Radical Biology & Medicine*, *107*, 13–34. DOI: 10.1016/j.freeradbiomed.2016.12.049 PMID: 28057600

Cai, Z., Apolinário, S., Baião, A. R., Pacini, C., Sousa, M. D., Vinga, S., Reddel, R. R., Robinson, P. J., Garnett, M. J., Zhong, Q., & Gonçalves, E. (2024). Synthetic augmentation of cancer cell line multi-omic datasets using unsupervised deep learning. *Nature Communications*, *15*(1), 10390. DOI: 10.1038/s41467-024-54771-4 PMID: 39614072

Cai, Z., Poulos, R. C., Liu, J., & Zhong, Q. (2022). Machine learning for multi-omics data integration in cancer. *iScience*, *25*(2), 103798. DOI: 10.1016/j.isci.2022.103798 PMID: 35169688

Calafat, A. M., Weuve, J., Ye, X., Jia, L. T., Hu, H., Ringer, S., Huttner, K., & Hauser, R. (2009). Exposure to bisphenol A and other phenols in neonatal intensive care unit premature infants. *Environmental Health Perspectives*, *117*(4), 639–644. DOI: 10.1289/ehp.0800265 PMID: 19440505

Callahan, B. J., McMurdie, P. J., Rosen, M. J., Han, A. W., Johnson, A. J. A., & Holmes, S. P. (2016). DADA2: High-resolution sample inference from Illumina amplicon data. *Nature Methods*, *13*(7), 581–583. DOI: 10.1038/nmeth.3869 PMID: 27214047

Candura, S. M., Manzo, L., Castoldi, A. F., & Costa, L. G. (2020). Metabolism and toxicity of occupational neurotoxicants: genetic, physiological, and environmental determinants. In *Occupational neurotoxicology* (pp. 21–48). CRC Press. DOI: 10.1201/9780429281044-2

Cannon, J. R., Vachaspati, P., & Yuan, Y. (2022). A Comprehensive Picture of Biotransformation in Drug Discovery. *Drug Metabolism Handbook: Concepts and Applications in Cancer Research*, *1*, 41–101. DOI: 10.1002/9781119851042.ch4

Capone, P., Chiarella, P., & Sisto, R. (2024). Advanced technologies in genomic toxicology: Current trend and future directions. *Current Opinion in Toxicology*, *37*, 100444. DOI: 10.1016/j.cotox.2023.100444

Carbone, M., Adusumilli, P. S., Alexander, H. R.Jr, Baas, P., Bardelli, F., Bononi, A., Bueno, R., Felley-Bosco, E., Galateau-Salle, F., Jablons, D., Mansfield, A. S., Minaai, M., De Perrot, M., Pesavento, P., Rusch, V., Severson, D. T., Taioli, E., Tsao, A., Woodard, G., & Pass, H. I. (2019). Mesothelioma: Scientific clues for prevention, diagnosis, and therapy. *CA: a Cancer Journal for Clinicians*, *69*(5), 402–429. DOI: 10.3322/caac.21572 PMID: 31283845

Carra, D., Maas, S. C. E., Seoane, J. A., & Alonso-Curbelo, D. (2025). Exposomal determinants of non-genetic plasticity in tumor initiation. *Trends in Cancer*, *0*(0), 295–308. Advance online publication. DOI: 10.1016/j.trecan.2025.01.010 PMID: 40023688

Carter, S. E., Ong, M. L., Simons, R. L., Gibbons, F. X., Lei, M. K., & Beach, S. R. H. (2019). The effect of early discrimination on accelerated aging among African Americans. *Health Psychology*, *38*(11), 1010–1013. DOI: 10.1037/hea0000788 PMID: 31343220

Cassotta, M., Cianciosi, D., Elexpuru-Zabaleta, M., Pascual, I. E., Cano, S. S., Giampieri, F., & Battino, M. (2024). Human-based new approach methodologies to accelerate advances in nutrition research. *Food Frontiers*, *5*(3), 1031–1062. DOI: 10.1002/fft2.369

Cata, J. P., Bachmann, D., & Pedraza, R. (2020). Perioperative inflammatory response and cancer recurrence risk. *Anesthesia and Analgesia*, *130*(6), 1686–1695. DOI: 10.1213/ANE.0000000000004711 PMID: 32384350

Cesario, A., D'Oria, M., Calvani, R., Picca, A., Pietragalla, A., Lorusso, D., Daniele, G., Lohmeyer, F. M., Boldrini, L., Valentini, V., Bernabei, R., Auffray, C., & Scambia, G. (2021). The Role of Artificial Intelligence in Managing Multimorbidity and Cancer. *Journal of Personalized Medicine*, *11*(4), 314. DOI: 10.3390/jpm11040314 PMID: 33921621

Chandra, G. V. S. A., Biradar, S., & Raghavan, R. (2025). Recent Trends in Soft Robotics for Assistive Technologies. *Assistive Technology Solutions for Aging Adults and Individuals With Disabilities*, 119–144. DOI: 10.4018/979-8-3693-6308-9.ch006

Chapadgaonkar, S. S., Bajpai, S. S., & Godbole, M. S. (2023). Gut microbiome influences incidence and outcomes of breast cancer by regulating levels and activity of steroid hormones in women. *Cancer Reports*, *6*(11), e1847. DOI: 10.1002/cnr2.1847 PMID: 37311575

Chapman, K. E., Wilde, E. C., Chapman, F. M., Verma, J. R., Shah, U.-K., Stannard, L. M., Seager, A. L., Tonkin, J. A., Brown, M. R., Doherty, A. T., Johnson, G. E., Doak, S. H., & Jenkins, G. J. S. (2021). Multiple-endpoint in vitro carcinogenicity test in human cell line TK6 distinguishes carcinogens from non-carcinogens and highlights mechanisms of action. *Archives of Toxicology*, *95*(1), 321–336. DOI: 10.1007/s00204-020-02902-3 PMID: 32910239

Charmsaz, S., Collins, D. M., Perry, A. S., & Prencipe, M. (2019). Novel Strategies for Cancer Treatment: Highlights from the 55th IACR Annual Conference. *Cancers (Basel)*, *11*(8), 1125. DOI: 10.3390/cancers11081125 PMID: 31394729

Chatterjee, G., Negi, S., Basu, S., Faintuch, J., O'donovan, A., & Shukla, P. (2022). Microbiome systems biology advancements for natural well-being. *The Science of the Total Environment*, *838*, 155915. DOI: 10.1016/j.scitotenv.2022.155915 PMID: 35568180

Chee, W. J. Y., Chew, S. Y., & Than, L. T. L. (2020). Vaginal microbiota and the potential of Lactobacillus derivatives in maintaining vaginal health. *Microbial Cell Factories*, *19*(1), 203. DOI: 10.1186/s12934-020-01464-4 PMID: 33160356

Chen, C. X., Park, H. S., Price, H., & Wax, A. (2021). Automated Classification of Breast Cancer Cells Using High-Throughput Holographic Cytometry. *Frontiers in Physics (Lausanne)*, *9*, 759142. Advance online publication. DOI: 10.3389/fphy.2021.759142

Chen, F., Wang, J., Wu, Y., Gao, Q., & Zhang, S. (2022). Potential Biomarkers for Liver Cancer Diagnosis Based on Multi-Omics Strategy. *Frontiers in Oncology*, *12*, 822449. DOI: 10.3389/fonc.2022.822449 PMID: 35186756

Cheng, T., Gamage, S. M. K., Lu, C.-T., Aktar, S., Gopalan, V., & Lam, A. K. (2022). Polymorphisms in PAH metabolising enzyme CYP1A1 in colorectal cancer and their clinicopathological correlations. *Pathology, Research and Practice*, *231*, 153801. DOI: 10.1016/j.prp.2022.153801 PMID: 35180652

Cheng, Y., Wang, T., Li, T., & Yan, Y. (2021). Challenges and opportunities of circulating tumor DNA detection using next-generation sequencing. *Frontiers in Medicine*, *8*, 674474. DOI: 10.3389/fmed.2021.674474

Chen, K., Zhang, F., Ding, J., Liang, Y., Zhan, Z., Zhan, Y., Chen, L., & Ding, Y. (2017). Histone Methyltransferase SETDB1 Promotes the Progression of Colorectal Cancer by Inhibiting the Expression of TP53. *Journal of Cancer*, *8*(16), 3318–3330. DOI: 10.7150/jca.20482 PMID: 29158805

Chen, L., Zhu, Y., Hou, X., Yang, L., & Chu, H. (2022). The Role of Gut Bacteria and Fungi in Alcohol-Associated Liver Disease. *Frontiers in Medicine*, *9*, 840752. DOI: 10.3389/fmed.2022.840752 PMID: 35308525

Chen, L., Zuo, M., Zhou, Q., & Wang, Y. (2023). Oncolytic virotherapy in cancer treatment: Challenges and optimization prospects. *Frontiers in Immunology*, *14*, 1308890. Advance online publication. DOI: 10.3389/fimmu.2023.1308890 PMID: 38169820

Chen, N., Liang, H., Huang, T., & Huang, N. (2022). Exposome approach for identifying modifiable factors for the prevention of colorectal cancer. *Scientific Reports, 12*(1), 21615. Advance online publication. DOI: 10.1038/s41598-022-25832-9 PMID: 36517625

Chen, Q. Y., DesMarais, T., & Costa, M. (2019). Metals and mechanisms of carcinogenesis. In *Annual Review of Pharmacology and Toxicology* (Vol. 59, pp. 537–554). Annual Reviews Inc. DOI: 10.1146/annurev-pharmtox-010818-021031

Chen, R., Caserto, J. S., & Chiu, D. (2021). RNA-based immune signatures for predicting response to immunotherapy in cancer patients. *Nature Communications, 12*(1), 1878. DOI: 10.1038/s41467-021-22129-x PMID: 33767163

Chen, Y., Xu, R., Ruze, R., Yang, J., Wang, H., Song, J., You, L., Wang, C., & Zhao, Y. (2021). Construction of a prognostic model with histone modification-related genes and identification of potential drugs in pancreatic cancer. *Cancer Cell International, 21*(1), 291. DOI: 10.1186/s12935-021-01928-6 PMID: 34090418

Chetwynd, A. J., Louyer, M.-V., Mercier, F., Bessonneau, V., & David, A. (2024). Polar organic pollutants, micro-nano plastics and nanomaterials: Analytical techniques to reveal the still invisible human physico-chemical exposome. *Trends in Analytical Chemistry, 177*, 117816. DOI: 10.1016/j.trac.2024.117816

Chiu, C. Y., & Miller, S. A. (2019). Clinical metagenomics. *Nature Reviews. Genetics, 20*(6), 341–355. DOI: 10.1038/s41576-019-0113-7 PMID: 30918369

Chiu, K., Warner, G., Nowak, R. A., Flaws, J. A., & Mei, W. (2020). The Impact of Environmental Chemicals on the Gut Microbiome. *Toxicological Sciences, 176*(2), 253–284. DOI: 10.1093/toxsci/kfaa065 PMID: 32392306

Chu, A. H., Lin, K., Croker, H., Kefyalew, S., Becerra-Tomás, N., Dossus, L., González-Gil, E. M., Ahmadi, N., Park, Y., Krebs, J., Weijenberg, M. P., Baskin, M. L., Copson, E., Lewis, S. J., Seidell, J. C., Chowdhury, R., Hill, L., Chan, D. S., Lee, D. H., & Giovannucci, E. L. (2025). Dietary patterns and colorectal cancer risk: Global Cancer Update Programme (CUP Global) systematic literature review. *The American Journal of Clinical Nutrition, 121*(5), 999–1016. Advance online publication. DOI: 10.1016/j.ajcnut.2025.02.021 PMID: 40010692

Chung, M., Lee, S., Lee, B. J., Son, K., Jeon, N. L., & Kim, J. H. (2018). Wet-AMD on a Chip: Modeling Outer Blood-Retinal Barrier In Vitro. *Advanced Healthcare Materials, 7*(2), 1700028. Advance online publication. DOI: 10.1002/adhm.201700028 PMID: 28557377

Clerici, M., Colombo, G., Secundo, F., Gagliano, N., Colombo, R., Portinaro, N., Giustarini, D., Milzani, A., Rossi, R., & Dalle-Donne, I. (2014). Cigarette smoke induces alterations in the drug-binding properties of human serum albumin. *Blood Cells, Molecules & Diseases*, *52*(4), 166–174. DOI: 10.1016/j.bcmd.2013.12.001 PMID: 24388826

Colwell, M. L., Townsel, C., Petroff, R. L., Goodrich, J. M., & Dolinoy, D. C. (2023). Epigenetics and the exposome: DNA methylation as a proxy for health impacts of prenatal environmental exposures. *Exposome*, *3*(1), osad001. Advance online publication. DOI: 10.1093/exposome/osad001 PMID: 37333730

Combarnous, Y., & Nguyen, T. M. D. (2019). Comparative Overview of the Mechanisms of Action of Hormones and Endocrine Disruptor Compounds. *Toxics*, *7*(1), 5. DOI: 10.3390/toxics7010005 PMID: 30682876

Corcos, C., Brey, J., & Corcos, L. (2002). The nuclear receptors CAR and PXR control induction of cytochromes P450 by phenobarbital. In *Medecine/Sciences* (Vol. 18, pp. 429–437). Elsevier Masson SAS. DOI: 10.1051/medsci/2002184429

Cordier, T., Alonso-Sáez, L., Apothéloz-Perret-Gentil, L., Aylagas, E., Bohan, D. A., Bouchez, A., & Pawlowski, J. (2019). Ecosystems monitoring powered by environmental genomics: A review of current strategies with an implementation roadmap. *Molecular Ecology*, *28*(14), 2937–2954. DOI: 10.1111/mec.15176 PMID: 32416615

Corning, B., Copland, A. P., & Frye, J. W. (2018). The Esophageal Microbiome in Health and Disease. *Current Gastroenterology Reports*, *20*(8), 39. DOI: 10.1007/s11894-018-0642-9 PMID: 30069679

Costa, E. C., Moreira, A. F., de Melo-Diogo, D., Gaspar, V. M., Carvalho, M. P., & Correia, I. J. (2016). 3D tumor spheroids: an overview on the tools and techniques used for their analysis. In *Biotechnology Advances* (Vol. 34, pp. 1427–1441). Elsevier Inc. DOI: 10.1016/j.biotechadv.2016.11.002

Coste, A., Bailey, H. D., Kartal-Kaess, M., Renella, R., Berthet, A., & Spycher, B. D. (2020). Parental occupational exposure to pesticides and risk of childhood cancer in Switzerland: A census-based cohort study. *BMC Cancer*, *20*(1), 819. DOI: 10.1186/s12885-020-07319-w PMID: 32859175

Creamer, B. A., Sloan, S. N. B., Dennis, J. F., Rogers, R., Spencer, S., McCuen, A., Persaud, P., & Staudinger, J. L. (2020). Associations between Pregnane X Receptor and Breast Cancer Growth and Progression. *Cells*, *9*(10), 2295. DOI: 10.3390/cells9102295 PMID: 33076284

Cristescu, M. E., & Hebert, P. D. N. (2018). Uses and misuses of environmental DNA in biodiversity science and conservation. *Annual Review of Ecology, Evolution, and Systematics*, *49*(1), 209–230. DOI: 10.1146/annurev-ecolsys-110617-062306

Crost, E. H., Coletto, E., Bell, A., & Juge, N. (2023). Ruminococcus gnavus: Friend or foe for human health. *FEMS Microbiology Reviews*, *47*(2), fuad014. Advance online publication. DOI: 10.1093/femsre/fuad014 PMID: 37015876

Cummings, J. H., & Macfarlane, G. T. (2002). Gastrointestinal effects of prebiotics. *British Journal of Nutrition*, *87*(S2), S145–S151. DOI: 10.1079/BJN/2002530 PMID: 12088511

Dahiya, D., & Nigam, P. S. (2023). Antibiotic-Therapy-Induced Gut Dysbiosis Affecting Gut Microbiota-Brain Axis and Cognition: Restoration by Intake of Probiotics and Synbiotics. *International Journal of Molecular Sciences*, *24*(4), 3074. DOI: 10.3390/ijms24043074 PMID: 36834485

Dai, W., Qiao, X., Fang, Y., Guo, R., Bai, P., Liu, S., Li, T., Jiang, Y., Wei, S., Na, Z., Xiao, X., & Li, D. (2024). Epigenetics-targeted drugs: Current paradigms and future challenges. *Signal Transduction and Targeted Therapy*, *9*(1), 332. DOI: 10.1038/s41392-024-02039-0 PMID: 39592582

Danieli, M. G., Casciaro, M., Paladini, A., Bartolucci, M., Sordoni, M., Shoenfeld, Y., & Gangemi, S. (2024). Exposome: Epigenetics and autoimmune diseases. In *Autoimmunity Reviews* (Vol. 23). Elsevier B.V. DOI: 10.1016/j.autrev.2024.103584

Das, P., Banka, R., Ghosh, J., Singh, K., Choudhury, S. R., & Koner, S. (2024). Synergism of Diet, Genetics, and Microbiome on Health. In *Nutrition Controversies and Advances in Autoimmune Disease* (pp. 131–189). IGI Global. DOI: 10.4018/979-8-3693-5528-2.ch006

David, L. A., Maurice, C. F., Carmody, R. N., Gootenberg, D. B., Button, J. E., Wolfe, B. E., Ling, A. V., Devlin, A. S., Varma, Y., Fischbach, M. A., Biddinger, S. B., Dutton, R. J., & Turnbaugh, P. J. (2014). Diet rapidly and reproducibly alters the human gut microbiome. *Nature*, *505*(7484), 559–563. DOI: 10.1038/nature12820 PMID: 24336217

Dayyih, W. A., Al-Ani, I., Hailat, M., Alarman, S. M., Zakaraya, Z., Assab, M. A., & Alkhader, E. (2024). Review of grapefruit juice-drugs interactions mediated by intestinal CYP3A4 inhibition. *Journal of Applied Pharmaceutical Science, 14*(5), 59-68. DOI: 10.7324/JAPS.2024.160197 de Abreu, V. A. C., Perdigão, J., & Almeida, S. (2021). Metagenomic Approaches to Analyze Antimicrobial Resistance: An Overview. *Frontiers in Genetics*, *11*, 575592. DOI: 10.3389/fgene.2020.575592 PMID: 33537056

De Almeida, A. J. P. O., de Oliveira, J. C. P. L., da Silva Pontes, L. V., de Souza Júnior, J. F., Gonçalves, T. A. F., Dantas, S. H., de Almeida Feitosa, M. S., Silva, A. O., & de Medeiros, I. A. (2022). ROS: Basic concepts, sources, cellular signaling, and its implications in aging pathways. *Oxidative Medicine and Cellular Longevity*, *2022*(1), 1225578. DOI: 10.1155/2022/1225578 PMID: 36312897

De Filippis, F., Valentino, V., Sequino, G., Borriello, G., Riccardi, M. G., Pierri, B., Cerino, P., Pizzolante, A., Pasolli, E., Esposito, M., Limone, A., & Ercolini, D. (2024). Exposure to environmental pollutants selects for xenobiotic-degrading functions in the human gut microbiome. *Nature Communications*, *15*(1), 4482. DOI: 10.1038/s41467-024-48739-7 PMID: 38802370

Deb, P., Bhan, A., Hussain, I., Ansari, K. I., Bobzean, S. A., Pandita, T. K., Perrotti, L. I., & Mandal, S. S. (2016). Endocrine disrupting chemical, bisphenol-A, induces breast cancer associated gene HOXB9 expression in vitro and in vivo. *Gene*, *590*(2), 234–243. DOI: 10.1016/j.gene.2016.05.009 PMID: 27182052

DeFilipp, Z., Bloom, P. P., Torres Soto, M., Mansour, M. K., Sater, M. R. A., Huntley, M. H., Turbett, S., Chung, R. T., Chen, Y.-B., & Hohmann, E. L. (2019). Drug-Resistant *E. coli* Bacteremia Transmitted by Fecal Microbiota Transplant. *The New England Journal of Medicine*, *381*(21), 2043–2050. DOI: 10.1056/NEJMoa1910437 PMID: 31665575

Dehghanbanadaki, H., Jimbo, M., Fendereski, K., Kunisaki, J., Horns, J. J., Ramsay, J. M., Gross, K. X., Pastuszak, A. W., & Hotaling, J. M. (2024). Transgenerational effects of paternal exposures: The role of germline de novo mutations. *Andrology*, *n/a*(n/a). DOI: 10.1111/andr.13609

Deiner, K., Bik, H. M., Mächler, E., Seymour, M., Lacoursière-Roussel, A., Altermatt, F., & Bernatchez, L. (2017). Environmental DNA metabarcoding: Transforming how we survey animal and plant communities. *Molecular Ecology*, *26*(21), 5872–5895. DOI: 10.1111/mec.14350 PMID: 28921802

Del Giudice, G., Serra, A., Pavel, A., Torres Maia, M., Saarimäki, L. A., Fratello, M., Federico, A., Alenius, H., Fadeel, B., & Greco, D. (2024). A network toxicology approach for mechanistic modelling of nanomaterial hazard and adverse outcomes. *Advancement of Science*, *11*(32), 2400389. DOI: 10.1002/advs.202400389 PMID: 38923832

Del Pozo, S., Gómez-Martínez, S., Díaz, L. E., Nova, E., Urrialde, R., & Marcos, A. (2022). Potential effects of sucralose and saccharin on gut microbiota: A review. *Nutrients, 14*(8), 1682. DOI: 10.3390/nu14081682 PMID: 35458244

Delfosse, V., Grimaldi, M., Pons, J.-L., Boulahtouf, A., Le Maire, A., Cavailles, V., Labesse, G., Bourguet, W., & Balaguer, P. (2012). Structural and mechanistic insights into bisphenols action provide guidelines for risk assessment and discovery of bisphenol A substitutes. *Proceedings of the National Academy of Sciences of the United States of America, 109*(37), 14930–14935. DOI: 10.1073/pnas.1203574109 PMID: 22927406

den Besten, G., van Eunen, K., Groen, A. K., Venema, K., Reijngoud, D.-J., & Bakker, B. M. (2013). The role of short-chain fatty acids in the interplay between diet, gut microbiota, and host energy metabolism. *Journal of Lipid Research, 54*(9), 2325–2340. DOI: 10.1194/jlr.R036012 PMID: 23821742

Deonarine, A., Batwara, A., Wada, R., Sharma, P., Loscalzo, J., Ojikutu, B., & Hall, K. (2025). De Novo exposomic geospatial assembly of chronic disease regions with machine learning & network analysis. *EBioMedicine, 112*, 105575. Advance online publication. DOI: 10.1016/j.ebiom.2025.105575 PMID: 39891994

Deo, P. N., & Deshmukh, R. (2019). Oral microbiome: Unveiling the fundamentals. *Journal of Oral and Maxillofacial Pathology : JOMFP, 23*(1), 122–128. DOI: 10.4103/jomfp.JOMFP_304_18 PMID: 31110428

Desai, S., Morimoto, L. M., Kang, A. Y., Miller, M. D., Wiemels, J. L., Winestone, L. E., & Metayer, C. (2025). Pre- and Postnatal Exposures to Residential Pesticides and Survival of Childhood Acute Lymphoblastic Leukemia. *Cancers (Basel), 17*(6), 6. Advance online publication. DOI: 10.3390/cancers17060978 PMID: 40149312

Dharmarathne, G., Kazi, S., King, S., & Jayasinghe, T. N. (2024). The Bidirectional Relationship Between Cardiovascular Medications and Oral and Gut Microbiome Health: A Comprehensive Review. *Microorganisms, 12*(11), 2246. DOI: 10.3390/microorganisms12112246 PMID: 39597635

di Magliano, M. P., & Logsdon, C. D. (2013). Roles for KRAS in Pancreatic Tumor Development and Progression. *Gastroenterology, 144*(6), 1220–1229. DOI: 10.1053/j.gastro.2013.01.071 PMID: 23622131

Di Renzo, L., Gualtieri, P., Frank, G., Cianci, R., Caldarelli, M., Leggeri, G., Raffaelli, G., Pizzocaro, E., Cirillo, M., & De Lorenzo, A. (2024). Exploring the Exposome Spectrum: Unveiling Endogenous and Exogenous Factors in Non-Communicable Chronic Diseases. *Diseases (Basel, Switzerland), 12*(8), 176. DOI: 10.3390/diseases12080176 PMID: 39195175

Diallo, A., Deschasaux, M., Latino-Martel, P., Hercberg, S., Galan, P., Fassier, P., Allès, B., Guéraud, F., Pierre, F. H., & Touvier, M. (2018). Red and processed meat intake and cancer risk: Results from the prospective NutriNet-Santé cohort study. *International Journal of Cancer, 142*(2), 230–237. DOI: 10.1002/ijc.31046 PMID: 28913916

Dimunová, D., Matoušková, P., Podlipná, R., Boušová, I., & Skálová, L. (2022). The role of UDP-glycosyltransferases in xenobioticresistance. *Drug Metabolism Reviews, 54*(3), 282–298. DOI: 10.1080/03602532.2022.2083632 PMID: 35635097

Di, S., Petch, J., Gerstein, H. C., Zhu, R., & Sherifali, D. (2022). Optimizing Health Coaching for Patients With Type 2 Diabetes Using Machine Learning: Model Development and Validation Study. *JMIR Formative Research, 6*(9), e37838. DOI: 10.2196/37838 PMID: 36099006

Dixit, A., Gupta, A. K., Chaplot, N., & Bharti, V. (2024). Emoji Support Predictive Mental Health Assessment Using Machine Learning: Unveiling Personalized Intervention Avenues. *International Journal of Experimental Research and Review, 42*, 228–240. DOI: 10.52756/ijerr.2024.v42.020

Dizdaroglu, M. (2015). Oxidatively induced DNA damage and its repair in cancer. *Mutation Research/Reviews in Mutation Research, 763*, 212–245. DOI: 10.1016/j.mrrev.2014.11.002 PMID: 25795122

Dong, Y., Xiao, Y., Shi, Q., & Jiang, C. (2020). Dysregulated lncRNA-miRNA-mRNA Network Reveals Patient Survival-Associated Modules and RNA Binding Proteins in Invasive Breast Carcinoma. *Frontiers in Genetics, 10*, 1284. DOI: 10.3389/fgene.2019.01284 PMID: 32010179

Dostert, C., Pétrilli, V., Van Bruggen, R., Steele, C., Mossman, B. T., & Tschopp, J. (2008). Innate Immune Activation Through Nalp3 Inflammasome Sensing of Asbestos and Silica. *Science, 320*(5876), 674–677. DOI: 10.1126/science.1156995 PMID: 18403674

Duarte-Mata, D. I., & Salinas-Carmona, M. C. (2023). Antimicrobial peptides´ immune modulation role in intracellular bacterial infection. *Frontiers in Immunology, 14*, 1119574. Advance online publication. DOI: 10.3389/fimmu.2023.1119574 PMID: 37056758

Dudas, B., & Miteva, M. A. (2024). Computational and artificial intelligence-based approaches for drug metabolism and transport prediction. *Trends in Pharmacological Sciences, 45*(1), 39–55. Advance online publication. DOI: 10.1016/j.tips.2023.11.001 PMID: 38072723

Durník, R., Šindlerová, L., Babica, P., & Jurček, O. (2022). Bile acids transporters of enterohepatic circulation for targeted drug delivery. *Molecules (Basel, Switzerland)*, *27*(9), 2961. DOI: 10.3390/molecules27092961 PMID: 35566302

Duvallet, C., Gibbons, S. M., Gurry, T., Irizarry, R. A., & Alm, E. J. (2017). Meta-analysis of gut microbiome studies identifies disease-specific and shared responses. *Nature Communications*, *8*(1), 1784. DOI: 10.1038/s41467-017-01973-8 PMID: 29209090

Dzierżyński, E., Gawlik, P. J., Puźniak, D., Flieger, W., Jóźwik, K., Teresiński, G., Forma, A., Wdowiak, P., Baj, J., & Flieger, J. (2024). Microplastics in the Human Body: Exposure, Detection, and Risk of Carcinogenesis: A State-of-the-Art Review. *Cancers (Basel)*, *16*(21), 3703. Advance online publication. DOI: 10.3390/cancers16213703 PMID: 39518141

Eberharter, A., & Becker, P. B. (2002). Histone acetylation: A switch between repressive and permissive chromatin: Second in review series on chromatin dynamics. *EMBO Reports*, *3*(3), 224–229. DOI: 10.1093/embo-reports/kvf053 PMID: 11882541

Edo, G. I., Samuel, P. O., Oloni, G. O., Ezekiel, G. O., Ikpekoro, V. O., Obasohan, P., Ongulu, J., Otunuya, C. F., Opiti, A. R., Ajakaye, R. S., Essaghah, A. E. A., & Agbo, J. J. (2024). Environmental persistence, bioaccumulation, and ecotoxicology of heavy metals. *Chemistry and Ecology*, *40*(3), 322–349. DOI: 10.1080/02757540.2024.2306839

Eisenstein, M. (2022). p53: An anticancer protein's chequered past and promising future. *Nature*, *603*(7899), S1–S1. DOI: 10.1038/d41586-022-00565-x PMID: 35236979

Emanowicz, P., Średnicka, P., Wójcicki, M., Roszko, M., & Juszczuk-Kubiak, E. (2024). Mitigating Dietary Bisphenol Exposure Through the Gut Microbiota: The Role of Next-Generation Probiotics in Bacterial Detoxification. *Nutrients*, *16*(21), 3757. DOI: 10.3390/nu16213757 PMID: 39519589

Ernawati, K., Burhan, A., Albar, A. S., Al Khaliel, A. T., & Al Fatich, A. S. F. (2024). *Professional Development of Environmental Health Workers*. DOI: 10.4018/979-8-3693-4334-0.ch010

Ernawati, K., Nugroho, B. S., Suryana, C., Riyanto, A., & Fatmawati, E. (2022). advantages of digital applications in public health services on automation era. *International Journal of Health Sciences*, *6*(1), 174–186. DOI: 10.53730/ijhs.v6n1.3684

Eslami-S, Z., Majidzadeh-A, K., Halvaei, S., Babapirali, F., & Esmaeili, R. (2020). Microbiome and Breast Cancer: New Role for an Ancient Population. *Frontiers in Oncology*, *10*, 120. DOI: 10.3389/fonc.2020.00120 PMID: 32117767

Ezez, D., Birhanu, H., Shamena, S., & Engidaw, S. (2024). Bioaccumulation of heavy metals, assessment of carcinogenic and non-carcinogenic health risk in various spices. *Journal of Hazardous Materials Advances*, *15*, 100441. Advance online publication. DOI: 10.1016/j.hazadv.2024.100441

Fakharian, F., Asgari, B., Nabavi-Rad, A., Sadeghi, A., Soleimani, N., Yadegar, A., & Zali, M. R. (2022). The interplay between Helicobacter pylori and the gut microbiota: An emerging driver influencing the immune system homeostasis and gastric carcinogenesis. *Frontiers in Cellular and Infection Microbiology*, *12*, 953718. DOI: 10.3389/fcimb.2022.953718 PMID: 36046747

Fan, C., Jin, M., Chen, K., Zhang, Y., Zhang, S., & Liu, B. (2007). Case-only study of interactions between metabolic enzymes and smoking in colorectal cancer. *BMC Cancer*, *7*(1), 115. DOI: 10.1186/1471-2407-7-115 PMID: 17603900

Farhang Doost, N., & Srivastava, S. K. (2024). A Comprehensive Review of Organ-on-a-Chip Technology and Its Applications. In *Biosensors* (Vol. 14). Multidisciplinary Digital Publishing Institute (MDPI). DOI: 10.3390/bios14050225

Farrukh, M., Shahzadi, S., & Irfan, M. (2024). Drug Metabolism: Phase I and Phase II Metabolic Pathways. In *Drug Metabolism and Pharmacokinetics*. IntechOpen. DOI: 10.5772/intechopen.112854

Feitelson, M. A., Arzumanyan, A., Medhat, A., & Spector, I. (2023). Short-chain fatty acids in cancer pathogenesis. *Cancer and Metastasis Reviews*, *42*(3), 677–698. DOI: 10.1007/s10555-023-10117-y PMID: 37432606

Fellah, S. (2024). *Stratégies thérapeutiques permettant de limiter l'agression chimique des xénobiotiques : ciblage du long ARN non codant DNM3OS et du récepteur à l'adénosine A2A*. https://doi.org/HALId:tel-04642293https://theses.hal.science/tel-04642293v1

Fenech, M., Amaya, I., Valpuesta, V., & Botella, M. A. (2018). Vitamin C Content in Fruits: Biosynthesis and Regulation. *Frontiers in Plant Science*, *9*, 2006. DOI: 10.3389/fpls.2018.02006 PMID: 30733729

Feng, C., Li, R., Shamim, A. A., Ullah, M. B., Li, M., Dev, R., Wang, Y., Zhao, T., Liao, J., Du, Z., Ling, Y., Lai, Y., & Hao, Y. (2021). High-resolution mapping of reproductive tract infections among women of childbearing age in Bangladesh: A spatial-temporal analysis of the demographic and health survey. *BMC Public Health, 21*(1), 342. DOI: 10.1186/s12889-021-10360-4 PMID: 33579253

Feng, J., Rubbi, L., Kianian, R., Mills, J. N., Osadchiy, V., Sigalos, J. T., Eleswarapu, S. V., & Pellegrini, M. (2024). Epigenetic aging of semen is associated with inflammation. *Epigenetics, 19*(1), 2436304. DOI: 10.1080/15592294.2024.2436304 PMID: 39637179

Feng, Z. (2010). P53 Regulation of the IGF-1/AKT/mTOR Pathways and the Endosomal Compartment. *Cold Spring Harbor Perspectives in Biology, 2*(2), a001057–a001057. DOI: 10.1101/cshperspect.a001057 PMID: 20182617

Ferrante, M., Cristaldi, A., & Oliveri Conti, G. (2021). Oncogenic Role of miRNA in Environmental Exposure to Plasticizers: A Systematic Review. *Journal of Personalized Medicine, 11*(6), 500. DOI: 10.3390/jpm11060500 PMID: 34199666

Fetse, J., Olawode, E. O., & Deb, S. (2024). Personalized Medicine Approach to Proteomics and Metabolomics of Cytochrome P450 Enzymes: A Narrative Review. *European Journal of Drug Metabolism and Pharmacokinetics, 49*(6), 661–676. DOI: 10.1007/s13318-024-00912-5 PMID: 39269556

Flemer, B., Warren, R. D., Barrett, M. P., Cisek, K., Das, A., Jeffery, I. B., & O'Toole, P. W. (2017). The oral microbiota in colorectal cancer is distinctive and predictive. *Gut, 67*(4), 1454–1463. DOI: 10.1136/gutjnl-2016-313173 PMID: 28988196

Foreman, A. L., Warth, B., Hessel, E. V. S., Price, E. J., Schymanski, E. L., Cantelli, G., Parkinson, H., Hecht, H., Klánová, J., Vlaanderen, J., Hilscherova, K., Vrijheid, M., Vineis, P., Araujo, R., Barouki, R., Vermeulen, R., Lanone, S., Brunak, S., Sebert, S., & Karjalainen, T. (2024). Adopting Mechanistic Molecular Biology Approaches in Exposome Research for Causal Understanding. *Environmental Science & Technology, 58*(17), 7256–7269. DOI: 10.1021/acs.est.3c07961 PMID: 38641325

Foronjy, R. F., Mirochnitchenko, O., Propokenko, O., Lemaitre, V., Jia, Y., Inouye, M., Okada, Y., & D'Armiento, J. M. (2006). Superoxide Dismutase Expression Attenuates Cigarette Smoke– or Elastase-generated Emphysema in Mice. *American Journal of Respiratory and Critical Care Medicine, 173*(6), 623–631. DOI: 10.1164/rccm.200506-850OC PMID: 16387805

Forsythe, S. D., Devarasetty, M., Shupe, T., Bishop, C., Atala, A., Soker, S., & Skardal, A. (2018). Environmental toxin screening using human-derived 3D bioengineered liver and cardiac organoids. *Frontiers in Public Health, 6*, 103. Advance online publication. DOI: 10.3389/fpubh.2018.00103 PMID: 29755963

França, G. S., Baron, M., King, B. R., Bossowski, J. P., Bjornberg, A., Pour, M., Rao, A., Patel, A. S., Misirlioglu, S., Barkley, D., Tang, K. H., Dolgalev, I., Liberman, D. A., Avital, G., Kuperwaser, F., Chiodin, M., Levine, D. A., Papagiannakopoulos, T., Marusyk, A., & Yanai, I. (2024). Cellular adaptation to cancer therapy along a resistance continuum. *Nature, 631*(8022), 876–883. DOI: 10.1038/s41586-024-07690-9 PMID: 38987605

Frank, S. A., & Yanai, I. (2024). The origin of novel traits in cancer. *Trends in Cancer, 10*(10), 880–892. DOI: 10.1016/j.trecan.2024.07.005 PMID: 39112299

Furlong, M. A., Paul, K. C., Parra, K. L., Fournier, A. J., Ellsworth, P. C., Cockburn, M. G., Arellano, A. F., Bedrick, E. J., Beamer, P. I., & Ritz, B. (2024). Pre-Conception And First Trimester Exposure To Pesticides And Associations With Stillbirth. *American Journal of Epidemiology*, kwae198. Advance online publication. DOI: 10.1093/aje/kwae198 PMID: 39013781

Fu, X., Cai, Q., Yang, Y., Xu, Y., Zhao, F., Yang, J., Qiao, L., Yao, L., & Li, W. (2022). Application of Mobile Monitoring to Study Characteristics of Air Pollution in Typical Areas of the Yangtze River Delta Eco-Green Integration Demonstration Zone, China. *Sustainability (Basel), 15*(1), 205. DOI: 10.3390/su15010205

Fu, Y., Moscoso, D. I., Porter, J., Krishnareddy, S., Abrams, J. A., Seres, D., Chong, D. H., & Freedberg, D. E. (2020). Relationship Between Dietary Fiber Intake and Short-Chain Fatty Acid-Producing Bacteria During Critical Illness: A Prospective Cohort Study. *JPEN. Journal of Parenteral and Enteral Nutrition, 44*(3), 463–471. DOI: 10.1002/jpen.1682 PMID: 31385326

Gagliardi, A., Bajraktari-Sylejmani, G., Barocelli, E., Weiss, J., & Rigalli, J. P. (2023). Extracellular vesicles as surrogates for drug metabolism and clearance: Promise vs. reality. *Life (Chicago, Ill.), 13*(8), 1745. DOI: 10.3390/life13081745 PMID: 37629602

Gaither, K. A., Yue, G., Singh, D. K., Trudeau, J., Ponraj, K., Davydova, N. Y., Lazarus, P., Davydov, D. R., & Prasad, B. (2025). Effects of Chronic Alcohol Intake on the Composition of the Ensemble of Drug-Metabolizing Enzymes and Transporters in the Human Liver. *Journal of Xenobiotics, 15*(1), 20. DOI: 10.3390/jox15010020 PMID: 39997363

Galateanu, B., Hudita, A., Biru, E. I., Iovu, H., Zaharia, C., Simsensohn, E., Costache, M., Petca, R. C., & Jinga, V. (2022). Applications of Polymers for Organ-on-Chip Technology in Urology. In *Polymers* (Vol. 14). MDPI., DOI: 10.3390/polym14091668

Gao, B., Shu, Z., Ren, S., & Gao, D. (2022). Biobanking: A foundation of life-science research and advancement. *Biosafety and Health*, *4*(5), 285–289. DOI: 10.1016/j.bsheal.2022.09.003

Gao, J., Shi, W., Wang, J., Guan, C., Dong, Q., Sheng, J., Zou, X., Xu, Z., Ge, Y., Yang, C., Li, J., Bao, H., Zhong, X., & Cui, Y. (2024). Research progress and applications of epigenetic biomarkers in cancer. *Frontiers in Pharmacology*, *15*, 1308309. DOI: 10.3389/fphar.2024.1308309 PMID: 38681199

Garcia, M., Thirouard, L., Sedès, L., Monrose, M., Holota, H., Caira, F., Volle, D. H., & Beaudoin, C. (2018). Nuclear receptor metabolism of bile acids and xenobiotics: A coordinated detoxification system with impact on health and diseases. *International Journal of Molecular Sciences*, *19*(11), 3630. DOI: 10.3390/ijms19113630 PMID: 30453651

Garcia, W. L., Miller, C. J., Lomas, G. X., Gaither, K. A., Tyrrell, K. J., Smith, J. N., Brandvold, K. R., & Wright, A. T. (2022). Profiling How the Gut Microbiome Modulates Host Xenobiotic Metabolism in Response to Benzo[*a*]pyrene and 1-Nitropyrene Exposure. *Chemical Research in Toxicology*, *35*(4), 585–596. DOI: 10.1021/acs.chemrestox.1c00360 PMID: 35347982

Garrett, W. S. (2015). Cancer and the microbiota. *Science*, *348*(6230), 80–86. DOI: 10.1126/science.aaa4972 PMID: 25838377

Gearhart-Serna, L. M., Davis, J. B., Jolly, M. K., Jayasundara, N., Sauer, S. J., Di Giulio, R. T., & Devi, G. R. (2020). A polycyclic aromatic hydrocarbon-enriched environmental chemical mixture enhances AhR, antiapoptotic signaling and a proliferative phenotype in breast cancer cells. *Carcinogenesis*, *41*(12), 1648–1659. DOI: 10.1093/carcin/bgaa047 PMID: 32747956

Gebrayel, P., Nicco, C., Al Khodor, S., Bilinski, J., Caselli, E., Comelli, E. M., Egert, M., Giaroni, C., Karpinski, T. M., Loniewski, I., Mulak, A., Reygner, J., Samczuk, P., Serino, M., Sikora, M., Terranegra, A., Ufnal, M., Villeger, R., Pichon, C., & Edeas, M. (2022). Microbiota medicine: Towards clinical revolution. *Journal of Translational Medicine*, *20*(1), 111. DOI: 10.1186/s12967-022-03296-9 PMID: 35255932

Geissler, F., Nesic, K., Kondrashova, O., Dobrovic, A., Swisher, E. M., Scott, C. L., & Wakefield, J., M. (. (2024). The role of aberrant DNA methylation in cancer initiation and clinical impacts. *Therapeutic Advances in Medical Oncology, 16*, 17588359231220511. DOI: 10.1177/17588359231220511 PMID: 38293277

Ghai, R., Mittal, A., Pandey, D., Alam, M. S., Kaushik, S., Ishtiyaq, P., Kaushik, Y., & Mishra, S. K. (2024). Role of Personalized Medicine in Clinical Practice: An Overview of Current and Future Perspectives. *Biomedical & Pharmacology Journal, 17*(4), 2111–2133. DOI: 10.13005/bpj/3011

Ghantous, A., Hernandez-Vargas, H., Byrnes, G., Dwyer, T., & Herceg, Z. (2015). Characterising the epigenome as a key component of the fetal exposome in evaluating in utero exposures and childhood cancer risk. In *Mutagenesis* (Vol. 30, pp. 733–742). Oxford University Press. DOI: 10.1093/mutage/gev010

Gholami, H., Chmiel, J. A., Burton, J. P., & Maleki Vareki, S. (2023). The Role of Microbiota-Derived Vitamins in Immune Homeostasis and Enhancing Cancer Immunotherapy. *Cancers (Basel), 15*(4), 1300. DOI: 10.3390/cancers15041300 PMID: 36831641

Gibbons, D. L., Byers, L. A., & Kurie, J. M. (2014). Smoking, p53 Mutation, and Lung Cancer. *Molecular Cancer Research, 12*(1), 3–13. DOI: 10.1158/1541-7786.MCR-13-0539 PMID: 24442106

Gibney, E. R., & Nolan, C. M. (2010). Epigenetics and gene expression. *Heredity, 105*(1), 4–13. DOI: 10.1038/hdy.2010.54 PMID: 20461105

Gill, P. A., Inniss, S., Kumagai, T., Rahman, F. Z., & Smith, A. M. (2022). The Role of Diet and Gut Microbiota in Regulating Gastrointestinal and Inflammatory Disease. *Frontiers in Immunology, 13*, 866059. DOI: 10.3389/fimmu.2022.866059 PMID: 35450067

Giri, A. K., & Aittokallio, T. (2019). DNMT Inhibitors Increase Methylation in the Cancer Genome. *Frontiers in Pharmacology, 10*, 385. DOI: 10.3389/fphar.2019.00385 PMID: 31068808

Goey, A. K., Sissung, T. M., Peer, C. J., & Figg, W. D. (2016). Pharmacogenomics and Histone Deacetylase Inhibitors. *Pharmacogenomics, 17*(16), 1807–1815. DOI: 10.2217/pgs-2016-0113 PMID: 27767376

Gong, P., Guo, Z., Wang, S., Gao, S., & Cao, Q. (2025). Histone Phosphorylation in DNA Damage Response. *International Journal of Molecular Sciences, 26*(6), 6. Advance online publication. DOI: 10.3390/ijms26062405 PMID: 40141048

Gong, Y., Lv, J., Pang, X., Zhang, S., Zhang, G., Liu, L., Wang, Y., & Li, C. (2023). Advances in the metabolic mechanism and functional characteristics of equol. *Foods, 12*(12), 2334. DOI: 10.3390/foods12122334 PMID: 37372545

Goode, E. L., White, K. L., Vierkant, R. A., Phelan, C. M., Cunningham, J. M., Schildkraut, J. M., Berchuck, A., Larson, M. C., Fridley, B. L., Olson, J. E., Webb, P. M., Chen, X., Beesley, J., Chenevix-Trench, G., & Sellers, T. A.Ovarian Cancer Association Consortium. (2011). Xenobiotic-Metabolizing gene polymorphisms and ovarian cancer risk. *Molecular Carcinogenesis, 50*(5), 397–402. DOI: 10.1002/mc.20714 PMID: 21480392

Goodman, S., Chappell, G., Guyton, K. Z., Pogribny, I. P., & Rusyn, I. (2022). Epigenetic alterations induced by genotoxic occupational and environmental human chemical carcinogens: An update of a systematic literature review. *Mutation Research/Reviews in Mutation Research, 789*, 108408. DOI: 10.1016/j.mrrev.2021.108408 PMID: 35690411

Go, Y.-M., Weinberg, J., Teeny, S., Cirillo, P. M., Krigbaum, N. Y., Singer, G., Tran, V., Cohn, B. A., & Jones, D. P. (2023). Exposome epidemiology for suspect environmental chemical exposures during pregnancy linked to subsequent breast cancer diagnosis. *Environment International, 178*, 108112. DOI: 10.1016/j.envint.2023.108112 PMID: 37517180

Goyal, N., Do, C., Sridhar, J., Shaik, S., Thompson, A., Perry, T., Carter, L., & Foroozesh, M. (2023). Design, Synthesis, and Biological Studies of Flavone-Based Esters and Acids as Potential P450 2A6 Inhibitors. *Chemical Research in Toxicology, 36*(12), 1973–1979. DOI: 10.1021/acs.chemrestox.3c00249 PMID: 37963190

Grabherr, M. G., Haas, B. J., Yassour, M., Levin, J. Z., Thompson, D. A., Amit, I., Adiconis, X., Fan, L., Raychowdhury, R., Zeng, Q., Chen, Z., Mauceli, E., Hacohen, N., Gnirke, A., Rhind, N., di Palma, F., Birren, B. W., Nusbaum, C., Lindblad-Toh, K., & Regev, A. (2011). Full-length transcriptome assembly from RNA-Seq data without a reference genome. *Nature Biotechnology, 29*(7), 644–652. DOI: 10.1038/nbt.1883 PMID: 21572440

Gracia-Cazaña, T., González, S., Parrado, C., Juarranz, Á., & Gilaberte, Y. (2020). Influence of the Exposome on Skin Cancer. [English Edition]. *Actas Dermo-Sifiliográficas, 111*(6), 460–470. DOI: 10.1016/j.adengl.2020.04.011 PMID: 32507282

Greathouse, K. L., White, J. R., Vargas, A. J., Bliskovsky, V. V., Beck, J. A., von Muhlinen, N., Polley, E. C., Bowman, E. D., Khan, M. A., Robles, A. I., Cooks, T., Ryan, B. M., Padgett, N., Dzutsev, A. H., Trinchieri, G., Pineda, M. A., Bilke, S., Meltzer, P. S., Hokenstad, A. N., & Harris, C. C. (2018). Interaction between the microbiome and TP53 in human lung cancer. *Genome Biology*, *19*(1), 123. DOI: 10.1186/s13059-018-1501-6 PMID: 30143034

Greeson, K. W., Crow, K. M. S., Edenfield, R. C., & Easley, C. A.IV. (2023). Inheritance of paternal lifestyles and exposures through sperm DNA methylation. *Nature Reviews. Urology*, *20*(6), 356–370. DOI: 10.1038/s41585-022-00708-9 PMID: 36653672

Griep, L. M., Wolbers, F., De Wagenaar, B., Ter Braak, P. M., Weksler, B. B., Romero, I. A., Couraud, P. O., Vermes, I., Van Der Meer, A. D., & Van Den Berg, A. (2013). BBB on CHIP: Microfluidic platform to mechanically and biochemically modulate blood-brain barrier function. *Biomedical Microdevices*, *15*(1), 145–150. DOI: 10.1007/s10544-012-9699-7 PMID: 22955726

Grocholska, P., Popiel, D., Walter, M., Biernat, M., Cebrat, M., Kuczer, M., Modzel, M., Bąchor, R., & Kluczyk, A. (2022). Citius, Altius, Fortius—Advanced Mass Spectrometry in Service of Forensic Analysis. *Chemosensors (Basel, Switzerland)*, *10*(8), 324. DOI: 10.3390/chemosensors10080324

Guenat, O. T., & Berthiaume, F. (2018). Incorporating mechanical strain in organs-on-a-chip: Lung and skin. *Biomicrofluidics*, *12*(4), 042207. DOI: 10.1063/1.5024895 PMID: 29861818

Guengerich, F. P. (2006). Cytochrome P450s and other enzymes in drug metabolism and toxicity. *The AAPS Journal*, *8*(1), E101–E111. DOI: 10.1208/aapsj080112 PMID: 16584116

Gu, H., Yu, Y., Sisoudiya, S. D., Mishra, P., Li, H., Schraw, J. M., Scheurer, M. E., Muzny, D. M., Mitchell, D., Taylor, O., Jhangiani, S. N., Dugan-Perez, S., Wu, Y., Doddapaneni, H., Bhamidipati, S. V., Gingras, M.-C., Posey, J. E., Gibbs, R. A., Huff, C. D., & Sabo, A. (2025). An evaluation of genetic predisposition to congenital anomalies and pediatric cancer supports KAT6B as a novel neuroblastoma susceptibility gene. *Genetics in Medicine Open*, *3*, 101901. Advance online publication. DOI: 10.1016/j.gimo.2024.101901

Günther, A., Yasotharan, S., Vagaon, A., Lochovsky, C., Pinto, S., Yang, J., Lau, C., Voigtlaender-Bolz, J., & Bolz, S. S. (2010). A microfluidic platform for probing small artery structure and function. *Lab on a Chip*, *10*(18), 2341–2349. DOI: 10.1039/c004675b PMID: 20603685

Guo, Q., Jin, Y., Chen, X., Ye, X., Shen, X., Lin, M., Zeng, C., Zhou, T., & Zhang, J. (2024). NF-κB in biology and targeted therapy: New insights and translational implications. *Signal Transduction and Targeted Therapy*, *9*(1), 53. DOI: 10.1038/s41392-024-01757-9 PMID: 38433280

Gupta, G., Maurya, S., Jha, P. N., & Chauhan, P. S. (2024). Valorization of Mushroom Spent Mushroom Substrate: A Sustainable Approach to Remediation of Xenobiotic Compounds-A Comprehensive Review. *Groundwater for Sustainable Development*, *101290*. Advance online publication. DOI: 10.1016/j.gsd.2024.101290

Gupta, N. S., & Kumar, P. (2023). Perspective of artificial intelligence in healthcare data management: A journey towards precision medicine. *Computers in Biology and Medicine*, *162*, 107051. DOI: 10.1016/j.compbiomed.2023.107051 PMID: 37271113

Guth, M., Lefevre, M., Pilorget, C., Coste, A., Ahmadi, S., Danjou, A., Dananché, B., Praud, D., Koscinski, I., Papaxanthos, A., Blagosklonov, O., Fauque, P., Pérol, O., Schüz, J., Bujan, L., Olsson, A., Fervers, B., & Charbotel, B.TESTIS study group. (2023). Parental occupational exposure to solvents and risk of developing testicular germ cell tumors among sons: A French nationwide case-control study (TESTIS study). *Scandinavian Journal of Work, Environment & Health*, *49*(6), 405–418. DOI: 10.5271/sjweh.4102 PMID: 37649372

GVS, A. C., Ananthakumar, B., & Raghavan, R. (2025). Enhancing Assistive Technologies With Neuromorphic Computing. *Revolutionizing AI with Brain-Inspired Technology: Neuromorphic Computing*, 207–232. DOI: 10.4018/979-8-3693-6303-4.ch009

GVS, A. C., Biradar, S., & Raghavan, R. (2025). Neuroscience-Driven Solutions for Speech Impairment: Assistive Technologies for Speech Rehabilitation. *Advancing Medical Research Through Neuroscience*, 119–146. DOI: 10.4018/979-8-3693-5464-3.ch006

Gyaneshwari, U., Swati, K., Singh, A. K., Prakash, A., Pal, P., Kumari, B., & Pandey, B. (2023). Alcohol Dehydrogenase: Structural and Functional Diversity. In *Integrative Approaches to Biotechnology* (pp. 249-265). CRC Press. DOI: 10.1201/9781003324706-21

Hahm, J. Y., Park, J., Jang, E.-S., & Chi, S. W. (2022). 8-Oxoguanine: From oxidative damage to epigenetic and epitranscriptional modification. *Experimental & Molecular Medicine*, *54*(10), 1626–1642. DOI: 10.1038/s12276-022-00822-z PMID: 36266447

Haiser, H. J., Gootenberg, D. B., Chatman, K., Sirasani, G., Balskus, E. P., & Turnbaugh, P. J. (2013). Predicting and Manipulating Cardiac Drug Inactivation by the Human Gut Bacterium *Eggerthella lenta. Science, 341*(6143), 295–298. DOI: 10.1126/science.1235872 PMID: 23869020

Hao, Q., Wang, M., Sun, N., Zhu, C., Lin, Y., Li, C., Liu, F., & Zhu, W. (2020). Sulforaphane suppresses carcinogenesis of colorectal cancer through the ERK/ Nrf2-UDP glucuronosyltransferase 1A metabolic axis activation. *Oncology Reports*. Advance online publication. DOI: 10.3892/or.2020.7495 PMID: 32323779

Hart, X. M., Gründer, G., Ansermot, N., Conca, A., Corruble, E., Crettol, S., Cumming, P., Frajerman, A., Hefner, G., Howes, O., Jukic, M. M., Kim, E., Kim, S., Maniscalco, I., Moriguchi, S., Müller, D. J., Nakajima, S., Osugo, M., Paulzen, M., & Eap, C. B. (2024). Optimisation of pharmacotherapy in psychiatry through therapeutic drug monitoring, molecular brain imaging and pharmacogenetic tests: Focus on antipsychotics. *The World Journal of Biological Psychiatry, 25*(9), 451–536. DOI: 10.1080/15622975.2024.2366235 PMID: 38913780

Hasan, N., & Yang, H. (2019). Factors affecting the composition of the gut microbiota, and its modulation. *PeerJ, 7*, e7502. DOI: 10.7717/peerj.7502 PMID: 31440436

Hasegawa, K., Motoki, N., Inaba, Y., Toubou, H., Shibazaki, T., Nakayama, S. F., Kamijima, M., Tsukahara, T., & Nomiyama, T.Japan Environment and Children's Study Group. (2024). Maternal Exposure to Per- and Polyfluoroalkyl Substances and Offspring Chromosomal Abnormalities: The Japan Environment and Children's Study. *Environmental Health Perspectives, 132*(9), 097004. DOI: 10.1289/ EHP13617 PMID: 39258902

Hasin, Y., Seldin, M., & Lusis, A. (2017). Multi-omics approaches to disease. *Genome Biology, 18*(1), 83. DOI: 10.1186/s13059-017-1215-1 PMID: 28476144

Hayes, J. D., Flanagan, J. U., & Jowsey, I. R. (2005). Glutathione transferases. *Annual Review of Pharmacology and Toxicology, 45*(1), 51–88. DOI: 10.1146/ annurev.pharmtox.45.120403.095857 PMID: 15822171

Healy, C. M., & Moran, G. P. (2019). The microbiome and oral cancer: More questions than answers. *Oral Oncology, 89*, 30–33. DOI: 10.1016/j.oraloncology.2018.12.003 PMID: 30732955

Heavey, P. M., & Rowland, I. R. (2004). Gastrointestinal cancer. *Best Practice & Research. Clinical Gastroenterology, 18*(2), 323–336. DOI: 10.1016/j.bpg.2003.10.003 PMID: 15123073

Hecht, S. S. (2012). Lung carcinogenesis by tobacco smoke. *International Journal of Cancer, 131*(12), 2724–2732. DOI: 10.1002/ijc.27816 PMID: 22945513

Heitzer, E., Haque, I. S., Roberts, C. E. S., & Speicher, M. R. (2019). Current and future perspectives of liquid biopsies in genomics-driven oncology. *Nature Reviews. Genetics, 20*(2), 71–88. DOI: 10.1038/s41576-018-0071-5 PMID: 30410101

Heo, Y. J., Hwa, C., Lee, G.-H., Park, J.-M., & An, J.-Y. (2021). Integrative Multi-Omics Approaches in Cancer Research: From Biological Networks to Clinical Subtypes. *Molecules and Cells, 44*(7), 433–443. DOI: 10.14348/molcells.2021.0042 PMID: 34238766

Heppel, C. W., Heling, A.-K., & Richter, E. (2009). Ultrasensitive method for the determination of 4-hydroxy-1-(3-pyridyl)-1-butanone-releasing DNA adducts by gas chromatography–high resolution mass spectrometry in mucosal biopsies of the lower esophagus. *Analytical and Bioanalytical Chemistry, 393*(5), 1525–1530. DOI: 10.1007/s00216-008-2566-y PMID: 19104779

Herath, H. M. S. S., Herath, H. M. K. K. M. B., Madhusanka, B. G. D. A., & Guruge, L. G. P. K. (2024). Data protection challenges in the processing of sensitive data. In *Data Protection: The Wake of AI and Machine Learning* (pp. 155–179). Springer Nature Switzerland. DOI: 10.1007/978-3-031-76473-8_8

He, X., & Feng, S. (2015). Role of Metabolic Enzymes P450 (CYP) on Activating Procarcinogen and their Polymorphisms on the Risk of Cancers. *Current Drug Metabolism, 16*(10), 850–863. DOI: 10.2174/138920021610151210164501 PMID: 26652254

Hickman, B., Salonen, A., Ponsero, A. J., Jokela, R., Kolho, K.-L., de Vos, W. M., & Korpela, K. (2024). Gut microbiota wellbeing index predicts overall health in a cohort of 1000 infants. *Nature Communications, 15*(1), 8323. DOI: 10.1038/s41467-024-52561-6 PMID: 39333099

Hillegass, J. M., Miller, J. M., MacPherson, M. B., Westbom, C. M., Sayan, M., Thompson, J. K., Macura, S. L., Perkins, T. N., Beuschel, S. L., Alexeeva, V., Pass, H. I., Steele, C., Mossman, B. T., & Shukla, A. (2013). Asbestos and erionite prime and activate the NLRP3 inflammasome that stimulates autocrine cytokine release in human mesothelial cells. *Particle and Fibre Toxicology, 10*(1), 39. DOI: 10.1186/1743-8977-10-39 PMID: 23937860

Hillege, L. E., Stevens, M. A. M., Kristen, P. A. J., De Vos-Geelen, J., Penders, J., Redinbo, M. R., & Smidt, M. L. (2024). The role of gut microbial β-glucuronidases in carcinogenesis and cancer treatment: A scoping review. *Journal of Cancer Research and Clinical Oncology, 150*(11), 495. DOI: 10.1007/s00432-024-06028-2 PMID: 39537966

Himmel, L. E., Wilson, K. L., Santagostino, S. F., & Bolon, B. (2022). Genetically Engineered Animal Models in Toxicologic Research. In *Haschek and Rousseaux's Handbook of Toxicologic Pathology* (pp. 859–924). Academic Press. DOI: 10.1016/B978-0-12-821044-4.00024-8

Hjorth, M. F., Blædel, T., Bendtsen, L. Q., Lorenzen, J. K., Holm, J. B., Kiilerich, P., Roager, H. M., Kristiansen, K., Larsen, L. H., & Astrup, A. (2019). Prevotella-to-Bacteroides ratio predicts body weight and fat loss success on 24-week diets varying in macronutrient composition and dietary fiber: Results from a post-hoc analysis. *International Journal of Obesity, 43*(1), 149–157. DOI: 10.1038/s41366-018-0093-2 PMID: 29777234

Ho, S.-M., Tang, W.-Y., Belmonte De Frausto, J., & Prins, G. S. (2006). Developmental Exposure to Estradiol and Bisphenol A Increases Susceptibility to Prostate Carcinogenesis and Epigenetically Regulates Phosphodiesterase Type 4 Variant 4. *Cancer Research, 66*(11), 5624–5632. DOI: 10.1158/0008-5472.CAN-06-0516 PMID: 16740699

Hou, M., Tang, S., Zhang, F., Fu, S., Ding, H., Cha, Y., Ma, X., Shi, Y., & Cai, Y. (2025). Chemical exposure in females of childbearing age associated with sex hormones: Evidence from an untargeted exposomic approach. *Environment International, 197*, 109362. DOI: 10.1016/j.envint.2025.109362 PMID: 40054345

Howarth, M. V., & Eiser, A. R. (2023). Environmentally Mediated Health Disparities. *The American Journal of Medicine, 136*(6), 518–522. DOI: 10.1016/j.amjmed.2023.02.008 PMID: 36828212

Hsiao, Y.-C., Liu, C.-W., Chi, L., Yang, Y., & Lu, K. (2020). The Effects of Gut Microbiome on Carcinogenic DNA Damage. *Chemical Research in Toxicology, 33*(8), 2130–2138. DOI: 10.1021/acs.chemrestox.0c00142 PMID: 32677427

Hua, Z. L. (2024). Elucidating the Role of Cytochrome p450 Enzymes in Drug Metabolism and Interactions. *Clinical Journal for Medicine, Health and Pharmacy, 2*(3), 1-10. http://cjmhp.com/index.php/journal/article/view/2.3.01

Huang, C. Y., Xie, R. H., Li, P. H., Chen, C. Y., You, B. H., Sun, Y. C., Chou, C. K., Chang, Y. H., Lin, W. C., & Chen, G. Y. (2025). Environmental Exposure to Bisphenol A Enhances Invasiveness in Papillary Thyroid Cancer. *International Journal of Molecular Sciences*, *26*(2), 814. Advance online publication. DOI: 10.3390/ijms26020814 PMID: 39859529

Huang, S. X. L., Jaurand, M.-C., Kamp, D. W., Whysner, J., & Hei, T. K. (2011). Role of Mutagenicity in Asbestos Fiber-Induced Carcinogenicity and Other Diseases. *Journal of Toxicology and Environmental Health. Part B, Critical Reviews*, *14*(1–4), 179–245. DOI: 10.1080/10937404.2011.556051 PMID: 21534089

Huang, Y., Zhang, Y., Wu, K., Tan, X., Lan, T., & Wang, G. (2024). Role of Gut Microecology in the Pathogenesis of Drug-Induced Liver Injury and Emerging Therapeutic Strategies. *Molecules (Basel, Switzerland)*, *29*(11), 2663. DOI: 10.3390/molecules29112663 PMID: 38893536

Hu, C., Liu, X., Zeng, Y., Liu, J., & Wu, F. (2021). DNA methyltransferase inhibitors combination therapy for the treatment of solid tumor: Mechanism and clinical application. *Clinical Epigenetics*, *13*(1), 166. DOI: 10.1186/s13148-021-01154-x PMID: 34452630

Huerta-Cepas, J., Szklarczyk, D., Heller, D., Hernández-Plaza, A., Forslund, S. K., Cook, H., Mende, D. R., Letunic, I., Rattei, T., Jensen, L. J., von Mering, C., & Bork, P. (2019). eggNOG 5.0: A hierarchical, functionally and phylogenetically annotated orthology resource based on 5090 organisms and 2502 viruses. *Nucleic Acids Research*, *47*(D1), D309–D314. DOI: 10.1093/nar/gky1085 PMID: 30418610

Huh, D., Matthews, B. D., Mammoto, A., Montoya-Zavala, M., Yuan Hsin, H., & Ingber, D. E. (2010). Reconstituting organ-level lung functions on a chip. *Science*, *328*(5986), 1662–1668. DOI: 10.1126/science.1188302 PMID: 20576885

Huoi, C., Olsson, A., Lightfoot, T., Roman, E., Clavel, J., Lacour, B., Kaatsch, P., Kromhout, H., Vermeulen, R., Peters, S., Bailey, H. D., & Schüz, J. (2014). Parental occupational exposure and risk of childhood central nervous system tumors: A pooled analysis of case-control studies from Germany, France, and the UK. *Cancer Causes & Control*, *25*(12), 1603–1613. DOI: 10.1007/s10552-014-0465-4 PMID: 25281325

Huynh, K. (2017). Targeting inflammatory pathways to treat atherosclerosis and cancer. *Nature Reviews. Cardiology*, *14*(11), 629–629. DOI: 10.1038/nrcardio.2017.152 PMID: 28905870

IARC. (2006). *Mécanismes du développement tumoral.*

Inamura, K. (2021). Gut microbiota contributes towards immunomodulation against cancer: New frontiers in precision cancer therapeutics. *Seminars in Cancer Biology*, *70*, 11–23. DOI: 10.1016/j.semcancer.2020.06.006 PMID: 32580023

Inamura, K., Hamada, T., Bullman, S., Ugai, T., Yachida, S., & Ogino, S. (2022). Cancer as microenvironmental, systemic and environmental diseases: opportunity for transdisciplinary microbiomics science. In *Gut* (Vol. 71, pp. 2107–2122). BMJ Publishing Group., DOI: 10.1136/gutjnl-2022-327209

International Agency for Research on Cancer (IARC). (2020). *Global Cancer Observatory: Cancer Today*. The Global Cancer Observatory (GCO) World Health Organization. https://gco.iarc.fr/today(https://gco.iarc.fr/today

Iorio, M. V., & Croce, C. M. (2012). Causes and Consequences of MicroRNA Dysregulation. *Cancer Journal (Sudbury, Mass.)*, *18*(3), 215–222. DOI: 10.1097/PPO.0b013e318250c001 PMID: 22647357

Irigaray, P., & Belpomme, D. (2010). Basic properties and molecular mechanisms of exogenous chemical carcinogens. In *Carcinogenesis* (Vol. 31, pp. 135–148). DOI: 10.1093/carcin/bgp252

Isachesku, E., Braicu, C., Pirlog, R., Kocijancic, A., Busuioc, C., Pruteanu, L. L., Pandey, D. P., & Berindan-Neagoe, I. (2023). The Role of Non-Coding RNAs in Epigenetic Dysregulation in Glioblastoma Development. In *International Journal of Molecular Sciences* (Vol. 24). Multidisciplinary Digital Publishing Institute (MDPI). DOI: 10.3390/ijms242216320

Ishikawa, H., Akedo, I., Otani, T., Suzuki, T., Nakamura, T., Takeyama, I., Ishiguro, S., Miyaoka, E., Sobue, T., & Kakizoe, T. (2005). Randomized trial of dietary fiber andLactobacillus casei administration for prevention of colorectal tumors. *International Journal of Cancer*, *116*(5), 762–767. DOI: 10.1002/ijc.21115 PMID: 15828052

Islami, F., Baeker Bispo, J., Lee, H., Wiese, D., Yabroff, K. R., Bandi, P., Sloan, K., Patel, A. V., Daniels, E. C., Kamal, A. H., Guerra, C. E., Dahut, W. L., & Jemal, A. (2024). American Cancer Society's report on the status of cancer disparities in the United States, 2023. *CA: a Cancer Journal for Clinicians*, *74*(2), 136–166. DOI: 10.3322/caac.21812 PMID: 37962495

Islam, T., Majumder, M., Kalita, B., Bhattacharjee, A., Mukhopadhyay, R., & Mukherjee, A. K. (2020). Transcriptomic, proteomic, and biochemical analyses reveal a novel neuritogenesis mechanism of *Naja naja* venom α-elapitoxin post binding to TrkA receptor of rat pheochromocytoma cells. *Journal of Neurochemistry*, *155*(6), 612–637. DOI: 10.1111/jnc.15153 PMID: 33460153

Iungman, T., Khomenko, S., Barboza, E. P., Cirach, M., Gonçalves, K., Petrone, P., Erbertseder, T., Taubenböck, H., Chakraborty, T., & Nieuwenhuijsen, M. (2024). The impact of urban configuration types on urban heat islands, air pollution, CO2 emissions, and mortality in Europe: A data science approach. *The Lancet. Planetary Health*, *8*(7), e489–e505. DOI: 10.1016/S2542-5196(24)00120-7 PMID: 38969476

Izat, N., Bolleddula, J., Carione, P., Huertas Valentin, L., Jones, R. S., Kulkarni, P., Moss, D., Peterkin, V. C., Tian, D. D., Treyer, A., Venkatakrishnan, K., Zientek, M. A., Barber, J., Houston, J. B., Galetin, A., & Scotcher, D. (2025). Establishing a physiologically based pharmacokinetic framework for aldehyde oxidase and dual aldehyde oxidase-CYP substrates. *CPT: Pharmacometrics & Systems Pharmacology*, *14*(1), 164–178. DOI: 10.1002/psp4.13255 PMID: 39444174

Jadhav, R., Santucci-Pereira, J., Wang, Y., Liu, J., Nguyen, T., Wang, J., Jenkins, S., Russo, J., Huang, T., Jin, V., & Lamartiniere, C. (2017). DNA Methylation Targets Influenced by Bisphenol A and/or Genistein Are Associated with Survival Outcomes in Breast Cancer Patients. *Genes*, *8*(5), 144. DOI: 10.3390/genes8050144 PMID: 28505145

Jakobsson, T., & Forsum, U. (2007). Lactobacillus iners: A marker of changes in the vaginal flora? *Journal of Clinical Microbiology*, *45*(9), 3145. DOI: 10.1128/JCM.00558-07 PMID: 17652481

Jang, J., Yoo, D.-S., & Chun, B. C. (2021). Spatial epidemiologic analysis of the liver cancer and gallbladder cancer incidence and its determinants in South Korea. *BMC Public Health*, *21*(1), 2090. DOI: 10.1186/s12889-021-12184-8 PMID: 34774036

Jia, B. (2019). Commentary: Gut microbiome–mediated bile acid metabolism regulates liver cancer via NKT cells. *Frontiers in Immunology*, *10*, 282. Advance online publication. DOI: 10.3389/fimmu.2019.00282 PMID: 30842777

Jiang, C., Wang, X., Li, X., Inlora, J., Wang, T., Liu, Q., & Snyder, M. (2018). Dynamic Human Environmental Exposome Revealed by Longitudinal Personal Monitoring. *Cell*, *175*(1), 277–291.e31. DOI: 10.1016/j.cell.2018.08.060 PMID: 30241608

Jiang, G., Zhang, S., Yazdanparast, A., Li, M., Pawar, A. V., Liu, Y., Inavolu, S. M., & Cheng, L. (2016). Comprehensive comparison of molecular portraits between cell lines and tumors in breast cancer. *BMC Genomics*, *17*(S7), 525. DOI: 10.1186/s12864-016-2911-z PMID: 27556158

Jiang, J.-W., Chen, X.-H., Ren, Z., & Zheng, S.-S. (2019). Gut microbial dysbiosis associates hepatocellular carcinoma via the gut-liver axis. *Hepatobiliary & Pancreatic Diseases International, 18*(1), 19–27. DOI: 10.1016/j.hbpd.2018.11.002 PMID: 30527903

Jiang, Z., Wang, H., Mou, Y., Li, L., & Jin, W. (2022). Functions and clinical applications of exosomes in pancreatic cancer. *Molecular Biology Reports, 49*(11), 11037–11048. DOI: 10.1007/s11033-022-07765-8 PMID: 36097109

Jin, W.-B., Xiao, L., Jeong, M., Han, S.-J., Zhang, W., Yano, H., Shi, H., Arifuzzaman, M., Lyu, M., Wang, D., Tang, Y. A., Qiao, S., Yang, X., Yang, H. S., Fu, J., Sonnenberg, G. F., Collins, N., Artis, D., & Guo, C.-J. (2025). Microbiota-derived bile acids antagonize the host androgen receptor and drive anti-tumor immunity. *Cell, 188*(9), 2336–2353.e38. DOI: 10.1016/j.cell.2025.02.029 PMID: 40239649

Jin, Y., Wu, S., Zeng, Z., & Fu, Z. (2017). Effects of environmental pollutants on gut microbiota. *Environmental Pollution, 222*, 1–9. DOI: 10.1016/j.envpol.2016.11.045 PMID: 28086130

Jones, C. F. E., Di Cio, S., Connelly, J. T., & Gautrot, J. E. (2022). Design of an Integrated Microvascularized Human Skin-on-a-Chip Tissue Equivalent Model. *Frontiers in Bioengineering and Biotechnology, 10*, 915702. DOI: 10.3389/fbioe.2022.915702 PMID: 35928950

Juarez, M. N., McDermott, A., Wade, M. G., & Plante, I. (2024). Exposure to brominated flame retardants in utero and through lactation delays the development of DMBA-induced mammary cancer: Potential effects on subtypes? *Frontiers in Endocrinology, 15*, 1429142. DOI: 10.3389/fendo.2024.1429142 PMID: 39610845

Juarez, P. D., Hood, D. B., Song, M., & Ramesh, A. (2023). Applying an Exposome-wide Association Study (ExWAS) Approach to Latino Cancer Disparities. In *Advancing the Science of Cancer in Latinos* (pp. 17–32). Springer International Publishing. DOI: 10.1007/978-3-031-14436-3_2

Kalmar, L., Gupta, S., Kean, I. R. L., Ba, X., Hadjirin, N., Lay, E. M., de Vries, S. P. W., Bateman, M., Bartlet, H., Hernandez-Garcia, J., Tucker, A. W., Restif, O., Stevens, M. P., Wood, J. L. N., Maskell, D. J., Grant, A. J., & Holmes, M. A. (2022). HAM-ART: An optimised culture-free Hi-C metagenomics pipeline for tracking antimicrobial resistance genes in complex microbial communities. *PLOS Genetics, 18*(3), e1009776. DOI: 10.1371/journal.pgen.1009776 PMID: 35286304

Kaltsas, A., Markou, E., Kyrgiafini, M.-A., Zikopoulos, A., Symeonidis, E. N., Dimitriadis, F., Zachariou, A., Sofikitis, N., & Chrisofos, M. (2025). Oxidative-Stress-Mediated Epigenetic Dysregulation in Spermatogenesis: Implications for Male Infertility and Offspring Health. *Genes*, *16*(1), 1. Advance online publication. DOI: 10.3390/genes16010093 PMID: 39858640

Kalyanaraman, B., Cheng, G., & Hardy, M. (2024). The role of short-chain fatty acids in cancer prevention and cancer treatment. *Archives of Biochemistry and Biophysics*, *761*, 110172. DOI: 10.1016/j.abb.2024.110172 PMID: 39369836

Kamel, M., Aleya, S., Alsubih, M., & Aleya, L. (2024). Microbiome Dynamics: A Paradigm Shift in Combatting Infectious Diseases. *Journal of Personalized Medicine*, *14*(2), 217. DOI: 10.3390/jpm14020217 PMID: 38392650

Kanehisa, M., & Goto, S. (2000). KEGG: Kyoto Encyclopedia of Genes and Genomes. *Nucleic Acids Research*, *28*(1), 27–30. DOI: 10.1093/nar/28.1.27 PMID: 10592173

Kang, J. H., Kondo, F., & Katayama, Y. (2006). Human exposure to bisphenol A. In *Toxicology* (Vol. 226, pp. 79–89). DOI: 10.1016/j.tox.2006.06.009

Kang, Y. B. A., Sodunke, T. R., Lamontagne, J., Cirillo, J., Rajiv, C., Bouchard, M. J., & Noh, M. (2015). Liver sinusoid on a chip: Long-term layered co-culture of primary rat hepatocytes and endothelial cells in microfluidic platforms. *Biotechnology and Bioengineering*, *112*(12), 2571–2582. DOI: 10.1002/bit.25659 PMID: 25994312

Kanoh, S., & Rubin, B. K. (2010). Mechanisms of action and clinical application of macrolides as immunomodulatory medications. *Clinical Microbiology Reviews*, *23*(3), 590–615. DOI: 10.1128/CMR.00078-09 PMID: 20610825

Karalexi, M. A., Tagkas, C. F., Markozannes, G., Tseretopoulou, X., Hernández, A. F., Schüz, J., Halldorsson, T. I., Psaltopoulou, T., Petridou, E. T., Tzoulaki, I., & Ntzani, E. E. (2021). Exposure to pesticides and childhood leukemia risk: A systematic review and meta-analysis. *Environmental Pollution (Barking, Essex: 1987)*, *285*, 117376. DOI: 10.1016/j.envpol.2021.117376

Karczewski, K. J., & Snyder, M. P. (2018). Integrative omics for health and disease. *Nature Reviews. Genetics*, *19*(5), 299–310. DOI: 10.1038/nrg.2018.4 PMID: 29479082

Kasendra, M., Tovaglieri, A., Sontheimer-Phelps, A., Jalili-Firoozinezhad, S., Bein, A., Chalkiadaki, A., Scholl, W., Zhang, C., Rickner, H., Richmond, C. A., Li, H., Breault, D. T., & Ingber, D. E. (2018). Development of a primary human Small Intestine-on-a-Chip using biopsy-derived organoids. *Scientific Reports*, *8*(1), 2871. Advance online publication. DOI: 10.1038/s41598-018-21201-7 PMID: 29440725

Katiyar, S. K., Singh, T., Prasad, R., Sun, Q., & Vaid, M. (2012). Epigenetic Alterations in Ultraviolet Radiation-Induced Skin Carcinogenesis: Interaction of Bioactive Dietary Components on Epigenetic Targets†. *Photochemistry and Photobiology, 88*(5), 1066–1074. DOI: 10.1111/j.1751-1097.2011.01020.x PMID: 22017262

Kawanishi, S., Ohnishi, S., Ma, N., Hiraku, Y., & Murata, M. (2017). Crosstalk between DNA Damage and Inflammation in the Multiple Steps of Carcinogenesis. *International Journal of Molecular Sciences, 18*(8), 1808. DOI: 10.3390/ijms18081808 PMID: 28825631

Kaye, J., Whitley, E. A., Lund, D., Morrison, M., Teare, H., & Melham, K. (2018). Data sharing in genomics—Re-shaping scientific practice. *Nature Reviews. Genetics, 19*(2), 111. PMID: 19308065

Kay, J., Thadhani, E., Samson, L., & Engelward, B. (2019). Inflammation-induced DNA damage, mutations and cancer. *DNA Repair, 83*, 102673. DOI: 10.1016/j.dnarep.2019.102673 PMID: 31387777

Kensler, T. W., Ng, D., Carmella, S. G., Chen, M., Jacobson, L. P., Muñoz, A., Egner, P. A., Chen, J. G., Qian, G. S., Chen, T. Y., Fahey, J. W., Talalay, P., Groopman, J. D., Yuan, J.-M., & Hecht, S. S. (2012). Modulation of the metabolism of airborne pollutants by glucoraphanin-rich and sulforaphane-rich broccoli sprout beverages in Qidong, China. *Carcinogenesis, 33*(1), 101–107. DOI: 10.1093/carcin/bgr229 PMID: 22045030

Khalil, S. M., MacKenzie, K. R., Maletic-Savatic, M., & Li, F. (2024). Metabolic bioactivation of antidepressants: Advance and underlying hepatotoxicity. *Drug Metabolism Reviews, 56*(2), 97–126. DOI: 10.1080/03602532.2024.2313967 PMID: 38311829

Khani, N., Soleimani, R. A., & Rad, A. H. (2025). Potential of Postbiotics for the Biodegradation of Xenobiotics: A Review. *Current Nutrition and Food Science, 21*(6), 653–670. Advance online publication. DOI: 10.2174/0115734013325225241211033631

Khelaifia, S., Caputo, A., Djossou, F., & Raoult, D. (2016). Draft genome sequence of a human-associated isolate of Haloferax alexandrinus strain Arc-hr, an extremely halophilic archaea. *New Microbes and New Infections, 15*, 44–45. DOI: 10.1016/j.nmni.2016.11.012 PMID: 28018603

Khmaissa, M., Zouari-Mechichi, H., Sciara, G., Record, E., & Mechichi, T. (2024). Pollution from livestock farming antibiotics an emerging environmental and human health concern: A Review. *Journal of Hazardous Materials Advances, 100410*, 100410. Advance online publication. DOI: 10.1016/j.hazadv.2024.100410

Khosravi, A., & Mazmanian, S. K. (2013). Disruption of the gut microbiome as a risk factor for microbial infections. *Current Opinion in Microbiology, 16*(2), 221–227. DOI: 10.1016/j.mib.2013.03.009 PMID: 23597788

Kim, D., Paggi, J. M., Park, C., Bennett, C., & Salzberg, S. L. (2019). Graph-based genome alignment and genotyping with HISAT2 and HISAT-genotype. *Nature Biotechnology, 37*(8), 907–915. DOI: 10.1038/s41587-019-0201-4 PMID: 31375807

Kim, H. G., Sung, J.-Y., Na, K., & Kim, S.-W. (2020). Low H3K9me3 Expression Is Associated With Poor Prognosis in Patients With Distal Common Bile Duct Cancer. *In Vivo (Athens, Greece), 34*(6), 3619–3626. DOI: 10.21873/invivo.12207 PMID: 33144476

Kim, K.-H., Lee, S. J., Kim, J., & Moon, Y. (2024). Leveraging Xenobiotic-Responsive Cancer Stemness in Cell Line-Based Tumoroids for Evaluating Chemoresistance: A Proof-of-Concept Study on Environmental Susceptibility. *International Journal of Molecular Sciences, 25*(21), 11383. DOI: 10.3390/ijms252111383 PMID: 39518936

Kim, S. T., Kim, S. Y., Klempner, S. J., Yoon, J., Kim, N., Ahn, S., Bang, H., Kim, K.-M., Park, W., Park, S. H., Park, J. O., Park, Y. S., Lim, H. Y., Lee, S. H., Park, K., Kang, W. K., & Lee, J. (2017). Rapamycin-insensitive companion of mTOR (RICTOR) amplification defines a subset of advanced gastric cancer and is sensitive to AZD2014-mediated mTORC1/2 inhibition. *Annals of Oncology : Official Journal of the European Society for Medical Oncology, 28*(3), 547–554. DOI: 10.1093/annonc/mdw669 PMID: 28028034

Kish, L., Hotte, N., Kaplan, G. G., Vincent, R., Tso, R., Gänzle, M., Rioux, K. P., Thiesen, A., Barkema, H. W., Wine, E., & Madsen, K. L. (2013). Environmental Particulate Matter Induces Murine Intestinal Inflammatory Responses and Alters the Gut Microbiome. *PLoS One, 8*(4), e62220. DOI: 10.1371/journal.pone.0062220 PMID: 23638009

Klega, K., Imamovic-Tuco, L., & An, E. (2018). Clinical applications of cell-free RNA sequencing in pediatric oncology. *Pediatric Blood & Cancer, 65*(5), e26936. DOI: 10.1002/pbc.26936 PMID: 29286573

Kleino, I., Frolovaitė, P., Suomi, T., & Elo, L. L. (2022). Computational solutions for spatial transcriptomics. *Computational and Structural Biotechnology Journal, 20*, 4870–4884. DOI: 10.1016/j.csbj.2022.08.043 PMID: 36147664

Knoppers, B. M., & Chadwick, R. (2021). Human genetics and genomics: A new paradigm. *Annual Review of Genomics and Human Genetics, 22*, 1–24.

Koehn, L. M. (2022). ABC Transporters: An Overview. In Talevi, A. (Ed.), *The ADME Encyclopedia*. Springer., DOI: 10.1007/978-3-030-84860-6_76

Kogevinas, M. (2001). Human health effects of dioxins: Cancer, reproductive and endocrine system effects. *Human Reproduction Update*, *7*(3), 331–339. DOI: 10.1093/humupd/7.3.331 PMID: 11392380

Koning, J. J., Rodrigues Neves, C. T., Schimek, K., Thon, M., Spiekstra, S. W., Waaijman, T., de Gruijl, T. D., & Gibbs, S. (2021). A Multi-Organ-on-Chip Approach to Investigate How Oral Exposure to Metals Can Cause Systemic Toxicity Leading to Langerhans Cell Activation in Skin. *Frontiers in Toxicology*, *3*, 824825. Advance online publication. DOI: 10.3389/ftox.2021.824825 PMID: 35295125

Kopylova, E., Noé, L., & Touzet, H. (2012). SortMeRNA: Fast and accurate filtering of ribosomal RNAs in metatranscriptomic data. *Bioinformatics (Oxford, England)*, *28*(24), 3211–3217. DOI: 10.1093/bioinformatics/bts611 PMID: 23071270

Korolenko, A. A., Noll, S. E., & Skinner, M. K. (2023). Epigenetic Inheritance and Transgenerational EnvironmentalJustice. *The Yale Journal of Biology and Medicine*, *96*(2), 241–250. DOI: 10.59249/FKWS5176 PMID: 37396986

Korrapati, C., Yaraladdi, A. B., Vaddi, H., & Raghavan, R. (2024). Applications of the Saffron European Kitchen Spice Crocus sativus. *Therapeutic and Pharmacological Applications of Ethnobotany*, 98–127. DOI: 10.4018/979-8-3693-1986-4.ch005

Kostic, A. D., Gevers, D., Pedamallu, C. S., Michaud, M., Duke, F., Earl, A. M., Ojesina, A. I., Jung, J., Bass, A. J., Tabernero, J., Baselga, J., Liu, C., Shivdasani, R. A., Ogino, S., Birren, B. W., Huttenhower, C., Garrett, W. S., & Meyerson, M. (2012). Genomic analysis identifies association of Fusobacterium with colorectal carcinoma. *Genome Research*, *22*(2), 292–298. DOI: 10.1101/gr.126573.111 PMID: 22009990

Koual, M., Tomkiewicz, C., Cano-Sancho, G., Antignac, J.-P., Bats, A.-S., & Coumoul, X. (2020). Environmental chemicals, breast cancer progression and drug resistance. *Environmental Health : A Global Access Science Source*, *19*(1), 117. DOI: 10.1186/s12940-020-00670-2 PMID: 33203443

Krausová, M., Braun, D., Buerki-Thurnherr, T., Gundacker, C., Schernhammer, E., Wisgrill, L., & Warth, B. (2023). Understanding the Chemical Exposome During Fetal Development and Early Childhood: A Review. *Annual Review of Pharmacology and Toxicology*, *63*(1), 517–540. DOI: 10.1146/annurev-pharmtox-051922-113350 PMID: 36202091

Kuiper, G. G. J. M., Carlsson, B., Grandien, K., Enmark, E., Häggblad, J., Nilsson, S., & Gustafsson, J.-Å. (1997). Comparison of the Ligand Binding Specificity and Transcript Tissue Distribution of Estrogen Receptors α and β. *Endocrinology*, *138*(3), 863–870. DOI: 10.1210/endo.138.3.4979 PMID: 9048584

Kulis, M., & Esteller, M. (2010). DNA Methylation and Cancer. In *Advances in Genetics* (Vol. 70, pp. 27–56). Elsevier., DOI: 10.1016/B978-0-12-380866-0.60002-2

Kumar, V., Vashishta, M., Kong, L., Wu, X., Lu, J. J., Guha, C., & Dwarakanath, B. S. (2021). The Role of Notch, Hedgehog, and Wnt Signaling Pathways in the Resistance of Tumors to Anticancer Therapies. In *Frontiers in Cell and Developmental Biology* (Vol. 9). Frontiers Media S.A. DOI: 10.3389/fcell.2021.650772

Kurogi, K., Suiko, M., & Sakakibara, Y. (2024). Evolution and multiple functions of sulfonation and cytosolic sulfotransferases across species. *Bioscience, Biotechnology, and Biochemistry*, *88*(4), 368–380. DOI: 10.1093/bbb/zbae008 PMID: 38271594

L'Hermitte, A., Pham, S., Cadoux, M., Couchy, G., Caruso, S., Anson, M., Crain-Denoyelle, A.-M., Celton-Morizur, S., Yamagoe, S., Zucman-Rossi, J., Desdouets, C., & Couty, J.-P. (2019). Lect2 Controls Inflammatory Monocytes to Constrain the Growth and Progression of Hepatocellular Carcinoma. *Hepatology (Baltimore, Md.)*, *69*(1), 160–178. DOI: 10.1002/hep.30140 PMID: 30070727

Lakshmaiah, A., Korrapati, C., Suresh, C., & Raghavan, R. (2025). Synthetic Biology and AI. *Spatially Variable Genes in Cancer*, 265–290. DOI: 10.4018/979-8-3693-7728-4.ch010

Langenbach, T. (2013). Persistence and Bioaccumulation of Persistent Organic Pollutants (POPs). In *Applied Bioremediation - Active and Passive Approaches*. InTech. DOI: 10.5772/56418

Lapin, A., Perfahl, H., Jain, H. V., & Reuss, M. (2022). Integrating a dynamic central metabolism model of cancer cells with a hybrid 3D multiscale model for vascular hepatocellular carcinoma growth. *Scientific Reports*, *12*(1), 12373. DOI: 10.1038/s41598-022-15767-6 PMID: 35858953

Lattimer, J. M., & Haub, M. D. (2010). Effects of dietary fiber and its components on metabolic health. *Nutrients*, *2*(12), 1266–1289. DOI: 10.3390/nu2121266 PMID: 22254008

Lauby-Secretan, B., Scoccianti, C., Loomis, D., Grosse, Y., Bianchini, F., & Straif, K. (2016). Body Fatness and Cancer—Viewpoint of the IARC Working Group. *The New England Journal of Medicine*, *375*(8), 794–798. DOI: 10.1056/NEJMsr1606602 PMID: 27557308

Lauri, G., Mills, K., Majumder, S., & Capurso, G. (2025). The exposome as a target for primary prevention and a tool for early detection of pancreatic cancer. *Best Practice & Research. Clinical Gastroenterology*, *101991*, 101991. Advance online publication. DOI: 10.1016/j.bpg.2025.101991 PMID: 40210335

Ledda, C. (2018). Cadmium exposure and prostate cancer insights mechanisms and perspectives. *Frontiers in Bioscience*, *23*(9), 1687–1700. DOI: 10.2741/4667 PMID: 29293457

Lee, D. G., Schuetz, J. M., Lai, A. S., Burstyn, I., Brooks-Wilson, A., Aronson, K. J., & Spinelli, J. J. (2022). Interactions between exposure to polycyclic aromatic hydrocarbons and xenobiotic metabolism genes, and risk of breast cancer. *Breast Cancer (Tokyo, Japan)*, *29*(1), 38–49. DOI: 10.1007/s12282-021-01279-0 PMID: 34351578

Lee, H.-J., Lee, Y., & Yun, J. (2020). Factors Associated with Physical Activity in Older Adults by Region: Based on the 2017 Community Health Survey. *Journal of Korean Academy of Community Health Nursing*, *31*(Suppl), 563. DOI: 10.12799/jkachn.2020.31.S.563

Lee, J. S., Romero, R., Han, Y. M., Kim, H. C., Kim, C. J., Hong, J. S., & Huh, D. (2016). Placenta-on-A-chip: A novel platform to study the biology of the human placenta. *The Journal of Maternal-Fetal & Neonatal Medicine*, *29*(7), 1046–1054. DOI: 10.3109/14767058.2015.1038518 PMID: 26075842

Lee, K. K., McCauley, H. A., Broda, T. R., Kofron, M. J., Wells, J. M., & Hong, C. I. (2018). Human stomach-on-a-chip with luminal flow and peristaltic-like motility. *Lab on a Chip*, *18*(20), 3079–3085. DOI: 10.1039/C8LC00910D PMID: 30238091

Lee, S., Yun, Y., Kim, S., Lee, E.-J., Chang, Y., Ryu, S., Shin, H., Kim, H.-L., Kim, H.-N., & Lee, J. (2018). Association between Cigarette Smoking Status and Composition of Gut Microbiota: Population-Based Cross-Sectional Study. *Journal of Clinical Medicine*, *7*(9), 282. DOI: 10.3390/jcm7090282 PMID: 30223529

Lei, L., Yang, J., Zhang, J., & Zhang, G. (2021). The lipid peroxidation product EKODE exacerbates colonic inflammation and colon tumorigenesis. *Redox Biology*, *42*, 101880. DOI: 10.1016/j.redox.2021.101880 PMID: 33541845

Leng, D., Zheng, L., Wen, Y., Zhang, Y., Wu, L., Wang, J., Wang, M., Zhang, Z., He, S., & Bo, X. (2022). A benchmark study of deep learning-based multi-omics data fusion methods for cancer. *Genome Biology*, *23*(1), 171. DOI: 10.1186/s13059-022-02739-2 PMID: 35945544

Lesina, M., Kurkowski, M. U., Ludes, K., Rose-John, S., Treiber, M., Klöppel, G., Yoshimura, A., Reindl, W., Sipos, B., Akira, S., Schmid, R. M., & Algül, H. (2011). Stat3/Socs3 Activation by IL-6 Transsignaling Promotes Progression of Pancreatic Intraepithelial Neoplasia and Development of Pancreatic Cancer. *Cancer Cell, 19*(4), 456–469. DOI: 10.1016/j.ccr.2011.03.009 PMID: 21481788

Lettieri, M., Rodda, M., & Carlucci, V. (2024). Machine Learning in Early Prediction of Metabolism of Drugs. In *Computational Toxicology: Methods and Protocols* (pp. 275–291). Springer US., DOI: 10.1007/978-1-0716-4003-6_13

Leung, A., & Pang, K. M. (2020). Utilizing deep learning to predict cancer diagnoses from gene expression profiles. *Scientific Reports, 10*(1), 1–11. DOI: 10.1038/s41598-020-67447-6 PMID: 31913322

Leung, C. M., de Haan, P., Ronaldson-Bouchard, K., Kim, G. A., Ko, J., Rho, H. S., Chen, Z., Habibovic, P., Jeon, N. L., Takayama, S., Shuler, M. L., Vunjak-Novakovic, G., Frey, O., Verpoorte, E., & Toh, Y. C. (2022). A guide to the organ-on-a-chip. In *Nature Reviews Methods Primers* (Vol. 2). Springer Nature., DOI: 10.1038/s43586-022-00118-6

Lewandowska, A., Rudzki, M., Rudzki, S., Lewandowski, T., & Laskowska, B. (2019a). Environmental risk factors for cancer – review paper. *Annals of Agricultural and Environmental Medicine, 26*(1), 1–7. DOI: 10.26444/aaem/94299 PMID: 30922021

Li, B., Wang, D., Zhang, C., Wang, Y., Huang, Z., Yang, L., Yang, H., Liang, N., Li, S., & Liu, Z. (2024). Role of respiratory system microbiota in development of lung cancer and clinical application. *iMeta, 3*(5), e232. DOI: 10.1002/imt2.232 PMID: 39429871

Libbrecht, M. W., & Noble, W. S. (2015). Machine learning applications in genetics and genomics. *Nature Reviews. Genetics, 16*(6), 321–332. DOI: 10.1038/nrg3920 PMID: 25948244

Li, D., Yun, Y., & Gao, R. (2019). Oxygenated Polycyclic aromatic hydrocarbons (Oxy-PAHs) facilitate lung cancer metastasis by epigenetically regulating the epithelial-to-mesenchymal transition (EMT). *Environmental Pollution, 255*, 113261. DOI: 10.1016/j.envpol.2019.113261 PMID: 31580991

Lim, D. (2015). *Rôle du récepteur des hydrocarbures aromatiques chez les cellules T auxiliaires dans le contrôle de la réponse immunitaire*. Https://Www.Semanticscholar.Org/Paper/R%C3%B4le-Du-R%C3%A9cepteur-Des-Hydrocarbures-Aromatiques-Les-Lim/2acbff8244f316a8a47469d7625c0a4817cc5376

Li, M., Wang, M., & Donovan, S. M. (2014). Early development of the gut microbiome and immune-mediated childhood disorders. *Seminars in Reproductive Medicine, 32*(1), 74–86. DOI: 10.1055/s-0033-1361825 PMID: 24390924

Lima, S. F., Pires, S., Rupert, A., Oguntunmibi, S., Jin, W.-B., Marderstein, A., Funez-dePagnier, G., Maldarelli, G., Viladomiu, M., Putzel, G., Yang, W., Tran, N., Xiang, G., Grier, A., Guo, C.-J., Lukin, D., Mandl, L. A., Scherl, E. J., & Longman, R. S. (2024). The gut microbiome regulates the clinical efficacy of sulfasalazine therapy for IBD-associated spondyloarthritis. *Cell Reports Medicine, 5*(3), 101431. DOI: 10.1016/j.xcrm.2024.101431 PMID: 38378002

Lim, C. H., & Seo, D. S. (2024). Assessment of the carcinogenic potential of particulate matter generated from 3D printing devices in Balb/c 3T3-1-1 cells. *Scientific Reports, 14*(1), 23981. DOI: 10.1038/s41598-024-75491-1 PMID: 39402095

Lin, B., Ye, Z., Ye, Z., Wang, M., Cao, Z., Gao, R., & Zhang, Y. (2023). Gut microbiota in brain tumors: An emerging crucial player. *CNS Neuroscience & Therapeutics, 29*(S1, Suppl 1), 84–97. DOI: 10.1111/cns.14081 PMID: 36627748

Lipenga, T., Matumba, L., Vidal, A., Herceg, Z., McCormack, V., De Saeger, S., & De Boevre, M. (2021). A concise review towards defining the exposome of oesophageal cancer in sub-Saharan Africa. In *Environment International* (Vol. 157). Elsevier Ltd. DOI: 10.1016/j.envint.2021.106880

Li, S., Duan, Y., Luo, S., Zhou, F., Wu, Q., & Lu, Z. (2025). Short-chain fatty acids and cancer. *Trends in Cancer, 11*(2), 154–168. DOI: 10.1016/j.trecan.2024.11.003 PMID: 39638744

Li, S., Jiang, Z., & Wei, S. (2024). Interaction of heavy metals and polycyclic aromatic hydrocarbons in soil-crop systems: The effects and mechanisms. *Environmental Research, 120035*, 120035. Advance online publication. DOI: 10.1016/j.envres.2024.120035 PMID: 39313170

Liu, C.-H., Chen, Z., Chen, K., Liao, F.-T., Chung, C.-E., Liu, X., Lin, Y.-C., Keohavong, P., Leikauf, G. D., & Di, Y. P. (2021). Lipopolysaccharide-Mediated Chronic Inflammation Promotes Tobacco Carcinogen-Induced Lung Cancer and Determines the Efficacy of Immunotherapy. *Cancer Research, 81*(1), 144–157. DOI: 10.1158/0008-5472.CAN-20-1994 PMID: 33122306

Liu, F., Li, J., Guan, Y., Lou, Y., Chen, H., Xu, M., Deng, D., Chen, J., Ni, B., Zhao, L., Li, H., Sang, H., & Cai, X. (2019). Dysbiosis of the Gut Microbiome is associated with Tumor Biomarkers in Lung Cancer. *International Journal of Biological Sciences, 15*(11), 2381–2392. DOI: 10.7150/ijbs.35980 PMID: 31595156

Liu, L., Wu, Q., Miao, X., Fan, T., Meng, Z., Chen, X., & Zhu, W. (2022). Study on toxicity effects of environmental pollutants based on metabolomics: A review. *Chemosphere*, *286*, 131815. DOI: 10.1016/j.chemosphere.2021.131815 PMID: 34375834

Liu, X. (2019). ABC Family Transporters. In Liu, X., & Pan, G. (Eds.), *Drug Transporters in Drug Disposition, Effects and Toxicity. Advances in Experimental Medicine and Biology* (Vol. 1141). Springer. DOI: 10.1007/978-981-13-7647-4_2

Liu, Y., Zhang, S., Zhou, W., Hu, D., Xu, H., & Ji, G. (2022). Secondary Bile Acids and Tumorigenesis in Colorectal Cancer. *Frontiers in Oncology*, *12*, 813745. DOI: 10.3389/fonc.2022.813745 PMID: 35574393

Liu, Z., Ren, Y., Weng, S., Xu, H., Li, L., & Han, X. (2022). A New Trend in Cancer Treatment: The Combination of Epigenetics and Immunotherapy. *Frontiers in Immunology*, *13*, 809761. DOI: 10.3389/fimmu.2022.809761 PMID: 35140720

Li, W. X., Liang, G. T., Yan, W., Zhang, Q., Wang, W., Zhou, X. M., & Liu, D. Y. (2013). Artificial uterus on a microfluidic chip. *Fenxi Huaxue. Chinese Journal of Analytical Chemistry*, *41*(4), 467–472. DOI: 10.1016/S1872-2040(13)60639-8

Li, X., Brejnrod, A. D., Ernst, M., Rykær, M., Herschend, J., Olsen, N. M. C., Dorrestein, P. C., Rensing, C., & Sørensen, S. J. (2019). Heavy metal exposure causes changes in the metabolic health-associated gut microbiome and metabolites. *Environment International*, *126*, 454–467. DOI: 10.1016/j.envint.2019.02.048 PMID: 30844581

Li, Y. (2025). Cellular Antioxidants and Phase 2 Proteins. *Molecular Basis of Oxidative Stress: Chemistry, Toxicology, Disease Pathogenesis. Diagnostics and Therapeutics*, 113–127. DOI: 10.1002/9781119790419.ch5

Li, Y., Steppi, A., Zhou, Y., Mao, F., Miller, P. C., He, M. M., Zhao, T., Sun, Q., & Zhang, J. (2017). Tumoral expression of drug and xenobiotic metabolizing enzymes in breast cancer patients of different ethnicities with implications to personalized medicine. *Scientific Reports*, *7*(1), 4747. DOI: 10.1038/s41598-017-04250-2 PMID: 28684774

Li, Z., Kwon, S. M., Li, D., Li, L., Peng, X., Zhang, J., Sueyoshi, T., Raufman, J.-P., Negishi, M., Wang, X. W., & Wang, H. (2022). Human constitutive androstane receptor represses liver cancer development and hepatoma cell proliferation by inhibiting erythropoietin signaling. *The Journal of Biological Chemistry*, *298*(5), 101885. DOI: 10.1016/j.jbc.2022.101885 PMID: 35367211

Li, Z., Ma, J., Li, X., Chan, M. T. V., Wu, W. K. K., Wu, Z., & Shen, J. (2019). Aberrantly expressed long non-coding RNAs in air pollution-induced congenital defects. *Journal of Cellular and Molecular Medicine*, *23*(11), 7717–7725. DOI: 10.1111/jcmm.14645 PMID: 31557384

Li, Z., Romanoff, L., Bartell, S., Pittman, E. N., Trinidad, D. A., McClean, M., Webster, T. F., & Sjödin, A. (2012). Excretion Profiles and half-lives of ten urinary polycyclic aromatic hydrocarbon metabolites after dietary exposure. *Chemical Research in Toxicology*, *25*(7), 1452–1461. DOI: 10.1021/tx300108e PMID: 22663094

Lobo, V., Patil, A., Phatak, A., & Chandra, N. (2010). Free radicals, antioxidants and functional foods: Impact on human health. *Pharmacognosy Reviews*, *4*(8), 118–126. DOI: 10.4103/0973-7847.70902 PMID: 22228951

Long, J., Zhang, C.-J., Zhu, N., Du, K., Yin, Y.-F., Tan, X., Liao, D.-F., & Qin, L. (2018). Lipid metabolism and carcinogenesis, cancer development. In *Am J Cancer Res* (Vol. 8, Issue 5). www.ajcr.us/ISSN:2156-6976/ajcr0076971

Louis, P., Hold, G. L., & Flint, H. J. (2014). The gut microbiota, bacterial metabolites and colorectal cancer. *Nature Reviews. Microbiology*, *12*(10), 661–672. DOI: 10.1038/nrmicro3344 PMID: 25198138

Luan, Z. L., Zhang, C., Ming, W. H., Huang, Y. Z., Guan, Y. F., & Zhang, X. Y. (2022). Nuclear receptors in renal health and disease. *EBioMedicine*, *76*, 103855. Advance online publication. DOI: 10.1016/j.ebiom.2022.103855 PMID: 35123268

Lu, C., Thompson, J. R., & Schwartz, A. G. (2020). Hereditary cancer risk assessment in clinical oncology. *The Lancet. Oncology*, *21*(2), 189–200. DOI: 10.1016/S1470-2045(19)30735-5 PMID: 31838012

Ludovini, V., Chiari, R., Tomassoni, L., Antonini, C., Baldelli, E., Baglivo, S., Siggillino, A., Tofanetti, F. R., Bellezza, G., Hodge, K. A., Petricoin, E., Pierobon, M., Crinò, L., & Bianconi, F. (2017). Reverse phase protein array (RPPA) combined with computational analysis to unravel relevant prognostic factors in non- small cell lung cancer (NSCLC): A pilot study. *Oncotarget*, *8*(47), 83343–83353. DOI: 10.18632/oncotarget.18480 PMID: 29137348

Lu, L., Cheng, Y., Wu, W., Wang, L., Li, S., Li, Q., Chen, L., Zhang, J., Chen, R., Tan, X., Hong, Y., Yang, L., & Song, Y. (2024). Paternal p,p′-DDE exposure and pre-pubertal high-fat diet increases the susceptibility to fertility impairment and sperm *Igf2* DMR2 hypo-methylation in male offspring. *Ecotoxicology and Environmental Safety*, *271*, 115999. DOI: 10.1016/j.ecoenv.2024.115999 PMID: 38262096

Lunshof, J. E., Church, G. M., & Prainsack, B. (2017). From genetic privacy to open consent. *Nature Reviews. Genetics*, *18*(8), 512. PMID: 18379574

Lupo, P. J., Archer, N. P., Harris, R. D., Marengo, L. K., Schraw, J. M., Hoyt, A. T., Tanksley, S., Lee, R., Drummond-Borg, M., Freedenberg, D., Shetty, P. B., Agopian, A. J., Shumate, C., Rasmussen, S. A., Langlois, P. H., & Canfield, M. A. (2024). Newborn screening analytes and structural birth defects among 27,000 newborns. *PLoS One*, *19*(7), e0304238. DOI: 10.1371/journal.pone.0304238 PMID: 38968308

Lu, X., Zhang, L., Lin, G. M., Lu, J. G., & Cui, Z. B. (2024). Analysis of Differential Gene Expression under Acute Lead or Mercury Exposure in Larval Zebrafish Using RNA-Seq. *Animals (Basel)*, *14*(19), 2877. DOI: 10.3390/ani14192877 PMID: 39409826

Lyu, S. I., Fretter, C., Eckel, H. N. C., Knipper, K., Schultheis, A. M., Büttner, R., Quaas, A., Klussmann, J. P., & Simon, A. G. (2025). High expression of H2AX/γ-H2AX is associated with distinct biological pathway alterations and shorter survival in oropharyngeal squamous cell carcinoma. *Oral Oncology*, *161*, 107171. DOI: 10.1016/j.oraloncology.2024.107171 PMID: 39756240

Ma, C., Han, M., Heinrich, B., Fu, Q., Zhang, Q., Sandhu, M., Agdashian, D., Terabe, M., Berzofsky, J. A., Fako, V., Ritz, T., Longerich, T., Theriot, C. M., McCulloch, J. A., Roy, S., Yuan, W., Thovarai, V., Sen, S. K., Ruchirawat, M., & Greten, T. F. (2018). Gut microbiome-mediated bile acid metabolism regulates liver cancer via NKT cells. *Science*, *360*(6391), eaan5931. Advance online publication. DOI: 10.1126/science.aan5931 PMID: 29798856

Madrigal, J. M., Pruitt, C. N., Fisher, J. A., Liao, L. M., Graubard, B. I., Gierach, G. L., Silverman, D. T., Ward, M. H., & Jones, R. R. (2024). Carcinogenic industrial air pollution and postmenopausal breast cancer risk in the National Institutes of Health AARP Diet and Health Study. *Environment International*, *191*, 108985. DOI: 10.1016/j.envint.2024.108985 PMID: 39226766

Mahanayak, B. (2024). Biotransformation reactions of xenobiotics: Mechanisms and implications for environmental and human health. *World Journal of Biology Pharmacy and Health Sciences*, *19*(1), 158–164. DOI: 10.30574/wjbphs.2024.19.1.0406

Maitre, L., Bustamante, M., Hernández-Ferrer, C., Thiel, D., Lau, C.-H. E., Siskos, A. P., Vives-Usano, M., Ruiz-Arenas, C., Pelegrí-Sisó, D., Robinson, O., Mason, D., Wright, J., Cadiou, S., Slama, R., Heude, B., Casas, M., Sunyer, J., Papadopoulou, E. Z., Gutzkow, K. B., & Vrijheid, M. (2022). Multi-omics signatures of the human early life exposome. *Nature Communications*, *13*(1), 7024. DOI: 10.1038/s41467-022-34422-2 PMID: 36411288

Majeed, A., & Rust, T. (2025). Antimicrobial Stewardship in Patients With Cancer: Interventions and Future Directions to Combat the Rise of Antimicrobial Resistance. *JCO Oncology Practice*, *0*, OP-25–OP-00124. DOI: 10.1200/OP-25-00124 PMID: 40080740

Makmor Bakry, M., Huri, Z. H., Suppiah, V., Toh, G. T., Chua, E. W., Tan, S. L. J., & Yow, H. Y. (2024). Interplay Between Genetic Variants and Morphine: Toward Personalized Medicine in Cancer Pain Management. In: *Interdisciplinary Cancer Research*. Springer, Cham. DOI: 10.1007/16833_2024_333

Maksymchuk, O., & Kashuba, V. (2019). Dietary lipids and environmental xenobiotics as risk factors for prostate cancer: The role of cytochrome P450. *Pharmacological Reports*, *71*(5), 826–832. DOI: 10.1016/j.pharep.2019.04.011 PMID: 31382168

Ma, L., Zhang, Y., Xu, J., Yu, Y., Zhou, P., Liu, X., & Guan, H. (2025). Effects of Ionizing Radiation on DNA Methylation Patterns and Their Potential as Biomarkers. *International Journal of Molecular Sciences*, *26*(7), 7. Advance online publication. DOI: 10.3390/ijms26073342 PMID: 40244232

Mandal, A., Biswas, N., & Alam, M. N. (2023). Implications of xenobiotic-response element(s) and aryl hydrocarbon receptor in health and diseases. *Human Cell*, *36*(5), 1638–1655. DOI: 10.1007/s13577-023-00931-5 PMID: 37329424

Mansoori, B., Mohammadi, A., Davudian, S., Shirjang, S., & Baradaran, B. (2017). The Different Mechanisms of Cancer Drug Resistance: A Brief Review. *Advanced Pharmaceutical Bulletin*, *7*(3), 339–348. DOI: 10.15171/apb.2017.041 PMID: 29071215

Manz, K. E., Feerick, A., Braun, J. M., Feng, Y. L., Hall, A., Koelmel, J., Manzano, C., Newton, S. R., Pennell, K. D., Place, B. J., Godri Pollitt, K. J., Prasse, C., & Young, J. A. (2023). Non-targeted analysis (NTA) and suspect screening analysis (SSA): a review of examining the chemical exposome. In *Journal of Exposure Science and Environmental Epidemiology* (Vol. 33, pp. 524–536). Springer Nature. DOI: 10.1038/s41370-023-00574-6

Maoz, B. M. (2021). Brain-on-a-Chip: Characterizing the next generation of advanced in vitro platforms for modeling the central nervous system. *APL Bioengineering*, *5*(3), 030902. DOI: 10.1063/5.0055812 PMID: 34368601

Marant Micallef, C., Shield, K. D., Baldi, I., Charbotel, B., Fervers, B., Gilg Soit Ilg, A., Guénel, P., Olsson, A., Rushton, L., Hutchings, S. J., Straif, K., & Soerjomataram, I. (2018). Occupational exposures and cancer: A review of agents and relative risk estimates. *Occupational and Environmental Medicine*, *75*(8), 604–614. DOI: 10.1136/oemed-2017-104858 PMID: 29735747

Mardinoglu, A., & Palsson, B. Ø. (2025). Genome-scale models in human metabologenomics. *Nature Reviews. Genetics*, *26*(2), 123–140. DOI: 10.1038/s41576-024-00768-0 PMID: 39300314

Marfo, A., & Obeng-Gyasi, E. (2024). *Empowering communities: The role of wearable devices in environmental justice*. DOI: 10.22541/au.170965072.20316399/v1

Maria, O. M., Weronika, P. K., Beata, B.-D., Ewa, G.-I., & Bożena, K.-N. (2023). Congenital glioblastoma – prenatal diagnosis becoming a diagnostic challenge after birth: A case report. *Case Reports in Perinatal Medicine*, *12*(1), 20230008. Advance online publication. DOI: 10.1515/crpm-2023-0008 PMID: 40041279

Marsano, A., Conficconi, C., Lemme, M., Occhetta, P., Gaudiello, E., Votta, E., Cerino, G., Redaelli, A., & Rasponi, M. (2016). Beating heart on a chip: A novel microfluidic platform to generate functional 3D cardiac microtissues. *Lab on a Chip*, *16*(3), 599–610. DOI: 10.1039/C5LC01356A PMID: 26758922

Masson, L. F., Sharp, L., Cotton, S. C., & Little, J. (2005). Cytochrome P-450 1A1 Gene Polymorphisms and Risk of Breast Cancer: A HuGE Review. *American Journal of Epidemiology*, *161*(10), 901–915. DOI: 10.1093/aje/kwi121 PMID: 15870154

Mastrangelo, G., Fedeli, U., Fadda, E., Valentini, F., Agnesi, R., Magarotto, G., Marchì, T., Buda, A., Pinzani, M., & Martines, D. (2004). Increased Risk of Hepatocellular Carcinoma and Liver Cirrhosis in Vinyl Chloride Workers: Synergistic Effect of Occupational Exposure with Alcohol Intake. *Environmental Health Perspectives*, *112*(11), 1188–1192. DOI: 10.1289/ehp.6972 PMID: 15289165

Mathis, C., Gebel, S., Poussin, C., Belcastro, V., Sewer, A., Weisensee, D., Hengstermann, A., Ansari, S., Wagner, S., Peitsch, M. C., & Hoeng, J. (2015). A Systems Biology Approach Reveals the Dose- and Time-Dependent Effect of Primary Human Airway Epithelium Tissue Culture after Exposure to Cigarette Smoke in Vitro. *Bioinformatics and Biology Insights, 9. Bioinformatics and Biology Insights, S19908*, BBI.S19908. Advance online publication. DOI: 10.4137/BBI.S19908 PMID: 25788831

Matus, P., Urquidi, C., Cárcamo, M., & Vidal, V. (2024). Integrating the exposome and one health approach to national health surveillance: An opportunity for Latin American countries in health preventive management. *Frontiers in Public Health*, *12*, 1376609. Advance online publication. DOI: 10.3389/fpubh.2024.1376609 PMID: 39211902

Matza Porges, S., & Shamriz, O. (2022). Genetics of Immune Dysregulation and Cancer Predisposition: Two Sides of the Same Coin. *Clinical and Experimental Immunology*, *210*(2), 114–127. DOI: 10.1093/cei/uxac089 PMID: 36165533

May, M., & Abrams, J. A. (2018). Emerging Insights into the Esophageal Microbiome. *Current Treatment Options in Gastroenterology*, *16*(1), 72–85. DOI: 10.1007/s11938-018-0171-5 PMID: 29350339

McKenna, A., Hanna, M., Banks, E., Sivachenko, A., Cibulskis, K., Kernytsky, A., Garimella, K., Altshuler, D., Gabriel, S., Daly, M., & DePristo, M. A. (2010). The genome analysis toolkit: A MapReduce framework for analyzing next-generation DNA sequencing data. *Genome Research*, *20*(9), 1297–1303. DOI: 10.1101/gr.107524.110 PMID: 20644199

Merk, O., & Speit, G. (1998). Significance of formaldehyde-induced DNA–protein crosslinks for mutagenesis. *Environmental and Molecular Mutagenesis*, *32*(3), 260–268. DOI: 10.1002/(SICI)1098-2280(1998)32:3<260::AID-EM9>3.0.CO;2-M PMID: 9814441

Mertins, P., Mani, D. R., Ruggles, K. V., Gillette, M. A., Clauser, K. R., Wang, P., Wang, X., Qiao, J. W., Cao, S., Petralia, F., Kawaler, E., Mundt, F., Krug, K., Tu, Z., Lei, J. T., Gatza, M. L., Wilkerson, M., Perou, C. M., Yellapantula, V., & Carr, S. A. (2016). Proteogenomics connects somatic mutations to signalling in breast cancer. *Nature*, *534*(7605), 55–62. DOI: 10.1038/nature18003 PMID: 27251275

Messelmani, T., Morisseau, L., Sakai, Y., Legallais, C., Le Goff, A., Leclerc, E., & Jellali, R. (2022). Liver organ-on-chip models for toxicity studies and risk assessment. In *Lab on a Chip* (Vol. 22, pp. 2423–2450). Royal Society of Chemistry. DOI: 10.1039/D2LC00307D

Miglani, R., Parveen, N., Kumar, A., Ansari, M. A., Khanna, S., Rawat, G., Panda, A. K., Bisht, S. S., Upadhyay, J., & Ansari, M. N. (2022). Degradation of xenobiotic pollutants: An environmentally sustainable approach. *Metabolites*, *12*(9), 818. DOI: 10.3390/metabo12090818 PMID: 36144222

Mills, G., Shand, A., Kennedy, D., Lowe, S., Bilsland, V., Cutts, B., McBride, B., Brown, W., Bolisetty, S., Wegner, E. A., & Kidson-Gerber, G. (2025). Position statement on the diagnosis and management of acute leukaemia and aggressive lymphomas in pregnancy. *The Lancet. Haematology*, *12*(2), e151–e162. DOI: 10.1016/S2352-3026(24)00309-0 PMID: 39761682

Milner, D. A.Jr, & Lennerz, J. K. (2024). Technology and Future of Multi-Cancer Early Detection. *Life (Chicago, Ill.)*, *14*(7), 833. DOI: 10.3390/life14070833 PMID: 39063587

Min, S., Lee, B., & Yoon, S. (2017). Deep learning in bioinformatics. *Briefings in Bioinformatics*, *18*(5), 851–869. DOI: 10.1093/bib/bbw068 PMID: 27473064

Mohan, S., Heitzer, E., Ulz, P., Lafer, I., Lax, S., Auer, M., & Speicher, M. R. (2022). Beyond the blood: Circulating tumor DNA in the liquid biopsies of other body fluids. *Nature Reviews. Clinical Oncology, 19*(9), 600–618. DOI: 10.1038/s41571-022-00660-y PMID: 35915225

Mohr, A. E., Ortega-Santos, C. P., Whisner, C. M., Klein-Seetharaman, J., & Jasbi, P. (2024). Navigating challenges and opportunities in multi-omics integration for personalized healthcare. *Biomedicines, 12*(7), 1496. DOI: 10.3390/biomedicines12071496 PMID: 39062068

Mokhosoev, I. M., Astakhov, D. V., Terentiev, A. A., & Moldogazieva, N. T. (2024). Human Cytochrome P450 Cancer-Related Metabolic Activities and Gene Polymorphisms: A Review. *Cells, 13*(23), 1958. DOI: 10.3390/cells13231958 PMID: 39682707

Mokrani, S., Houali, K., Yadav, K. K., Arabi, A. I. A., Eltayeb, L. B., AwjanAlreshidi, M., Benguerba, Y., Cabral-Pinto, M. M. S., & Nabti, E. (2024). Bioremediation techniques for soil organic pollution: Mechanisms, microorganisms, and technologies-A comprehensive review. *Ecological Engineering, 207*, 107338. DOI: 10.1016/j.ecoleng.2024.107338

Molina-García, M., Malvehy, J., Granger, C., Garre, A., Trullàs, C., & Puig, S. (2022). Exposome and Skin. Part 2. The Influential Role of the Exposome, Beyond UVR, in Actinic Keratosis, Bowen's Disease and Squamous Cell Carcinoma: A Proposal. In *Dermatology and Therapy* (Vol. 12, Issue 2, pp. 361–380). Adis. DOI: 10.1007/s13555-021-00644-3

Molina-Montes, E., Ubago-Guisado, E., Petrova, D., Amiano, P., Chirlaque, M.-D., Agudo, A., & Sánchez, M.-J. (2021). The Role of Diet, Alcohol, BMI, and Physical Activity in Cancer Mortality: Summary Findings of the EPIC Study. *Nutrients, 13*(12), 4293. DOI: 10.3390/nu13124293 PMID: 34959845

Mollah, S. A., & Subramaniam, S. (2020). Histone Signatures Predict Therapeutic Efficacy in Breast Cancer. *IEEE Open Journal of Engineering in Medicine and Biology, 1*, 74–82. DOI: 10.1109/OJEMB.2020.2967105 PMID: 32412527

Moon, Y. J., Wang, X., & Morris, M. E. (2006). Dietary flavonoids: Effects on xenobiotic and carcinogen metabolism. *Toxicology In Vitro, 20*(2), 187–210. DOI: 10.1016/j.tiv.2005.06.048 PMID: 16289744

Morandeira, N. S., Castesana, P. S., Cardo, M. V., Salomone, V. N., Vadell, M. V., & Rubio, A. (2019). An interdisciplinary approach to assess human health risk in an urban environment: A case study in temperate Argentina. *Heliyon, 5*(10), e02555. DOI: 10.1016/j.heliyon.2019.e02555 PMID: 31687482

Motsinger-Reif, A. A., Reif, D. M., Akhtari, F. S., House, J. S., Campbell, C. R., Messier, K. P., Fargo, D. C., Bowen, T. A., Nadadur, S. S., Schmitt, C. P., Pettibone, K. G., Balshaw, D. M., Lawler, C. P., Newton, S. A., Collman, G. W., Miller, A. K., Merrick, B. A., Cui, Y., Anchang, B., & Woychik, R. (2024). Gene-environment interactions within a precision environmental health framework. *Cell Genomics, 4*(7), 100591. Advance online publication. DOI: 10.1016/j.xgen.2024.100591 PMID: 38925123

Mousa, S., Sarfraz, M., & Mousa, W. K. (2023). The interplay between gut microbiota and oral medications and its impact on advancing precision medicine. *Metabolites, 13*(5), 674. DOI: 10.3390/metabo13050674 PMID: 37233715

Mowat, C., Dhatt, J., Bhatti, I., Hamie, A., & Baker, K. (2023a). Short chain fatty acids prime colorectal cancer cells to activate antitumor immunity. *Frontiers in Immunology, 14*, 1190810. DOI: 10.3389/fimmu.2023.1190810 PMID: 37304266

Msallem, E., Pacquement, H., Olivier, L., Brugières, L., Landman Parker, J., Garnier, N., Lambilliotte, A., Faure, L., Clavel, J., & Bonaventure, A. (2025). Association Between Perinatal Factors and Childhood Lymphoma—A Pooled Analysis of the ESCALE and ES LE Studies (SFCE). *Pediatric Blood & Cancer, 72*(2), e31439. DOI: 10.1002/pbc.31439 PMID: 39579109

Mulware, S. J. (2013). The Mammary Gland Carcinogens: The Role of Metal Compounds and Organic Solvents. *International Journal of Breast Cancer, 2013*, 1–10. DOI: 10.1155/2013/640851 PMID: 23762568

Mungi, C., Lai, D., & Du, X. L. (2019). Spatial Analysis of Industrial Benzene Emissions and Cancer Incidence Rates in Texas. *International Journal of Environmental Research and Public Health, 16*(15), 2627. DOI: 10.3390/ijerph16152627 PMID: 31344779

Munteanu, C., & Schwartz, B. (2024). Interactions between Dietary Antioxidants, Dietary Fiber and the Gut Microbiome: Their Putative Role in Inflammation and Cancer. *International Journal of Molecular Sciences, 25*(15), 8250. DOI: 10.3390/ijms25158250 PMID: 39125822

Murphy, C. C., Wang, J. S., Betts, A. C., Lupo, P. J., Shay, L. A., Allicock, M. A., Kirk, C. L., & Pruitt, S. L. (2025). Childbirth after cancer among 42 896 male adolescents and young adults: A population-based study. *Journal of the National Cancer Institute, 117*(5), djae347. Advance online publication. DOI: 10.1093/jnci/djae347 PMID: 39752327

Musah, S., Dimitrakakis, N., Camacho, D. M., Church, G. M., & Ingber, D. E. (2018). Directed differentiation of human induced pluripotent stem cells into mature kidney podocytes and establishment of a Glomerulus Chip. *Nature Protocols, 13*(7), 1662–1685. DOI: 10.1038/s41596-018-0007-8 PMID: 29995874

Nagashri, N., Archana, L., & Raghavan, R. (2024). Microbial Volatile Compounds (MVOCs) in Food Industries and Food Safety Applications. *Innovations, Securities, and Case Studies Across Healthcare, Business, and Technology*, 75–96. DOI: 10.4018/979-8-3693-1906-2.ch005

Nagini, S., Kallamadi, P. R., Tanagala, K. K. K., & Reddy, G. B. (2024). Aldo-keto reductases: Role in cancer development and theranostics. *Oncology Research, 32*(8), 1287–1308. DOI: 10.32604/or.2024.049918 PMID: 39055885

Nakano, M., Gi, M., Toyooka, T., Suzuki, S., Wanibuchi, H., & Takebayashi, T. (2025). Occupational health topics series on the effects of chemicals: Epidemiological and toxicological risk assessments of ortho-toluidine for bladder cancer. *Journal of Occupational Health, 67*(1), uiaf005. Advance online publication. DOI: 10.1093/joccuh/uiaf005 PMID: 39930727

Nandi, D., Parida, S., & Sharma, D. (2023). The gut microbiota in breast cancer development and treatment: The good, the bad, and the useful! *Gut Microbes, 15*(1), 2221452. DOI: 10.1080/19490976.2023.2221452 PMID: 37305949

Narendra, G., Choudhary, S., Raju, B., Verma, H., & Silakari, O. (2022). Role of genetic polymorphisms in drug-metabolizing enzyme-mediated toxicity and pharmacokinetic resistance to anti-cancer agents: A review on the pharmacogenomics aspect. *Clinical Pharmacokinetics, 61*(11), 1495–1517. DOI: 10.1007/s40262-022-01174-7 PMID: 36180817

Nault, J.-C. (2015). *Spécialité : Bases Fondamentales de l'Oncogenèse Présentée par Identification de nouveaux mécanismes de carcinogenèse et facteurs pronostiques des tumeurs hépatocellulaires.*

Neagu, A.-N., Bruno, P., Johnson, K. R., Ballestas, G., & Darie, C. C. (2024). Biological Basis of Breast Cancer-Related Disparities in Precision Oncology Era. *International Journal of Molecular Sciences, 25*(7), 4113. DOI: 10.3390/ijms25074113 PMID: 38612922

Neagu, A.-N., Jayaweera, T., Corrice, L., Johnson, K., & Darie, C. (2024). Breast Cancer Exposomics. *Life (Chicago, Ill.), 14*(3), 402. DOI: 10.3390/life14030402 PMID: 38541726

Nichols, T. A., Einarsson, A., & Willerslev, E. (2018). Contamination and DNA degradation in ancient DNA. *Science and Technology of Archaeological Research, 4*(1), 63–73.

Nieminen, M. T., & Salaspuro, M. (2018). Local Acetaldehyde-An Essential Role in Alcohol-Related Upper Gastrointestinal Tract Carcinogenesis. *Cancers (Basel), 10*(1), 11. DOI: 10.3390/cancers10010011 PMID: 29303995

Nitsche, K. S., Müller, I., Malcomber, S., Carmichael, P. L., & Bouwmeester, H. (2022). Implementing organ-on-chip in a next-generation risk assessment of chemicals: a review. In *Archives of Toxicology* (Vol. 96, Issue 3, pp. 711–741). Springer Science and Business Media Deutschland GmbH. DOI: 10.1007/s00204-022-03234-0

Nogacka, A., Gómez-Martín, M., Suárez, A., González-Bernardo, O., De Los Reyes-Gavilán, C., & González, S. (2019). Xenobiotics Formed during Food Processing: Their Relation with the Intestinal Microbiota and Colorectal Cancer. *International Journal of Molecular Sciences, 20*(8), 2051. DOI: 10.3390/ijms20082051 PMID: 31027304

Non, A. L. (2025). The eighth annual US DOHAD meeting: Promising approaches in epigenetics research of early life exposures. *Epigenomics, 17*(4), 209–211. DOI: 10.1080/17501911.2025.2459550 PMID: 39874076

Nowak, A., & Libudzisz, Z. (2006). Influence of phenol, p-cresol and indole on growth and survival of intestinal lactic acid bacteria. *Anaerobe, 12*(2), 80–84. DOI: 10.1016/j.anaerobe.2005.10.003 PMID: 16701619

O'Keefe, S. J. D. (2016). Diet, microorganisms and their metabolites, and colon cancer. *Nature Reviews. Gastroenterology & Hepatology, 13*(12), 691–706. DOI: 10.1038/nrgastro.2016.165 PMID: 27848961

Obtulowicz, T., Swoboda, M., Speina, E., Gackowski, D., Rozalski, R., Siomek, A., Janik, J., Janowska, B., Ciesla, J. M., Jawien, A., Banaszkiewicz, Z., Guz, J., Dziaman, T., Szpila, A., Olinski, R., & Tudek, B. (2010). Oxidative stress and 8-oxoguanine repair are enhanced in colon adenoma and carcinoma patients. *Mutagenesis, 25*(5), 463–471. DOI: 10.1093/mutage/geq028 PMID: 20534734

Ogidi, O. I. (2024). Recent advances in anticancer activity and Bioinformatics Approach from Potential Plants. In: Computational Approaches in Biomaterials, Bioinformatics and Biomedical Engineering Applications. *CRC Press, Taylor and Francis Group, Florida, USA*. DOI: 10.1201/9781003354437-3

Ogidi, O. I., & Ajoko, I. (2024). Neuroprotective Potentials of Phytochemicals. In: M.S. Rajput, T. Sarachana, P.D. Sarkar, M. Raval (eds) NeuroPhytomedicine. *CRC Press, Routledge Taylor and Francis Group.*

Ogidi, O. I., & Emaikwu, N. G. (2024). Plant Phenolic compound isolation and its Bioinformatics Approaches of Molecular Mechanisms in Antimicrobial activities and Resistance. In: Computational Approaches in Biomaterials, Bioinformatics and Biomedical Engineering Applications. *CRC Press, Taylor and Francis Group, Florida, USA.* DOI: 10.1201/9781003354437-8

Ogidi, O. I., Chukwunonso, O. A., Afakwu-Adimoha, H. C., & Barwant, M. M. (2025c). Ethical Considerations in Generative Artificial Intelligence in Healthcare. In: Generative Artificial Intelligence in Healthcare: Current Practice and Future Development. *CRC Press, Taylor and Francis Group, Florida, USA.* DOI: 10.1201/9781003488255-5

Ogidi, O. I., Ogoun, T. R., Alex, E. I., Edward, R. B., Joshua, M. T., & Bunu, E. M. (2024b). Radiogenomics and Genetic Diversity of Glioblastoma Characterization. In: Radiomics and Radiogenomics in Neuro-Oncology: An Artificial Intelligence Paradigm- volume 2: Genetics and clinical applications. *Elsevier.* DOI: 10.1016/B978-0-443-18509-0.00002-5

Ogidi, O. I. (2025). Natural Products Modulating Mitophagy: Implications for Cancer Therapy. In Pandurangan, A. (Ed.), *Roles of Mitophagy in Cancer Regulation* (pp. 325–358). IGI Global Scientific Publishing, DOI: 10.4018/979-8-3693-3836-0.ch012

Ogidi, O. I., Ajoko, I. T., & Tawariowei, A. M. (2024c). Sustainable Application of Genetic Ecotoxicological Techniques. In *Biomonitoring For Environmental Sustainability. In: Biomonitoring of Pollutants in the Global South.* Springer Nature Singapore Pte Ltd. DOI: 10.1007/978-981-97-1658-6_19

Ogidi, O. I., Barwant, M. M., & Okara, E. (2024a). Biomarker Discovery: Protein Phosphorylation State. In *Spatially Variable Genes in Cancer: Development, Progression, and Treatment Response.* IGI Global. DOI: 10.4018/979-8-3693-7728-4.ch005

Ogidi, O. I., Erho, S. A., & Omu, O. (2025a). Reactive Oxygen Species in Cancer. In Prabhakar, P. (Ed.), *The Role of Reactive Oxygen Species in Human Health and Disease* (pp. 339–376). IGI Global Scientific Publishing. DOI: 10.4018/979-8-3693-7919-6.ch010

Ogidi, O. I., Ijere, N. D., & Sogoi, P. B. (2025b). Neural and Endocrine Regulation of Immunity. In Reddy, K. (Ed.), *Research Methodologies and Practical Applications in Psychoneuroimmunology* (pp. 17–42). IGI Global Scientific Publishing. DOI: 10.4018/979-8-3693-7432-0.ch002

Ogidi, O. I., Onwuagba, C. G., & Richard-Nwachukwu, N. (2024d). Biomonitoring Tools, Techniques and Approaches For Environmental Assessments. In *Biomonitoring of Pollutants in the Global South*. Springer Nature Singapore Pte Ltd. DOI: 10.1007/978-981-97-1658-6_7

Ogidi, O. I., & Tawariowei, A. M. (2023). Endocrine Disrupting Chemicals and their Role in Cancer-A review. *Molecular Sciences And Applications.*, *3*, 5–14. DOI: 10.37394/232023.2023.3.2

Ogidi, O. I., & Tobia, P. S. (2024). Harnessing Artificial Intelligence (AI) Techniques for the prevention of Microbial Disease in Humans. In *Artificial Intelligence in Microbiology: scopes and Challenges*. Elsevier.

Ogunjobi, T. T., Ohaeri, P. N., Akintola, O. T., Atanda, D. O., Orji, F. P., Adebayo, J. O., Abdul, S. O., Eji, C. A., Asebebe, A. B., Shodipe, O. O., & Adedeji, O. O. (2024). *Bioinformatics Applications in Chronic Diseases: A Comprehensive Review of Genomic, Transcriptomics, Proteomic, Metabolomics, and Machine Learning Approaches*. Medinformatics., DOI: 10.47852/bonviewMEDIN42022335

Okwan-Duodu, D., Pandiri, A. R., & Adams, D. J. (2024). Not All Carcinogens Are Directly Mutagenic: A Holistic View of the Environmental Exposure–Cancer Connection. *Annual Review of Cancer Biology*. Advance online publication. DOI: 10.1146/annurev-cancerbio-060424-052905

Oladosu, J. I., & Flaws, J. A. (2024). The Impact of Neonicotinoid Pesticides on Reproductive Health. *Toxicological Sciences*, kfae138. Advance online publication. DOI: 10.1093/toxsci/kfae138 PMID: 39460954

Ollberding, N. J., Wilkens, L. R., Henderson, B. E., Kolonel, L. N., & Le Marchand, L. (2012). Meat consumption, heterocyclic amines and colorectal cancer risk: The Multiethnic Cohort Study. *International Journal of Cancer*, *131*(7). Advance online publication. DOI: 10.1002/ijc.27546 PMID: 22438055

Olmedo-Suárez, M. Á., Ramírez-Díaz, I., Pérez-González, A., Molina-Herrera, A., Coral-García, M. Á., Lobato, S., Sarvari, P., Barreto, G., & Rubio, K. (2022). Epigenetic Regulation in Exposome-Induced Tumorigenesis: Emerging Roles of ncRNAs. *Biomolecules*, *12*(4), 513. Advance online publication. DOI: 10.3390/biom12040513 PMID: 35454102

Onyije, F. M., Dolatkhah, R., Olsson, A., Bouaoun, L., & Schüz, J. (2024). Environmental risk factors of Wilms tumour: A systematic review and meta-analysis. *EJC Paediatric Oncology*, *4*, 100178. Advance online publication. DOI: 10.1016/j.ejcped.2024.100178 PMID: 39678930

Onyije, F. M., Olsson, A., Erdmann, F., Magnani, C., Petridou, E., Clavel, J., Miligi, L., Bonaventure, A., Ferrante, D., Piro, S., Peters, S., Vermeulen, R., Kromhout, H., & Schüz, J. (2022). Parental occupational exposure to combustion products, metals, silica and asbestos and risk of childhood leukaemia: Findings from the Childhood Cancer and Leukaemia International Consortium (CLIC). *Environment International*, *167*, 107409. DOI: 10.1016/j.envint.2022.107409 PMID: 35908390

Orešič, M., McGlinchey, A., Wheelock, C. E., & Hyötyläinen, T. (2020). Metabolic Signatures of the Exposome—Quantifying the Impact of Exposure to Environmental Chemicals on Human Health. *Metabolites*, *10*(11), 454. DOI: 10.3390/metabo10110454 PMID: 33182712

Ouma, R. B., Ngari, S. M., & Kibet, J. K. (2024). A review of the current trends in computational approaches in drug design and metabolism. *Discover Public Health*, *21*(1), 108. DOI: 10.1186/s12982-024-00229-3

Ozbek, O., Genc, D. E., & Ulgen, O., K. (. (2024). Advances in Physiologically Based Pharmacokinetic (PBPK) Modeling of Nanomaterials. *ACS Pharmacology & Translational Science*, *7*(8), 2251–2279. DOI: 10.1021/acsptsci.4c00250 PMID: 39144562

Pal, S., & Firdous, S. M. (2024). Unraveling the role of heavy metals xenobiotics in cancer: A critical review. *Discover. Oncology*, *15*(1), 615. DOI: 10.1007/s12672-024-01417-y PMID: 39495398

Panda, C., Komarnytsky, S., Fleming, M. N., Marsh, C., Barron, K., Le Brun-Blashka, S., & Metzger, B. (2023). Guided Metabolic Detoxification program supports phase II detoxification enzymes and antioxidant balance in healthy participants. *Nutrients*, *15*(9), 2209. DOI: 10.3390/nu15092209 PMID: 37432335

Pandey, H., Tang, D. W. T., Wong, S. H., & Lal, D. (2023). Gut Microbiota in Colorectal Cancer: Biological Role and Therapeutic Opportunities. *Cancers (Basel)*, *15*(3), 866. DOI: 10.3390/cancers15030866 PMID: 36765824

Panebianco, C., Andriulli, A., & Pazienza, V. (2018). Pharmacomicrobiomics: Exploiting the drug-microbiota interactions in anticancer therapies. *Microbiome*, *6*(1), 1–13. DOI: 10.1186/s40168-018-0483-7 PMID: 29789015

Pant, A., Maiti, T. K., Mahajan, D., & Das, B. (2023). Human gut microbiota and drug metabolism. *Microbial Ecology*, *86*(1), 97–111. DOI: 10.1007/s00248-022-02081-x PMID: 35869999

Parida, S., & Sharma, D. (2019). The Microbiome-Estrogen Connection and Breast Cancer Risk. *Cells*, *8*(12), 1642. DOI: 10.3390/cells8121642 PMID: 31847455

Park, A. S., Ritz, B., Ling, C., Cockburn, M., & Heck, J. E. (2017). Exposure to ambient dichloromethane in pregnancy and infancy from industrial sources and childhood cancers in California. *International Journal of Hygiene and Environmental Health, 220*(7), 1133–1140. DOI: 10.1016/j.ijheh.2017.06.006 PMID: 28720343

Park, H. E., Jo, S. H., Lee, R. H., Macks, C. P., Ku, T., Park, J., Lee, C. W., Hur, J. K., & Sohn, C. H. (2023). Spatial transcriptomics: Technical aspects of recent developments and their applications in neuroscience and cancer research. *Advancement of Science, 10*(16), 2206939. DOI: 10.1002/advs.202206939 PMID: 37026425

Park, H.-M., Kim, H., Lee, K.-H., & Cho, J.-Y. (2020). Analysis of opposing histone modifications H3K4me3 and H3K27me3 reveals candidate diagnostic biomarkers for TNBC and gene set prediction combination. *BMB Reports, 53*(5), 266–271. DOI: 10.5483/BMBRep.2020.53.5.045 PMID: 32317088

Parkinson, L. V., Geueke, B., & Muncke, J. (2024). Potential mammary carcinogens used in food contact articles: Implications for policy, enforcement, and prevention. *Frontiers in Toxicology, 6*, 1440331. DOI: 10.3389/ftox.2024.1440331 PMID: 39381597

Parris, B. A., O'Farrell, H. E., Fong, K. M., & Yang, I. A. (2019). Chronic obstructive pulmonary disease (COPD) and lung cancer: Common pathways for pathogenesis. *Journal of Thoracic Disease, 11*(S17), S2155–S2172. DOI: 10.21037/jtd.2019.10.54 PMID: 31737343

Patangia, D. V., Anthony Ryan, C., Dempsey, E., Paul Ross, R., & Stanton, C. (2022). Impact of antibiotics on the human microbiome and consequences for host health. *MicrobiologyOpen, 11*(1), e1260. DOI: 10.1002/mbo3.1260 PMID: 35212478

Patnaik, S., & Anupriya, . (2019). Drugs Targeting Epigenetic Modifications and Plausible Therapeutic Strategies Against Colorectal Cancer. *Frontiers in Pharmacology, 10*, 588. DOI: 10.3389/fphar.2019.00588 PMID: 31244652

Patro, R., Duggal, G., Love, M. I., Irizarry, R. A., & Kingsford, C. (2017). Salmon provides fast and bias-aware quantification of transcript expression. *Nature Methods, 14*(4), 417–419. DOI: 10.1038/nmeth.4197 PMID: 28263959

Paul, A., Danjou, A. M. N., Deygas, F., Guth, M., Coste, A., Lefevre, M., Dananché, B., Kromhout, H., Spinosi, J., Béranger, R., Pérol, O., Boyle, H., Hersant, C., Loup-Cabaniols, V., Veau, S., Bujan, L., Olsson, A., Schüz, J., Fervers, B., & Charbotel, B. (2023). Parental occupations at birth and risk of adult testicular germ cell tumors in offspring: A French nationwide case-control study. *Frontiers in Public Health, 11*, 1303998. DOI: 10.3389/fpubh.2023.1303998 PMID: 38292387

Pauwels, I., Versporten, A., Drapier, N., Vlieghe, E., Goossens, H., Koraqi, A., Hoxha, I., Tafaj, S., Cornistein, W., Quiros, R., Hojman, M., Ghazaryan, L., Horne, K., Cairns, K., Doukas, F., Gottlieb, T., Sermijn, E., Verhamme, K., Brands, C., & Lindholm, D. A. (2021). Hospital antibiotic prescribing patterns in adult patients according to the WHO Access, Watch and Reserve classification (AWaRe): Results from a worldwide point prevalence survey in 69 countries. *The Journal of Antimicrobial Chemotherapy*, *76*(6), 1614–1624. DOI: 10.1093/jac/dkab050 PMID: 33822971

Pawlowski, J., Audic, S., Adl, S., Bass, D., Belbahri, L., Berney, C., & de Vargas, C. (2018). CBOL protist working group: Barcoding eukaryotic richness beyond the animal, plant, and fungal kingdoms. *PLoS Biology*, *16*(10), e2005849. DOI: 10.1371/journal.pbio.2005849 PMID: 23139639

Pecori Giraldi, F., Ferraù, F., Ragonese, M., & Cannavò, S. (2024). Endocrine disruptors, aryl hydrocarbon receptor and cortisol secretion. *Journal of Endocrinological Investigation*, *47*(10), 1–13. DOI: 10.1007/s40618-024-02371-w PMID: 38637430

Pelkonen, O., Abass, K., Parra Morte, J. M., Panzarea, M., Testai, E., Rudaz, S., Louisse, J., Gundert-Remy, U., Wolterink, G., Jean-Lou Cm, D., Coecke, S., & Bernasconi, C. (2023). Metabolites in the regulatory risk assessment of pesticides in the EU. *Frontiers in Toxicology*, *5*, 1304885. DOI: 10.3389/ftox.2023.1304885 PMID: 38188093

Pellegrini, L., Xue, J., Larson, D., Pastorino, S., Jube, S., Forest, K. H., Saad-Jube, Z. S., Napolitano, A., Pagano, I., Negi, V. S., Bianchi, M. E., Morris, P., Pass, H. I., Gaudino, G., Carbone, M., & Yang, H. (2017). HMGB1 targeting by ethyl pyruvate suppresses malignant phenotype of human mesothelioma. *Oncotarget*, *8*(14), 22649–22661. DOI: 10.18632/oncotarget.15152 PMID: 28186988

Peng, C., He, M., Cutrona, S. L., Kiefe, C. I., Liu, F., & Wang, Z. (2020). Theme Trends and Knowledge Structure on Mobile Health Apps: Bibliometric Analysis. *JMIR mHealth and uHealth*, *8*(7), e18212. DOI: 10.2196/18212 PMID: 32716312

Penning, T. M., Su, A. L., & El-Bayoumy, K. (2022). Nitroreduction: A critical metabolic pathway for drugs, environmental pollutants, and explosives. *Chemical Research in Toxicology*, *35*(10), 1747–1765. DOI: 10.1021/acs.chemrestox.2c00175 PMID: 36044734

Perri, A. M., Agosti, V., Olivo, E., Concolino, A., De Angelis, M., Tammè, L., Fiumara, C. V., Cuda, G., & Scumaci, D. (2019). Histone proteomics reveals novel post-translational modifications in breast cancer. *Aging (Albany NY)*, *11*(23), 11722–11755. DOI: 10.18632/aging.102577 PMID: 31816600

Phillips, D. H. (1999). Polycyclic aromatic hydrocarbons in the diet. *Mutation Research/Genetic Toxicology and Environmental Mutagenesis, 443*(1–2), 139–147. DOI: 10.1016/S1383-5742(99)00016-2 PMID: 10415437

Pinu, F. R., Beale, D. J., Paten, A. M., Kouremenos, K., Swarup, S., Schirra, H. J., & Wishart, D. (2019). Systems Biology and Multi-Omics Integration: Viewpoints from the Metabolomics Research Community. *Metabolites, 9*(4), 76. DOI: 10.3390/metabo9040076 PMID: 31003499

Pisoschi, A. M., & Pop, A. (2015). The role of antioxidants in the chemistry of oxidative stress: A review. *European Journal of Medicinal Chemistry, 97*, 55–74. DOI: 10.1016/j.ejmech.2015.04.040 PMID: 25942353

Pizzino, G., Irrera, N., Cucinotta, M., Pallio, G., Mannino, F., Arcoraci, V., Squadrito, F., Altavilla, D., & Bitto, A. (2017). Oxidative Stress: Harms and Benefits for Human Health. *Oxidative Medicine and Cellular Longevity, 2017*(1), 8416763. DOI: 10.1155/2017/8416763 PMID: 28819546

Pool, M., De Boer, H. R., Hooge, M. N. L., Van Vugt, M. A. T. M., & De Vries, E. G. E. (2017). Harnessing Integrative Omics to Facilitate Molecular Imaging of the Human Epidermal Growth Factor Receptor Family for Precision Medicine. *Theranostics, 7*(7), 2111–2133. DOI: 10.7150/thno.17934 PMID: 28638489

Poschl, G. (2004). ALCOHOL AND CANCER. *Alcohol and Alcoholism, 39*(3), 155–165. DOI: 10.1093/alcalc/agh057 PMID: 15082451

Pramana, C., Peranawengrum, K. B., & Juliani, V. (2020). Maternal characteristics and perinatal outcomes in women with severe preeclampsia. *Systematic Reviews in Pharmacy, 11*, 549–553.

Prasad, A. S. (2014). Zinc: an antioxidant and anti-inflammatory agent: role of zinc in degenerative disorders of aging. *Journal of Trace Elements in Medicine and Biology, 28*(4), 364–371. DOI: 10.1016/j.jtemb.2014.07.019 PMID: 25200490

Pristner, M., & Warth, B. (2020). Drug–Exposome Interactions: The Next Frontier in Precision Medicine. In *Trends in Pharmacological Sciences* (Vol. 41, pp. 994–1005). Elsevier Ltd. DOI: 10.1016/j.tips.2020.09.012

Priya, A. K., Muruganandam, M., Kumar, A., Senthilkumar, N., Shkir, M., Pandit, B., Imran, M., Prakash, C., & Ubaidullah, M. (2024). Recent advances in microbial-assisted degradation and remediation of xenobiotic contaminants; challenges and future prospects. *Journal of Water Process Engineering, 60*, 105106. DOI: 10.1016/j.jwpe.2024.105106

Priyadarshini, B. I.B. Indira Priyadarshini. (2024). Deep Learning for Predictive Toxicology Assessment Early Detection of Adverse Drug Reactions. *Power System Technology*, *48*(1), 680–697. DOI: 10.52783/pst.322

Priyadarshini, M., Kotlo, K. U., Dudeja, P. K., & Layden, B. T. (2018). Role of Short Chain Fatty Acid Receptors in Intestinal Physiology and Pathophysiology. *Comprehensive Physiology*, *8*(3), 1091–1115. DOI: 10.1002/j.2040-4603.2018.tb00038.x PMID: 29978895

Przanowska, R. K., Labban, N., Przanowski, P., Hawes, R. B., Atkins, K. A., Showalter, S. L., & Janes, K. A. (2024). Patient-derived response estimates from zero-passage organoids of luminal breast cancer. BioRxiv *: The Preprint Server for Biology*.

Qin, N., He, W., Liu, W., Kong, X., Xu, F., & Giesy, J. P. (2020). Tissue distribution, bioaccumulation, and carcinogenic risk of polycyclic aromatic hydrocarbons in aquatic organisms from Lake Chaohu, China. *The Science of the Total Environment*, *749*, 141577. Advance online publication. DOI: 10.1016/j.scitotenv.2020.141577 PMID: 32829278

Qin, T., Zhang, X., Guo, T., Yang, T., Gao, Y., Hao, W., & Xiao, X. (2021). Epigenetic Alteration Shaped by the Environmental Chemical Bisphenol A. *Frontiers in Genetics*, *11*, 618966. DOI: 10.3389/fgene.2020.618966 PMID: 33505438

Qriouet, Z., Qmichou, Z., Bouchoutrouch, N., Mahi, H., Cherrah, Y., & Sefrioui, H. (2019). Analytical methods used for the detection and quantification of benzodiazepines. *Journal of Analytical Methods in Chemistry*, *2019*(1), 2035492. DOI: 10.1155/2019/2035492 PMID: 31583157

Quast, C., Pruesse, E., Yilmaz, P., Gerken, J., Schweer, T., Yarza, P., Peplies, J., & Glöckner, F. O. (2013). The SILVA ribosomal RNA gene database project: Improved data processing and web-based tools. *Nucleic Acids Research*, *41*(D1), D590–D596. DOI: 10.1093/nar/gks1219 PMID: 23193283

Rafter, J. (2003). Probiotics and colon cancer. *Best Practice & Research. Clinical Gastroenterology*, *17*(5), 849–859. DOI: 10.1016/S1521-6918(03)00056-8 PMID: 14507593

Rahbar, M. H., Samms-Vaughan, M., Kim, S., Saroukhani, S., Bressler, J., Hessabi, M., Grove, M. L., Shakspeare-Pellington, S., & Loveland, K. A. (2022). Detoxification Role of Metabolic Glutathione S-Transferase (GST) Genes in Blood Lead Concentrations of Jamaican Children with and without Autism Spectrum Disorder. *Genes*, *13*(6), 975. DOI: 10.3390/genes13060975 PMID: 35741737

Rahman, M., Irmler, M., Introna, M., Beckers, J., Palmberg, L., Johanson, G., Upadhyay, S., & Ganguly, K. (2022). Insight into the pulmonary molecular toxicity of heated tobacco products using human bronchial and alveolar mucosa models at air–liquid interface. *Scientific Reports*, *12*(1), 16396. DOI: 10.1038/s41598-022-20657-y PMID: 36180488

Rai, M., Paudel, N., Sakhrie, M., Gemmati, D., Khan, I. A., Tisato, V., Kanase, A., Schulz, A., & Singh, A. V. (2023). Perspective on quantitative structure–toxicity relationship (QSTR) models to predict hepatic biotransformation of xenobiotics. *Livers*, *3*(3), 448–462. DOI: 10.3390/livers3030032

Rampášek, L., Hidru, D., Smirnov, P., Haibe-Kains, B., & Goldenberg, A. (2019). Dr.VAE: Drug Response Variational Autoencoder. *bioRxiv*. DOI: 10.1101/602607

Rappoport, N., Safra, R., & Shamir, R. (2020). MONET: Multi-omic module discovery by omic selection. *PLoS Computational Biology*, *16*(9), e1008182. DOI: 10.1371/journal.pcbi.1008182 PMID: 32931516

Ratnasekhar, C. H., Rathor, P., Rakwal, P., Verma, A. K., & Khan, S. (2024). Analytical platforms in metabolomics of health and disease. In *Comprehensive Analytical Chemistry* (Vol. 104, pp. 1–20). Elsevier. DOI: 10.1016/bs.coac.2023.09.007

Raufaste-Cazavieille, V., Santiago, R., & Droit, A. (2022). Multi-omics analysis: Paving the path toward achieving precision medicine in cancer treatment and immuno-oncology. *Frontiers in Molecular Biosciences*, *9*, 962743. DOI: 10.3389/fmolb.2022.962743 PMID: 36304921

Ren, Y., Wu, J., Wang, Y., Zhang, L., Ren, J., Zhang, Z., Chen, B., Zhang, K., Zhu, B., Liu, W., Li, S., & Li, X. (2023). Lifestyle patterns influence the composition of the gut microbiome in a healthy Chinese population. *Scientific Reports*, *13*(1), 14425. DOI: 10.1038/s41598-023-41532-4 PMID: 37660184

Reszka, E., Wasowicz, W., & Gromadzinska, J. (n.d.). *Genetic polymorphism of xenobiotic metabolising enzymes, diet and cancer susceptibility*. DOI: 10.1079/BJN20061878

Rezazadegan, M., Forootani, B., Hoveyda, Y., Rezazadegan, N., & Amani, R. (2025). Major heavy metals and human gut microbiota composition: A systematic review with nutritional approach. *Journal of Health, Population and Nutrition*, *44*(1), 21. DOI: 10.1186/s41043-025-00750-4 PMID: 39871318

Režen, T., Rozman, D., Kovács, T., Kovács, P., Sipos, A., Bai, P., & Mikó, E. (2022). The role of bile acids in carcinogenesis. *Cellular and Molecular Life Sciences : CMLS*, *79*(5), 243. DOI: 10.1007/s00018-022-04278-2 PMID: 35429253

Rigat-Brugarolas, L. G., Elizalde-Torrent, A., Bernabeu, M., De Niz, M., Martin-Jaular, L., Fernandez-Becerra, C., Homs-Corbera, A., Samitier, J., & Del Portillo, H. A. (2014). A functional microengineered model of the human splenon-on-a-chip. *Lab on a Chip, 14*(10), 1715–1724. DOI: 10.1039/C3LC51449H PMID: 24663955

Rineh, A., Kelso, M. J., Vatansever, F., Tegos, G. P., & Hamblin, M. R. (2014). Clostridium difficile infection: Molecular pathogenesis and novel therapeutics. *Expert Review of Anti-Infective Therapy, 12*(1), 131–150. DOI: 10.1586/14787210.2014.866515 PMID: 24410618

Riquelme, M. A., Cardenas, E. R., & Jiang, J. X. (2020). Osteocytes and Bone Metastasis. *Frontiers in Endocrinology, 11*, 567844. DOI: 10.3389/fendo.2020.567844 PMID: 33162934

Rivas-Domínguez, A., Pastor, N., Martínez-López, L., Colón-Pérez, J., Bermúdez, B., & Orta, M. L. (2021). The Role of DNA Damage Response in Dysbiosis-Induced Colorectal. *Cancer Cells (Cold Spring Harbor, N.Y.), 10*(8), 1934. DOI: 10.3390/cells10081934 PMID: 34440703

Rodríguez, A. T. (2024). Clinically important pharmacokinetic drug-drug interactions with antibacterial agents. *Revista Española de Quimioterapia, 37*(4), 299–322. DOI: 10.37201/req/037.2024 PMID: 38840420

Roje, B., Zhang, B., Mastrorilli, E., Kovačić, A., Sušak, L., Ljubenkov, I., Ćosić, E., Vilović, K., Meštrović, A., Vukovac, E. L., Bučević-Popović, V., Puljiz, Ž., Karaman, I., Terzić, J., & Zimmermann, M. (2024). Gut microbiota carcinogen metabolism causes distal tissue tumours. *Nature, 632*(8027), 1137–1144. DOI: 10.1038/s41586-024-07754-w PMID: 39085612

Rossman, T. (2003). Mechanism of arsenic carcinogenesis: An integrated approach. *Mutation Research. Fundamental and Molecular Mechanisms of Mutagenesis, 533*(1–2), 37–65. DOI: 10.1016/j.mrfmmm.2003.07.009 PMID: 14643412

Ruiz-Saavedra, S., Zapico, A., Del Rey, C. G., Gonzalez, C., Suárez, A., Díaz, Y., De Los Reyes-Gavilán, C. G., & González, S. (2022). Dietary Xenobiotics Derived from Food Processing: Association with Fecal Mutagenicity and Gut Mucosal Damage. *Nutrients, 14*(17), 3482. DOI: 10.3390/nu14173482 PMID: 36079735

Ruiz, V. E., Battaglia, T., Kurtz, Z. D., Bijnens, L., Ou, A., Engstrand, I., Zheng, X., Iizumi, T., Mullins, B. J., Müller, C. L., Cadwell, K., Bonneau, R., Perez-Perez, G. I., & Blaser, M. J. (2017). A single early-in-life macrolide course has lasting effects on murine microbial network topology and immunity. *Nature Communications, 8*(1), 518. DOI: 10.1038/s41467-017-00531-6 PMID: 28894149

Sadee, B. A., Zebari, S. M. S., Galali, Y., & Saleem, M. F. (2025). A review on arsenic contamination in drinking water: Sources, health impacts, and remediation approaches. *RSC Advances, 15*(4), 2684–2703. DOI: 10.1039/D4RA08867K PMID: 39871983

Safarlou, C. W., Jongsma, K. R., & Vermeulen, R. (2024). Reconceptualizing and Defining Exposomics within Environmental Health: Expanding the Scope of Health Research. *Environmental Health Perspectives, 132*(9), 095001. DOI: 10.1289/EHP14509 PMID: 39331035

Sahoo, R., Pattnaik, S., Mohanty, B., Mir, S. A., & Behera, B. (2025). Aryl hydrocarbon receptor (AHR) signalling: A double-edged sword guiding both cancer progression and cancer therapy. *Biochimica et Biophysica Acta (BBA) -. Biochimica et Biophysica Acta. G, General Subjects, 1869*(6), 130805. DOI: 10.1016/j.bbagen.2025.130805 PMID: 40222634

Saini, S., PSA, K. L. K., & PCA3. (2018). Non-coding RNA in prostate cancer: Molecular functions and clinical implications. *The Prostate, 78*(14), 1057–1074. DOI: 10.1002/pros.23673

Salazar-González, R. A., Doll, M. A., & Hein, D. W. (2023). N-acetyltransferase 2 genetic polymorphism modifies genotoxic and oxidative damage from new psychoactive substances. *Archives of Toxicology, 97*(1), 189–199. DOI: 10.1007/s00204-022-03383-2 PMID: 36138126

Salim, S. Y., Kaplan, G. G., & Madsen, K. L. (2014). Air pollution effects on the gut microbiota: A link between exposure and inflammatory disease. *Gut Microbes, 5*(2), 215–219. DOI: 10.4161/gmic.27251 PMID: 24637593

Sampsell, K., Hao, D., & Reimer, R. A. (2020). The Gut Microbiota: A Potential Gateway to Improved Health Outcomes in Breast Cancer Treatment and Survivorship. *International Journal of Molecular Sciences, 21*(23), 9239. DOI: 10.3390/ijms21239239 PMID: 33287442

Sarbassov, D. D., Guertin, D. A., Ali, S. M., & Sabatini, D. M. (2005). Phosphorylation and Regulation of Akt/PKB by the Rictor-mTOR Complex. *Science, 307*(5712), 1098–1101. DOI: 10.1126/science.1106148 PMID: 15718470

Sarlak, S. (2021). *Exposome du cancer : reprogrammation métabolique du cancer du poumon par les nitrosamines spécifiques de la fumée de tabac*. Https://Hal.Science/Tel-04138441/

Saucy, A., Coloma, F., Olmos, S., Åström, C., Blay, N., Boer, J. M. A., Dadvand, P., de Bont, J., de Cid, R., de Hoogh, K., Dimakopoulou, K., Gehring, U., Huss, A., Ibi, D., Katsouyanni, K., Koppelman, G., Ljungman, P., Melén, E., Nieuwenhuijsen, M., & Tonne, C. (2024). Socioeconomic Inequalities in the External Exposome in European Cohorts: The EXPANSE Project. *Environmental Science & Technology*, *58*(37), 16248–16257. DOI: 10.1021/acs.est.4c01509 PMID: 39237108

Savin, M., Mihailescu, C.-M., Avramescu, V., Dinulescu, S., Firtat, B., Craciun, G., Brasoveanu, C., Pachiu, C., Romanitan, C., Serban, A.-B., Ion, A. C., & Moldovan, C. (2021). A New Hybrid Sensitive PANI/SWCNT/Ferrocene-Based Layer for a Wearable CO Sensor. *Sensors (Basel)*, *21*(5), 1801. DOI: 10.3390/s21051801 PMID: 33807640

Sayyed, Y., Rehman, K., Akash, M. S. H., Kamran, S. H., & Badran, M. (2022). Xenobiotics and drug-metabolizing enzymes: Challenges and strategies. In *Biochemistry of Drug Metabolizing Enzymes* (pp. 305–321). Academic Press., DOI: 10.1016/B978-0-323-95120-3.00007-5

Schirmer, M., Smeekens, S. P., Vlamakis, H., Jaeger, M., Oosting, M., Franzosa, E. A., ter Horst, R., Jansen, T., Jacobs, L., Bonder, M. J., Kurilshikov, A., Fu, J., Joosten, L. A. B., Zhernakova, A., Huttenhower, C., Wijmenga, C., Netea, M. G., & Xavier, R. J. (2016). Linking the Human Gut Microbiome to Inflammatory Cytokine Production Capacity. *Cell*, *167*(4), 1125–1136.e8. DOI: 10.1016/j.cell.2016.10.020 PMID: 27814509

Schnekenburger, M., Karius, T., & Diederich, M. (2014). Regulation of epigenetic traits of the glutathione S-transferase P1 gene: From detoxification toward cancer prevention and diagnosis. *Frontiers in Pharmacology*, *5*. Advance online publication. DOI: 10.3389/fphar.2014.00170 PMID: 25076909

Schraw, J. M., Tark, J. Y., Desrosiers, T. A., Chambers, T. M., Shumate, C. J., Nembhard, W. N., Yazdy, M. M., Nestoridi, E., Malone, M. F. W., Laetsch, T. W., Widemann, B. C., Janitz, A. E., Tanner, J. P., Kirby, R. S., Salemi, J. L., Spector, L. G., Huff, C. D., Plon, S. E., & Lupo, P. J. (2025). Risk of carcinomas among children and adolescents with birth defects. *Cancer Epidemiology*, *95*, 102748. DOI: 10.1016/j.canep.2025.102748 PMID: 39848200

Schulz, C., Schütte, K., Mayerle, J., & Malfertheiner, P. (2019). The role of the gastric bacterial microbiome in gastric cancer: Helicobacter pylori and beyond. *Therapeutic Advances in Gastroenterology*, *12*, 1756284819894062. DOI: 10.1177/1756284819894062 PMID: 31897087

Schwabe, R. F., & Jobin, C. (2013). The microbiome and cancer. *Nature Reviews. Cancer, 13*(11), 800–812. DOI: 10.1038/nrc3610 PMID: 24132111

Sędzikowska, A., & Szablewski, L. (2021). Human Gut Microbiota in Health and Selected Cancers. *International Journal of Molecular Sciences, 22*(24), 13440. DOI: 10.3390/ijms222413440 PMID: 34948234

Seekatz, A. M., Safdar, N., & Khanna, S. (2022). The role of the gut microbiome in colonization resistance and recurrent Clostridioides difficile infection. *Therapeutic Advances in Gastroenterology, 15*, 17562848221134396. DOI: 10.1177/17562848221134396 PMID: 36425405

Sender, R., Fuchs, S., & Milo, R. (2016). Revised Estimates for the Number of Human and Bacteria Cells in the Body. *PLoS Biology, 14*(8), e1002533. DOI: 10.1371/journal.pbio.1002533 PMID: 27541692

Senghor, B., Sokhna, C., Ruimy, R., & Lagier, J.-C. (2018). Gut microbiota diversity according to dietary habits and geographical provenance. *Human Microbiome Journal, 7–8*, 1–9. DOI: 10.1016/j.humic.2018.01.001

Seo, S.-S., Oh, H. Y., Lee, J.-K., Kong, J.-S., Lee, D. O., & Kim, M. K. (2016). Combined effect of diet and cervical microbiome on the risk of cervical intraepithelial neoplasia. *Clinical Nutrition (Edinburgh, Lothian), 35*(6), 1434–1441. DOI: 10.1016/j.clnu.2016.03.019 PMID: 27075319

Shang, Y., Zhang, Z., Liu, Z., Feng, B., Ren, G., Li, K., Zhou, L., Sun, Y., Li, M., Zhou, J., An, Y., Wu, K., Nie, Y., & Fan, D. (2014). miR-508-5p regulates multidrug resistance of gastric cancer by targeting ABCB1 and ZNRD1. *Oncogene, 33*(25), 3267–3276. DOI: 10.1038/onc.2013.297 PMID: 23893241

Shanti, A., Hallfors, N., Petroianu, G. A., Planelles, L., & Stefanini, C. (2021). Lymph Nodes-On-Chip: Promising Immune Platforms for Pharmacological and Toxicological Applications. *Frontiers in Pharmacology, 12*, 711307. DOI: 10.3389/fphar.2021.711307 PMID: 34483920

Shao, K., Pu, W., Zhang, J., Guo, S., Qian, F., Glurich, I., Jin, Q., Ma, Y., Ju, S., Zhang, Z., & Ding, W. (2021). DNA hypermethylation contributes to colorectal cancer metastasis by regulating the binding of CEBPB and TFCP2 to the CPEB1 promoter. *Clinical Epigenetics, 13*(1), 89. DOI: 10.1186/s13148-021-01071-z PMID: 33892791

Sharifi-Noghabi, H., Zolotareva, O., Collins, C. C., & Ester, M. (2019). MOLI: Multi-omics late integration with deep neural networks for drug response prediction. *Bioinformatics (Oxford, England)*, *35*(14), i501–i509. DOI: 10.1093/bioinformatics/btz318 PMID: 31510700

Sharma, P., Siwan, D., & Rudrapal, M. (2024). Introductory Chapter: Pharmacokinetics and Drug Metabolism with Special Reference to Herbal Formulations. In *Drug Metabolism and Pharmacokinetics*. IntechOpen. DOI: 10.5772/intechopen.112889

Sharma, A. D., McCoy, L., Jacobs, E., Willey, H., Behn, J. Q., Nguyen, H., Bolon, B., Curley, J. L., & Moore, M. J. (2019). Engineering a 3D functional human peripheral nerve in vitro using the Nerve-on-a-Chip platform. *Scientific Reports*, *9*(1), 8921. Advance online publication. DOI: 10.1038/s41598-019-45407-5 PMID: 31222141

Sharma, K., Dhar, N., Thacker, V. V., Simonet, T. M., Signorino-Gelo, F., Knott, G., & McKinney, J. D. (2021). Dynamic persistence of intracellular bacterial communities of uropathogenic escherichia coli in a human bladder-chip model of urinary tract infections. *eLife*, *10*. Advance online publication. DOI: 10.7554/eLife.66481 PMID: 34219648

Sheller, M. J., Edwards, B., Reina, G. A., Martin, J., Pati, S., Kotrotsou, A., Milchenko, M., Xu, W., Marcus, D., Colen, R. R., & Bakas, S. (2020). Federated learning in medicine: Facilitating multi-institutional collaborations without sharing patient data. *Scientific Reports*, *10*(1), 12598. DOI: 10.1038/s41598-020-69250-1 PMID: 32724046

Shendure, J., Balasubramanian, S., Church, G. M., Gilbert, W., Rogers, J., Schloss, J. A., & Waterston, R. H. (2017). DNA sequencing at 40: Past, present, and future. *Nature*, *550*(7676), 345–353. DOI: 10.1038/nature24286 PMID: 29019985

Sherif, Z. A., Ogunwobi, O. O., & Ressom, H. W. (2025). Mechanisms and technologies in cancer epigenetics. *Frontiers in Oncology*, *14*, 1513654. Advance online publication. DOI: 10.3389/fonc.2024.1513654 PMID: 39839798

Shi, C., Cheng, L., Yu, Y., Chen, S., Dai, Y., Yang, J., Zhang, H., Chen, J., & Geng, N. (2024). Multi-omics integration analysis: Tools and applications in environmental toxicology. *Environmental Pollution*, *124675*, 124675. Advance online publication. DOI: 10.1016/j.envpol.2024.124675 PMID: 39103035

Shik Mun, K., Arora, K., Huang, Y., Yang, F., Yarlagadda, S., Ramananda, Y., Abu-El-Haija, M., Palermo, J. J., Appakalai, B. N., Nathan, J. D., & Naren, A. P. (2019). Patient-derived pancreas-on-a-chip to model cystic fibrosis-related disorders. *Nature Communications*, *10*(1), 3124. Advance online publication. DOI: 10.1038/s41467-019-11178-w PMID: 31311920

Shimada, T. (2006). Xenobiotic-Metabolizing Enzymes Involved in Activation and Detoxification of Carcinogenic Polycyclic Aromatic Hydrocarbons. *Drug Metabolism and Pharmacokinetics*, *21*(4), 257–276. DOI: 10.2133/dmpk.21.257 PMID: 16946553

Shimizu, T., LoRusso, P. M., Papadopoulos, K. P., Patnaik, A., Beeram, M., Smith, L. S., Rasco, D. W., Mays, T. A., Chambers, G., Ma, A., Wang, J., Laliberte, R., Voi, M., & Tolcher, A. W. (2014). Phase I First-in-Human Study of CUDC-101, a Multitargeted Inhibitor of HDACs, EGFR, and HER2 in Patients with Advanced Solid Tumors. *Clinical Cancer Research*, *20*(19), 5032–5040. DOI: 10.1158/1078-0432.CCR-14-0570 PMID: 25107918

Shi, Y. S., Zhao, Y., Li, X. N., Li, M. Z., & Li, J. L. (2023). Xenobiotic-sensing nuclear receptors as targets for phthalates-induced lung injury and antagonism of lycopene. *Chemosphere*, *312*, 137265. DOI: 10.1016/j.chemosphere.2022.137265 PMID: 36403809

Shi, Z., & Han, S. (2025). Personalized statin therapy: Targeting metabolic processes to modulate the therapeutic and adverse effects of statins. *Heliyon*, *11*(1), e41629. Advance online publication. DOI: 10.1016/j.heliyon.2025.e41629 PMID: 39866414

Show, S., & Halder, G. (2024). Biodegradation of Anti-Inflammatory, Non-Steroidal, Pharmaceutical Active Compounds. In *Biodegradation of Toxic and Hazardous Chemicals* (pp. 14–29). CRC Press. DOI: 10.1201/9781003391487-2

Shreenidhi, K. S., Vigneshwar, R., Sv, S. R., Maline, M., Roy, S., & Geetha, V. (2024). A Study on Toxicity Mechanisms of Xenobiotics Using Network Pharmacology Approach. *Current Trends in Biotechnology and Pharmacy*, *18*(4s), 138–151. DOI: 10.5530/ctbp.2024.4s.11

Sieber, S., Wirth, L., Cavak, N., Koenigsmark, M., Marx, U., Lauster, R., & Rosowski, M. (2018). Bone marrow-on-a-chip: Long-term culture of human haematopoietic stem cells in a three-dimensional microfluidic environment. *Journal of Tissue Engineering and Regenerative Medicine*, *12*(2), 479–489. DOI: 10.1002/term.2507 PMID: 28658717

Sillé, F. C. M., Busquet, F., Fitzpatrick, S., Herrmann, K., Leenhouts-Martin, L., Luechtefeld, T., Maertens, A., Miller, G. W., Smirnova, L., Tsaioun, K., & Hartung, T. (2024). The Implementation Moonshot Project for Alternative Chemical Testing (IMPACT) toward a Human Exposome Project. *ALTEX*, *41*(3), 344–362. DOI: 10.14573/altex.2407081 PMID: 39016082

Silva, J., Oliveira, P. A., Duarte, J. A., & Faustino-Rocha, A. I. (2025). Mammary Cancer Models: An Overview from the Past to the Future. *In Vivo (Athens, Greece)*, *39*(1), 1–16. DOI: 10.21873/invivo.13800 PMID: 39740866

Simner, P. J., Miller, S., & Carroll, K. C. (2017). Understanding the promises and hurdles of metagenomic next-generation sequencing as a diagnostic tool for infectious diseases. *Clinical Infectious Diseases*, *66*(5), 778–788. DOI: 10.1093/cid/cix881 PMID: 29040428

Singh, D. D. (2024). Epigenetic Mechanisms of Endocrine-Disrupting Chemicals in Breast Cancer and Their Impact on Dietary Intake. *Journal of Xenobiotics*, *15*(1), 1. DOI: 10.3390/jox15010001 PMID: 39846533

Singh, L. K., Kumar, A., Siddiqi, N. J., & Sharma, B. (2024). Heavy metals altered the xenobiotic metabolism of rats by targeting the GST enzyme: An in vitro and in silico study. *Toxicology*, *509*, 153946. DOI: 10.1016/j.tox.2024.153946 PMID: 39270966

Singh, M., Mishra, R. C., Shah, I., Wadhwa, V., & Mor, V. (2023a). Xenobiotics: Sources, Pathways, Degradation, and Risk Associated with Major Emphasis on Pharmaceutical Compounds. In *Xenobiotics in Urban Ecosystems: Sources, Distribution and Health Impacts* (pp. 87–106). Springer International Publishing. DOI: 10.1007/978-3-031-35775-6_5

Singh, R. D., Avadhesh, A., Sharma, G., Dholariya, S., Shah, R. B., Goyal, B., & Gupta, S. C. (2023). Potential of Cytochrome P450, a Family of Xenobiotic Metabolizing Enzymes, in Cancer Therapy. *Antioxidants & Redox Signaling*, *38*(10–12), 853–876. DOI: 10.1089/ars.2022.0116 PMID: 36242099

Singh, S., & Li, S. S.-L. (2012). Epigenetic Effects of Environmental Chemicals Bisphenol A and Phthalates. *International Journal of Molecular Sciences*, *13*(8), 10143–10153. DOI: 10.3390/ijms130810143 PMID: 22949852

Singh, S., Sarma, D. K., Verma, V., Nagpal, R., & Kumar, M. (2023b). Unveiling the future of metabolic medicine: Omics technologies driving personalized solutions for precision treatment of metabolic disorders. *Biochemical and Biophysical Research Communications*, *682*, 1–20. Advance online publication. DOI: 10.1016/j.bbrc.2023.09.064 PMID: 37788525

Singh, S., Sharma, P., Pal, N., Kumawat, M., Shubham, S., Sarma, D. K., Tiwari, R. R., Kumar, M., & Nagpal, R. (2022). Impact of Environmental Pollutants on Gut Microbiome and Mental Health via the Gut–Brain Axis. *Microorganisms*, *10*(7), 1457. DOI: 10.3390/microorganisms10071457 PMID: 35889175

Siravegna, G., Marsoni, S., Siena, S., & Bardelli, A. (2017). Integrating liquid biopsies into the management of cancer. *Nature Reviews. Clinical Oncology*, *14*(9), 531–548. DOI: 10.1038/nrclinonc.2017.14 PMID: 28252003

Si, W., Shen, J., Zheng, H., & Fan, W. (2019). The role and mechanisms of action of microRNAs in cancer drug resistance. *Clinical Epigenetics*, *11*(1), 25. DOI: 10.1186/s13148-018-0587-8 PMID: 30744689

Skonberg, C., & Olsen, J. (2023). A review of the synthesis, bioanalysis, and chemical reactivity of xenobiotic acyl-coenzyme a thioesters. *Medicinal Chemistry Research*, *32*(9), 2001–2015. DOI: 10.1007/s00044-023-03129-4

Smith, C. C., Selitsky, S. R., Chai, S., Liu, W., Busman-Sahay, K., & Parker, J. S. (2020). Long-read sequencing for improved detection of oncogenic fusions in acute leukemia. *Leukemia*, *34*(3), 799–810. DOI: 10.1038/s41375-019-0677-9 PMID: 31628430

Smith, J. N., Gaither, K. A., & Pande, P. (2022). Competitive Metabolism of Polycyclic Aromatic Hydrocarbons (PAHs): An Assessment Using In Vitro Metabolism and Physiologically Based Pharmacokinetic (PBPK) Modeling. *International Journal of Environmental Research and Public Health*, *19*(14), 8266. DOI: 10.3390/ijerph19148266 PMID: 35886113

Smith, M. T., Guyton, K. Z., Gibbons, C. F., Fritz, J. M., Portier, C. J., Rusyn, I., DeMarini, D. M., Caldwell, J. C., Kavlock, R. J., Lambert, P. F., Hecht, S. S., Bucher, J. R., Stewart, B. W., Baan, R. A., Cogliano, V. J., & Straif, K. (2016). Key characteristics of carcinogens as a basis for organizing data on mechanisms of carcinogenesis. In *Environmental Health Perspectives* (Vol. 124, pp. 713–721). Public Health Services, US Dept of Health and Human Services. DOI: 10.1289/ehp.1509912

Somala, C. S., Sathyapriya, S., Bharathkumar, N., Anand, T., Mathangi, D. C., & Saravanan, K. M. (2025). Therapeutic Potential of FTO Demethylase in Metabolism and Disease Pathways. *The Protein Journal*, *44*(1), 21–34. DOI: 10.1007/s10930-025-10250-3 PMID: 39923206

Sonnenburg, J. L., & Bäckhed, F. (2016). Diet–microbiota interactions as moderators of human metabolism. *Nature*, *535*(7610), 56–64. DOI: 10.1038/nature18846 PMID: 27383980

Srinivas, U. S., Tan, B. W. Q., Vellayappan, B. A., & Jeyasekharan, A. D. (2019). ROS and the DNA damage response in cancer. *Redox Biology*, *25*, 101084. DOI: 10.1016/j.redox.2018.101084 PMID: 30612957

Stanley, L. A. (2024). Drug metabolism. In *Pharmacognosy* (pp. 597–624). Academic Press. DOI: 10.1016/B978-0-443-18657-8.00029-3

Stepanov, I., Muzic, J., Le, C. T., Sebero, E., Villalta, P., Ma, B., Jensen, J., Hatsukami, D., & Hecht, S. S. (2013). Analysis of 4-Hydroxy-1-(3-pyridyl)-1-butanone (HPB)-Releasing DNA Adducts in Human Exfoliated Oral Mucosa Cells by Liquid Chromatography–Electrospray Ionization–Tandem Mass Spectrometry. *Chemical Research in Toxicology*, *26*(1), 37–45. DOI: 10.1021/tx300282k PMID: 23252610

Stewart, C. A., Gay, C. M., Xi, Y., Sivajothi, S., Sivakumar, S., Fujimoto, J., & Wistuba, I. I. (2021). Single-cell analyses reveal increased intratumoral heterogeneity after the onset of therapy resistance in small-cell lung cancer. *Nature Cancer*, *2*(4), 404–421. DOI: 10.1038/s43018-021-00184-1 PMID: 33521652

Stone, L. (2023). A vagina on a chip to model microbiome–host interactions. In *Nature Reviews Urology* (Vol. 20, p. 64). Nature Research., DOI: 10.1038/s41585-022-00717-8

Subramanian, I., Verma, S., Kumar, S., Jere, A., & Anamika, K. (2020). Multi-omics Data Integration, Interpretation, and Its Application. *Bioinformatics and Biology Insights*, *14*, 117793221989905. DOI: 10.1177/1177932219899051 PMID: 32076369

Suez, J., Zmora, N., Zilberman-Schapira, G., Mor, U., Dori-Bachash, M., Bashiardes, S., Zur, M., Regev-Lehavi, D., Ben-Zeev Brik, R., Federici, S., Horn, M., Cohen, Y., Moor, A. E., Zeevi, D., Korem, T., Kotler, E., Harmelin, A., Itzkovitz, S., Maharshak, N., & Elinav, E. (2018). Post-Antibiotic Gut Mucosal Microbiome Reconstitution Is Impaired by Probiotics and Improved by Autologous FMT. *Cell*, *174*(6), 1406–1423.e16. DOI: 10.1016/j.cell.2018.08.047 PMID: 30193113

Sun, C., Wang, A., Zhou, Y., Chen, P., Wang, X., Huang, J., Gao, J., Wang, X., Shu, L., Lu, J., Dai, W., Bu, Z., Ji, J., & He, J. (2023). Spatially resolved multi-omics highlights cell-specific metabolic remodeling and interactions in gastric cancer. *Nature Communications*, *14*(1), 2692. DOI: 10.1038/s41467-023-38360-5 PMID: 37164975

Sun, J., Chen, F., & Wu, G. (2023). Potential effects of gut microbiota on host cancers: Focus on immunity, DNA damage, cellular pathways, and anticancer therapy. *The ISME Journal*, *17*(10), 1535–1551. DOI: 10.1038/s41396-023-01483-0 PMID: 37553473

Sun, L., Yang, H., Cai, Y., Li, W., Liu, G., & Tang, Y. (2019). *In Silico* Prediction of Endocrine Disrupting Chemicals Using Single-Label and Multilabel Models. *Journal of Chemical Information and Modeling*, *59*(3), 973–982. DOI: 10.1021/acs.jcim.8b00551 PMID: 30807141

Sun, Y., Zhang, Y., Qi, X., Zhou, Y., & Yu, J. (2021). Helicobacter pylori-induced DNA methylation alterations in gastric carcinogenesis: A pathway-based analysis of whole-genome methylation sequencing data. *Frontiers in Oncology, 11*, 654230. DOI: 10.3389/fonc.2021.654230

Su, Q., & Liu, Q. (2021). Factors Affecting Gut Microbiome in Daily Diet. *Frontiers in Nutrition, 8*, 644138. DOI: 10.3389/fnut.2021.644138 PMID: 34041257

Surendradoss, J., Varghese, A., & Deb, S. (2023). Drug metabolism: Detoxification and xenobiotic biotransformation. In *Biologically Active Small Molecules* (pp. 287–332). Apple Academic Press. DOI: 10.1201/9781003283119-17

Szabo, C., Coletta, C., Chao, C., Módis, K., Szczesny, B., Papapetropoulos, A., & Hellmich, M. R. (2013). Tumor-derived hydrogen sulfide, produced by cystathionine-β-synthase, stimulates bioenergetics, cell proliferation, and angiogenesis in colon cancer. *Proceedings of the National Academy of Sciences of the United States of America, 110*(30), 12474–12479. DOI: 10.1073/pnas.1306241110 PMID: 23836652

Takata, A., Yamauchi, H., Yamashita, K., Aminaka, M., Hitomi, T., Toya, T., & Kohyama, N. (2025). Mesothelioma carcinogenesis of chrysotile and forsterite compared and validated by intraperitoneal injection in rat. *Industrial Health, 63*(1), 14–28. Advance online publication. DOI: 10.2486/indhealth.2024-0025

Talevi, A., & Bellera, C. L. (2022). Organic anion transporters and organic anion transporting polypeptides. In *The ADME Encyclopedia: A Comprehensive Guide on Biopharmacy and Pharmacokinetics* (pp. 739–745). Springer International Publishing. DOI: 10.1007/978-3-030-84860-6_84

Tamási, V., Monostory, K., Prough, R. A., & Falus, A. (2011). Role of xenobiotic metabolism in cancer: Involvement of transcriptional and miRNA regulation of P450s. *Cellular and Molecular Life Sciences : CMLS, 68*(7), 1131–1146. DOI: 10.1007/s00018-010-0600-7 PMID: 21184128

Tamer, F., & Yuksel, M. E. (2020). Colonoscopy in patients with psoriasis before the initiation of treatment with biological agents. *Dermatologic Therapy, 33*(4). Advance online publication. DOI: 10.1111/dth.13720 PMID: 32506694

Tantengco, O. A. G., Richardson, L., Radnaa, E., Kammala, A. K., Kechichian, T., Ganguly, E., Kim, S., Han, A., Medina, P. M., & Menon, R. (2022). Cervix-on-a-chip for investigating ascending Ureaplasma parvum infection in pregnancy. *American Journal of Obstetrics and Gynecology, 226*(1), S12–S13. DOI: 10.1016/j.ajog.2021.11.068

Taş, İ., Varlı, M., Pulat, S., Sim, H. B., Kim, J.-J., & Kim, H. (2024). TDO2 inhibition counters Benzo[a]pyrene-induced immune evasion and suppresses tumorigenesis in lung adenocarcinoma. *Cancer & Metabolism, 12*(1), 36. DOI: 10.1186/s40170-024-00365-z PMID: 39593177

Taylor, J. L., Debost, J.-C. P. G., Morton, S. U., Wigdor, E. M., Heyne, H. O., Lal, D., Howrigan, D. P., Bloemendal, A., Larsen, J. T., Kosmicki, J. A., Weiner, D. J., Homsy, J., Seidman, J. G., Seidman, C. E., Agerbo, E., McGrath, J. J., Mortensen, P. B., Petersen, L., Daly, M. J., & Robinson, E. B. (2019). Paternal-age-related de novo mutations and risk for five disorders. *Nature Communications, 10*(1), 3043. DOI: 10.1038/s41467-019-11039-6 PMID: 31292440

Tedaldi, A. M., Behrouzi, P., & Grootswagers, P. (2025). Diet, lifestyle and telomere length: Using Copula Graphical Models on NHANES data. *Aging (Albany NY), 17*(2), 329–356. DOI: 10.18632/aging.206194 PMID: 39883078

Tekpli, X., Zienolddiny, S., Skaug, V., Stangeland, L., Haugen, A., & Mollerup, S. (2012). DNA methylation of the CYP1A1 enhancer is associated with smoking-induced genetic alterations in human lung. *International Journal of Cancer, 131*(7), 1509–1516. DOI: 10.1002/ijc.27421 PMID: 22213191

Telkmann, K., Gudi-Mindermann, H., Bogers, R., Ahrens, J., Tönnies, J., van Kamp, I., Vrijkotte, T., & Bolte, G. (2025). Identification of exposome clusters based on societal, social, built and natural environment – results of the ABCD cohort study. *Environment International, 197*, 109335. DOI: 10.1016/j.envint.2025.109335 PMID: 39983415

Terrazas-Salgado, L., García-Gasca, A., Betancourt-Lozano, M., Llera-Herrera, R., Alvarado-Cruz, I., & Yáñez-Rivera, B. (2022). Epigenetic transgenerational modifications induced by xenobiotic exposure in zebrafish. *Frontiers in Cell and Developmental Biology, 10*, 832982. DOI: 10.3389/fcell.2022.832982 PMID: 35281093

Thomas, R. M., Gharaibeh, R. Z., Gauthier, J., Beveridge, M., Pope, J. L., Guijarro, M. V., Yu, Q., He, Z., Ohland, C., Newsome, R., Trevino, J., Hughes, S. J., Reinhard, M., Winglee, K., Fodor, A. A., Zajac-Kaye, M., & Jobin, C. (2018). Intestinal microbiota enhances pancreatic carcinogenesis in preclinical models. *Carcinogenesis, 39*(8), 1068–1078. DOI: 10.1093/carcin/bgy073 PMID: 29846515

Thu, M. S., Ondee, T., Nopsopon, T., Farzana, I. A. K., Fothergill, J. L., Hirankarn, N., Campbell, B. J., & Pongpirul, K. (2023). Effect of Probiotics in Breast Cancer: A Systematic Review and Meta-Analysis. *Biology (Basel), 12*(2), 280. DOI: 10.3390/biology12020280 PMID: 36829557

Thum, T., Erpenbeck, V. J., Moeller, J., Hohlfeld, J. M., Krug, N., & Borlak, J. (2006). Expression of Xenobiotic Metabolizing Enzymes in Different Lung Compartments of Smokers and Nonsmokers. *Environmental Health Perspectives, 114*(11), 1655–1661. DOI: 10.1289/ehp.8861 PMID: 17107849

Tomkiewicz, C., Coumoul, X., Nioche, P., Barouki, R., & Blanc, E. B. (2024). Costs of molecular adaptation to the chemical exposome: A focus on xenobiotic metabolism pathways. *Philosophical Transactions of the Royal Society of London. Series B, Biological Sciences, 379*(1898), 20220510. Advance online publication. DOI: 10.1098/rstb.2022.0510 PMID: 38310928

Tomonaga, T., Izumi, H., Yoshiura, Y., Nishida, C., Yatera, K., & Morimoto, Y. (2021). Examination of Surfactant Protein D as a Biomarker for Evaluating Pulmonary Toxicity of Nanomaterials in Rat. *International Journal of Molecular Sciences, 22*(9), 4635. DOI: 10.3390/ijms22094635 PMID: 33924924

Toraño, E. G., García, M. G., Fernández-Morera, J. L., Niño-García, P., & Fernández, A. F. (2016). The Impact of External Factors on the Epigenome: *In Utero* and over Lifetime. *BioMed Research International, 2016*, 1–17. DOI: 10.1155/2016/2568635 PMID: 27294112

Tortolero, G. A., Betts, A. C., Suragh, T. A., Pruitt, S. L., Roth, M. E., & Murphy, C. C. (2024). Social vulnerability and survival in 112000 adolescents and young adults with cancer: A population-based study. *Journal of the National Cancer Institute, 116*(12), 2003–2008. DOI: 10.1093/jnci/djae170 PMID: 39084675

Towle, K. M., Benson, S. M., Egnot, N. S., & Marsh, G. M. (2021). An Ecological Evaluation of Vinyl Chloride Exposure and Liver Cancer Incidence and Mortality in Texas. *Journal of Clinical and Translational Hepatology, 000*(000), 1–7. DOI: 10.14218/JCTH.2020.00073 PMID: 33604260

Truhn, D., Tayebi Arasteh, S., Saldanha, O. L., Müller-Franzes, G., Khader, F., Quirke, P., West, N. P., Gray, R., Hutchins, G. G. A., James, J. A., Loughrey, M. B., Salto-Tellez, M., Brenner, H., Brobeil, A., Yuan, T., Chang-Claude, J., Hoffmeister, M., Foersch, S., Han, T., & Kather, J. N. (2024). Encrypted federated learning for secure decentralized collaboration in cancer image analysis. *Medical Image Analysis, 92*, 103059. DOI: 10.1016/j.media.2023.103059 PMID: 38104402

Tsai, Y.-S., Jou, Y.-C., Cheong, I. S., Tung, H.-T., Hsu, L.-N., Tsai, H.-T., & Tzai, T.-S. (2025). Phthalate exposure induces microRNA-5010/Nrf2-EGR1/GDF15 signaling expression in prostate cancer. *Ecotoxicology and Environmental Safety, 290*, 117759. DOI: 10.1016/j.ecoenv.2025.117759 PMID: 39837010

Tseng, C.-H., Tsuang, B.-J., Chiang, C.-J., Ku, K.-C., Tseng, J.-S., Yang, T.-Y., Hsu, K.-H., Chen, K.-C., Yu, S.-L., Lee, W.-C., Liu, T.-W., Chan, C.-C., & Chang, G.-C. (2019). The Relationship Between Air Pollution and Lung Cancer in Non-smokers in Taiwan. *Journal of Thoracic Oncology*, *14*(5), 784–792. DOI: 10.1016/j.jtho.2018.12.033 PMID: 30664991

Tundjungsari, V., Ernawati, K., & Mutia, N. (2020). *Public Health Surveillance to Promote Clean and Healthy Life Behaviours Using Big Data Approach (An Indonesian Case Study)* (pp. 761–775). DOI: 10.1007/978-3-030-23162-0_69

Turner, N. D., & Lupton, J. R. (2021). Dietary Fiber. *Advances in Nutrition*, *12*(6), 2553–2555. DOI: 10.1093/advances/nmab116 PMID: 34687531

Uyar, B., Ronen, J., Franke, V., Gargiulo, G., & Akalin, A. (2021). Multi-omics and deep learning provide a multifaceted view of cancer. *Bioinformatics (Oxford, England)*. Advance online publication. DOI: 10.1101/2021.09.29.462364

Vasan, N., Baselga, J., & Hyman, D. M. (2019). A view on drug resistance in cancer. *Nature*, *575*(7782), 299–309. DOI: 10.1038/s41586-019-1730-1 PMID: 31723286

Vázquez-Gómez, G., Petráš, J., Dvořák, Z., & Vondráček, J. (2023). Aryl hydrocarbon receptor (AhR) and pregnane X receptor (PXR) play both distinct and common roles in the regulation of colon homeostasis and intestinal carcinogenesis. In *Biochemical Pharmacology* (Vol. 216). Elsevier Inc. DOI: 10.1016/j.bcp.2023.115797

Vermeulen, R., Schymanski, E. L., Barabási, A.-L., & Miller, G. W. (2020). The exposome and health: Where chemistry meets biology. *Science*, *367*(6476), 392–396. DOI: 10.1126/science.aay3164 PMID: 31974245

Vicidomini, C., Palumbo, R., Moccia, M., & Roviello, G. N. (2024). Oxidative Processes and Xenobiotic Metabolism in Plants: Mechanisms of Defense and Potential Therapeutic Implications. *Journal of Xenobiotics*, *14*(4), 1541–1569. DOI: 10.3390/jox14040084 PMID: 39449425

Villanueva, A., Chiang, D. Y., Newell, P., Peix, J., Thung, S., Alsinet, C., Tovar, V., Roayaie, S., Minguez, B., Sole, M., Battiston, C., Van Laarhoven, S., Fiel, M. I., Di Feo, A., Hoshida, Y., Yea, S., Toffanin, S., Ramos, A., Martignetti, J. A., & Llovet, J. M. (2008). Pivotal Role of mTOR Signaling in Hepatocellular Carcinoma. *Gastroenterology*, *135*(6), 1972–1983.e11. DOI: 10.1053/j.gastro.2008.08.008 PMID: 18929564

Vineis, P., & Dagnino, S. (2024). An evolutionary perspective for the exposome. *Exposome*, *4*(1), osae008. Advance online publication. DOI: 10.1093/exposome/osae008 PMID: 39867564

Vineis, P., Schatzkin, A., & Potter, J. D. (2010). Models of carcinogenesis: An overview. *Carcinogenesis, 31*(10), 1703–1709. DOI: 10.1093/carcin/bgq087 PMID: 20430846

VoPham, T., White, A. J., & Jones, R. R.VoPham. (2024). Geospatial Science for the Environmental Epidemiology of Cancer in the Exposome Era. *Cancer Epidemiology, Biomarkers & Prevention, 33*(4), 451–460. DOI: 10.1158/1055-9965.EPI-23-1237 PMID: 38566558

Vuong, T. P. (2022). Research on the Relationship between Exposure to Dioxins and Cancer Incidence in Vietnam. *Toxics, 10*(7), 384. DOI: 10.3390/toxics10070384 PMID: 35878289

Walboomers, J. M., Jacobs, M. V., Manos, M. M., Bosch, F. X., Kummer, J. A., Shah, K. V., & Meijer, C. J. (1999). Human papillomavirus is a necessary cause of invasive cervical cancer worldwide. *The Journal of Pathology, 189*(1), 12–19. DOI: 10.1002/(SICI)1096-9896(199909)189:1<12::AID-PATH431>3.0.CO;2-F PMID: 10451482

Waldum, H., & Fossmark, R. (2023). Inflammation and Digestive Cancer. *International Journal of Molecular Sciences, 24*(17), 13503. DOI: 10.3390/ijms241713503 PMID: 37686307

Wang, F., Zhuang, Z., Gao, F., He, R., Zhang, S., Wang, L., Liu, J., & Li, Y. (2024). TMO-Net: An explainable pretrained multi-omics model for multi-task learning in oncology. *Genome Biology, 25*(1), 149. DOI: 10.1186/s13059-024-03293-9 PMID: 38845006

Wang, L., Zhu, R., Huang, Z., Li, H., & Zhu, H. (2013). Lipopolysaccharide-induced toll-like receptor 4 signaling in cancer cells promotes cell survival and proliferation in hepatocellular carcinoma. *Digestive Diseases and Sciences, 58*(8), 2223–2236. DOI: 10.1007/s10620-013-2745-3 PMID: 23828139

Wang, W., Rong, Z., Wang, G., Hou, Y., Yang, F., & Qiu, M. (2023). Cancer metabolites: Promising biomarkers for cancer liquid biopsy. *Biomarker Research, 11*(1), 66. DOI: 10.1186/s40364-023-00507-3 PMID: 37391812

Wang, W., Zhen, S., Ping, Y., Wang, L., & Zhang, Y. (2024). Metabolomic biomarkers in liquid biopsy: Accurate cancer diagnosis and prognosis monitoring. *Frontiers in Oncology, 14*, 1331215. DOI: 10.3389/fonc.2024.1331215 PMID: 38384814

Wang, X., Guan, P., You, L., Qin, W., Li, Q., Wang, X., Chen, Q., Yu, D., Ye, Y., Wang, T., Liu, X., Fan, J., & Xu, G. (2025). Risk of serum circulating environmental chemical residues to esophageal squamous cell carcinoma: A nested case–control metabolome-wide association study. *Analytical and Bioanalytical Chemistry*, *417*(13), 2783–2795. Advance online publication. DOI: 10.1007/s00216-025-05784-5 PMID: 39939416

Wang, X., Qi, Y., & Zheng, H. (2022). Dietary Polyphenol, Gut Microbiota, and Health Benefits. *Antioxidants*, *11*(6), 1212. DOI: 10.3390/antiox11061212 PMID: 35740109

Wan, J. C. M., Massie, C., Garcia-Corbacho, J., Mouliere, F., Brenton, J. D., Caldas, C., & Rosenfeld, N. (2020). Liquid biopsies come of age: Towards implementation of circulating tumor DNA. *Nature Reviews. Cancer*, *17*(4), 223–238. DOI: 10.1038/nrc.2017.7 PMID: 28233803

Wan, M., Simonin, E. M., Johnson, M. M., Zhang, X., Lin, X., Gao, P., Patel, C. J., Yousuf, A., Snyder, M. P., Hong, X., Wang, X., Sampath, V., & Nadeau, K. C. (2025). Exposomics: A review of methodologies, applications, and future directions in molecular medicine. *EMBO Molecular Medicine*, *17*(4), 1–10. DOI: 10.1038/s44321-025-00191-w PMID: 39870881

Wan, Y., Ding, J., Jia, Z., Hong, Y., Tian, G., Zheng, S., Pan, P., Wang, J., & Liang, H. (2024). Current trends and research topics regarding organoids: A bibliometric analysis of global research from 2000 to 2023. *Heliyon*, *10*(12), e32965. DOI: 10.1016/j.heliyon.2024.e32965 PMID: 39022082

Wei, X., Huang, Z., Jiang, L., Li, Y., Zhang, X., Leng, Y., & Jiang, C. (2022). Charting the landscape of the environmental exposome. In *iMeta* (Vol. 1). John Wiley and Sons Inc. DOI: 10.1002/imt2.50

Weinberg, B. A., Murphy, C. C., Freyer, D. R., Greathouse, K. L., Blancato, J. K., Stoffel, E. M., Drewes, J. L., Blaes, A., Salsman, J. M., You, Y. N., Arem, H., Mukherji, R., Kanth, P., Hu, X., Fabrizio, A., Hartley, M. L., Giannakis, M., & Marshall, J. L. (2025). Rethinking the rise of early-onset gastrointestinal cancers: A call to action. *JNCI Cancer Spectrum*, *9*(1), pkaf002. Advance online publication. DOI: 10.1093/jncics/pkaf002 PMID: 39814070

Wen, L., & Han, Z. (2021). Identification and validation of xenobiotic metabolism-associated prognostic signature based on five genes to evaluate immune microenvironment in colon cancer. *Journal of Gastrointestinal Oncology*, *12*(6), 2788–2802. DOI: 10.21037/jgo-21-655 PMID: 35070407

Wheeler, M. A., & Quintana, F. J. (2025). The neuroimmune connectome in health and disease. *Nature*, *638*(8050), 333–342. DOI: 10.1038/s41586-024-08474-x PMID: 39939792

Wiese, D., DuBois, T. D., Sorice, K. A., Fang, C. Y., Ragin, C., Daly, M., Reese, A. C., Henry, K. A., & Lynch, S. M. (2024). An exploratory analysis of the impact of area-level exposome on geographic disparities in aggressive prostate cancer. *Scientific Reports*, *14*(1), 16900. DOI: 10.1038/s41598-024-63726-0 PMID: 39075110

Wijaya, A. P., Nugraha, A. L., Sukmono, A., & Firdaus, H. S. (2022). Study on the analysis of demographic data based on spatial information systems. *IOP Conference Series. Earth and Environmental Science*, *1098*(1), 012029. DOI: 10.1088/1755-1315/1098/1/012029

Wild, C. P. (2005). Complementing the genome with an "exposome": The outstanding challenge of environmental exposure measurement in molecular epidemiology. In *Cancer Epidemiology Biomarkers and Prevention* (Vol. 14, pp. 1847–1850). DOI: 10.1158/1055-9965.EPI-05-0456

Williams, J. A., & Phillips, D. H. (n.d.). *Mammary Expression of Xenobiotic Metabolizing Enzymes and Their Potential Role in Breast Cancer.*

Wilson, I. D., & Nicholson, J. K. (2017). Gut microbiome interactions with drug metabolism, efficacy, and toxicity. *Translational Research; the Journal of Laboratory and Clinical Medicine*, *179*, 204–222. DOI: 10.1016/j.trsl.2016.08.002 PMID: 27591027

Winz, C., Zong, W., & Suh, N. (2023). Endocrine-disrupting compounds and metabolomic reprogramming in breast cancer. *Journal of Biochemical and Molecular Toxicology*, *37*(12), e23506. DOI: 10.1002/jbt.23506 PMID: 37598318

Wong, S. H., & Yu, J. (2019). Gut microbiota in colorectal cancer: Mechanisms of action and clinical applications. *Nature Reviews. Gastroenterology & Hepatology*, *16*(11), 690–704. DOI: 10.1038/s41575-019-0209-8 PMID: 31554963

Wong, S. H., Zhao, L., Zhang, X., Nakatsu, G., Han, J., Xu, W., Xiao, X., Kwong, T. N. Y., Tsoi, H., Wu, W. K. K., Zeng, B., Chan, F. K. L., Sung, J. J. Y., Wei, H., & Yu, J. (2017). Gavage of Fecal Samples From Patients With Colorectal Cancer Promotes Intestinal Carcinogenesis in Germ-Free and Conventional Mice. *Gastroenterology*, *153*(6), 1621–1633.e6. DOI: 10.1053/j.gastro.2017.08.022 PMID: 28823860

Wright, A. T., Hudson, L. A., & Garcia, W. L. (2023). Activity-Based Protein Profiling–Enabling Phenotyping of Host-Associated and Environmental Microbiomes. *Israel Journal of Chemistry*, *63*(3-4), e202200099. DOI: 10.1002/ijch.202200099

Wu, D., Zhang, K., Guan, K., Khan, F. A., Pandupuspitasari, N. S., Negara, W., Sun, F., & Huang, C. (2024). Future in the past: Paternal reprogramming of offspring phenotype and the epigenetic mechanisms. *Archives of Toxicology, 98*(6), 1685–1703. DOI: 10.1007/s00204-024-03713-6 PMID: 38460001

Wu, Y., Rong, X., Pan, M., Wang, T., Yang, H., Chen, X., Xiao, Z., & Zhao, C. (2022). Integrated Analysis Reveals the Gut Microbial Metabolite TMAO Promotes Inflammatory Hepatocellular Carcinoma by Upregulating POSTN. *Frontiers in Cell and Developmental Biology, 10*, 840171. DOI: 10.3389/fcell.2022.840171 PMID: 35676936

Xiao, S., Cui, J., Cao, Y., Zhang, Y., Yang, J., Zheng, L., Zhao, F., Liu, X., Zhou, Z., Liu, D., & Wang, P. (2024). Adolescent exposure to organophosphate insecticide malathion induces spermatogenesis dysfunction in mice by activating the HIF-1/MAPK/PI3K pathway. *Environmental Pollution, 363*, 125209. DOI: 10.1016/j.envpol.2024.125209 PMID: 39476999

Xiaoyi, Z., Yang, H., Kumar, N., Bhutto, M. H., Kun, W., & Hu, T. (2023). Assessing Chinese Textile and Apparel Industry Business Sustainability: The Role of Organization Green Culture, Green Dynamic Capabilities, and Green Innovation in Relation to Environmental Orientation and Business Sustainability. *Sustainability (Basel), 15*(11), 8588. Advance online publication. DOI: 10.3390/su15118588

Xie, G., Si, Q., Zhang, G., Fan, Y., Li, Q., Leng, P., Qiao, F., Liang, S., Yu, R., & Wang, Y. (2024). The role of imprinting genes' loss of imprints in cancers and their clinical implications. *Frontiers in Oncology, 14*, 1365474. Advance online publication. DOI: 10.3389/fonc.2024.1365474 PMID: 38812777

Xie, M. Z., Liu, J. L., Gao, Q. Z., Bo, D. Y., Wang, L., Zhou, X. C., Zhao, M. M., Zhang, Y. C., Zhang, Y. J., Zhao, G. A., & Jiao, L. Y. (2022). Proteomics-based evaluation of the mechanism underlying vascular injury via DNA interstrand cross-links, glutathione perturbation, mitogen-activated protein kinase, and Wnt and ErbB signaling pathways induced by crotonaldehyde. *Clinical Proteomics, 19*(1), 33. DOI: 10.1186/s12014-022-09369-7 PMID: 36002804

Xie, Y., Geng, Y., Yao, J., Ji, J., Chen, F., Xiao, J., Hu, X., & Ma, L. (2023). N-nitrosamines in processed meats: Exposure, formation and mitigation strategies. *Journal of Agriculture and Food Research, 13*, 100645. DOI: 10.1016/j.jafr.2023.100645

Xue, B., Zhao, J., Feng, P., Xing, J., Wu, H., & Li, Y. (2019). Epigenetic mechanism and target therapy of UHRF1 protein complex in malignancies. *OncoTargets and Therapy, 12*, 549–559. DOI: 10.2147/OTT.S192234 PMID: 30666134

Xu, H., & Li, H. (2019). Acne, the Skin Microbiome, and Antibiotic Treatment. *American Journal of Clinical Dermatology*, *20*(3), 335–344. DOI: 10.1007/s40257-018-00417-3 PMID: 30632097

Xu, M.-Q., Pan, F., Peng, L.-H., & Yang, Y.-S. (2024). Advances in the isolation, cultivation, and identification of gut microbes. *Military Medical Research*, *11*(1), 34. DOI: 10.1186/s40779-024-00534-7 PMID: 38831462

Xu, S., Lan, H., Huang, C., Ge, X., & Zhu, J. (2024). Mechanisms and emerging strategies for irinotecan-induced diarrhea. *European Journal of Pharmacology*, *176614*, 176614. Advance online publication. DOI: 10.1016/j.ejphar.2024.176614 PMID: 38677535

Xu, W. S., Parmigiani, R. B., & Marks, P. A. (2007). Histone deacetylase inhibitors: Molecular mechanisms of action. *Oncogene*, *26*(37), 5541–5552. DOI: 10.1038/sj.onc.1210620 PMID: 17694093

Xu, Y., Morales, A. J., Towlerton, A. M. H., Akilesh, S., Miller, C. P., Tykodi, S. S., & Warren, E. H. (2022). Integrated TCR repertoire analysis and single-cell transcriptomic profiling of tumor-infiltrating T cells in renal cell carcinoma identifies shared and tumor-restricted expanded clones with unique phenotypes. *Frontiers in Oncology*, *12*, 952252. DOI: 10.3389/fonc.2022.952252 PMID: 36185254

Yamada, H., Odagiri, M., Yamakita, K., Chiba, A., Ukai, A., Yasui, M., Honma, M., Sugiyama, K.-I., Ura, K., & Sassa, A. (2025). Dual-directional epi-genotoxicity assay for assessing chemically induced epigenetic effects utilizing the housekeeping TK gene. *Scientific Reports*, *15*(1), 7780. DOI: 10.1038/s41598-025-92121-6 PMID: 40044744

Yang, C. S. (2015). Influences of Dietary and Other Factors on Xenobiotic Metabolism and Carcinogenesis—A Review Article in Memory of Dr. Allan H. Conney (1930–2013). *Nutrition and Cancer*, *67*(8), 1209–1215. DOI: 10.1080/01635581.2015.1081010 PMID: 26474329

Yang, H., Rivera, Z., Jube, S., Nasu, M., Bertino, P., Goparaju, C., Franzoso, G., Lotze, M. T., Krausz, T., Pass, H. I., Bianchi, M. E., & Carbone, M. (2010). Programmed necrosis induced by asbestos in human mesothelial cells causes high-mobility group box 1 protein release and resultant inflammation. *Proceedings of the National Academy of Sciences of the United States of America*, *107*(28), 12611–12616. DOI: 10.1073/pnas.1006542107 PMID: 20616036

Yang, H., Yu, F., Qian, Z., Huang, T., Peng, T., & Hu, Z. (2024). Cytochrome P450 for environmental remediation: Catalytic mechanism, engineering strategies and future prospects. *World Journal of Microbiology & Biotechnology*, *40*(1), 33. DOI: 10.1007/s11274-023-03823-w PMID: 38057619

Yang, R., Lu, Y., Yin, N., & Faiola, F. (2023). Transcriptomic Integration Analyses Uncover Common Bisphenol A Effects Across Species and Tissues Primarily Mediated by Disruption of JUN/FOS, EGFR, ER, PPARG, and P53 Pathways. *Environmental Science & Technology*, *57*(48), 19156–19168. DOI: 10.1021/acs.est.3c02016 PMID: 37978927

Yang, Y., Chen, Y., Xu, S., Guo, X., Jia, G., Ping, J., Shu, X., Zhao, T., Yuan, F., Wang, G., Xie, Y., Ci, H., Liu, H., Qi, Y., Liu, Y., Liu, D., Li, W., Ye, F., Shu, X.-O., & Long, J. (2024). Integrating muti-omics data to identify tissue-specific DNA methylation biomarkers for cancer risk. *Nature Communications*, *15*(1), 6071. DOI: 10.1038/s41467-024-50404-y PMID: 39025880

Yan, M., Zou, X., Wang, Y., Wang, C., Wang, Y., Liu, Z., Shang, L., Cui, X., & Cao, B. (2024). Impact of Metagenomic Next-Generation Sequencing of Bronchoalveolar Lavage Fluid on Antimicrobial Stewardship in Patients With Lower Respiratory Tract Infections: A Retrospective Cohort Study. *The Journal of Infectious Diseases*, *229*(1), 223–231. DOI: 10.1093/infdis/jiad296 PMID: 37506257

Youn, C. K., Koh, J. W., Lee, J.-H., & Park, S.-J. (2025). P53-binding Protein Inhibits Intracellular Reactive Oxygen Species by Increasing the Expression of Metallothioneins. *Anticancer Research*, *45*(4), 1535–1545. DOI: 10.21873/anticanres.17535 PMID: 40155029

Young, A. S., Mullins, C. E., Sehgal, N., Vermeulen, R. C. H., Kolijn, P. M., Vlaanderen, J., Rahman, M. L., Birmann, B. M., Barupal, D., Lan, Q., Rothman, N., & Walker, D. I. (2025). The need for a cancer exposome atlas: A scoping review. *JNCI Cancer Spectrum*, *9*(1), pkae122. Advance online publication. DOI: 10.1093/jncics/pkae122 PMID: 39700422

Yu, F., Liu, Y., Zhang, R., Zhu, L., Zhang, T., & Shi, Y. (2022a). Recent advances in circadian-regulated pharmacokinetics and its implications for chronotherapy. *Biochemical Pharmacology*, *203*, 115185. DOI: 10.1016/j.bcp.2022.115185 PMID: 35902039

Yu, H., Lin, L., Zhang, Z., Zhang, H., & Hu, H. (2020). Targeting NF-κB pathway for the therapy of diseases: Mechanism and clinical study. *Signal Transduction and Targeted Therapy*, *5*(1), 209. DOI: 10.1038/s41392-020-00312-6 PMID: 32958760

Yu, H., Meng, H., Zhou, F., Ni, X., Shen, S., & Das, U. N. (2015). Clinical research Urinary microbiota in patients with prostate cancer and benign prostatic hyperplasia. *Archives of Medical Science : AMS, 11*, 385–394. DOI: 10.5114/aoms.2015.50970 PMID: 25995756

Yu, W., Zhang, Y., & Sang, W. (2022b). Integration of transcriptomic and metabolomic reveals metabolic pathway alteration in earthworms (*Eisenia fetida*) under copper exposure. *Comparative Biochemistry and Physiology. Toxicology & Pharmacology : CBP, 260*, 109400. DOI: 10.1016/j.cbpc.2022.109400 PMID: 35753647

Zafar H, Saier MH Gut Bacteroides species in health and disease. Gut Microbes 13:1848158. DOI: 10.1080/19490976.2020.1848158

Zambrano, E., & Ibáñez, C. A. (2025). Celebrating 280 birth years of Lamarck: Revisiting his legacy in the concept of Developmental Origins of Health and Disease. *Journal of Developmental Origins of Health and Disease, 16*, e8. DOI: 10.1017/S2040174425000030 PMID: 39950302

Zemskov, E. A., Wu, X., Aggarwal, S., Yegambaram, M., Gross, C., Lu, Q., Wang, H., Tang, H., Wang, T., & Black, S. M. (2021). Nitration of protein kinase G-Iα modulates cyclic nucleotide crosstalk via phosphodiesterase 3A: Implications for acute lung injury. *The Journal of Biological Chemistry, 297*(2), 100946. DOI: 10.1016/j.jbc.2021.100946 PMID: 34252457

Zhang, P., Carlsten, C., Chaleckis, R., Hanhineva, K., Huang, M., Isobe, T., Koistinen, V. M., Meister, I., Papazian, S., Sdougkou, K., Xie, H., Martin, J. W., Rappaport, S. M., Tsugawa, H., Walker, D. I., Woodruff, T. J., Wright, R. O., & Wheelock, C. E. (2021). Defining the Scope of Exposome Studies and Research Needs from a Multidisciplinary Perspective. In *Environmental Science and Technology Letters* (Vol. 8, Issue 10, pp. 839–852). American Chemical Society. DOI: 10.1021/acs.estlett.1c00648

Zhang, A., Luo, X., Li, Y., Yan, L., Lai, X., Yang, Q., Zhao, Z., Huang, G., Li, Z., Wu, Q., & Wang, J. (2024). Epigenetic changes driven by environmental pollutants in lung carcinogenesis: A comprehensive review. *Frontiers in Public Health, 12*, 1420933. DOI: 10.3389/fpubh.2024.1420933 PMID: 39440184

Zhang, H., & Fu, L. (2021). The role of ALDH2 in tumorigenesis and tumor progression: Targeting ALDH2 as a potential cancer treatment. *Acta Pharmaceutica Sinica. B, 11*(6), 1400–1411. DOI: 10.1016/j.apsb.2021.02.008 PMID: 34221859

Zhang, P. (2022). Influence of Foods and Nutrition on the Gut Microbiome and Implications for Intestinal Health. *International Journal of Molecular Sciences, 23*(17), 9588. DOI: 10.3390/ijms23179588 PMID: 36076980

Zhang, P., Zheng, P., & Liu, Y. (2019). Amplification of the CD24 Gene Is an Independent Predictor for Poor Prognosis of Breast Cancer. *Frontiers in Genetics, 10*, 560. DOI: 10.3389/fgene.2019.00560 PMID: 31244889

Zhao, L.-Y., Mei, J.-X., Yu, G., Lei, L., Zhang, W.-H., Liu, K., Chen, X.-L., Kołat, D., Yang, K., & Hu, J.-K. (2023a). Role of the gut microbiota in anticancer therapy: From molecular mechanisms to clinical applications. *Signal Transduction and Targeted Therapy, 8*(1), 1–27. DOI: 10.1038/s41392-023-01406-7 PMID: 37179402

Zhao, M., Chu, J., Feng, S., Guo, C., Xue, B., He, K., & Li, L. (2023b). Immunological mechanisms of inflammatory diseases caused by gut microbiota dysbiosis: A review. *Biomedicine and Pharmacotherapy, 164*, 114985. DOI: 10.1016/j.biopha.2023.114985 PMID: 37311282

Zhao, M., & Simon, R. (2020). Identification of cancer subtypes using unsupervised clustering and cancer gene expression data. *Cancers (Basel), 12*(10), 2767. DOI: 10.3390/cancers12102767 PMID: 32992445

Zheng, D., Liwinski, T., & Elinav, E. (2020). Interaction between microbiota and immunity in health and disease. *Cell Research, 30*(6), 492–506. DOI: 10.1038/s41422-020-0332-7 PMID: 32433595

Zheng, J. H., Nguyen, V. H., Jiang, S.-N., Park, S.-H., Tan, W., Hong, S. H., Shin, M. G., Chung, I.-J., Hong, Y., Bom, H.-S., Choy, H. E., Lee, S. E., Rhee, J. H., & Min, J.-J. (2017). Two-step enhanced cancer immunotherapy with engineered Salmonella typhimurium secreting heterologous flagellin. *Science Translational Medicine, 9*(376), eaak9537. Advance online publication. DOI: 10.1126/scitranslmed.aak9537 PMID: 28179508

Zhi, M.-X., & Wang, J.-S. (2024). [Advances in the applications of exposomics in the identification of environmental pollutants and their health hazards]. *Se Pu =. Se Pu = Chinese Journal of Chromatography, 42*(2), 142–149. DOI: 10.3724/SP.J.1123.2023.12011 PMID: 38374594

Zhou, H., Yuan, Y., Wang, H., Xiang, W., Li, S., Zheng, H., Wen, Y., Ming, Y., Chen, L., & Zhou, J. (2021). Gut Microbiota: A Potential Target for Cancer Interventions. *Cancer Management and Research, 13*, 8281–8296. DOI: 10.2147/CMAR.S328249 PMID: 34764691

Zhou, Y., Lv, J., Jin, S., Fu, C., Liu, B., Shen, Y., Li, M., Zhang, Y., & Feng, N. (2024). Gut microbiota derived metabolite trimethylamine N-oxide influences prostate cancer progression via the p38/HMOX1 pathway. *Frontiers in Pharmacology, 15*, 1526051. DOI: 10.3389/fphar.2024.1526051 PMID: 39850572

Zhu, J., Wu, Y., Ji, P., Qi, J., Yang, X., Pocha, C., Tustumi, F., & Biachi De Castria, T. (2024). Identification of a prognostic disulfidptosis-related gene signature in hepatocellular cancer. *Journal of Gastrointestinal Oncology*, *15*(4), 1647–1656. DOI: 10.21037/jgo-24-522 PMID: 39279954

Zhu, J., Zou, Z., Nie, P., Kou, X., Wu, B., Wang, S., Song, Z., & He, J. (2016). Downregulation of microRNA-27b-3p enhances tamoxifen resistance in breast cancer by increasing NR5A2 and CREB1 expression. *Cell Death & Disease*, *7*(11), e2454–e2454. DOI: 10.1038/cddis.2016.361 PMID: 27809310

Zitvogel, L., Ma, Y., Raoult, D., Kroemer, G., & Gajewski, T. F. (2018). The microbiome in cancer immunotherapy: Diagnostic tools and therapeutic strategies. *Science*, *359*(6382), 1366–1370. DOI: 10.1126/science.aar6918 PMID: 29567708

Zou, C., & Mallampalli, R. K. (2014). Regulation of histone modifying enzymes by the ubiquitin–proteasome system. *Biochimica et Biophysica Acta (BBA) -. Biochimica et Biophysica Acta. Molecular Cell Research*, *1843*(4), 694–702. DOI: 10.1016/j.bbamcr.2013.12.016 PMID: 24389248

About the Contributors

Ramya Raghavan is Assistant Professor at Sri Sathya Sai University for Human Excellence, India. Dr Raghavan's research interests include Genetics, Biostatistics, Biophotons, Epigenetic factors Intellectual disability, Assistive Technologies. Her recent editorial work on a book dedicated to advancing cancer treatment through spatial omics approaches underscores her commitment to innovation. As an experienced editor specializing in medical and scientific publications, Dr. Raghavan possesses a unique ability to bridge complex scientific concepts with broader societal impact. Her expertise extends to the critical intersection of the exposome and Social Determinants of Health (SDOH). Dr. Raghavan's work underscores how a holistic understanding of environmental exposures, from the molecular level to population-wide influences. Currently working on various early developmental programming projects, aligning with the Developmental Origins of Health and Disease (DOHaD) paradigm and also addressing health disparities and equitable approach to disease prevention.

***

Majdeldin Ehab Abdelgilil is a Projects Manager specializing in bioinformatics and computational biology. He holds a BSc in Applied Biotechnology from the Faculty of Science, Ain Shams University, and a Postgraduate Diploma from Nile University's School of Computer and Information Technology. He has published two articles in Q1 journals. ORCID: 0009-0002-7378-5083.

Tania Aich obtained her BSc degree in Biotechnology from JIS University, Kolkata -India in 2024. Currently she is pursuing masters in Biotechnology from Adamas University, Kolkata. One of the highlights of her academic journey was her researchwork on "Plant-based Bio-coagulats" from Cucurbita pepo and Cicer arietinum seeds, aimed at improving water quality. This led to a publication in the

"International Journal of Agriculture, Environment and Biotechnology". She also exhibited a poster on a review paper entitled "Prospects of Natural Coagulants in Treating Drinking Water"at International Seminar entitled "Recent Advances in Biological Sciences", organized by Scottish Church College, Kolkata (IQAC). To deepen her practical knowledge, she actively participated in several workshops and training programs covering topics such as protein purification, in silico data analysis and multi-omics techniques.

Anass Belbachir is a Professor of Pathological Anatomy at the Faculty of Medicine and Pharmacy of Marrakech and the Director of the Center for Regenerative Medicine. His research focuses on cancer, the use of biomaterials, and stem cells for clinical applications, aiming to advance therapeutic strategies in regenerative medicine and cancer treatment.

Ankur Bhardwaj (Ph.D.) is working as Assistant professor in the Department of Biotechnology, Shri Vaishnav Institute of Sciences, Shri Vaishnav Vidyapeeth Vishwavidyalaya, Indore. He obtained Ph.D. (2021) in Molecular Biology and Microbiology from Mangalayatan University, Aligarh, Uttar Pradesh, India. He started his career as a Lecturer in Department of Biotechnology and Life Sciences, Mangalayatan University, Aligarh in 2014 and served there for more than 05 years. He has more than 10 years of teaching and research experience. He prominently has worked in the field of plant Biotechnology, Molecular Biology, Immuno-informatics and Microbiology. He has published more than 11 research papers in peer reviewed Journals and 14 book chapters. From 2017 to 2024 he received 03 young scientist award and best thesis award in 2021. Dr. Bhardwaj has successfully guided more than 10 master's students in their final year project. Dr. Bhardwaj is a lifetime member of the Scholars Academic and Scientific Society and American Chemical Society and have published more than 05 conference abstracts. Recently Dr. Bhardwaj served as an editor for the book entitled "Exploring the Mycology and Parasitology of Plant Life: Roots and Rivals", that is going to be published by Cambridge Scholars Publisher, UK and received Prof. M.L. Khorana IJPS Best Paper Award in the area of Pharmaceutical & Medicinal Synthetic Chemistry and was a keynote speaker in National webinar series entitled "Current Trends in Infectious disease, Diagnosis and Therapeutics".

Dicky Budiman, Ph.D., is an internationally recognized global health security and pandemic preparedness expert, with more than 20 years of experience in infectious disease control, epidemiology, and public health strategy. He holds a Ph.D. in Global Health Security from Griffith University, Australia, where his research focused on health system resilience and pandemic risk governance. As a medical doctor and public health specialist, Dr. Budiman has advised governments, global institutions, and multilateral organizations including the World Health Organization (WHO), UNICEF, and the Indonesian Ministry of Health on epidemic response strategies and health system strengthening. Dr. Budiman has an active scientific portfolio as a principal investigator and co-author in numerous peer-reviewed publications, particularly in the areas of pandemic preparedness, risk communication, and the social dimensions of health crises. His scholarly work bridges empirical research and policy formulation, with publications featured in high-impact international journals and conference proceedings. He is frequently invited as a keynote speaker and panel expert in global health summits, and serves as a reviewer for several scientific journals in the fields of public health and infectious diseases. In addition to his academic and policy contributions, Dr. Budiman is a prominent scientific communicator, widely recognized for translating complex health science into accessible public knowledge. He is affiliated with leading global think tanks and continues to mentor public health professionals, contributing to capacity building in low- and middle-income countries. His multidimensional expertise uniquely positions him at the nexus of science, policy, and community engagement in global health.

Joyjyoti Das obtained his Ph.D degree in Biotechnology from the Indian Institute of Technology, Kharagpur- India in 2019. He then joined the University of Kalyani in a temporary position as a faculty for the M.Sc.course in Nanoscience & Nanotechnology. In 2021, he joined Adamas University as a regular faculty of the Biotechnology Department and is currently a Grade II Assistant Professor. His research domains of interest are cancer biology, autophagy, nanobiotechnology, microfludic sensors, and food packaging. Currently, he is working on the development of food adulterant sensors and smart food packaging systems. He has authored 22 research/review articles in journals of international repute and 5 SCI/ Scopus- indexed book chapters.

Ritika Halder is an undergraduate student currently pursuing a Bachelor of Science (Hons) in Biotechnology from Adamas University, India. With a keen interest in the fields of allergen research and cancer biology, She has actively engaged in academic and practical learning. She completed her internship at Presidency University, and gained valuable hands-on experience in advanced biological research techniques. Driven by curiosity and a passion for scientific discovery, she aspires to contribute meaningfully to the field of biological sciences.

Fatima Ezzahra Elamrani is a PhD student in Biology, specializing in Cellular Biology and Oncology Cadi Ayyad University. Her research focuses on cellular studies to enhance cancer diagnosis and treatment. She is particularly interested in integrating cutting-edge technologies, such as digital pathology, omics, and AI, to advance precision medicine.

Kholis Ernawati, S.Si, S.Ag, M.Kes., is a scholar in Environmental Health, Public Health, and Digital Health, with interdisciplinary interests in environmental science, tech-based healthcare services, and Islamic perspectives on health. She is a faculty member at the Faculty of Medicine, Universitas YARSI, Indonesia. She is known for contributing to health promotion strategies, digital health innovation, and integrating Islamic ethics into public health education. Dr. Ernawati holds a B.Sc. in Chemistry and an M.P.H. from Universitas Airlangga, a Doctorate in Environmental Health (cum laude) from Universitas Indonesia, and a B.A. in Islamic Studies (cum laude) from STIU Darul Hikmah Bekasi. She has authored over 130 publications, with 1,250+ citations, an H-index of 25, and a SINTA score of 1,558. Her research appears in international journals (Q2–Q4), covering dengue prevention, COVID-19, and big data in health surveillance. Dr. Ernawati work fosters technology-driven, culturally sensitive, and ethically grounded health practices, advancing sustainable public health in Indonesia and beyond. ID ORCID: https://orcid.org/0000-0002-3582-5294 Web of Science ResearcherID: AAD-4716-2021 Scopus: https://www.scopus.com/authid/detail.uri?authorId=57210110753.

Surendra Prakash Gupta is working as Associate professor in the Department of Biotechnology, SVIS, Shri Vaishnav Vidyapeeth Vishwavidyalaya, Indore. He received Doctorate degree in Biological Science from Dayalbagh Educational Institute, Deemed University, Agra, INDIA. He has 16 years of academic experience under various capacities in university. He has worked in Drug-DNA interactions, Bioenergy, and Computational Biology. He qualified for GATE in 2006 in Life Science. He has published 05 research papers in peer reviewed Journals, 12 book chapters, 04 conference papers and more than 30 conference abstracts. He has supervised B. Tech and M.Sc. Biotechnology students successfully and currently supervising two Doctoral students. He is also a member of several reputed professional bodies like, IAENG, Education and Development Research and ASR etc. and Lifetime Member of IARA, and ISTD, Indore Chapter.

Hafsa Gwidah is an undergraduate student in biotechnology and bioinformatics at the Faculty of Science, Tanta University. She has published a paper in bioinformatics and works as a research assistant in the genetics lab. Her research interests focus on cancer genetics and precision oncology. ORCID: 0009-0001-8040-849X.

Yaser Hassan is an undergraduate student in biotechnology and bioinformatics with expertise in molecular docking. He has received national awards, published in Q1 and Q2 journals, and presented his work at AUC's 2025 Undergraduate Research Conference. His accomplishments reflect strong research potential and a solid foundation in STEM. ORCID: 0009-0008-0061-739X.

Youssef Hassan is a Teaching Assistant and an MSc candidate in Molecular Applied Biotechnology Ain Shams University. With two years of experience, his expertise spans CRISPR-based diagnostics, biosensors, and molecular diagnostics, with published work in forensics and biomedical research. His professional interests include advancing diagnostic technologies for cancer and infectious diseases and integrating AI and bioinformatics in healthcare. ORCID: 0009-0005-3615-4137.

Sai Priyanka J. is a Research Scholar in Sri Sathya Sai University for Human Excellence, India.

Ahmed Mohamed is a BSc student in the Applied Biotechnology Program at the Faculty of Science, Ain Shams University. He is passionate about cancer biology and is expanding his expertise into bioinformatics, particularly cancer transcriptomics and molecular modeling. He has published a review article in a Q2-ranked journal. ORCID: 0009-0007-1093-2695.

Odangowei Inetiminebi Ogidi is a Lecturer, Acting Head, Department of Biochemistry and Sub-Dean, Faculty of Basic Medical Sciences, Bayelsa Medical University, Yenagoa, Bayelsa State, Nigeria. He holds a Bachelor of Science degree in Biochemistry, Master of Science and Doctor of Philosophy degrees in Biotechnology. He has also served as a Lecturer, Head of Departments of Science Laboratory Technology and Biochemistry, and Deputy Director, Centre for Continuing Education in Federal Polytechnic Ekowe, Bayelsa State. He has authored over 80 peer-reviewed academic articles in reputable local and international journals, published over 50 book chapters and presented over 40 conference papers. He is a member of various Journal Editorial Boards. He is indexed in World Scientist and University Ranking (AD Scientific Index ID https://www.adscientificindex.com/scientist/ogidi-odangowei-inetiminebi/4306173) amongst other international bodies. He have supervised over 30 ND and HND students and currently supervising over 20 undergraduate students. His research interest has been Medical/Pharmaceutical and Environmental Biotechnology/Biochemistry, Phytomedicine, Phytochemistry, Human and Environmental health risk assessments and ecotoxicology amongst others. He is a member of West Africa Society of Toxicology, Nigerian Society of Biochemistry and Molecular Biology, Foundation for African Development through International Biotechnology and Nigerian Environmental Society. Details of his research output can be found in Google scholar: https://scholar.google.com/citations?user=umwO5DAAAAAJ&hl=en, Orcid: https://orcid.org/0000-0002-9961-893X, Scopus: https://www.scopus.com/authid/detail.uri?authorId=57204760143 and Research gate: https://www.researchgate.net/profile/Odangowei-Ogidi among others.

Bandana Padhan is an Assistant Professor in the Department of Biotechnology at Adamas University, India. She holds a Ph.D. in Molecular Biology and Plant Biotechnology, with her research centered on the sustainable utilization of plant bioresources. Her current focus lies in the fields of nutraceuticals, bioactive compounds, and the development of intelligent food packaging films.Dr. Padhan has over four years of research experience, during which she has significantly contributed to plant tissue culture, bio-fertilizer production, and phytoremediation. Her recent work emphasizes the extraction and analysis of bioactive phytochemicals from underutilized plants for use in health-promoting nutraceuticals. Additionally, she explores the use of natural polymers to develop biodegradable, antimicrobial packaging materials, aiming to enhance food safety and reduce plastic waste.She has been recognized with multiple honors, including the Best Biotechnology Student Award and several Best Poster Awards. A committed academic and researcher, Dr. Padhan continues to contribute to the advancement of plant biotechnology through innovative, sustainable solutions and student mentorship.

Swetashree Purohit is an Assistant Professor of Zoology at the Department of Agriculture and Allied Sciences, C.V. Raman Global University, Bhubaneswar. She holds a Ph.D. in Biodiversity and Conservation of Natural Resources from the Central University of Odisha, with academic training in Zoology from Utkal University and OUAT. Her research focuses on wildlife biology, particularly avian ecology, biodiversity, and the impacts of anthropogenic stressors such as noise and chemical pollution on ecosystem health. She has conducted extensive fieldwork in the Eastern Ghats, studying how habitat disturbances and environmental contaminants affect wildlife behavior and distribution. Dr. Purohit has authored multiple peer-reviewed publications spanning avian biology, herpetology, and conservation. She is also a strong advocate for citizen science and environmental education, serving as a regional reviewer for eBird and Regional Coordinator for Bird Count India in Odisha. She leads initiatives like The Bhubaneswar Bird Walks and contributes to wildlife census efforts and interpretation center development at Nandankanan Zoological Park. An avid birdwatcher, nature photographer, and writer, she blends scientific research with creative outreach to promote biodiversity conservation.

Anjali Sadhukhan obtained her Bachelor's degree in Biotechnology from Adamas University in 2024 and is currently pursuing her Master's from the same. Her research experience includes a bachelor's thesis on recent advances in lung cancer vaccines and internships at Woodlands Multispecialty Hospital in the Department of Pathology & Phlebotomy. She had a publication in a UGC care journal and an Indian patent under processing for a cost-effective purifier used in waste water treatment. Her research interest lies in the field of cancer biology, immunology and genetics. Currently, she is working on developing a chip-based diagnostic tool for detecting a specific type of lung cancer. She posseses strong analytical skills in various laboratory techniques and is dedicated to explore advanced and cutting-edge technologies to improve cancer diagnosis and treatment.

Mahmoud Salah is a multi-passionate student at Ain Shams University with a keen interest in biological sciences, bioinformatics, and programming. ORCID: 0009-0006-8648-7957.

Abdulrahman Shalaby is a BSc student in the Applied Biotechnology Program at the Faculty of Science, Ain Shams University. He is an aspiring biotechnology entrepreneur with a focus on synthetic biology and innovative waste-to-value solutions. ORCID: 0009-0001-8672-854X.

Ahmad Rusdan Handoyo Utomo, Ph.D., is a leading expert in molecular medicine, specializing in cancer genetics, immunology, and molecular diagnostics. His groundbreaking research has contributed significantly to advancements in precision medicine and immunotherapy. Dr. Utomo earned his Ph.D. in Molecular Medicine from the University of Texas Health Science Center at San Antonio, TX, USA (1995–2003) and completed a Postdoctoral Fellowship in Pathology at Harvard Medical School, Boston, USA (2003–2007). He holds a B.Sc. in Chemistry (Magna Cum Laude) from Angelo State University, TX, USA (1991–1995). Currently affiliated with Universitas YARSI, Dr. Utomo has an extensive publication record, with 75 research articles indexed on Google Scholar and 22 articles indexed on Scopus. His work has been cited over 1,600 times, and he holds an H-index of 17, reflecting the impact of his contributions to biomedical research2. His contributions extend to book authorship and pioneering patented innovations in molecular diagnostics and cancer treatment. Through his research and academic leadership, Dr. Utomo continues to shape the future of biomedical science, driving forward new discoveries in personalized medicine and diagnostic methodologies. https://orcid.org/0000-0003-3092-3714.

Mohamed Waly is a BSc. Biotechnology student, Helwan University with a strong passion for bioinformatics, particularly structural bioinformatics. He has published a research paper in the field and continues to explore computational approaches in biology. ORCID: 0009-0002-6529-6570.

Dian Widiyanti, PhD, is a microbiologist and a member of the teaching staff at the Faculty of Medicine, Universitas YARSI, Indonesia. She has a special interest in research on microbial genetics, particularly microorganisms related to human diseases and antimicrobial resistance. Several of her achievements have been published in high-impact factor journals. https://orcid.org/0000-0002-6642-4864.

Index

E

G

H

I

L

M

O

P

R

S

T

W

X

www.ingramcontent.com/pod-product-compliance
Lightning Source LLC
LaVergne TN
LVHW062328300926
849161LV00007B/1622